Terminology *for* Health Professionals

Sixth Edition

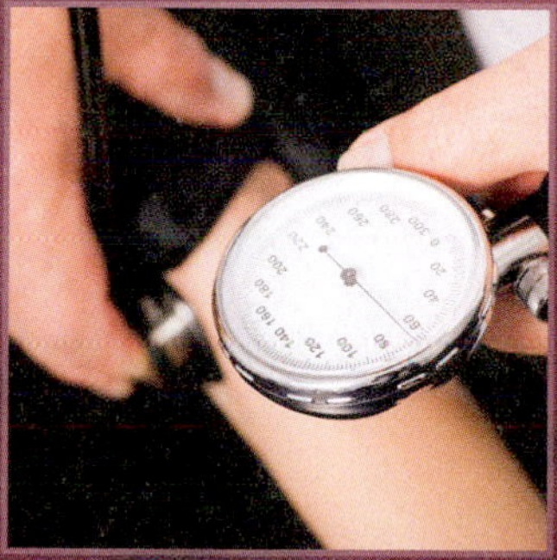
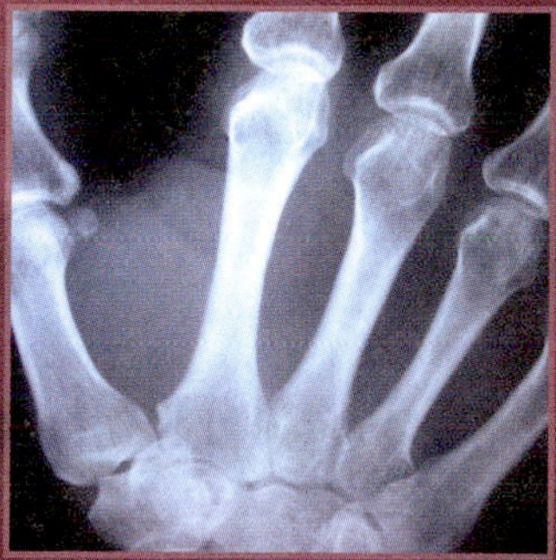
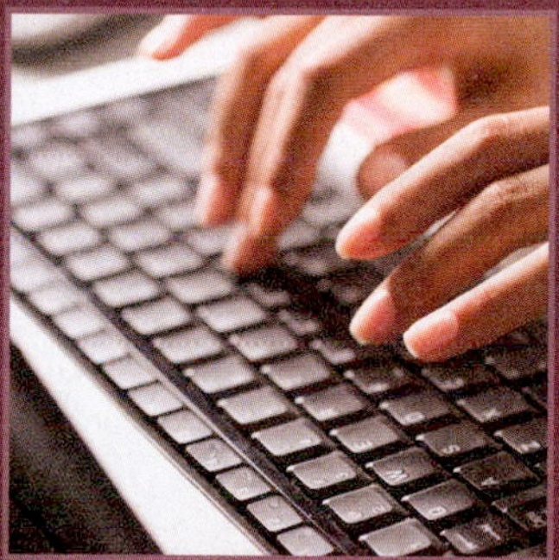
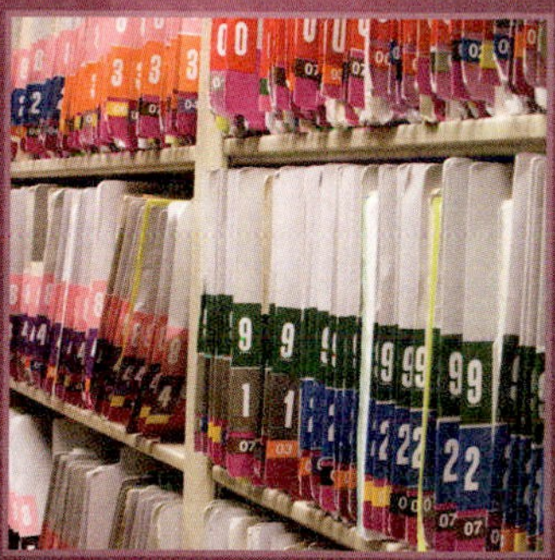

Carolee Sormunen, Ph.D.

Educational Consultant

Professor Emerita, Ball State University, Muncie, Indiana

Research and technical assistance from
RONALD F. JONES

DELMAR
CENGAGE Learning

Australia • Brazil • Japan • Korea • Mexico • Singapore • Spain • United Kingdom • United States

DELMAR
CENGAGE Learning™

Terminology for Health Professionals, Sixth Edition

Carolee Sormunen, Ph.D.

Vice President, Career and Professional Editorial: Dave Garza

Director of Learning Solutions: Matthew Kane

Acquisitions Editor: Matthew Seeley

Managing Editor: Marah Bellegarde

Senior Product Manager: Debra Myette-Flis

Editorial Assistant: Samantha Zullo

Vice President, Career and Professional Marketing: Jennifer McAvey

Executive Marketing Manager: Wendy Mapstone

Senior Marketing Manager: Michele McTighe

Marketing Coordinator: Scott Chrysler

Production Director: Carolyn S. Miller

Content Project Manager: Thomas Heffernan

Senior Art Director: Jack Pendleton

Technology Project Manager: Benjamin Knapp

Library of Congress Control Number: 2009927996

ISBN 13: 978-1-428-37634-2
ISBN 10: 1-4283-7634-8

Delmar
5 Maxwell Drive
Clifton Park, NY 12065-2919
USA

Cengage Learning is a leading provider of customized learning solutions with office locations around the globe, including Singapore, the United Kingdom, Australia, Mexico, Brazil, and Japan. Locate your local office at:
international.cengage.com/region

Cengage Learning products are represented in Canada by Nelson Education, Ltd.

To learn more about Delmar, visit **www.cengage.com/delmar**
Purchase any of our products at your local college store or at our preferred online store
www.ichapters.com

Notice to the Reader

Publisher does not warrant or guarantee any of the products described herein or perform any independent analysis in connection with any of the product information contained herein. Publisher does not assume, and expressly disclaims, any obligation to obtain and include information other than that provided to it by the manufacturer. The reader is expressly warned to consider and adopt all safety precautions that might be indicated by the activities described herein and to avoid all potential hazards. By following the instructions contained herein, the reader willingly assumes all risks in connection with such instructions. The publisher makes no representations or warranties of any kind, including but not limited to, the warranties of fitness for particular purpose or merchantability, nor are any such representations implied with respect to the material set forth herein, and the publisher takes no responsibility with respect to such material. The publisher shall not be liable for any special, consequential, or exemplary damages resulting, in whole or part, from the readers' use of, or reliance upon, this material.

Printed in the United States of America
1 2 3 4 5 6 7 12 11 10 09

Contents

Preface

Terminology for Health Professionals, sixth edition, is designed to integrate the entire spectrum of information need by health professionals who must understand medical terminology.

PHILOSOPHY

Terminology for Health Professionals focuses on successful learning by applying information in the context in which it is used in a medical environment.

A simple-to-complex instructional design begins in Chapter 1 with an introduction to the word elements—roots, prefixes, and suffixes—which are used in constructing medical terms. In each subsequent chapter more word elements and medical terms are presented as they relate to the specific body system or medical support area being discussed. By the end of the text, more than 600 word elements and 800 medical terms will have been defined.

The text contains a mix of anatomy (the body systems), physiology (how the body works), and pathophysiology (the effect of disease on the body) combined with information about the medical records in which the medical terms appear.

The instructional material begins with introductory chapters on terminology, basic anatomy, and medical history reports. This is followed with the opening discussion of body systems in Chapters 5 and 6. The rest of the book follows this general pattern of a chapter or two on support systems and then one or two on body systems.

Each of the body system chapters has a section called Working Practice which illustrates how medical terminology is used in the medical environment. This section has three basic parts: diagnostic procedures, diagnoses, and treatment procedures. In most cases there also is a subsection providing related abbreviations, medications, and other system-specific material.

Specialty chapters, such as Pharmacology, Oncology, Radiology and Nuclear Medicine, and Mental Health, provide added knowledge, dimension, and depth to your learning experience. This will help you in your efforts to secure employment.

To reinforce the chapter discussions and to give a clearer meaning to the complexities of the various medical topics, more than 235 illustrations and photographs are woven through the book. Many terms in the text are numbered to coincide with a number in the related anatomical illustration. Where practical, these numbers move clockwise around the illustration to make it easier to locate a particular point.

In addition, all chapters end with a summary and a series of exercises concerning the terminology and word elements introduced. The Working Practice has a separate exercise section. These exercises may be any mix of matching, fill-in, brief discussion and other questions. Completion of these activities will give you an opportunity to highlight important information so that you can better focus review efforts in mastering the content.

The health care industry has used a variety of terms to describe patient health information, but in recent years, *legal health record* has emerged as the key term to identify the patient's entire health documentation. Medical history and physical examinations, surgical notes, radiology reports, discharge summaries, pathology reports, and autopsies are the basic six types of reports found in legal health records. Introduction to each of these report types is not done until they have been discussed in the textual material. In other words, history and physical report first appear as an example in Chapter 3, surgical notes are not used as examples until Chapter 7, radiology reports in Chapter 11, and so forth for the other kinds of reports.

Dictionary Exercises are included in each chapter. Medical transcriptionists suggested many of the words used in these exercises, drawing on the terminology commonly found in dictation in their specialty offices.

Medical reports have been provided from a variety of offices to give an in-depth exposure to the more common formats found in a medical environment. The reports have been carefully dictated as "Listening Exercises" on the accompanying StudyWARE™ CD-ROM so that the terminology can be heard in a "live" situation. They are also provided in printed form so you follow along as you listen.

Listening to these recordings will allow you to experience just how the medical terms you have learned sound in the context of a medical report thus helping you in your transition to the workplace.

This text and its supporting materials encourage you to develop critical thinking skills. This is a skill that employers look for. They want individuals who can take that step beyond memorizing lists of words to using them confidently and to interact comfortably with the medical professionals who use them.

The sixth edition of *Terminology for Health Professionals* retains its basic instructional design, but has been carefully reviewed by the author and a panel of consulting physicians so that each chapter reflects the latest in medical developments.

Major revisions to this edition include the following:

- A StudyWARE™ CD-ROM was added. This interactive software packaged with the book offers an exciting way to gain additional practice (while having fun) through games, quizzes and animations. (See "How To Use the StudyWARE™" on page xvi for details.)
- The Listening Exercises are included on the StudyWARE™ CD-ROM rather than on a separate audio CD.
- The StudyWARE™ Connection feature encourage learners to go to their interactive CD-ROM to watch animations, perform a labeling activity, hear medical reports read, play interactive games or complete a practice quiz related to the chapter.
- Chapter 1 was expanded to introduce more roots, prefixes, and suffixes earlier.
- Chapter 10, Oncology, was substantially rewritten to reflect the continued expansion of knowledge in this area.
- Chapter 11, Radiology, was rewritten to include developments in noninvasive radiology and diagnostic imaging.
- In the body system chapters, the Word Element Review and Practice Exercises were moved with the Key Terminology Review and Practice Exercise section
- More than 50 new or updated illustrations and photos support text discussion.
- Frequently used terms that describe information pertinent to each system, often in the Working Practice, were updated with cooperation from the specific medical offices involved.
- Activities that introduce helpful and relevant Internet web sites were checked for accuracy and were replaced when new, more pertinent sites became available.
- All review activities were evaluated for relevance and expanded for coverage of added content.

REFERENCES

In addition to the nineteen physicians and clinical professionals identified in the Special Acknowledgement section, the primary source used to clarify information was *Taber's Cyclopedic Medical Dictionary*. Extensive use was made of the Internet for research on various diseases, conditions, diagnostic and treatment procedures, medications, and other information. For style, resources are available through the Association for Healthcare Documentation, 4230 Kleman Avenue, Suite 130, Modesto, CA 95356, (800) 982-2182, or on the net at **www.ahdionline.org**.

FLASHCARDS

Improve your knowledge and test yourself by with over 900 flashcards. Packaged separately, these cards are an effective study aid for use even when you only have a small amount of time.

ISBN 1-4283-7638-0

INSTRUCTOR RESOURCES

Instructor Resources is a robust computerized tool for your instructional needs! A must-have for all instructors, this comprehensive and convenient CD-ROM contains:

- **The Instructors Manual** includes information on teaching and learning strategies, evaluations, and helpful suggestions based on the author's experience; a critical thinking tip in each chapter designed to help learners develop this highly desirable work skill; optional exercises such as charting exercises based on the listening exercises in Chapters 3, 7, 11, 14, and 18; and suggestions for assignments using the Internet to find chapter related information
- **Exam View® Computerized Testbank** contains 1000 questions. You can use these questions to create your own review materials or tests. This versatile program enables you to create your own tests and to write additional questions.
- **Instructor Slides created in PowerPoint®**, including animations, are designed to aid you in planning your class presentations.
- **Answers to Review Exercises** in the text.

ISBN 1-4283-7635-6

WEBTUTOR ADVANTAGE™

Designed to complement the text, WebTutor Advantage™ is a content-rich, web-based teaching and learning aid that reinforces and clarifies complex concepts. The WebCT™ and Blackboard™ platforms also provide rich communication tools to instructors and students, including a course calendar, chat, e-mail, and threaded discussions.

WebTutor Advantage on WebCT™ (ISBN 1-4283-7637-2)
Text Bundled with WebTutor Advantage on WebCT™ (ISBN 1-4283-5036-5)
WebTutor Advantage on Blackboard™ (ISBN 1-4283-7636-4)
Text Bundled with WebTutor Advantage on Blackboard™ (ISBN 1-4283-7257-1)

ADDITIONAL RESOURCES

DELMAR'S MEDICAL TERMINOLOGY STUDENT THEATER: AN INTERACTIVE VIDEO PROGRAM

Organized by body system, this CD-ROM is invaluable to learners trying to master the complex world of medical terminology. The program is designed for allied health and nursing students who are enrolled in medical terminology courses. A series of video clips leads learners through the various concepts, interspersing lectures with illustrations to emphasize key points. Quizzes and games allow learners to assess their understanding of the video content.

ISBN: 1-4283-1863-1

DELMAR LEARNING'S ANATOMY AND PHYSIOLOGY IMAGE LIBRARY CD-ROM, THIRD EDITION

This CD-ROM includes over 1,050 graphic files. These files can be incorporated into a Power Point®, Microsoft® Word presentation, used directly from the CD-ROM in a classroom presentation, or used to make color transparencies. The Image Library is organized around body systems and medical specialties. The library includes various anatomy, physiology, and pathology graphics of different levels of complexity. Instructors can search and select the graphics that best apply to their teaching situation. This is an ideal resource to enhance your teaching presentation of medical terminology or anatomy and physiology.

ISBN: 1-4180-3928-4

DELMAR'S MEDICAL TERMINOLOGY AUDIO LIBRARY

This extensive audio library of medical terminology includes four Audio CDs with over 3,700 terms pronounced, and a software CD-ROM. The CD-ROM presents terms organized by body systems, medical specialty, and general medical term categories. The user can search for a specific term by typing in the term or key words, or click on a category to view an alphabetical list of all terms within the category. The user can hear the correct pronunciation of one term or listen to each term on the list pronounced automatically. Definitions can be viewed after hearing the pronunciation of terms.

Institutional Version, ISBN: 1-4018-3223-7
Individual Version, ISBN: 1-4018-3222-9

DELMAR'S MEDICAL TERMINOLOGY CD-ROM (INSTITUTIONAL VERSION)

This exciting interactive reference, practice, and assessment tool complements any medical terminology program. Features include the extensive use of multimedia—animations, video, graphics, and activities—to present terms and word-building features. Difficult functions, processes, and procedures are included, so learners can more effectively learn from a textbook.

CD-ROM, Institutional Version, ISBN 0-7668-0979-X

DELMAR'S MEDICAL TERMINOLOGY FLASH!: COMPUTERIZED FLASHCARDS

Learn and review over 1,500 medical terms using this unique electronic flashcard program. Flash! is a computerized flashcard-type question-and-answer program designed to help users learn correct spellings, definitions, and pronunciations. The use of graphics and audio clips makes it a fun and easy way for users to learn and test their knowledge of medical terminology.

CD-ROM, ISBN 0-7668-4320-3

FUNDAMENTALS OF ANATOMY AND PHYSIOLOGY ONLINE COURSE

This fully developed online course introduces learners with little or no prior biology knowledge to the complex and exciting world of anatomy and physiology. The course is a complete interactive online learning solution. Chapter content is organized around body systems and focuses on how each system works together to promote homeostasis. Full-color art, 3D anatomical animations, audio, and "bite-size" chunks of content fully engage the learner. Interactive games such as image labeling, concentration, and championship reinforce learning. Powerful customization tools allow administrators to individualize the course and assessment tools, while extensive tracking features allow administrators to monitor learner performance and progress.

Anatomy & Physiology Online—Academic Individual Access Code, ISBN 1-4180-0131-7
Anatomy & Physiology Online—Academic Institutional Access Code, ISBN 1-4180-0130-9

ABOUT THE AUTHOR

The author brings a unique combination of experiences to the development of this edition of the textbook. As an instructional design and training specialist, the author applies her expertise to provide a solid instructional program for you. This expertise has been enhanced by her own experience in the medical environment, as well as her working relationship with individuals in a variety of positions in clinics, physician's offices, and hospitals. These experiences have resulted in a practical approach to preparing you for a variety of opportunities as an allied health professional.

ACKNOWLEDGMENTS

This text represents the efforts of many people. I am indebted to those reviewers who reviewed the manuscript drafts of the fifth edition and provided valuable suggestions.

Debra Biddle, MS, RTR
Instructor
Portland Community College
Portland, Oregon
Cathy Kelley-Arney, CMA, MLTC, BSHS, AS
Health Care Education
Amy B. Mori, MBA-HCM
Associate Dean of Instruction
Bryant & Stratton College
Albany, New York
Sally Nichols, RHIT, MS
Office Administration Instructor
Crowder College
Neosho, Missouri
Joy RenFro, EdD, RHIA, CMA, CCS-P
Professor/Program Director
Eastern Kentucky University
Richmond, Kentucky
Marta E. Urdaneta, PhD
Program Director, Health Science
Program Coordinator, Health Services Administration
Keiser University
Fort Lauderdale, Florida
Valerie Weiss, MD, MS
Associate Professor
Chair, Health Studies Program
Hodges University
Naples, Florida
Stacey Wilson, MHA, MT, CMA
Program Coordinator
Cabarrus College of Health Sciences
Concord, North Carolina

In addition to the medically related professional individuals and physicians identified on the following pages, I am indebted to staff members in the offices of the Marquette Medical Center and Marquette General Hospital, Marquette, Michigan, for their assistance.

Ronald F. Jones, my unofficial partner in this project, deserves special recognition for his valuable assistance with the revision of the text. He is a stalwart contributor who researched and verified portions of the text. His willingness to commit a significant amount of time, his technical writing skills, and his excellent editing skills added immeasurably to the creative process.

I appreciate the strong support I have had for this edition from Matthew Seeley, acquisitions editor, and Debra Myette-Flis, senior product manager, at Delmar Cengage Learning. Because a project of this nature is enriched by the efforts of each individual who assists in its completion, I wish to acknowledge the significant contributions all of you have made. Without that help, this book would not have been possible.

SPECIAL ACKNOWLEDGMENTS

I would like to thank the following contributors for their assistance in developing this text.

Y. Haroon Ahmed, M.D.
Arizona Oncology, Tucson, Arizona
Cary M. Bjork, M.D., F.A.C.P.
Marquette Internal Medicine and Pediatric Associates, P.C.
Robert H. Blotter, M.D.
Fellow, American Academy of Orthopaedic Surgeons
Assistant Clinical Professor, Michigan State University College of Human Medicine, E. Lansing, Michigan
Marquette General Hospital, Marquette, Michigan

Michael K. Conley, M.D.
Fellow, American College of Obstetricians and Gynecologists
Fellow, American College of Surgeons
Assistant Clinical Professor, Obstetrics and Gynecology, Michigan State University College of Human Medicine, E. Lansing, Michigan

John K. DiBaise, M.D., SACG
Professor of Medicine, Division of Gastroenterology and Hepatology, Mayo Clinic, Scottsdale, Arizona

Randy J. Folker, M.D.
Board Certified Otolaryngologist

Mark L. Griswold, D.O., F.A.C.D.O.
Board Certified Ophthalmologist
Griswold Eye Care, Oro Valley, Arizona

J. Marc Himes, M.D.
Staff Nephrologist and Medical Director of Hemodialysis, Marquette General Hospital, Marquette, Michigan
Clinical Associate Professor, Department of Medicine, Michigan State College of Human Medicine, E. Lansing, Michigan

Joyce E. Honorof, M.D.
American Board of Internal Medicine

James B. Keplinger, M.D.
American Board of Surgery

Karl B. Kern, M.D. FACC
Professor of Medicine, University of Arizona
Director, Cardiac Catheterization Laboratories and Interventional Cardiology Fellowship Program

Ross Lane, Ph.D., H.S.P.P.
Licensed Psychologist

Ethelbert Lara, M.D.
Diagnostic Radiology

James H. Mering III, M.D.
Diplomate, American Board of Urology

Debra J. Morley, M.D., Ph.D.
Diplomate, American Board of Psychiatry and Neurology
Clinical Assistant Professor, Michigan State University College of Human Medicine, E. Lansing, Michigan
Chief of Staff, Marquette General Hospital, Marquette, Michigan
Adjunct Faculty, Department of Biology, Northern Michigan University, Marquette, Michigan

Reid Nishikawa, Pharm.D., B.C.N.S.P., F.L.S.H.P.
Director of Research and Coordinator of Clinical Services, Nutrishare, Inc., Elk Grove, California

Aaron P. Scholnik, M.D., F.A.C.P.
American Subspecialty Board in Medical Oncology
American Subspecialty Board in Hematology
Director of Cancer Research, Marquette General Cancer Center, Marquette, Michigan

Martha Short, M.D.
Board Certified Internal Medicine
Marquette Internal Medicine and Pediatrics, Marquette, Michigan

Milton D. Soderberg, M.D.
Diplomate, American Academy of Dermatology
Associate Clinical Professor, Michigan State University College of Human Medicine, E. Lansing, Michigan

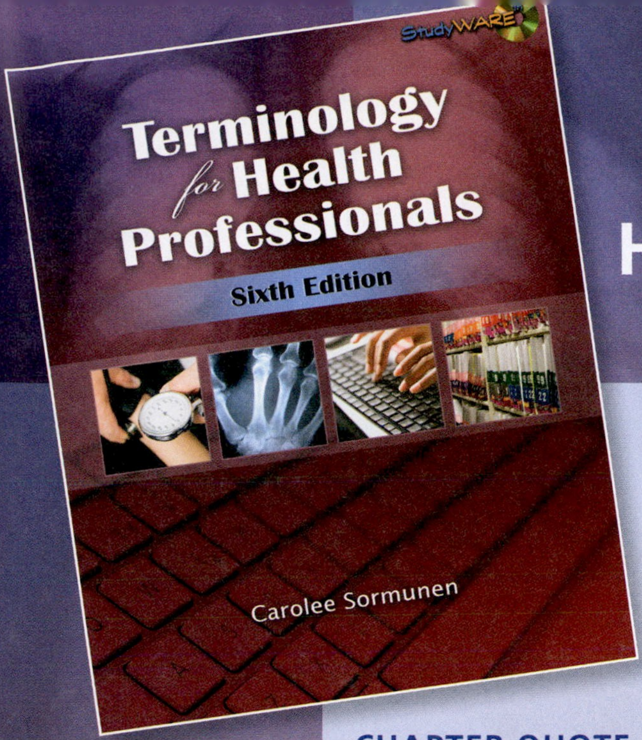

How to Use This Book

Terminology for Health Professionals, sixth edition, focuses on successful learning by applying information in the context in which it is used in the medical environment. The following features are integrated throughout the text to assist you in learning and mastering medical terminology.

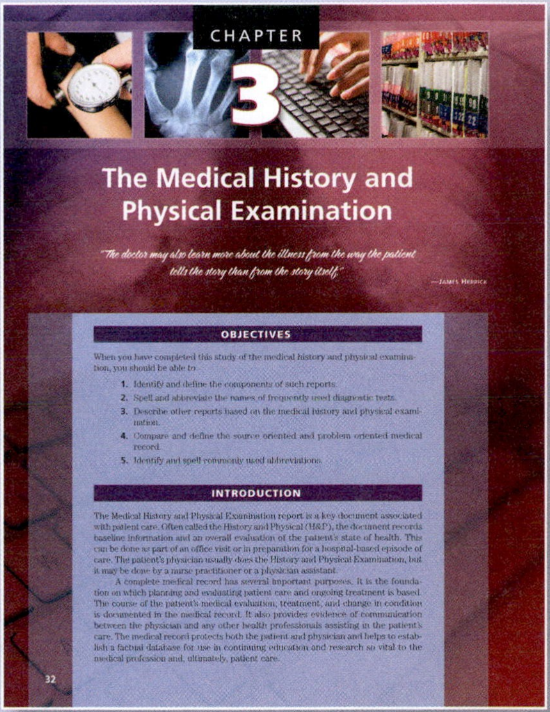

CHAPTER QUOTE

The quotation at the beginning of each chapter can be used to stimulate discussion and develop critical thinking. Reflect on the relevance of the quote in relation to the chapter material.

OBJECTIVES

Chapter objectives help you focus on key concepts presented in the chapter. The objectives are achieved through a combination of written and listening exercises, using a multisensory approach to learning.

INTRODUCTION

The introduction provides you with an overview of important concepts you will learn in the chapter.

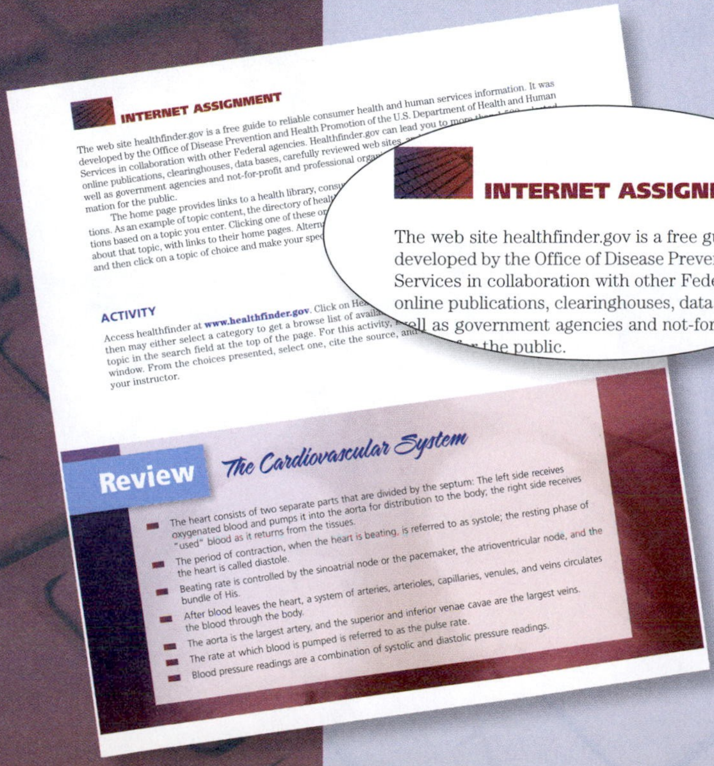

INTERNET ASSIGNMENT

These brief assignments help you improve your research and Internet skills. Through the exploration of various web sites, you gain experience in locating chapter-related information.

REVIEW

The review helps you assess your understanding of key facts presented in the chapter.

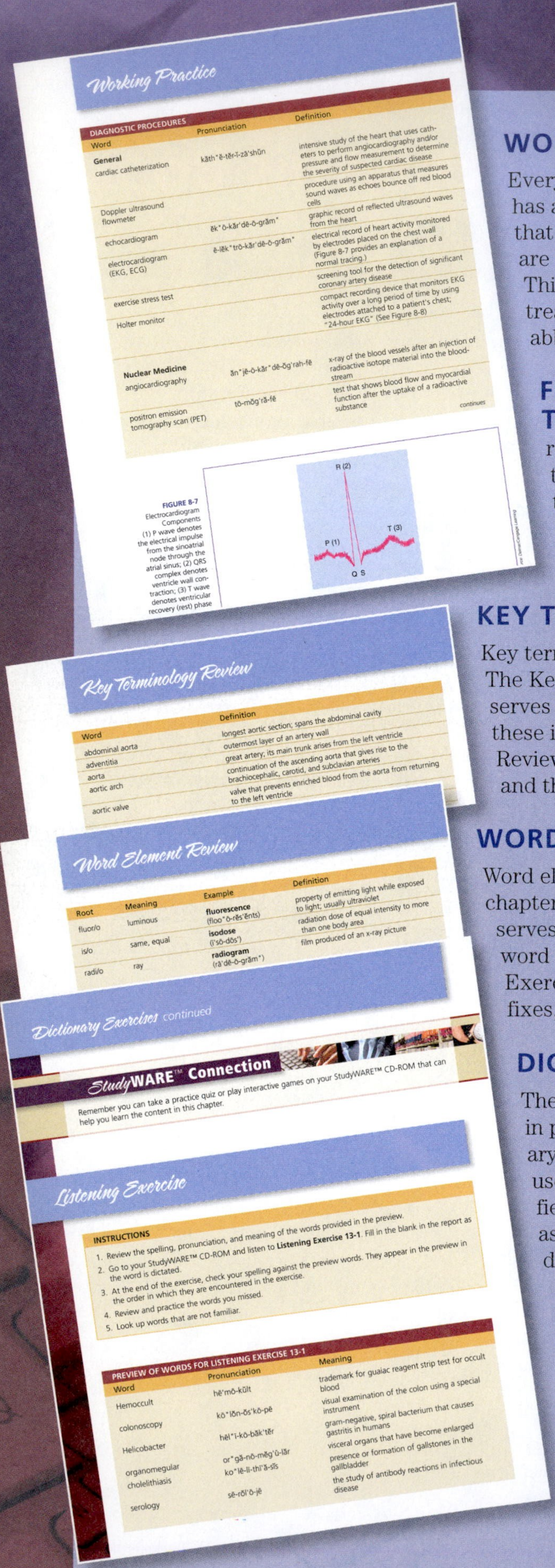
Working Practice

DIAGNOSTIC PROCEDURES Word	Pronunciation	Definition
General		
cardiac catheterization	kăth″ĕ-tĕr-ĭ-zā′shŭn	intensive study of the heart that uses catheters to perform angiocardiography and/or pressure and flow measurement to determine the severity of suspected cardiac disease
Doppler ultrasound flowmeter		procedure using an apparatus that measures sound waves as echoes bounce off red blood cells
echocardiogram	ĕk″ō-kăr′dē-ō-grăm″	graphic record of reflected ultrasound waves from the heart
electrocardiogram (EKG, ECG)	ē-lĕk″trō-kăr′dē-ō-grăm″	electrical record of heart activity monitored by electrodes placed on the chest wall (Figure 8-7 provides an explanation of a normal tracing.)
exercise stress test		screening tool for the detection of significant coronary artery disease
Holter monitor		compact recording device that monitors EKG activity over a long period of time by using electrodes attached to a patient's chest; "24-hour EKG" (See Figure 8-8)
Nuclear Medicine		
angiocardiography	ăn″jē-ō-kăr″dē-ŏg′rah-fē	x-ray of the blood vessels after an injection of radioactive isotope material into the bloodstream
positron emission tomography scan (PET)	tō-mŏg′rā-fē	test that shows blood flow and myocardial function after the uptake of a radioactive substance

continues

FIGURE 8-7 Electrocardiogram Components (1) P wave denotes the electrical impulse from the sinoatrial node through the atrial sinus; (2) QRS complex denotes ventricle wall contraction; (3) T wave denotes ventricular recovery (rest) phase

R (2)
P (1)
T (3)
Q S

Key Terminology Review

Word	Definition
abdominal aorta	longest aortic section; spans the abdominal cavity
adventitia	outermost layer of an artery wall
aorta	great artery; its main trunk arises from the left ventricle
aortic arch	continuation of the ascending aorta that gives rise to the brachiocephalic, carotid, and subclavian arteries
aortic valve	valve that prevents enriched blood from the aorta from returning to the left ventricle

Word Element Review

Root	Meaning	Example	Definition
fluor/o	luminous	**fluorescence** (floo″ō-rĕs′ĕnts)	property of emitting light while exposed to light; usually ultraviolet
is/o	same, equal	**isodose** (ī′sō-dōs″)	radiation dose of equal intensity to more than one body area
radi/o	ray	**radiogram** (rā′dē-ō-grăm″)	film produced of an x-ray picture

Dictionary Exercises continued

*Study*WARE™ Connection

Remember you can take a practice quiz or play interactive games on your StudyWARE™ CD-ROM that can help you learn the content in this chapter.

Listening Exercise

INSTRUCTIONS
1. Review the spelling, pronunciation, and meaning of the words provided in the preview.
2. Go to your StudyWARE™ CD-ROM and listen to **Listening Exercise 13-1**. Fill in the blank in the report as the word is dictated.
3. At the end of the exercise, check your spelling against the preview words. They appear in the preview in the order in which they are encountered in the exercise.
4. Review and practice the words you missed.
5. Look up words that are not familiar.

PREVIEW OF WORDS FOR LISTENING EXERCISE 13-1 Word	Pronunciation	Meaning
Hemoccult	hē′mō-kŭlt	trademark for guaiac reagent strip test for occult blood
colonoscopy	kō″lŏn-ŏs′kō-pē	visual examination of the colon using a special instrument
Helicobacter	hĕl″ĭ-kō-băk′tĕr	gram-negative, spiral bacterium that causes gastritis in humans
organomegular	or″gă-nō-mĕg′ū-lăr	visceral organs that have become enlarged
cholelithiasis	kō″lē-lĭ-thī′ă-sĭs	presence or formation of gallstones in the gallbladder
serology	sē-rŏl′ō-jē	the study of antibody reactions in infectious disease

WORKING PRACTICE

Every chapter related to body systems has a section called Working Practice that allows you to learn how the terms are used in medical environments. This section presents diagnostic and treatment procedures, diagnoses, abbreviations, and medications.

FULL-COLOR ILLUSTRATIONS of anatomical structures reinforce the terms used to describe them. Full-color illustrations in the Working Practice section reinforce diagnostic and treatment procedures.

KEY TERMINOLOGY REVIEW

Key terms within chapters are **boldface**. The Key Terminology Review section serves as a chapter-level glossary of these important terms. Key Terminology Review Exercises reinforce the terms and their meanings.

WORD ELEMENT REVIEW

Word elements are integrated into each chapter. The Word Element Review serves as a chapter-level glossary of word elements. Word Element Review Exercises help you review roots, prefixes, and suffixes.

DICTIONARY EXERCISES

The Dictionary Exercises guide you in practicing using a medical dictionary effectively. Many of the words used in these exercises were identified by medical transcriptionists as terminology commonly found in dictation in their specialty offices.

LISTENING EXERCISES

The Listening Exercises, taken from actual medical documents, expose you to the most common formats in medical environments. The exercises allow you to *see* medical words in context. Listen to "real-life dictation" on the StudyWARE™ CD in the back of the book and *hear* words in the context in which they are used. Listening to the correct pronunciation of the words and phrases as they are used in the context of a medical report provides "live" experience that will ease your move into the workplace.

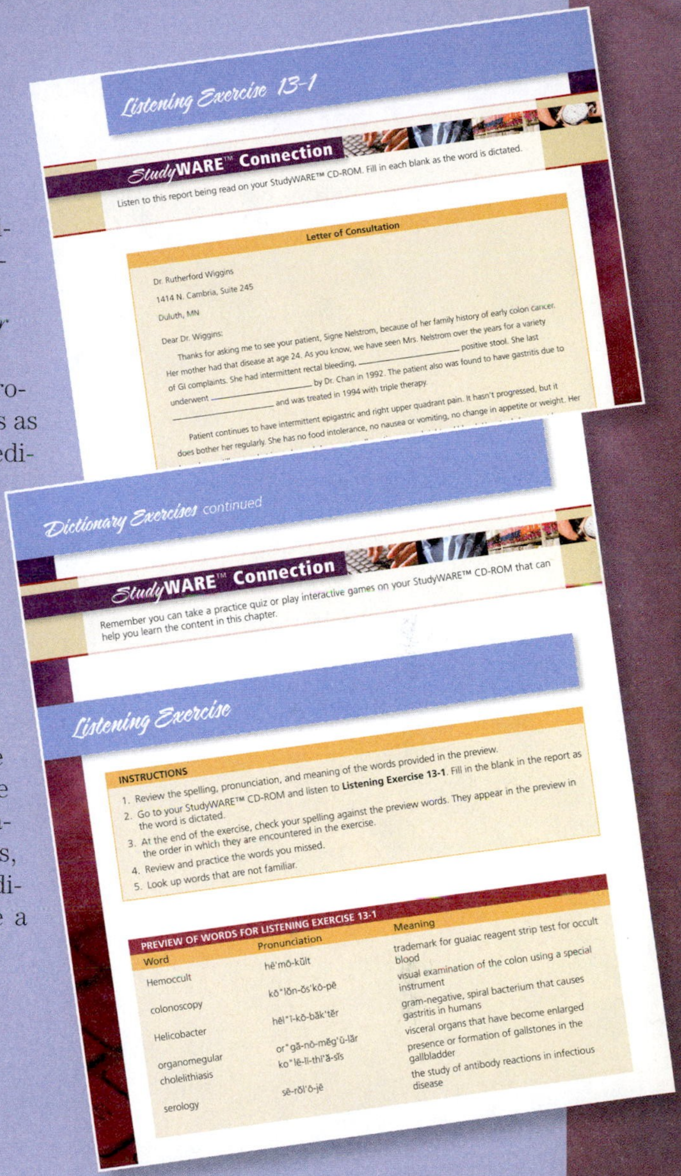

NEW STUDYWARE™ CONNECTION feature

encourages learners to go to the accompanying CD-ROM for additional activities that can enhance their learning. On this interactive CD-ROM learners can watch animations, label anatomical illustrations, play interactive games, listen to medical reports being read or complete a practice quiz related to the chapter.

HOW TO USE STUDYWARE™ TO ACCOMPANY *TERMINOLOGY FOR HEALTH PROFESSIONALS, SIXTH EDITION*

Minimum System Requirements

- Operating systems: Microsoft Windows XP w/SP 2, Windows Vista w/SP 1
- Processor: Minimum required by Operating System
- Memory: Minimum required by Operating System

Hard Drive Space: 450 MB
Screen resolution: 800 x 600 pixels
CD-ROM drive
Sound card & listening device required for audio features
Flash Player 9. The Adobe Flash Player is free, and can be downloaded from http://www.adobe.com/products/flashplayer/

Setup Instructions

1. Insert disc into CD-ROM drive. The StudyWare™ installation program should start automatically. If it does not, go to step 2.
2. From My Computer, double-click the icon for the CD drive.
3. Double-click the *setup.exe* file to start the program.

Technical Support

Telephone: 1-800-648-7450
8:30 A.M.-6:30 P.M. Eastern Time
E-mail: delmar.help@cengage.com

StudyWare™ is a trademark used herein under license.
Microsoft® and Windows® are registered trademarks of the Microsoft Corporation.
Pentium® is a registered trademark of the Intel Corporation.

The StudyWARE™ software helps you learn terms and concepts in *Terminology for Health Professionals, Sixth Edition.* As you study each chapter in the text, be sure to explore the activities in the corresponding chapter in the software. Use StudyWARE™ as your own private tutor to help you learn medical terminology content.

Getting started is easy. Install the software by inserting the CD-ROM into your computer's CD-ROM drive and following the on-screen instructions. When you open the software, enter your first and last name so the software can store your quiz results. Then choose a chapter from the menu to take a quiz or explore one of the activities.

Menus

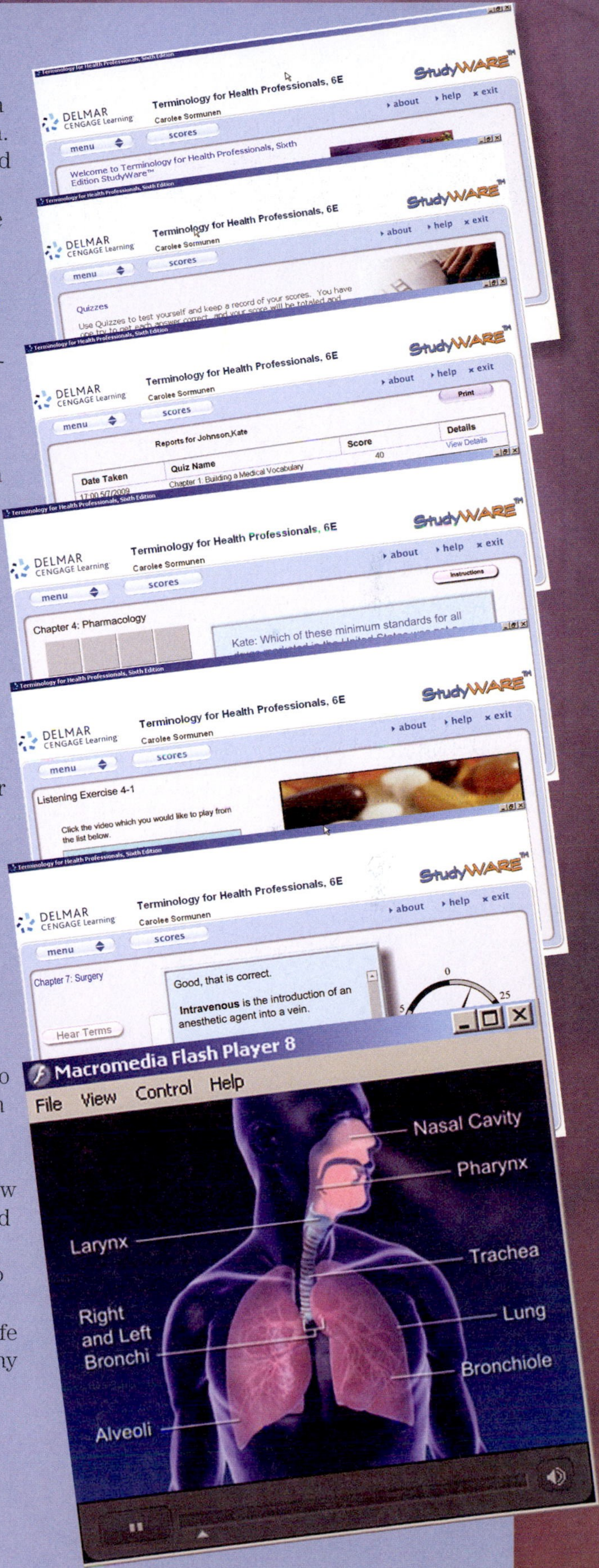

You can access the menus from wherever you are in the program. The menus include Quizzes and other Activities.

Quizzes. Quizzes include multiple choice, true/false, and fill-in-the-blank questions. You can take the quizzes in both practice mode and quiz mode. Use practice mode to improve your mastery of the material. You have multiple tries to get the answers correct. Instant feedback tells you whether you're right or wrong and helps you learn quickly by explaining why an answer was correct or incorrect. Use quiz mode when you are ready to test yourself and keep a record of your scores. In quiz mode, you have one try to get the answers right, but you can take each quiz as many times as you want.

Scores. You can view your last scores for each quiz and print your results to hand in to your instructor.

Activities. Activities include image labeling, concentration, hangman, spelling bee, and a Championship game. Have fun while increasing your knowledge!

Listening Exercises. The Listening Exercises are used in conjunction with your textbook. To begin, first read the instructions in your text, then listen to the audio on your StudyWARE™ CD-ROM. This activity allows you to hear how terms learned in the chapter sound in the context of a medical report, and helps ease your transition into the workplace.

Animations. Animations bring to life difficult concepts related to anatomy and pathological conditions.

CHAPTER 1

Building a Medical Vocabulary

"Education isn't something you've had; it's something you're always getting."

—Franklin P. Jones

OBJECTIVES

When you have completed this chapter on building a medical vocabulary, you should be able to

1. Define medical terminology.
2. Define word elements, roots, combining forms, suffixes, and prefixes.
3. Create the singular and plural forms of commonly used medical terms.
4. Identify homonyms, eponyms, and other confusing terms used in medical reports.
5. Use a medical dictionary.
6. Identify and spell the word elements and determine their meaning.

INTRODUCTION

A medical vocabulary is the heart of a career in the allied health fields. It provides the means by which all individuals concerned with patient health care issues can share information. Whether in a one-physician office, a major clinic, or a centralized laboratory, a behind-the-scenes health care team provides a variety of services. A list follows of some of those representative health care positions identified in the Occupational Outlook Handbook:

Representative Health Care Positions

admissions clerk
cancer registrar
cardiovascular technologist
clinical laboratory technician
coding specialist
CT technologist
echocardiograph technician
health information management technician
histologist
licensed practical nurse
medical and health services manager

- medical transcriptionist
- MRI technologist
- nurse practitioner
- occupational therapist
- office manager
- paramedic
- pharmacist
- pharmacy aide
- pharmacy technician
- phlebotomist
- physical therapist
- physician's assistant
- psychologist
- radiographer
- registered nurse
- respiratory therapy technician
- ultrasound technician

Educational requirements for these positions may vary considerably, but the one requirement that cuts across all of these positions is the ability to understand medical terminology.

What is medical vocabulary or terminology? It is the collection of all of the terms used by physicians, scientists, and other medical personnel to describe their work in the allied health field. The collection, or language, of medical terminology is more extensive than that of many other technical specialties. And like all languages, it is constantly changing. Progress in science and technology continually contributes new words—and occasionally makes some obsolete. Advances in the use of lasers, nuclear medicine, noninvasive radiology, and computer technology have led to the addition of words that did not even exist just a few years ago.

Medical terminology consists of four major elements. Each of these elements will be addressed in this text.

Roots, prefixes, and suffixes. Medical terminology begins with a thorough understanding of roots, prefixes, and suffixes—referred to in this text as word elements—and how they can be combined in a variety of ways to create medical words. This includes knowing how to join the word elements to form medical terms; recognizing the difference between the adjective and noun form of a term; knowing the singular and plural form of a term; and knowing how to use eponyms and homonyms.

Anatomical terms. Because body parts frequently are referred to in the medical work environment, members of the health care team should be familiar with at least the most commonly used anatomical terms. Understanding how the systems of the body function helps to make sense of medical terms. Basic body structure is presented in Chapter 2; more detailed anatomy and associated terminology with each body system appears in subsequent chapters.

Regular words with specialized medical meanings. Some familiar, everyday words or phrases may actually have a special, even formal, medical meaning. For instance, the "thrill" noted in a medical report refers to a vibration felt when the hand is placed on the body, not the feeling you get when you win a prize. In other cases, informal regional and institutional terms have arisen that are not covered in medical reference books. These are learned as needed on the job. You will be introduced to some of the ordinary words with specialized medical meanings in the Listening Activities and other chapter-end activities.

Diagnostic procedures, diagnoses, and treatment procedures, including medications. Physicians record the names and results of diagnostic procedures that they order. These, as well as the resulting diagnoses, treatment procedures, and medications, must be recorded accurately. It is also helpful to know metric measures and abbreviations.

The knowledge you gain from this course of study will not only prepare you for a career in the allied health field but will also enable you to become an informed user of medical services, allowing you to make more intelligent choices about your personal health care.

WORD ELEMENTS

Although medical terminology is far more than knowledge of roots, prefixes, and suffixes, these word elements do provide a solid foundation upon which to build the vocabulary of medicine. Many of the word elements are derived from Greek or Latin. It is not necessary to know all of the word elements, but if you know those most commonly used, literally thousands of medical terms can be a part of your vocabulary.

For the purposes of this textbook, roots are the basic foundation of the words. Suffixes are word endings, and prefixes are word beginnings. When interpreting any given word, the process begins with the suffix, moves to the prefix, and finally attacks the root or roots and any combining vowels in the order in which they appear. However, for this discussion of the various word elements, let's begin with roots.

ROOTS

The foundation of a word is called the *root*. The root word in medical terminology usually indicates the part of the body under discussion and forms the main substance or meaning of the word. All medical words have at least one root, whose meaning does not change. The prefix or suffix, however, may change the meaning of the complete term. Sometimes a word element may be a medical word by itself. For instance, *-emesis* is a suffix, but *emesis* may stand alone as a word meaning vomiting.

In the following terms, note how the meaning of the root (shown in bold) is changed by the addition of a suffix.

EXAMPLES

Gastr- is the root meaning *stomach*.

Term	Suffix	Meaning
gastric	*-ic* is a suffix meaning *pertaining to*	pertaining to the stomach
gastrology	*-ology* is a suffix meaning *study of*	study of the function and diseases of the stomach
gastralgia	*-algia* is a suffix meaning *pain*	pain in the stomach
gastrectomy	*-ectomy* is a suffix meaning *surgical removal of all or part of*	surgical removal of all or part of the stomach
gastritis	*-itis* is a suffix meaning *inflammation*	inflammation of the stomach lining

Cardi- is the root meaning heart.

Term	Suffix	Meaning
cardiac	*-ac* is a suffix meaning pertaining to	pertaining to the heart
cardiology	*-ology* is a suffix meaning study of	study of the physiology and pathology of the heart
cardiogram	*-gram* is a suffix meaning graph or picture	graph of the electrical activity of the heart
cardiograph	*-graph* is a suffix meaning registering a record	a device for registering the electrical activity of the heart
cardiopathy	*-pathy* is a suffix meaning any disease	any disease of the heart

In this text, the majority of the roots are presented in the chapter where they are most likely to be used. For instance, the digestive system will include the roots in the section that presents anatomical information. All the roots, prefixes, and suffixes presented are reviewed in the Word Element Practice Exercises.

The following table presents some roots with which you may be familiar.

GREEK AND LATIN WORDS		
Root	Meaning	Example Words
morhp-	form	morphology
path-	feeling, suffering	pathology
ped, pedo-	child, children	pediatrician
pend-	to hang	appendix
phon-	sound	phonetics
port-	to carry	transport
scrib-, script-	to write	transcription, prescribe
tract-	to pull, drag, or draw	attract, traction

COMBINING FORMS

A combing form is a root with an added vowel (usually *o*), which is referred to as a combining vowel. The root with the addition of the *combining vowel* is called a *combining form*. Let's look at some examples and the rules that affect the way the word elements are combined.

The combining vowel *o* is added to the root. Note the ease in saying the word with the addition of the o. Sometimes the vowel *i* is used.

EXAMPLE

splenomegaly

splen- + o + -megaly = enlargement of the spleen

↓ ↓ ↓

root combining vowel suffix

Splen- is the root meaning spleen, *o* is the combining vowel, and *-megaly* is the suffix meaning enlargement. Interpreting from suffix to the root, the meaning becomes *enlargement of the spleen*.

EXAMPLE

gastrology

gastr- + o + -logy = study of the stomach

↓ ↓ ↓

root combining form suffix

Gastr- is the root meaning stomach, *o* is the combining vowel, and *-logy* is the suffix meaning study of. Interpreting from suffix to the root, the meaning is *study of the stomach*.

If the combining form and suffix brings two vowels together, the combining vowel at the end of the root is usually dropped. (The combining form is shown in bold.)

EXAMPLE

gastritis

gastro + -itis = inflammation of the stomach lining

↓ ↓

combining form suffix

In the aforementioned example, ***gastro*** is the combining form meaning stomach and *-itis* is the suffix meaning inflammation. Thus, interpreting from suffix to root, gastritis means *the inflammation of the stomach lining*. Because two vowels are brought together, the combining vowel at the end of the combining form (*gastro*) is dropped.

EXAMPLE

gastrectomy

gastro + -ectomy = surgical removal of all or part of the stomach
↓ ↓
combining form suffix

In the above example, ***gastro*** is the combining form meaning stomach and *-ectomy* is a suffix meaning surgical removal of all or part of. Interpreting from the suffix to the combining form, we have *surgical removal of all or part of the stomach*. The combining vowel at the end of the root is dropped because two vowels are brought together with the combining form and the suffix.

If two roots are joined bringing two vowels together, the combining vowel is retained.

EXAMPLE

gastroenteritis

gastr- + o + **enter-** + -itis
↓ ↓ ↓ ↓
root combining vowel root suffix

In this word, interpreting from the suffix *-itis*, meaning inflammation, to the two roots meaning stomach (***gastr-***) and intestines (***enter-***), we have inflammation of the stomach and intestines. The roots *gastr-* and *enter-* and the combining vowel *o* put the combining vowels *o* and *e* at the beginning of the second root *enter-* together. The vowel will be retained, thus spelling gastroenteritis.

A word may not end in a combining form. To make the word either a noun or adjective, the combining vowel must be dropped and a suffix added. In the aforementioned word, gastroenteritis, it would be incorrect to say "gasteroentero." The combining vowel *o* after *entero* is dropped and the suffix *-itis* turns the word into a noun.

In summary, the rules of joining roots and combining forms are as follows:

- **The combining vowel o is added to the root.**
- **If the combining form and suffix brings two vowels together, the combining vowel at the end of the root usually is dropped.**
- **If two roots are joined bringing two vowels together, the combining vowel is retained.**
- **A word may not end in a combining form.**

SUFFIXES

A *suffix* is added to the end of a word to further clarify the meaning of the root. Generally, when a suffix stands alone, a hyphen precedes it. For instance, use the root *gastr-*, which means stomach, and add the suffix *-ectomy*, which means removal of all or part of, as indicated to follow. The suffix in the example is shown in bold.

The root will attach directly to a suffix if the suffix begins with a vowel.

Otherwise, a combining vowel must be added to the root, as shown to follow:

EXAMPLE

gastrectomy

gastr + **-ectomy**
↓ ↓
root suffix

Because ***-ectomy*** is a suffix that begins with a vowel, the root gastr- will be joined directly to it. Interpreting from the suffix to the root, we have *surgical removal of all or part of the stomach*.

If a suffix begins with a consonant, add a combining vowel to the root. Note how this rule applies to the following example.

EXAMPLE

Cardiotherapy

Cardi +	o +	**-therapy**
↓	↓	↓
root	combining vowel	suffix

Because ***-therapy***, meaning treatment, is a suffix beginning with a consonant, the root, *cardi-*, needs a combining vowel *o*. Interpreting from the suffix to the root, we have *treatment of cardiac diseases*.

In summary, the rules of joining suffixes to roots are as follows:

- **The root will attach directly to a suffix if the suffix begins with a vowel.**
- **If a suffix begins with a consonant, add a combining vowel to the root.**

Another function of the suffix is to help indicate whether the word is a noun (person, place, or thing) or an adjective (noun modifier). This is helpful because knowing the proper form of a word is an important skill. Note the following example that uses non-medical terms.

EXAMPLE

noun	music
adjective	musical

In this case, music is the name of a thing and is thus considered a noun. Adding the suffix *-al* (meaning pertaining to) forms the adjective musical. Thus, a musical event would be an event that *pertains to music*.

In the language of medicine, the word ending also indicates whether the word is an adjective or noun, as in the following example:

EXAMPLE

noun	tonsil
adjective	tonsillar

Here, tonsil is the name of a thing, making it a noun. Adding the suffix -ar (meaning resembling) forms the adjective tonsillar. So, if tonsillar is used as a modifier of tissue (noun), a tonsillar tissue would mean *tissue that resembles the tonsils*.

The following list provides some common adjective suffixes, their meaning, and examples of each.

Adjective Suffixes	Meaning	Example
-ac	pertaining to	cardi**ac**
-al, -ial	pertaining to	pleur**al**
-ar	of, relating to, resembling	vascul**ar**
-ary	pertaining to	pulmon**ary**
-eal	pertaining to	periton**eal**
-iac	of, relating to	cel**iac**
-ic	pertaining to, relating to	gastr**ic**

continues

Adjective Suffixes	Meaning	Example
-ical	pertaining to	patholog**ical**
-ile	pertaining to, capable	febr**ile**
-oid	resembling	aden**oid**
-ory	pertaining to, relating to	supposit**ory**
-ose	pertaining to, glucose	adip**ose**
-ous	full of, possessing	cancer**ous**
-tic	pertaining to	narco**tic**

Common noun endings are *a, ia, um,* and *y*. Note the differences in the form of the following nouns and adjectives.

Noun Form	Adjective Form	Noun Form	Adjective Form
artery	arterial	mania	manic
bacteria	bacterial	pericardium	pericardial
cranium	cranial	septum	septal
derma	dermal	stigma	stigmatic
fascia	fascial	surgery	surgical

Some common noun suffixes and examples are as follows:

Noun Suffix	Example	Noun Suffix	Example
-ate	particul**ate**	-ist	podiat**rist**
-e	bronchoscop**e**	-megaly	cardio**megaly**
-emia	hyper**emia**	-ole	bronchi**ole**
-er	vom**er**	-osis	cyan**osis**
-esis	hyperem**esis**	-tion	micturi**tion**
-iatry	psych**iatry**	-ula	fist**ula**
-ion	vis**ion**	-ule	gran**ule**
-ism	alcohol**ism**	-us	vill**us**

PREFIXES

A prefix is placed at the beginning of a word and modifies its meaning. In general use, when a prefix stands alone, a hyphen follows it. For example, take the word *gastrectomy* (meaning surgical removal of the stomach) and add the *hemi-* (meaning half). The prefix is shown in bold in the following example:

EXAMPLE

hemigastrectomy

hemi- + gastr- + -ectomy
↓ ↓ ↓
prefix root suffix

In analyzing this word, start with *-ectomy*, which means surgical removal of all or part of. Add hemi, which means half, and then move to *gastr-*, which means stomach. We now have the *surgical removal of half of the stomach.*

The prefix of a word provides more specific information about the meaning of the term. They are used in everyday language probably more than is realized. The following table presents several examples of these common prefixes.

Prefix	Meaning	Example
bi-	two, double	**bi**annually
hemi-, semi-	half	**hemi**sphere, **semi**annually
hyper-	excessive	**hyper**ventilate
infra-	beneath, below, under	**infra**structure
pre-	before, in front of	**pre**test
retro-	backward, behind	**retro**active
tri-	three	**tri**mester

A list of some prefixes that will help you to being your journey into medical language follows.

Prefix	Meaning
a-, an-	not, without, away from
an, ana-	up, against, back
aut-, auto-	self
end-, endo-	within
ep, epi-	above, upon
iso-	equal
mal-	bad
neo-	new, recent
nulli-	none
tel, tele-	distant

A word of caution about interpreting roots, prefixes, and suffixes needs to be said. Sometimes it is necessary to check your dictionary for an exact meaning. An example is *cardiectomy. Cardi-* means heart and *-ectomy* means surgical removal of all or part. Thus, the surgical removal of all or part of the heart would appear to be the correct meaning. Actually, the term cardiectomy means the *surgical removal of the upper end of the stomach.* Check your dictionary frequently.

SINGULAR AND PLURAL FORMS OF WORDS

To use medical terminology correctly, you must also understand the plural and singular forms of words. Plurals of medical words can be either in English or another language. For instance, the plural form of appendix becomes *appendixes* in English, but the foreign plural is *appendices*. But note that despite the American Medical Association's suggestion to use the English rules, you will encounter a mix of both forms in the medical arena.

The list that follows contains examples of some of the basic rules for forming the plurals of medical terms. Most are derived from the Latin or Greek languages.

Singular Form		Plural Form	
Ending	Example	Ending	Example
a	ampulla	ae	ampullae
ax	thorax	aces	thoraces
en	lumen	ina	lumina
ex	apex	ices	apices
is	diagnosis	es	diagnoses
ix	cervix	ices	cervices
ma	stigma	mata	stigmata
on	criterion	a	criteria
um	bacterium	a	bacteria
us	bronchus	i	bronchi

As in any language, there are exceptions to the rules. For example, some words are always singular in usage (ascites, herpes), some are always plural (adnexa, genitalia), and some words retain the same form whether the usage is singular or plural (biceps, facies). Still other words are exceptions, such as

Singular	**Plural**
cornu	cornua
epididymis	epididymides
viscus	viscera

Always refer to a medical dictionary for proper guidance.

HOMONYMS AND OTHER WORDS THAT MAY CAUSE CONFUSION

In linguistics, a **homonym** is one of a group of words that share the same spelling or pronunciation (or both) but have different meanings. There is a great deal of confusion and contradiction in published sources about the distinction between homonyms, homographs, homophones, and heteronyms. *Homographs* are homonyms that share the same spelling. *Homophones* are homonyms that share the same pronunciation. Homophones may be spelled the same (in which case they are also homographs) or spelled differently (in which case they are heterographs). *Heteronyms* are homonyms that share the same spelling but have different pronunciations. Heteronyms are also sometimes called *heterophones*. Regardless of the term used, careful discrimination is required. Examples of words that commonly cause confusion in medical records are shown in the following table.

Word	Definition
bare	naked
bear	to produce, give birth, sustain
breath	respiration
breathe	to inhale and exhale
cancer	malignant tumor
canker	an ulceration
chancre	primary lesion of syphilis

continues

Word	Definition
die	to cease to live
dye	to stain
facial	pertaining to the face
fascial	pertaining to fascia (connective tissue)
perineal	pertaining to the anatomical region between the thighs at the lower end of the trunk
peritoneal	pertaining to a membrane
peroneal	pertaining to the region of the fibula or outer side of the leg
sight	vision
site	place
cite	to quote
villous	shaggy with soft hair
villus	small vascular protrusion

EPONYMS

An eponym is a name derived from the name of the person who discovered or perfected a particular medical disease, body part, or procedure. They are the only medical terms that are capitalized with the exception of trade names. Although the AMA recommends that a comparable medical term be used, eponyms are still commonly found in medical reports.

Some examples of eponyms with their comparable medical terms or definitions are as follows.

Eponym	Definition
Babinski's reflex	extension of the great toe with flexion of other toes on exciting the sole
Bell's palsy	peripheral facial paralysis
Dupuytren's contracture	flexion deformity of fingers
Graves' disease	exophthalmic (ek"sŏf-thal'mĭk) goiter
Hodgkin's disease	lymphogranulomatosis (lĭm"fō-grăn"ū-lō-mah-tō'sĭs)
Parkinson's disease	paralysis agitans (ăg'ĭ-tăns)
Romberg's sign	swaying of the body and an inability to stand when the eyes are closed and the feet are placed together

The possessive form of an eponym is acceptable and in use in many institutions. However, the growing trend is to eliminate the possessive form as in *Down syndrome* and *Alzheimer disease*. This trend is supported by the Association for Healthcare Documentation Integrity (AHDI) and the AMA.

MEDICAL DICTIONARIES

Knowledge of word elements, the ability to form plurals correctly, the ability to provide noun or adjective word endings, and knowledge of homonyms and eponyms will help you to learn medical terminology. However, there is one other skill you need to develop: how to use a medical dictionary.

A medical dictionary is a standard reference for a medical office because it includes terms from the basic sciences of anatomy, physiology, biochemistry, and pharmacology, as well as all the major specialties of clinical medicine and surgery.

To use a dictionary effectively, you should be familiar with its organization and the kinds of information it contains. In many medical dictionaries illustrations are placed within the text near the associated term. Some dictionaries include, as a separate section of the book, detailed anatomical plates (often in full color) that show the body in meaningful sections or by system. Other dictionaries have the plates integrated appropriately within the text.

When referencing a word or term, you will in most cases be able to quickly find it. However, sometimes—especially for phrases—you may need to determine the "key" word in the phrase to know where to look. For example, if you are looking for polycystic kidney disease, the key term is disease and is your starting point. Under *disease* there will be a list of phrases defining a specific disease where you should find *polycystic kidney d.* In some cases you may need to use your newfound word element knowledge to help in your search. Or you may need to reference a different dictionary, including a nonmedical dictionary or even the Internet.

Another important point about medical dictionaries is that most have a set of appendixes that provide additional useful information. It will be to your advantage to become familiar with the "extras" your dictionary provides.

Because many words sound different from their spelling, a variety of entries in the dictionary should be checked. Some examples of beginning letters that have a different sound are shown in this table.

Beginning Letters	Sounds Like	Example
ch	k	**ch**romatin
kn	n	**kn**ee
pn	n	**pn**eumonia
ps	s	**ps**ychiatry
pt	t	**pt**osis
sc	sk	**sc**lerosis
sch	sk	**sch**izoid
x	z	**x**anthoma

Some word beginnings sound alike but are spelled differently. The following are commonly encountered.

EXAMPLES

dys, dis, des sounds like dis   ker, cur sounds like ker
cy, si, sy, psy sounds like sy

The dictionary also includes pronunciation marks for medical words. Generally, pronunciation follows certain rules. These are

1. Words of two syllables are commonly accented on the first syllable.

EXAMPLES

renal (rē'năl)   ventral (vĕn'trăl)
ptosis (tō'sĭs)

2. In words of more than two syllables, the next to the last syllable is accented; the first syllable is rarely accented.

EXAMPLES

chromatic (krō-măt'ĭk)   orthoptic (or-thŏp'tĭk)

3. In the accented syllable, a vowel is short if it is followed by a consonant in the same syllable; if a vowel ends the accented syllable, it is long.

EXAMPLES

bronchoscopy (brong-kŏs'kō-pē)—accented syllable with short vowel

adrenal (ah-drē'năl)—accented syllable with long vowel

For the pronunciation of individual words, consult your medical dictionary. Read the notes or guidelines on the use of the dictionary that are usually found at the beginning of the reference source.

Practice in using the dictionary will build your skill in this area. Beginning with this chapter, exercises designed to acquaint you with the use of your dictionary are provided. Effective use of the dictionary will improve your production and effectiveness as an allied health professional.

INTERNET ASSIGNMENT

A wealth of medical information is available on the Internet. The challenge is knowing how and where to look for that one piece of information that fills your need, whether it be business or personal.

To give you some basic experience in finding "just the right" source, each chapter will introduce you to a web site and suggest an activity that will provide supplemental information about the topic of the chapter. For more practice, the Web Tutor Internet tool offers three additional web sites for each chapter.

An effort has been made to choose web sites that are well established and properly maintained and are likely to remain available for some time. However, over the life of this textbook, existing sites may be withdrawn—sometimes with little notice, other times with referrals to replacements—and new sites will be introduced. If an assigned web site is not available, your standing assignment is to find a suitable substitute.

Some web sites are limited in scope, often targeting a single topic. Others take a broad-brush approach, giving you overview information and then directing you to a wide range of specific subjects. This is the case with the site introduced in this chapter.

The National Institutes of Health (NIH) is one of the eight health agencies of the Public Health Services, which, in turn, is part of the U.S. Department of Health and Human Services. Its web site is located at **www.nih.gov**. The NIH has 27 separate components, which are mainly research institutes and centers. The mission of the NIH is to uncover new knowledge that will lead to better health for everyone. Its goal is to help prevent, detect, diagnose, and treat disease and disability, from the rarest genetic disorder to the common cold. This valuable site has information about health conditions, research studies, drug information, health literature references, and special programs and provides links to other federal agencies.

By accessing each of these institutes and centers, you can obtain specific information that relates to the various topics covered in the textbook. These include cancer; the eye; heart, lung, and blood; alcohol abuse and alcoholism; allergy and infectious diseases; arthritis and musculoskeletal and skin diseases; biomedical imaging; child health and human development; deafness and other communication disorders; diabetes and digestive and kidney diseases; drug abuse; mental health; neurological disorders and stroke; and complementary and alternative medicine.

The NIH site is also home to the National Library of Medicine, which includes electronic data bases such as MEDLINE and MEDLINEplus, used extensively throughout the world by both professionals and the general public.

ACTIVITY

Access the National Health Institutes at **www.nih.gov**. Click on Health Information and explore the hyperlinks listed. Write a short summary of your findings with respect to the kinds of information and aids available on this site. Submit it to your instructor.

Review *Building a Medical Vocabulary*

- To understand medical terminology requires knowledge of word elements, body structure, human anatomy, special medical meanings of otherwise familiar words, diagnostic and treatment procedures, medications, metric measures, and abbreviations.
- The language of medicine, derived primarily from Greek and Latin, is highly technical and extensive.
- The major word element is a root, which can be combined with a suffix, a prefix, or another root.
- The plural form of a word varies widely. The American Medical Association suggests using the English plural, but foreign plurals are used as well.
- Adjective and noun suffixes must be used appropriately in reports.
- Homonyms (words that sound alike but differ in meaning) and words that are spelled similarly or sound similar require careful discrimination by medical office workers.
- Eponyms combine a person's name with a disease or part of the body.
- Effective use of a medical dictionary is essential; be familiar with its contents.

Key Terminology Practice Exercises

COMPLETION

Complete the following statements.

1. A large portion of the language of medicine comes from the _____________ and _____________ languages.
2. The major word element is called a _____________.
3. An element placed at the end of a word that further defines the word is called a _____________.
4. An element placed at the beginning of a word that modifies the meaning of the word is called a _____________.
5. The root with the addition of the combining vowel is called a _____________.
6. A word is a/an _____________ when *-al*, *-ac*, *-ic*, *-ary*, *-eal*, or *-ous* is added as a suffix.
7. If two roots bring two vowels together, the combining vowel at the end of the first root is _____________.
8. *Romberg's sign* is an example of a/an _____________.
9. Words alike in sound but different in meaning are called _____________.
10. If a combining form and suffix bring two vowels together, the combining vowel at the end of the root is usually _____________.
11. Words of two syllables are commonly accented on the _____________ syllable.
12. Place the accent on the correct syllable for these words: re-nal; chro-mat-ic.
13. When the suffix of a word is *-a*, *-ia*, *-um*, or *-y*, the part of speech for the word is a/an _____________.
14. When a singular word ends in us, the plural form ends in _____________.

15. Dye and die are examples of ____________.
16. Words of more than two syllables are usually accented ____________the last syllable.
17. A website that is maintained by the U.S. Department of Health and Human Services is ____________.

PLURALS

Form the plural of each of the singular words provided.

1. viscus ____________
2. bacterium ____________
3. epididymis ____________
4. lumen ____________
5. diagnosis ____________
6. stigma ____________
7. criterion ____________
8. cornu ____________
9. bronchus ____________
10. ampulla ____________

CORRECT DEFINITION

Place a check next to the correct definition of the following words.

1. a place
   _____ site
   _____ sight
   _____ cite
2. an ulceration
   _____ cancer
   _____ canker
   _____ chancre
3. respiration
   _____ breath
   _____ breathe
4. pertaining to the face
   _____ facial
   _____ fascial
5. pertaining to a membrane
   _____ perineal
   _____ peritoneal
   _____ peroneal
6. shaggy with soft hair
   _____ villous
   _____ villus

NOUN/ADJECTIVE

Indicate whether the following words are nouns (N) or adjectives (A).

Word	N or A
1. adipose	____________
2. arterial	____________
3. bacteria	____________
4. cardiac	____________
5. surgical	____________

6. fascia ______________
7. mania ______________
8. narcotic ______________
9. pediatrist ______________
10. pericardium ______________
11. pleural ______________
12. pulmonary ______________
13. celiac ______________
14. septum ______________
15. cancerous ______________

Word Element Review

In each of the following chapters, you will learn some roots, prefixes, and suffixes. The roots will be shown with their combining vowel. Whenever possible, they are related to the subject matter of the text. Some of them, however, relate to many chapters.

Below are several basic prefixes and suffixes. A few root words with combining vowels are included to provide an opportunity for practice exercises.

Root	Meaning	Example	Definition
acr/o	extremity	**acrocyanosis** (ăk"rō-sī"ah-nō'sĭs)	bluish or reddish color in the fingers, wrists, and ankles
bas/o	base	**basic** (bā'sĭk)	pertaining to a base
cardi/o	heart	**cardiogenic** (kăr"dē-ō-jĕn'ĭk)	originating in the heart
cyan/o	blue	**cyanophil** (sī-ān'ō-fĭl)	cell easily stained with blue dyes
enter/o	intestine	**enteritis** (ĕn"tĕr-ī'tĭs)	inflammation of the intestine
gastr/o	stomach	**gastrology** (găs-trŏl'ō-jē)	study of the stomach
pharmac/o	drug	**pharmacology** (fahr"mah-kŏl'ō-jē)	study of drugs
physi/o	nature	**physiology** (fiz"ē-ŏl'ō-jē)	study of the function of cells, tissues, and organs of living organisms

continues

Root	Meaning	Example	Definition
splen/o	spleen	**splenectomy** (splē-nĕk'tō-mē)	surgical removal of the spleen
top/o	place	**topical** (tŏp'ĕ-kăl)	pertaining to place or surface
Prefix	**Meaning**	**Example**	**Definition**
a-, an-	without	**acardia** (ă-kăr'dē-ah)	congenital absence of the heart
ana-	backward, up, against	**anatropia** (ăn"ă-trō'-pē-ă)	tendency of eyeballs to turn inward
auto-	self	**autoactivation** (aw"tō-ăk"tĭ-vā'shŭn)	gland activation by its own secretion
end-, endo-	within	**endoscope** (ĕn'dō-skōp)	instrument used to look inside an organ
gran-	grain	**granule** (grăn'ūl)	small grain
hemi-	half	**hemigastrectomy** (hĕm"ē-găs-trĕk'tō-mē)	surgical removal of half of the stomach
nulli-	none	**nulliparous** (nŭl-lĭp'ăr-ŭs)	never having borne a child
Suffix	**Meaning**	**Example**	**Definition**
-ac, -al, -ar, -ary	pertaining to	**pulmonary** (pŭl'mō-nĕ-rē)	pertaining to the lungs
-crit	separate	**hematocrit** (hē-măt'ō-krĭt)	test that separates erythrocytes in total blood volume
-cyte	cell	**leukocyte** (loo'kō-sīt)	white blood cell
-ectomy	excision, surgical removal	**gastrectomy** (găs-trĕk'tō-mē)	surgical removal of all or part of the stomach
-gen	originate, produce	**antigen** (ăn'tĭ-jĕn)	any substance capable of inducing antibody formation
-globin	protein	**hemoglobin** (hē"mō-glō' bĭn)	primary carrier of oxygen in red blood cells
-gram	record, picture, tracing	**cardiogram** (kăr'dē-ō-grăm")	picture of the heart
-graph	instrument used for recording	**electrocardiograph** (ē-lĕk"trō-kăr'dē-ō-grăf)	instrument for recording electrical activity of the heart
-iac; -ic	pertaining to	**toxic** (tŏks'ĭk)	pertaining to poisons
-it is	inflammation of	**gastritis** (găs-trī'tĭs)	inflammation of the stomach
-megaly	enlargement	**cardiomegaly** (kăr"dē-ō-mĕg'ă-lē)	enlargement of the heart

continues

Suffix	Meaning	Example	Definition
-(o)logist	specialist in the study of the	**gastrologist** (găs-trŏl'ō-jĭst)	one who specializes in the study of the stomach
-(o)logy	study of	**cardiology** (kăr-dē-ŏl'ō-jē)	study of the heart
-osis	condition	**cyanosis** (sī"ah-nō'sĭs)	condition of blueness
-scope	instrument used for visual examination	**bronchoscope** (brŏng'kō-skōp)	instrument for visual examination of the bronchi
-scopy	visual examination	**gastroscopy** (găs-trŏs'kō-pē)	visual examination of the stomach
-therapy	treatment	**cardiotherapy** (kăr"dē-ō-thĕr'ă-pē)	treatment of cardiac diseases
-tocia	labor, birth	**dystocia** (dĭs-tō'sē-ă)	difficult labor
-tome	instrument to cut	**microtome** (mī'krō-tōm)	instrument that cuts thin sections of tissue
-tresia	opening	**atresia** (ă-trē'zē-ă)	congenital absence of a normal body opening
-version	act of turning	**cardioversion** (kăr'dē-ō-vĕr"zhŭn)	restoration of normal sinus heart rhythm by electrical or chemical means

Word Element Practice Exercises

ROOT, PREFIX, OR SUFFIX

Circle the root and underline the prefix or suffix in the following words from the Word Element Review.

1. cardiology
2. gastrology
3. physiology
4. pharmacology
5. basic
6. cyanosis
7. antigen
8. topical
9. gastrologist
10. acardia
11. granule
12. acrocyanosis
13. splenectomy
14. cardiogenic
15. cardiogram
16. gastroscopy
17. enteritis
18. nulliparous
19. leukocyte
20. hemoglobin
21. endoscope
22. cardioversion
23. microtome
24. toxic
25. hematocrit

WORD ENDING—NOUN OR ADJECTIVE

Circle the word ending and specify whether the word is a noun (N) or an adjective (A).

	Word	N or A
1.	cardiac	______
2.	basal	______
3.	pulmonary	______
4.	topical	______
5.	gastroscopy	______
6.	basic	______
7.	pericardium	______
8.	granule	______
9.	cardiogenic	______
10.	gastrologist	______
11.	nulliparous	______
12.	fistula	______
13.	podiatrist	______
14.	villus	______
15.	bronchiole	______
16.	toxic	______
17.	fascial	______
18.	bacteria	______
19.	adenoid	______
20.	manic	______

SPELLING

Rewrite the misspelled words.

1. cardiojenic ______
2. granull ______
3. cyanosis ______
4. antegen ______
5. acrocyinosis ______
6. physiology ______
7. acardia ______
8. bacteria ______
9. bronchis ______
10. apexs ______

PRONUNCIATIONS AND DEFINITIONS

Provide the pronunciation and definition for each of the following terms.

1. physiology ____________________
2. acardia ____________________
3. basic ____________________
4. granule ____________________
5. cyanosis ____________________
6. topical ____________________
7. acrocyanosis ____________________
8. cardiogram ____________________
9. gastrology ____________________
10. pharmacology ____________________
11. cardiogenic ____________________
12. cyanophil ____________________
13. antigen ____________________
14. gastrologist ____________________
15. gastroscopy ____________________
16. dystocia ____________________
17. microtome ____________________
18. hemoglobin ____________________
19. toxic ____________________
20. gastritis ____________________
21. hemigastrectomy ____________________
22. leukocyte ____________________
23. pulmonary ____________________
24. nulliparous ____________________
25. astresia ____________________
26. enteritis ____________________
27. autoactivation ____________________
28. cardioversion ____________________
29. splenectomy ____________________
30. hematocrit ____________________

WORD ELEMENT MEANINGS

Give the meaning of each word element. Then use your dictionary to find a new word that contains each of the word elements. Specify whether the new word is a noun or adjective by placing N or A in the last column.

Word Element	Meaning	Word	N or A
1. a-, an-			
2. ac-			
3. acr/o			
4. -al			
5. ana-			
6. -ar, -ary			
7. auto-			
8. bas/o			
9. cardi/o			
10. crit-			
11. cyan/o			
12. -cyte			
13. -ectomy			
14. end-/endo-			
15. enter/o			
16. gastr/o			
17. -gen			
18. -globin			
19. -gram			
20. gram-			
21. -graph			
22. hemi-			
23. -iac, -ic			
24. -itis			
25. -megaly			
26. nulli-			
27. -(o)logist			
28. -(o)logy			
29. -osis			
30. pharmac/o			
31. physi/o			
32. -scope			
33. -scopy			
34. splen/o			
35. -therapy			

36. -tocia ____ ____ ____
37. -tome ____ ____ ____
38. top/o ____ ____ ____
39. -tresia ____ ____ ____
40. -version ____ ____ ____

Dictionary Exercises

Each chapter contains exercises that will enable you to use your medical dictionary effectively. On occasion, you may have to use a regular dictionary, just as allied health professionals are required to do.

DICTIONARY EXERCISE 1

Use your dictionary to find the definitions for the following homonyms and look-alike/sound-alike terms.

	Word	Pronunciation	Definition
1.	cord	____	____
	chord	____	____
2.	gait	____	____
	gate	____	____
3.	humerus	____	____
	humorous	____	____
4.	facet	____	____
	faucet	____	____
5.	colic	____	____
	choleic	____	____
6.	wen	____	____
	when	____	____
7.	acidic	____	____
	acetic	____	____
	acinic	____	____
8.	form	____	____
	forum	____	____
9.	shocky	____	____
	shotty	____	____
	shoddy	____	____
10.	radical	____	____
	radicle	____	____

11. profusion ______________ ______________
    perfusion ______________ ______________
12. casual ______________ ______________
    causal ______________ ______________
13. feet ______________ ______________
    feat ______________ ______________
14. affect ______________ ______________
    effect ______________ ______________
15. callous ______________ ______________
    callus ______________ ______________

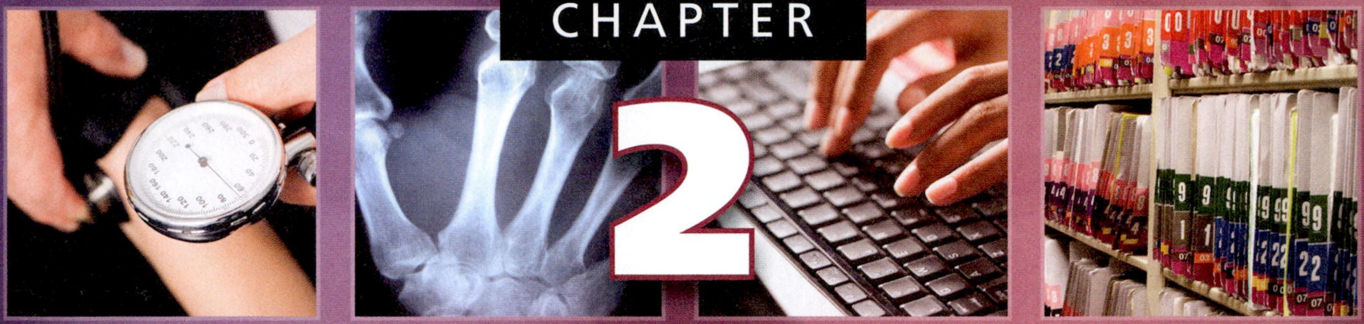

CHAPTER 2

Introduction to Body Structure

"You will have to learn many things . . . which you will forget the moment you have passed your final exam, but in anatomy it is better to have learned and lost than never to have learned at all."

—W. Somerset Maugham

OBJECTIVES

When you have completed this chapter on human anatomy, you should be able to

1. Spell and define the terms *cell*, *tissue*, *organ*, and *system* as they relate to the structure of living organisms.
2. Define the directions used in reference to the body structure.
3. Define the terms designated as planes of the body.
4. Define the cavities used to identify internal spaces of the body.
5. Name and define eleven systems of the body.
6. Identify the meanings of related word elements.

INTRODUCTION

Anatomy is defined as the science of the structure of living organisms. The study of human anatomy helps us to understand how our bodies work and is an important asset for anyone associated with the medical profession.

STRUCTURE OF THE BODY

a-	without	hypo-	beneath, less than
ana-	against, back	ne/o	new
dys-	bad, difficult, disordered	-plasia	formation, growth
hyper-	excessive		

Our bodies are marvelously intricate, delicate, and unique. Each part of the body has a purpose and function that fits into the total. Cells, tissues, organs, and systems are all part of the human anatomy.

CELLS

The smallest unit of life, the **cell**, is the basic structural unit of the body. Its contents are referred to collectively as **protoplasm** (prō'tō-plăzm). This thick, viscous colloidal material contains various organic and inorganic substances including, principally, the chemical elements oxygen, carbon, hydrogen, nitrogen, calcium, sulfur, and phosphorus.

Cells vary in size and purpose, as indicated in Figure 2-1. All have basic parts. The **cell membrane** is the outside covering. Next is the **cytoplasm** (sitō-plăzm"), which carries on the work of the cell and contains water, food particles, and pigment. Finally comes the **nucleus** (nu'klē-ŭs), the controlling structure of the cell. It normally contains 23 pairs of **chromosomes** (krō'mō-sōmz), small, threadlike structures that transmit genetic information. These in turn contain **genes**, which control heredity.

In a more general sense, there are three types of cells present in the body: **differentiated cells** (static cells), **undifferentiated cells** (expanding cells), and **stem cells** (renewing cells that give rise to other kinds of cells). The key difference between differentiated and undifferentiated cells is that undifferentiated cells can grow again, but differentiated cells cannot. An example of differentiated, or static, cells is muscle cells. Examples of undifferentiated, or expanding, cells are those of the skin, lining of the gut, or bone marrow. Stem, or renewing, cells die regularly and are replaced at regular intervals, as in the case of hair or the lining of your intestinal tract. Stem cells obey signals to stop growth, whereas cancer cells lack a control mechanism to switch off growth (see Figure 2-1).

TISSUES

Cells that are similar in nature group together to perform certain functions. Together they form **tissues**. These specialized cells make up four primary types of tissues: **epithelial** (ĕp"ĭ-thē'lē-ăl), **connective**, **muscular**, and **nervous**.

Epithelial Tissue

Epithelial tissue functions to protect, absorb, or secrete. This tissue may cover a surface, line a cavity, or form glandular structures. Epithelial tissues are classified by shape, arrangement, or function.

Shape. Shape-based classifications are squamous, cuboidal, and columnar cells. *Squamous* cells are flat, and slightly irregular epithelial cells found in the mouth, blood and lymph vessels, kidney tubules, throat, esophagus, anus, or skin and are designed to protect. *Cuboidal* cells are small cubes found in glands and linings or coverings of gland ducts whose purpose it is to secrete and protect, as well as to absorb in the kidney tubules. *Columnar* cells are tall and rectangular cells found in the ducts of certain glands and the bile duct of the liver, as well as in mucus-secreting tissues.

Arrangement. Arrangement-based classifications are simple, stratified, pseudostratified, and transitional. *Simple* arrangement is one cell layer thick, while *stratified* arrangement is several cell layers thick. *Pseudostratified*

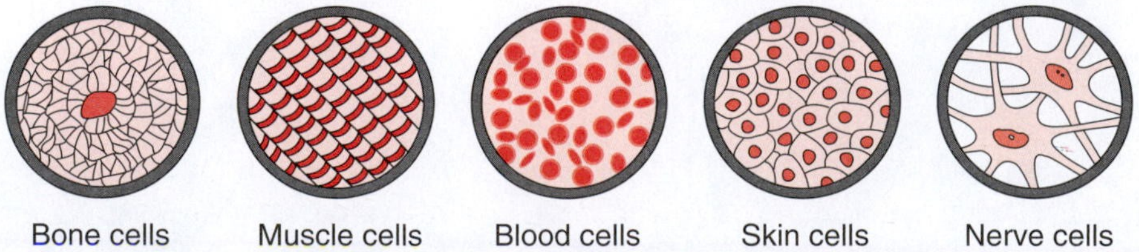

FIGURE 2-1
Types of Cells

arrangement is identified as all cells extending from the basement membrane to the outer surface of the cells. *Transitional* arrangement of the epithelium is several layers thick and closely packed, but flexible and stretchy.
Function. Function-based classifications are mucous membrane, glands, endothelium, and mesothelium. Mesothelium (or serous) tissue may take the form of pericardium, if it covers the heart; peritoneum, if it lines the abdominal cavity; or pleura, if it lines the thoracic cavity.

Connective Tissue

Connective tissue allows movement and provides support for the other types of tissues and holds the body together. It is subdivided into three groups. *Loose* connective tissue may be areolar (easily stretched without tearing), adipose (loaded with fat cells), or reticular (a fine network of fibers forming a framework of some organs). *Dense* connective tissue is tightly packed protein fibers that may have a regular arrangement such as tendons, ligaments, and aponeurosis (wide, flat tendons) or irregular arrangements such as muscle sheaths, the dermis skin layers, and the outer covering of the arteries. *Specialized* connective tissue has specific functions. Examples of this tissue type are cartilage (hyaline, fibrocartilage or elastic); bone and dentin; blood and hematopoietic tissue; lymphoid tissue; and synovial membranes.

Muscle Tissue

Muscle tissue has the ability to shorten, thicken, or contract, and is of three types. *Smooth* muscle tissue is involuntary: that is, it is not voluntarily controlled by an individual, but rather by the autonomic nervous system. An example is the digestive tract. *Striated* or *skeletal* muscle tissue, on the other hand, is voluntary. It is the tissue that causes movement of your body by pulling on bones. *Cardiac* muscle is found only in the heart and causes the contraction or beating of the heart.

Nervous Tissue

Nervous tissue conducts nerve impulses. It consists of neurons (conducting cells) and neuroglia (supporting cells). This tissue makes up the brain, spinal cord, and various nerves of the body and is the most highly organized tissue of the body. Nervous tissue is discussed in greater detail in Chapter 20.

Terms that relate to cellular growth include the following:

Anaplasia	loss of cellular differentiation and useful function
Aplasia	failure of tissue to develop normally
Dysplasia	abnormal development of tissue
Hyperplasia	excessive proliferation of normal cells in the normal arrangement of an organ
Hypoplasia	underdevelopment of a tissue organ or body
Neoplasia	development of growths that serve no useful function at the expense of the healthy organism

ORGANS

Two or more tissues combine to form an **organ**. Examples of cells and tissues grouped together to perform a certain function are the kidneys, heart, lungs, and liver. Internal organs are often referred to as **viscera** (vĭs'ĕr-ah).

SYSTEMS

Organs do not function independently. They work in combinations to form a **system**, which performs a function or a related group of functions. Systems of the body may be identified in a variety of ways. We will study them in the following framework.

System	Function
integumentary	The skin, hair, sweat, and sebaceous (sĕ-bā'shus) glands provide a covering and protection for the body.
musculoskeletal	Bones form the framework of the body, support organs, and provide a place to which muscles are attached; muscles permit motion and movement of the body.
blood and lymphatic	Blood carries oxygen and other substances to body parts; the lymph system furnishes protective mechanisms against infection.
cardiovascular	The heart pumps blood through the arteries and veins.
respiratory	The specialized organ group that transfers oxygen from air that is inhaled to the blood and transfers carbon dioxide from the blood to the air that is exhaled.
gastrointestinal	The alimentary canal transports and digests food, absorbs nutrients, and excretes waste products as necessary from the body.
urinary	The kidneys filter blood and excrete urine through the urinary tract.
reproductive	The function and composition of the male and female anatomies are designed for reproduction of the human race.
endocrine	The internal glands manufacture hormones.
nervous	The brain and nervous system integrate various intellectual and physical processes of the body.
sensory	The eyes, ears, nose, and throat provide information about the environment.

Each of these systems is presented later in this textbook.

BODY DIRECTION

Direction in the human body cannot be adequately managed using traditional terms. (Have you ever heard of the *eastern* part of your body?) A group of more definitive terms have been devised to designate specific regions of the body: anatomical position, body planes, and body cavities.

ANATOMICAL POSITION

The directional terms in the following table refers to the body when in the anatomical position, which is, body upright, face forward, and palms forward.

Direction	Pronunciation	Meaning	Example
anterior (ventral)	ăn-tēr'ē-or	toward the front	Both *anterior* cerebral arteries filled from the right side.
posterior (dorsal)	pōs-tēr'ē-or (dor'sal)	toward the back	The *posterior* wall of the disc space was excised.
medial	mē'dē-ăl	lying nearest the middle	A catheter was placed beneath the *medial* skin flap.
lateral	lăt'er-ăl	lying farthest from the median	The mass extended to the left *lateral* wall of the pelvis.
superior	soo-pē'rē-or	referring to the upper or head end	An extension of the tumor was found n the *superior* portion of the breast.
inferior	ĭn-fēr'ē-or	referring to the lower, away-from-the-head end	The *inferior* rectus muscle was detached from its insertion.
proximal	prŏk'sĭ-măl	that part closest to the source	The muscles were resected and reflected *proximally*.
distal	dĭs'tăl	that part farthest from the source	The *distal* portion of the common duct was thoroughly irrigated.
apex	ā'pĕks	tip, summit	The uppermost part of the lung is the *apex* of the lung.
base	bās	bottom, lower part	The fracture was at the *base* of the skull.
supine	soo'pīn	lying face up	The patient was placed in the *supine* position.
prone	prōn	lying face down	The operation was done with the patient in the *prone* position.

BODY PLANES

Another way to identify structures and areas of the body is to refer to planes. As displayed in Figure 2-2, the **median** or **mid-sagittal plane** (1) passes through the center of the head, chest, and pelvis, dividing the body into two equal right and left portions. The **sagittal** (săj'ĭ-tăl)**plane** (2) is parallel to the median plane, can be in any location, and divides the body into any two right and left portions. The **vertical** or **frontal plane** anterior (front) portion (3), also called the coronal plane, divides the body to create a posterior (back) and anterior (front) portion. This line is at right angles to the median (center) plane. Finally, the **transverse** or **horizontal plane** (4) divides the body horizontally into an upper and a lower portion.

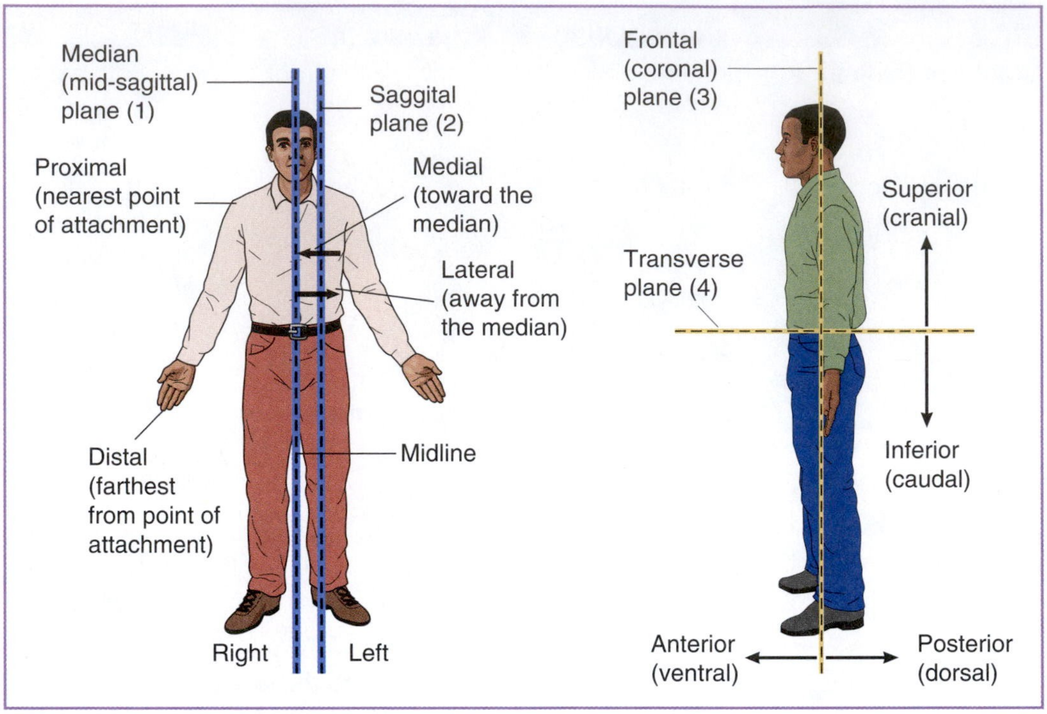

FIGURE 2-2
Planes of the Body

Source: Delmar/Cengage Learning

***StudyWARE™* Connection**

To watch an animation on **Body Planes**, go to your StudyWARE™ CD-ROM.

BODY CAVITIES

Sometimes the body is referred to in terms of a specific body cavity. Basically, as shown in Figure 2-3, there are two large internal spaces, which are called the **dorsal** (1) and **ventral** (8) **cavities**.

The two dorsal cavities are the **cranial cavity** (2), which contains the brain, and the **spinal cavity** (3), which encloses the spinal cord. Because they join, they are a continuous space.

The ventral cavities are much larger than the dorsal cavities and are not continuous. The **thoracic** (thō-răs'ĭk) **cavity** (4) is above and separated from the **abdominal cavity** (6) and the **pelvic cavity** (7) by a muscular membrane called the **diaphragm** (5). The thoracic cavity, shown in more detail in Figure 2-4, contains the heart, lungs, and large blood vessels. Included in this area are two smaller cavities, the **pleural** (ploo'răl) **cavity** and **mediastinum** (mē"dē-ah-stī'nŭm). The pleural cavity (one for each lung) is the space between the membranes that surround the lung, which is lined with a double-folded membrane called **pleura** (ploo'rah). The mediastinum is the area between the lungs that contains the heart and other organs. The abdominal cavity contains the stomach, intestines, kidney, liver, gallbladder, pancreas, and spleen. The pelvic cavity is joined with the abdominal cavity and contains the urinary bladder, rectum, and internal parts of the reproductive system.

Because the **abdominal cavity region** is so large, it is divided into nine divisions, as shown in Figure 2-5. The three central regions are the epigastrium (ĕp"ī -găs'trē-ŭm) (1), umbilical (ŭm-bĭl'ĭ-kal) (2), and hypogastric (hī "pō-gas'trĭk) (3). At each side are the right and left hypochondrium (hī "pōkon'drē-ŭm) regions (6), the right and left inguinal (ĭng'gwĭ -nal) (iliac [ĭl'ē-ak]) regions (4), and the right and left lumbar regions (5) near the waist. These directions allow a physician to identify specifically any area of the body.

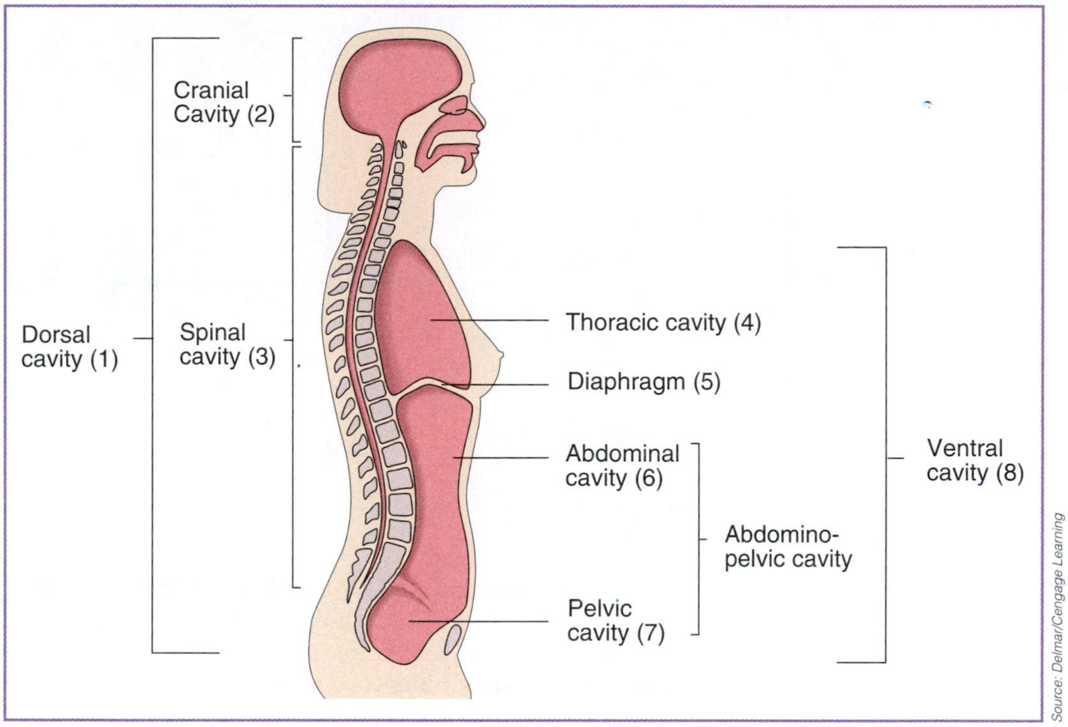

FIGURE 2-3
Cavities of the Body

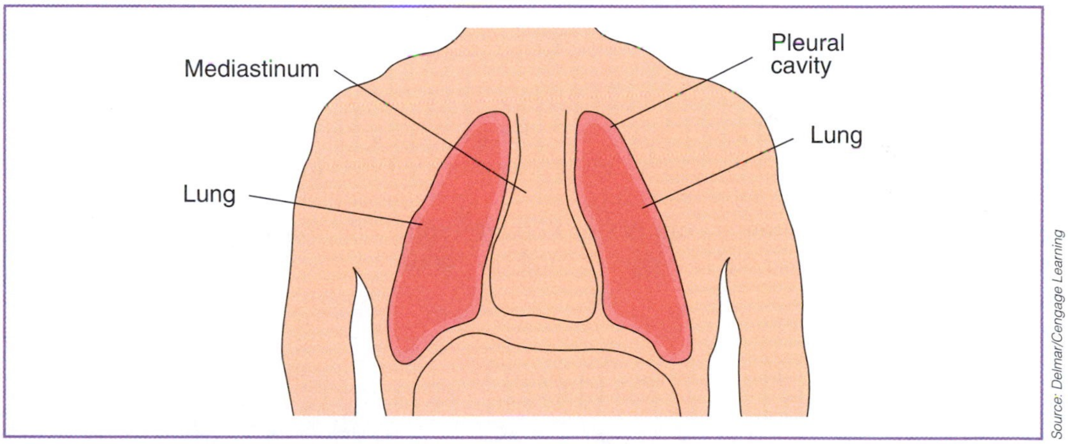

FIGURE 2-4
Divisons of the Thoracic Cavity

INTERNET ASSIGNMENT

When searching for medical information, a good source is a medical dictionary. The books have a complete list of terms, supporting photographs and anatomical drawings, and an encyclopedic list of informative appendices. Most of these dictionaries can be found on the Internet and many are available free (although some require a no-cost registration). Let's check a few of them.

Key in **www.medlineplus.gov** and you will be shown a list of general and specialty medical topics. Click on "Medical Encyclopedia" and you will be directed to *A.D.A.M. Medical Encyclopedia* which includes an extensive library of medical photographs and illustrations as well as terminology.

Another source is **www.medterms.com.** This site, a subset of Medinenet.com, is owned and operated by WebMD and is part of the WEB MD Network. Webster's New World Medical Dictionary is the medical reference for MedicineNet.com.

Miriam-Webster Online at **www.m-w.com** provides a medical term search function. Simply key in the word you wish to find and press enter.

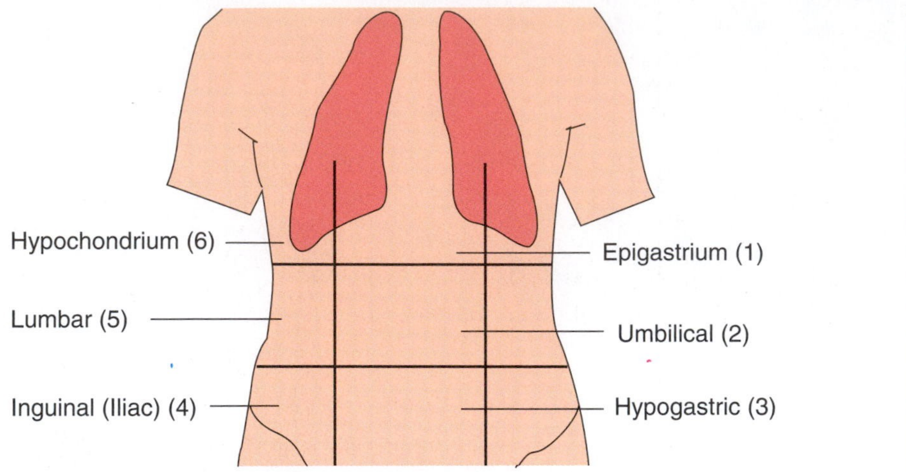

FIGURE 2-5 Divisons of the Abdominal Cavity

The Free Dictionary, found at **www.medical-dictionary.thefreedictionary.com**, uses *The American Heritage Stedman's Medical Dictionary* and *Dorland's Medical Dictionary for Health Care Consumers* as its main sources. Select "Medical Dictionary" from the *What's Inside* menu.

And finally, check **www.online-medical-dictionary.org** for a free online medical information search engine for definitions of medical terminology, pharmaceutical drugs, healthcare equipment, health conditions, medical devices, specialty terms, and medical abbreviations. Consider adding their free, continuously updated medical dictionary software to your computer.

ACTIVITY

Access *A.D.A.M. Medical Encyclopedia* to check out the anatomy available in it. Write a summary about the content. Next, access one of the other general medical dictionaries and summarize your investigation to the instructor. As an alternative assignment, use the keyword search function of your Internet service, your Internet browser, or search engine (**www.google.com** is a good one) to find a dictionary. Select three dictionaries and write a brief report to your instructor on their content and ease of use.

Review *Introduction to Body Structure*

- The body is composed of a progression of units beginning with a cell. Groups of specialized cells form tissues, which in turn form organs.
- Although organs are independent units, they usually are part of a system that serves a particular function.
- The systems of the body are integumentary, musculoskeletal, blood and lymphatic, cardiovascular, respiratory, gastrointestinal, urinary, reproductive, endocrine, nervous, and sensory.
- Body direction is identified by planes: median (mid-sagittal), sagittal, frontal (vertical), and transverse (horizontal).
- Two main body cavities are dorsal (containing the cranial and spinal cavities) and ventral (containing the abdominal, pelvic, and thoracic cavities).

Key Terminology Review

Word	Meaning
abdominal cavity	largest ventral cavity, containing the stomach, intestines, kidneys, liver, gallbladder, pancreas, and spleen
abdominal cavity regions	epigastrium, umbilical, hypogastric, right and left hypochondriac, right and regions left inguinal (iliac), and right and left lumbar regions
cell	smallest unit of life
cell membrane	outside covering of a cell
chromosome	threadlike structure that transmits genetic information; 1 of 23 pairs in a cell
connective tissue	groups of specialized cells that hold all parts of the body in place
cranial cavity	space that contains the brain; one of the dorsal cavities
cytoplasm	all substances of a cell other than the nucleus; carries on work of a cell
diaphragm	muscular membrane that separates ventral cavities
differentiated cells	static cells that cannot grow
dorsal cavity	large internal space containing the cranial and spinal cavities
epithelial tissue	tissue that forms glands, covers surfaces, and lines cavities
genes	blueprints that control heredity
median plane (mid-sagittal)	plane that passes through the center of the head, chest, and pelvis, dividing the body into two equal portions
mediastinum	middle portion of the thoracic cavity
muscular tissue	tissue composed of fibers that contract and cause or allow movement
nervous tissue	tissue that conducts nerve impulses
nucleus	controlling structure of a cell
organ	formed by two or more tissues working together to perform a certain function
pelvic cavity	bony hollow formed by the innominate bones, the sacrum, and the coccyx
pleura	double-folded membrane lining the pleural cavities
pleural cavities	right and left portions of the thoracic cavity; space between the membranes that surround each lung
protoplasm	collective name for the organic and inorganic substances that make up the contents of a cell
sagittal plane	plane that is parallel to the median plane in any location, dividing the body into any two portions, right and left spinal cavity dorsal cavity enclosing the spinal cord
stem cells	renewing cells that are replaced regularly
system	organs that combine to perform a function or related group of functions
thoracic cavity	uppermost section of the ventral cavity; contains heart, lungs, and large blood vessels as well as pleural cavities and mediastinum
tissues	groups of specialized cells that perform specific functions
transverse plane (horizontal)	plane that divides the body horizontally into two parts, upper and lower portions
undifferentiated cells	expanding cells that can grow again
ventral cavities	large cavities separated by the diaphragm
vertical plane (frontal)	plane that divides the body into a back and a front
viscera	name for internal organs

Key Terminology Practice Exercises

CHOICES

Circle the correct answer in each statement.

1. The (vertical, sagittal) plane divides the body into back and front portions.
2. The (vertical, transverse) plane divides the body horizontally into upper and lower portions.
3. The (sagittal, transverse) plane is parallel to the median plane, can be in any location, and divides the body into any two right and left portions.
4. The (median, sagittal) plane refers to a line from the center of the head through the center of the chest and pelvis and divides the body into two equal portions.
5. The tissues that form glands, cover surfaces, and line cavities are (epithelial, connective).
6. The tissue that holds body parts in place is (epithelial, connective).
7. Tissue that expands and contracts to allow movement is (connective, muscular).
8. The tissue that conducts nerve impulses is (nervous, epithelial).

COMPLETION

Complete the following statements.

1. The three ventral cavities are the _______________, _______________, and _______________.
2. Cells and tissues grouped together to perform certain functions are called ___________.
3. Internal organs are often referred to as the _______________.
4. The cavity that contains the urinary bladder, rectum, and internal parts of the reproductive system is called the _______________ cavity.
5. A continuous space that contains the cranial and spinal cavities is called the _______________ cavity.
6. The muscular membrane separating the thoracic cavity from the abdominal and pelvic cavities is the _______________.
7. The thoracic cavity has two smaller cavities: the _______________ and the _______________.
8. The abdominal cavity is divided into _______________ regions.
9. The central regions of the abdominal cavity are called _______________, _______________, and _______________ regions.
10. The right and left regions next to the three central regions are _______________, _______________, and _______________.
11. The difference between differentiated and undifferentiated cells is _______________.
12. Cells that are replaced on a regular basis are _______________ cells.

DEFINITIONS

Define the following body directions.

1. distal ____
2. proximal ____
3. inferior ____
4. lateral ____
5. anterior ____

MATCHING

Match the systems to their functions.

1. ___________ manufactures hormones
2. ___________ filters blood and excretes urine
3. ___________ covers and protects the body
4. ___________ forms the framework of the body; permits motion and movement of the body
5. ___________ handles the integration of intellectual and physical processes
6. ___________ transfers oxygen from the air we inhale to the blood and transfers carbon dioxide from the blood to the air we exhale
7. ___________ transports blood throughout the body through veins and arteries
8. ___________ transports and digests food, absorbs nutrients, and excretes waste products
9. ___________ provides for perpetuation of the human species
10. ___________ carries oxygen and other materials to body parts; furnishes protection against infection
11. ___________ provides the body with information about the environment

a. cardiovascular
b. endocrine
c. gastrointestinal
d. urinary
e. integumentary
f. blood, lymphatic
g. musculoskeletal
h. nervous
i. respiratory
j. reproductive
k. sensory

IDENTIFICATION

Identify the direction intended in the following phrases.

1. anterior cerebral artery ___________
2. medial skin flap ___________
3. superior portion of the breast ___________
4. distal portion of the common duct ___________
5. supine position ___________
6. in the prone position ___________
7. base of the organ ___________
8. apex of the organ ___________

DESCRIPTIONS

Describe each of the terms that are associated with a cell.

1. cell ___________
2. protoplasm ___________
3. cell membrane ___________
4. cytoplasm ___________
5. nucleus ___________
6. chromosomes ___________
7. genes ___________

Word Element Review

Root	Meaning	Example	Definition
cyt/o	cell	**cytology** (sī-tŏl'ō-jē)	study of cells
dors/o	back	**dorsal** (dor'săl)	pertaining to the back
end/o	inside	**endocardium** (ĕn"dō-kar'dē-ŭm)	innermost lining membrane of the heart
later/o	side	**lateral** (lăt"er-ăl)	pertaining to a side
ne/o	new	**neoplasm** (nē'ō-plăzm)	abnormal tissue growth, tumor
somat/o	body	**somatic** (sō-măt'ĭk)	pertaining to the body
viscer/o	internal organ	**visceral** (vĭs'er-ăl)	pertaining to the organs of the body

Prefix	Meaning	Example	Definition
a-	without	**aplasia** (ă-plā'zē-ă)	failure of tissue to develop normally
ana-	against, back	**anaplasia** (ăn"ă-plā'zē-ă)	loss of cellular differentiation and useful function
contra-	against	**contraindicated** (kŏn"trah-ĭn'dĭ-kā"tĕd)	not advisable; not recommended
dys-	bad, difficult	**dysplasia** (dĭs-plā'zē-ă)	abnormal development of tissue
ex-	out, away from	**excrete** (ĕks-krēt')	to throw off or eliminate
hyper-	excessive	**hyperplasia** (hī"pĕr-plā'zē-ă)	excessive proliferation of normal cells in the normal arrangement of an organ
hypo-	beneath, less than	**hypoplasia** (hī"pō-plā'zē-ă)	underdevelopment of a tissue organ or body
inter-	between	**intermuscular** (ĭn"ter-mŭs'kū-lăr)	between muscles
intra-	within	**intramuscular** (ĭn"trah-mŭs'kū-lăr)	within the muscle
peri-	about, around, surrounding	**pericardium** (pĕr"ĭ-kăr'dē-ŭm)	fibrous sac enclosing the heart
retro-	backward	**retrograde** (rĕt'rō-grād)	moving backward; degenerating to a worsened state
sub-	under, below	**subconscious** (sŭb-kŏn'shŭs) **subnormal**	below the level of conscious perception; below normal

continues

Prefix	Meaning	Example	Definition
trans-	through, across	**transplant**	to graft tissue from one place to another
Suffix	**Meaning**	**Example**	**Definition**
-plasia	formation, growth	**neoplasia** (nē"ō-plā'zē-ă)	development of growths that serve no useful purposescontinues

Word Element Practice Exercises

ROOT OR COMBINING FORM

Circle the root or combining form in the following words.

1. dorsolateral
2. cytology
3. lateral
4. somatic
5. visceral
6. endocardium
7. neoplasia

PREFIX

Circle the prefix in the following words.

1. dysplasia
2. transplant
3. retrograde
4. anaplasia
5. intermuscular
6. contraindicated
7. hyperplasia
8. excrete
9. pericardium
10. hypoplasia
11. intramuscular
12. subconscious

WORD ENDINGS—NOUN OR ADJECTIVE

Circle the word ending and specify whether the word is a noun (N) or an adjective (A).

1. visceral ____________________
2. somatic ____________________
3. subconscious ____________________
4. lateral ____________________
5. dorsal ____________________
6. pericardium ____________________

COMPLETION

Complete the following statements.

1. To graft tissue from one place to another is to ________________.
2. The study of cells is called ________________.
3. The failure of normal tissue development is ________________.
4. ________________ means pertaining to the side of the body.
5. The fibrous sac that surrounds the heart is the ________________.
6. ________________ means pertaining to the body.
7. ________________ means pertaining to the back.
8. In medical usage, ________________ means that something is not recommended.
9. ________________ means pertaining to the organs of the body.
10. ________________ means between muscles.
11. The innermost lining membrane of the heart is the ________________.
12. The abnormal formation of tissue is called a ________________.

MEANINGS

Give the meaning of the underscored words.

1. The <u>dorsal</u> lobes of the brain are the occipital lobes.

   ____

2. The little toes are <u>lateral</u> to the big toes.

   ____

3. Administering antibiotics is <u>contraindicated</u> at this time.

   ____

4. An <u>intramuscular</u> injection was given.

   ____

5. The body <u>excretes</u> urine through the bladder.

   ____

WORD ELEMENT MEANINGS

Give the meaning of each word element. Then use your dictionary to find a new word that contains each of the word elements. Specify whether the new word is a noun or adjective by placing N or A in the last column.

Word Element	Meaning	Word	N or A
1. a-			
2. ana-			
3. contra-			
4. cyt/o			
5. dors/o			
6. dys-			
7. end/o			
8. ex-			
9. hyper-			
10. hypo-			
11. inter-			
12. intra-			
13. later/o			
14. ne/o			
15. peri-			
16. -plasia			
17. retro-			
18. somato/o			
19. sub-			
20. trans-			
21. viscer/o			

Dictionary Exercises

DICTIONARY EXERCISE 1

Use your dictionary to find the pronunciation and definition of the following words.

Word	Pronunciation	Definition
1. metabolism		
2. histologist		
3. endogenous		

4. peritoneum	______________	______________
5. quadrant	______________	______________
6. superficial	______________	______________
7. catabolism	______________	______________
8. hypochondriac	______________	______________
9. megakaryocyte	______________	______________
10. mitochondria	______________	______________
11. viscera	______________	______________
12. retroflexion	______________	______________

DICTIONARY EXERCISE 2

Pronunciation of the words below is provided. Using your dictionary, find the correct spelling and definition of each word.

Word	Pronunciation	Definition
1. ______________	en"dō-kăr-dī'tĭs	______________
2. ______________	lăt"ĕr-ō-vĕr'shŭn	______________
3. ______________	trăns"thō-răs'ĭk	______________
4. ______________	rĕt"rō-ăk'shŭn	______________
5. ______________	sŭb-frĕn'ĭk	______________
6. ______________	vĭs"ĕr-ō-jĕn'ĭk	______________
7. ______________	si"tō-păth-ŏl'ō-jē	______________
8. ______________	dor"sō-vĕn'trăl	______________
9. ______________	sō"măt-ō-jĕn'ĭk	______________
10. ______________	ĭn"tĕr-mē'dē-ār-ē	______________
11. ______________	ĭn-tră-vē'nŭs	______________
12. ______________	ĕks-prĕs'	______________
13. ______________	skwā'mŭs	______________
14. ______________	kū-boyd'ăl	______________
15. ______________	soo-dō-străt'ĭ-fī d	______________
16. ______________	strī'ā-tĕd	______________

StudyWARE™ Connection

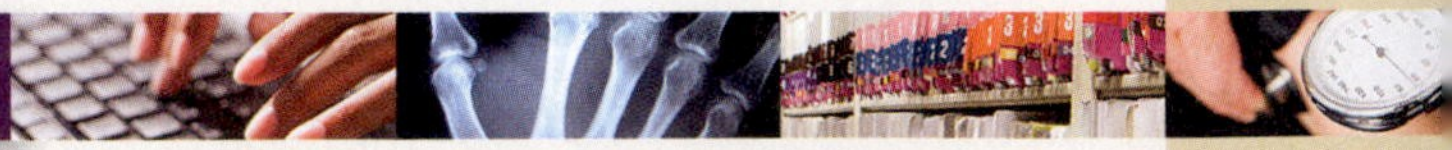

To play interactive games that reinforce the content in this chapter, go to your StudyWARE™ CD-ROM.

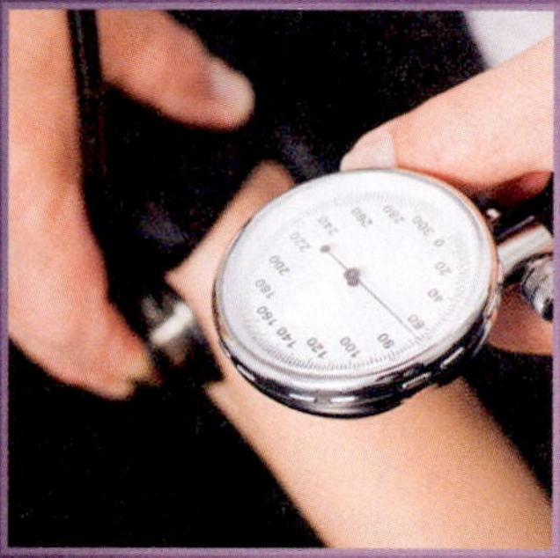

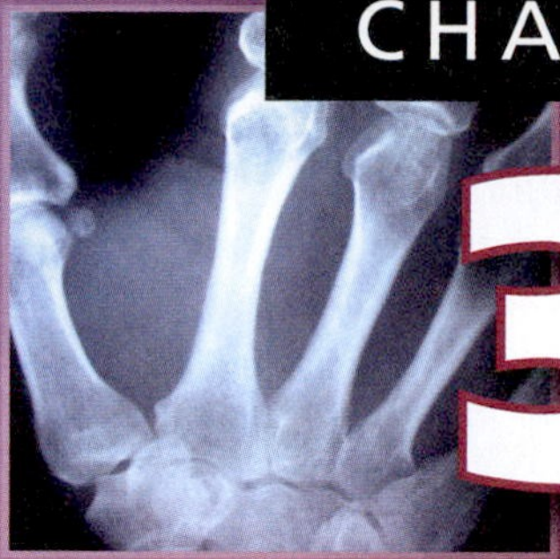

CHAPTER 3

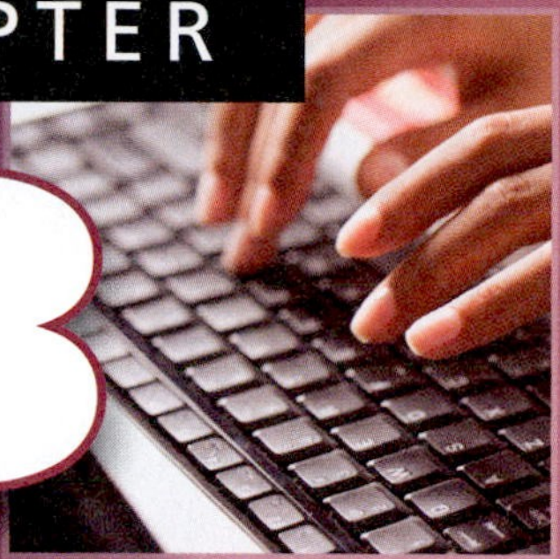

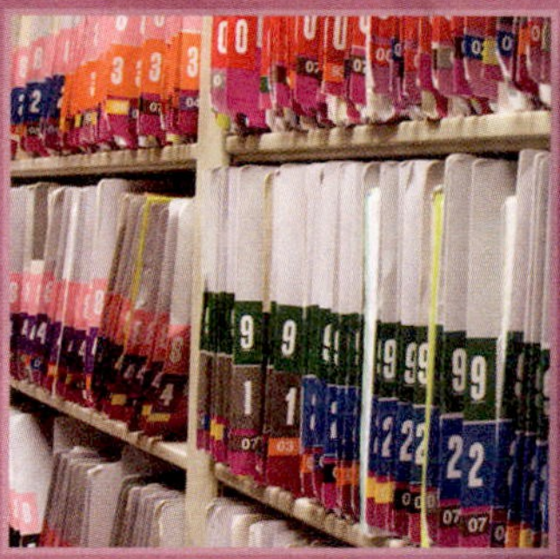

The Medical History and Physical Examination

"The doctor may also learn more about the illness from the way the patient tells the story than from the story itself."

—James Herrick

OBJECTIVES

When you have completed this study of the medical history and physical examination, you should be able to

1. Define the legal health record.
2. Identify the role of confidentiality with medical records.
3. Identify and define the components of the medical history and physical examination.
4. Identify and abbreviate the names of frequently used diagnostic tests.
5. Describe other reports based on the medical history and physical examination.
6. Define the source oriented and problem oriented medical records.
7. Identify and spell commonly used abbreviations used in medical history and physical examination records and in laboratory results.
8. Identify the meanings of related word elements.

INTRODUCTION

Historically, information about patients comprised merely paper documents, radiology films, or other imaging studies. Today, according to the American Health Information Management Association (AHIMA), the definition of the **legal health record** is the documentation of healthcare services provided to an individual, in any aspect of healthcare delivery by a healthcare provider organization. This expanded need for a more complete patient record has made the process more complex and time-consuming. Fortunately, this data collection and maintenance process has been eased somewhat with advent of electronic media, the Internet, and recognition of the role of consumers in compiling their own health information.

The legal health record contains data that are individually identifiable, stored on any medium, and directly used in documenting health care or status. It must meet standards identified by Centers for Medicare and Medicaid Services Conditions of Participation, federal regulations, state laws, standards of accrediting agencies such as the Joint Commission on Accreditation of Healthcare Organization, and policies of the healthcare providers themselves.

In this chapter you will be studying the medical history and physical examination record. As shown in Table 3-1, this is only one of several items that AHIMA considers part of the medical record.

TABLE 3-1 DATA AND DOCUMENTS CONSIDERED PART OF THE MEDICAL RECORD
Advance directives
Consent forms for care, treatment, and research
Diagnostic images
Discharge instructions
Discharge summaries
Emergency department records
Medical history and physical examination records
Medication orders
Nursing assignments
Pathology reports
Problem lists
Respiratory therapy, physical therapy, speech therapy, and occupational therapy records
Results of tests and studies from laboratory and radiology
Wave forms such as ECGs and EMGs from which interpretations are derived

All items are designed to support the decisions made in a patient's care, substantiate the revenue sought from third-party payers, and document the services provided as legal testimony regarding the patient's illness or injury, response to treatment, and caregiver decisions. Their website at **http://library.ahima.org** provides further discussion of the most recent guidelines about legal health records.

CONFIDENTIALITY OF MEDICAL RECORDS

Confidentiality is a very important factor when working in the medical environment. Both the information the patient shares with the physician and the physician's observations during the course of consultation or treatment are considered privileged communication. This information may be given to other members of the health care team if it pertains directly to the course of treatment, but to no one else without the express authorization of the patient.

Authorization may be made on a preprinted form (the AMA offers several variations) or as a simple letter. However, it must include certain specific items. For example, the release must specify exactly what information is to be disclosed, to whom it is to be disclosed, and the reason for the disclosure. It must also be signed and dated by the patient. The signed release form is kept in the patient's file.

There are a few exceptions to the physician-patient privileged communication. These primarily relate to court-ordered or other limited legal situations, which vary from state to state.

The need for confidentiality extends beyond the clinical staff, who deals directly with a patient, to include the support staff, who are privy to patient information. These employees are bound by the same moral and legal restrictions as a physician. Should a physician's employee repeat confidential information, not only the employee, but the physician, too, becomes liable for legal action by the patient. If for no other reason than this single example, *confidentiality is absolutely essential and must be maintained at all times.*

MEDICAL HISTORY AND PHYSICAL EXAMINATION REPORTS

The Medical History and Physical Examination report is a key document associated with patient care. Often called the History and Physical (H&P), the document records baseline information and an overall evaluation of the patient's state of health. This step can be performed as part of an office visit or in preparation for a hospital-based episode of care. The patient's physician usually completes the History and Physical Examination, but it may be undertaken by a nurse practitioner or a physician assistant.

The Medical History and Physical Examination contains both subjective and objective information. Symptoms and feelings that the patient describes to the physician are categorized as *subjective*. What the examiner can see, hear, or touch provides objective information. Test results also are considered *objective* information. For example, a young child may pull at his ear and say his head hurts. This is subjective information. When the physician looks into the ear canal and sees an inflamed, bulging eardrum, an ear infection can be objectively identified.

Although a health practitioner may complete the H&P examination and dictate the information to be included, members of another allied health profession will be responsible for producing the printed report. Understanding the document requires familiarity with the components of a history and physical examination report and the associated terminology.

The basic content of a H&P examination report is determined by convention. Various regulatory and statuary agencies require certain components, as do such groups as health insurance companies and health maintenance organizations (HMO). But because no one format is exactly right for every physician, every patient, or every situation, medical facilities often develop their own format and expect it to be used. For example, abbreviations indicated for each report component are acceptable in some offices and hospitals while others do not allow their use.

On the occasion that an error is noted in a completed medical report, there is a proper procedure to correct it to maintain the report's integrity. The person finding the error should draw a single line through the incorrect data, indicate what the error is, provide the corrected information, and then initial and date the notation.

COMPONENTS OF THE MEDICAL HISTORY AND PHYSICAL EXAMINATION

The history and physical report is usually treated as one document with two distinct arts—the Medical History and the Physical Examination. Although it is possible and acceptable to generate this report as two separate documents, the components remain the same. There is a signature block at the end of the Physical Examination. There may also be one at the end of the Medical History section. In this textbook, the History and Physical report will be treated as one document with two distinct parts.

HISTORY

The first section of the Medical History and Physical Examination is the patient's **history**. The section contains several headings: Chief Complaint, Present Illness, Past History, Family History, Social History, and Review of Systems. Each will be identified and defined.

Chief Complaint (CC)

The **Chief Complaint** is a subjective description of the symptom or **symptoms** that caused the patient to seek medical attention. These symptoms may be indications of disease as reported by the patient and should be listed in the order of importance. The primary symptoms are directly related to a disease and the secondary symptoms are the results or consequences of the disease process.

The information can be recorded as a series of words or as a phrase.

EXAMPLES

CHIEF COMPLAINT: Tiredness, headaches, increased thirst and hunger, frequency of urination, general **malaise*** (măl-āz').

CHIEF COMPLAINT: Severe pain of approximately eight hours' duration radiating into the groin from the right side.

Present Illness (PI)

Present Illness can also be called *History of Present Illness (HPI)*. The patient gives detailed information as to when the symptoms were first noticed, their extent and intensity, and the patient's opinion as to what caused the symptoms. To gather additional relevant information the physician may prompt the patient by asking questions about the symptoms. Any medications the patient is taking to relieve the symptoms, whether home remedy, over the counter, or prescription, should be listed. Essentially, the HPI should include location, duration, timing, severity, quality, content, modify factor, and associated signs and symptoms.

EXAMPLE

PRESENT ILLNESS: This is the first admission for this 70-year-old white male, a retired dockhand, who enters with the chief complaint of gradual loss of clear sight in his right eye over a period of 4 months. The left eye presents no problem. The patient describes his sight like "looking through a frosted window." He denies eye pain or discomfort, change in appearance, **diplopia** (dĭ-plō'pē-ah), discharge, or change in **lacrimation** (lăk"rĭ-mā'shŭn).

Past History (PH)

The **Past History** may also be called the *Past Medical History (PMH)*. The past history includes any childhood or adult diseases, surgical procedures, accidents, pregnancies, deliveries, previous illnesses, physical defects, treatments, medications, and allergies to medications or other items. Medications should include those recently taken, as well as those currently taken. The past medical history can be especially important for identification of allergies or patterns of disease. Any notation of allergies should be placed in a prominent location in the record.

EXAMPLE

PAST HISTORY: Patient had an appendectomy in 1995. No other history of surgery, disease, or accident. She does not take any medication and claims to have no allergies.

Family History (FH)

The **Family History** should include relevant medical information about family members. Many diseases are hereditary; others can be found in ethnic groups. Also include information about whether parents are living or deceased. If deceased, at what age and the cause of death may provide insightful information about the patient's current situation. A family history of breast cancer would be very significant for a female patient. A significant family history of diabetes or heart disease may alert the physician and the patient to begin preventive measures. The patient's marital status is sometimes included in this section.

EXAMPLE

FAMILY HISTORY: Father died at age 50 of prostate cancer; mother died as a result of heart disease. The patient has been married for 25 years. There are three children.

Social History (SH)

The purpose of the **Social History** is to summarize the patient's lifestyle and environment and determine whether something about the environment may be contributing to the disease. Recent foreign travel, recreation activities, or pets may also introduce environmental pathogens. The use of alcohol, tobacco, and drugs is of particular

*Words appearing in boldface in the examples are defined in the Key Terminology Review section of this chapter.

interest because these can be factors affecting a person's health. The patient's occupation should be included, especially in those cases where occupational hazards may occur. Sexual activity and number of sexual partners are also noted.

EXAMPLE

SOCIAL HISTORY: The patient reports occasional use of alcohol, no more than three times per week. Consumes six to twelve cups of coffee per day. She has worked for an asbestos removal company for the past ten years. Quit smoking approximately two years ago. Denies any drug use.

Review of Systems (ROS)

The **Review of Systems** is an exchange between the physician and the patient. The physician will ask specific questions and record significant responses. At this time, the presence or absence of signs and symptoms can be identified. A **sign** is an objective, observable, or measurable manifestation of a disease as noted or observed by the physician or health care practitioner. Signs are often accompanied by symptoms.

The order of the review usually starts with constitutional symptoms such as fever or weight loss, moves to the patient's head and continues down to the fingers and toes. The length and detail of this section will vary according to the patient's physical condition.

Several headings pertain to the names of body systems, which were discussed in Chapter 2. These headings, with representative narratives, are presented below. Some agencies allow the use of abbreviations to identify the headings. Those most commonly used are shown. HEENT is frequently used for the heading Head, Eyes, Ears, Nose, and Throat.

EXAMPLE

REVIEW OF SYSTEMS:

HEENT: Postnasal drip. Occasional sinus trouble. Migraine headaches about twice a month. No change in vision or hearing.

CARDIOVASCULAR: Denies prior history of chest pain, **murmurs**, or arrhythmias.

RESPIRATORY: No pneumonia, tuberculosis, pleurisy or **hemoptysis** (hē-mŏp'tĭ-sĭs). Has a dry cough occasionally productive of clear **sputum** (spū'tŭm).

GASTROINTESTINAL (GI): Mild, recurrent heartburn. Denies food intolerance or vomiting.

GENITOURINARY (GU): Recent urinary tract infection (UTI). Menstrual history is unremarkable.

MUSCULOSKELETAL: No complaints at this time.

INTEGUMENTARY: No reports of rashes, lesions, or other skin disorders.

NEUROLOGICAL: Denies **vertigo** (ver'tĭ-gō), weakness, or problems with coordination.

PSYCHIATRIC: Unremarkable.

ENDOCRINE: Reports thyroid nodules.

HEMATOLOGIC/LYMPHATIC: No complaints.

ALLERGIC/IMMUNOLOGY: No known allergies.

PHYSICAL EXAMINATION (PX, PE)

The **Physical Examination** is usually completed at the same time as the medical history, especially when the Medical History and Physical Examination report is generated as a single document with two distinct parts.

The Physical Examination is the objective assessment of the patient. It is most often completed by the patient's physician or other qualified practitioner. The physician uses general observation techniques as well as special or unique evaluation methods. These methods are defined in the following list.

Auscultation (aws"kŭl-tā'shŭn)
Listening for sounds within the body chiefly to determine the condition of thoracic or abdominal organs. Using a stethoscope achieves the best results with this technique.

Palpation (păl-pā'shŭn)
Feeling with fingers or hands to determine the physical characteristics of organs or tissues.

Percussion (per-kŭsh'ŭn)
Using the fingertips to tap the surface area of the body to produce sound, as shown in Figure 3-1. Solid and hollow areas will produce different tones. This information helps the physician determine size, position, and density of body organs and cavities.

Visualization or inspection
Using both observation and inspection to assess parts of the body that can be evaluated by sight alone.

General (or Constitutional)

The first part of the Physical Examination section is a general description of the patient. The description is based on the physician's observation and information that can be supported in an objective manner. The patient's vital signs and basic biometrics can be included under the general heading or may be documented as a separate heading.

Vital signs include temperature, blood pressure, pulse, and respiratory rate. **Basic biometrics** are height, weight, and pain intensity. General appearance includes the observations of the person taking the history, such as deafness, jaundice, cyanosis of the skin, development, nutritional state, body deformities, grooming, or emotional condition of patient.

EXAMPLE

GENERAL: This 40-year-old black female appears to be in no acute distress. **Vital signs** include oral temperature, 98.6°F; pulse rate, 80 beats per minute; blood pressure, 180/100; weight, 180 lb.; height, 5'6".

The physical examination continues with an objective assessment of each area or body system. As with the review of systems, the physician begins with the head and neck and proceeds all the way to the extremities. Although other headings may be included, the example presented here represents those most frequently employed. Formats will vary depending on patient need, physician training, and the documentation policies of the specific health care setting.

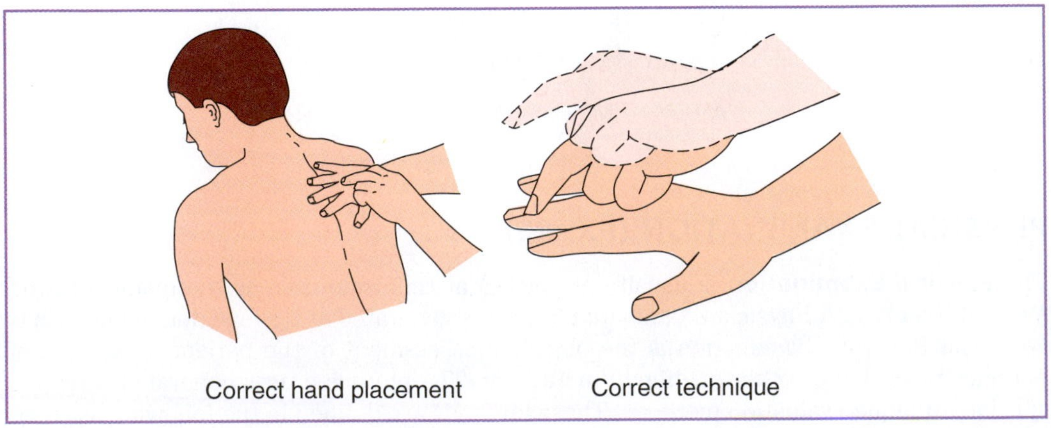

FIGURE 3-1
Percussion

EXAMPLE

HEAD AND NECK: Eyes: Pupils are equal, round, and react to light and accommodation. Normal **extraocular** (ĕks"trah-ŏk'ū-lar) movements. **Fundi** (fŭn'dī) are normal. Ears: External auditory canals are clear. **Tympanic** (tĭm-păn'ĭk) **membranes** are clear. Nose: Normal nasal mucosa. No **septal** (sĕp'tăl) deviation. Mouth and throat: No pathological findings. Neck: Supple. **Trachea** (trā'kē-ah) in midline. Thyroid gland not palpably enlarged. **Carotid** (kah-rŏt'ĭd) pulses are equal.

CHEST: Normal expansion. Breasts: No masses palpable. Heart: Not enlarged; no **thrills**; heart tones good; regular rhythm; no murmurs or **rubs**. Lungs: Clear to percussion and auscultation.

ABDOMEN: Soft, nontender; no rebound tenderness; no masses palpable. Bowel sounds are present. No **hepatosplenomegaly** (hĕp"ah-tō-splē"nō-mĕg'ah-lē). No inguinal hernia. **Femoral** (fĕm'or-ăl) pulses are equal.

EXTREMITIES: Symmetrical. No **edema** (ĕ-dē'mah). No varicose veins. No limitation of motion.

NEUROLOGICAL: Cranial nerves intact. Normal deep tendon reflexes. No Babinski's reflex. Romberg's sign negative.

Impressions/Diagnoses

Once the physical examination has been completed, the physician will state diagnostic conclusions in a section called **Impressions/Diagnoses**. A **diagnosis** is the identification of a disease or condition by a scientific evaluation of physical signs, symptoms, history, laboratory tests, and procedures. There are four types of diagnoses.

Clinical diagnosis
A diagnosis made on the basis of the knowledge obtained from the medical history and physical examination without the benefit of laboratory tests or radiological imaging.

Differential diagnosis
A diagnosis that distinguishes between two or more diseases with similar symptoms by systematically comparing their signs and symptoms.

Laboratory diagnosis
A diagnosis derived from the results of laboratory tests.

Physical diagnosis
A diagnosis supported by both the clinical diagnosis and the laboratory diagnosis.

This section may also be called *Impression, Diagnosis, Diagnostic Impression,* or *Findings*. The conclusions can be written in paragraph form or listed and enumerated.

EXAMPLE

IMPRESSION: Hypertension. Obesity. Rule out **atherosclerosis** (ăth"er-ō-sklĕ-rō'sĭs).

DIAGNOSES:
1. Hypertension
2. Obesity
3. Rule out atherosclerosis

Plan

Accrediting and regulatory agencies require the inclusion of a treatment plan that relates to the impressions or diagnoses. The **Plan** may include specific laboratory and diagnostic tests, referrals to specialists, specific instructions to the patient, and/or follow-up appointments as needed. The Plan may be written as a paragraph or in a list format.

EXAMPLE

PLAN: Consultation with the dietitian for a 1,500 calorie, low salt, reducing diet. Monitor blood pressure, weekly. Complete Blood Count (CBC) with **lipid** (lĭ'pĭd) profile.

Prognosis

The **Prognosis** indicates the probable outcome of the disease or injury and the prospect of recovery. In the case of an accident or an industrial injury, an estimate of whether disability will be partial or total is provided.

Refer to the listening exercise at the end of this chapter to examine a complete History and Physical report.

DIAGNOSTIC TESTS

Diagnostic tests help the physician to clarify or rule out suspected or provisional diagnoses. In the past, a physician ordered routine tests such as a complete blood count (CBC), urinalysis (UA), chest x-ray, and other blood chemistry tests so that the results would be available at the time of the annual physical examination. Today cost-containment regulations limit this practice. This may require the physician to order only those tests that specifically relate to the diagnostic findings documented in the physical examination.

If the physical examination is performed in preparation for a surgical or diagnostic procedure, the tests ordered would relate to both the diagnosis and procedure. Laboratory and diagnostic test terminology is included in each chapter of this text. Some of the more frequently used tests are identified and defined below.

COMPLETE BLOOD COUNT (CBC)

The complete blood count is one of the most frequently ordered blood tests. The CBC provides valuable information about the patient's state of health; it measures and evaluates the cellular component of blood. Some of the tests included in the CBC are as follows:

Red blood cell (RBC) count
Determines the number of red blood cells found in a cubic millimeter of blood.

Hemoglobin (Hgb)
A component of red blood cells necessary for transporting oxygen throughout the body. The CBC measures the amount of hemoglobin in the blood.

Hematocrit (Hct)
Determines the percentage of red blood cells contained in a volume of blood. Literally translated, it means to separate blood.

Red blood cell indices
A collective name for three separate diagnostic test results. The results are calculated by a mathematical formula using the hemoglobin, hematocrit, and red blood cell count. The tests are the mean corpuscular volume (MCV), mean corpuscular hemoglobin (MCH), and mean corpuscular hemoglobin concentration (MCHC). The purpose of these tests is to define the size and hemoglobin concentration of the red blood cell.

White blood cell (WBC) count
Determines the number of white blood cells found in a cubic millimeter of blood.

Differential white blood cell count (diff)
Determines the number of different types of circulating white blood cells. The test is often called the differential count.

Blood smear
Examines peripheral blood to determine variations and abnormalities in RBCs, WBCs, and platelets.

Platelet count
Measures the number of platelets per cubic milliliter of blood.

NOTE: A more complete presentation on blood cell terminology is found in Chapter 9.

BLOOD CHEMISTRY PROFILE

A **blood chemistry profile** is an analysis of the chemical components of the patient's blood. This type of test often is ordered as part of the physical assessment of the patient. This profile might include an analysis of electrolytes (sodium, potassium, chloride, and carbon dioxide) and glucose (blood sugar); a series of liver tests; and tests for uric acid, creatinine (a kidney function test), and albumin (a major protein in the blood). Different combinations may be used in different institutions. The abbreviation and unit of measure for some of the more common tests are as follows:

Element	Abbreviation	Unit of Measure
calcium	Ca	milligrams% (mg%)
cholesterol	Chol*	milligrams% (mg%)
creatinine	creat*	milligrams% (mg%)
glucose	glu*	milligrams% (mg%)
phosphorus	phos*	milligrams% (mg%)
total bilirubin	T bili*	milligrams% (mg%)
uric acid		milligrams% (mg%)
albumin	alb*	grams% (gm%)
total protein	TP*	grams% (gm%)
alkaline phosphatase	alk phos	IU/L (international units per liter)
lactic dehydrogenase	LDH	IU/L
aspartate aminotransferase	AST	IU/L

*These abbreviations will appear only on preprinted lab requisition slips or on automated lab report print-outs. They are not used in written or dictated medical reports.

MISCELLANEOUS BLOOD TESTS

Other blood tests taken may include sedimentation rate and coagulation prothrombin time. The **erythrocyte sedimentation rate** (ESR) is the rate at which red blood cells settle in a tube within a given amount of time to determine the degree of inflammation in the body. The **coagulation prothrombin time** measures the effectiveness of several blood-clotting factors. If there is insufficient quantity of any of these factors, prothrombin time is prolonged.

For those individuals with high cholesterol, a lipid profile measures **cholesterol** (kō-lĕs'tĕr-ōl), **triglycerides** (trī-glĭs'ĕr-īdz), low-density **lipoprotein** (lĭp"ō-prō'tēn) (LDL), and high-density lipoprotein (HDL) in the blood. These tests help to assess the risk of coronary artery disease, stroke, and myocardial infarction.

URINALYSIS

A routine urinalysis (UA) often is ordered in preparation for a diagnostic or surgical procedure or as a screening test for a physical examination. The test identifies various physical properties and chemical components of the patient's urine. On occasion, a twenty-four hour urine specimen may be called for. Color, specific gravity, and clarity may be indicators of problems, but microscopic laboratory examination will provide definitive analysis.

ELECTROCARDIOGRAM

An electrocardiogram (ECG, EKG) is a graphic recording of the electrical activity of the heart. A highly sensitive machine that uses electrodes is attached to the body to record the heart's electrical activity. The activity is recorded as tracings and can indicate cardiac abnormalities and changes in the heartbeat.

STOOL SPECIMEN

Blood in the stool (occult blood) can be an indicator of serious problems. Hemoccult SENSA is the trademark for a guaiac reagent strip that indicates the presence of blood and, consequently, the need for additional testing to determine the source of the blood. This test is given routinely to patients older than 40 years of age and for those who have a personal history of inflammatory bowel disease.

REPORTS BASED ON THE HISTORY AND PHYSICAL EXAMINATION

There are several other types of reports based on the History and Physical Examination. They are Interval History and Physical Examination, Short-Stay History and Physical Examination, Consultations, and Progress Notes. Each is used in specific circumstances, as discussed in the following sections.

INTERVAL HISTORY AND PHYSICAL EXAMINATION

When a patient is repeatedly hospitalized for the same condition, the physician may complete an **Interval History and Physical Examination** report. The use of this abbreviated format is governed by accrediting and regulatory standards, quality care issues, and physician training and preference. (Check with local agencies to determine the appropriate use of this format.) The Interval History and Physical Examination report must include a summary of what has happened to the patient since last being examined. Any changes in the patient's physical status must be thoroughly documented. Figure 3-2 is an example of the Interval History and Physical Examination.

SHORT-STAY HISTORY AND PHYSICAL EXAMINATION

With the explosion of ambulatory, same-day, and short-stay surgical interventions, there may be a limited amount of time to do a thorough history and physical examination during the hospitalization. In these situations, the History and Physical Examination may be completed in the physician's office, with a copy provided for the hospital record, or the physician may complete a shortened form of the History and Physical Examination called a **Short-Stay History and Physical Examination**. Figure 3-3 is an example of this abbreviated format.

CONSULTATIONS

There are situations when the patient's primary physician sometimes requests input from another physician. The most common situation is when a specialist is asked to evaluate a specific problem or condition or give a second opinion. Documentation of such a request is called a **Consultation** report. The Consultation report format varies from physician to physician. When the consultation occurs between physician offices, a letter format is used. If the consultation is part of a hospitalization, the hospital usually has a format that must be followed.

The consulting physician conducts an evaluation of the patient and records the results. Particular attention is given to the consultant's area of specialization. Impressions or diagnoses with treatment plans must be included in the report.

PROGRESS NOTES

After the initial physical examination, the physician generates brief notes about the patient's progress or lack of progress. The physician's **Progress Notes** will include updated information based on implementation of the treatment plan. The physician may also use the Progress Notes to change the course of treatment.

Although physician Progress Notes are often handwritten, the physician may dictate Progress Notes in some settings, including the physician's office progress note, nursing facility (long-term care) progress notes, and emergency department progress notes.

EXAMPLE

PROGRESS NOTE: March 5, 20—. Doing well. No further episodes of chest pain. Has not taken any nitroglycerin. Continue with digoxin 0.25 mg daily. Physical exam today reveals blood pressure of 150/88. Pulse is 72 and regular. No neck vein distention. Lungs are clear to percussion and auscultation. Heart perhaps slightly enlarged to the left, although this is equivocal. Heart tones are somewhat distant and of poor to fair quality. No murmurs heard. PLAN: Continue as stated. Return in three months. (Signature.)

INTERVAL HISTORY

NAME: Bruce Babbs

ADDRESS: 720 Bellaire Court
El Cajon, CA
92020-1808

DATE OF BIRTH: June 4, 19—

HOSPITAL NO.: 586072

PHYSICIAN: Henry Neal, M.D.

DATE: July 11, 20—

PRESENT COMPLAINT: This is a 45-year-old known diabetic for five years who was admitted July 6 after being found unconscious in the men's room at work. At that time he was in ketoacidosis and was in the hospital for four days to regulate his diet control. Two days after discharge, he began to experience general malaise. He is presently complaining of some occasional dyspnea with mild exertion, tension headaches, nocturia, increased thirst, and lack of energy. Patient is being admitted for diet and medication regulation and additional tests.

PAST HISTORY: Unchanged from admission of (date). See previous record.

PHYSICAL EXAMINATION: Patient is a well-developed, well-nourished male in no acute distress. Blood pressure is 140/90; pulse 85; temperature, 98.6F.

HEENT: Normal. Eyes: React to light and accommodation.

LUNGS: Clear to percussion and auscultation.

HEART: Normal sinus rythm. No cardiomegaly. No murmurs, rubs, or gallops.

ABDOMEN: No masses present.

EXREMITIES: Negative.

IMPRESSION: Diabetes mellitus.

RECOMMENDATIONS: 1) Supervision of prescribed diet.
2) Increase insulin to 40 units NPH subcu daily.

Henry Neal, M.D.

DD: 7-12-20—
DT: 7-12-20—

FIGURE 3-2
An Interval History

HILLCREST Medical Center

SHORT-STAY HISTORY

NAME: Jamie Holtz

ADDRESS: 363 Poe Drive
Winter Haven, FL
33880-1225

DATE OF BIRTH: August 29, 20—

HOSPITAL NO.: 383490

PHYSICIAN: Clara Stewart, M.D.

DATE: February 25, 20—

PRESENT COMPLAINT: This 10-month-old child comes in with a history of ear infections occurring about every three weeks since she was born. She has been on multiple antibiotics and decongestants and is just finishing a course of Ceclor. Examination in the office has revealed bilateral serous otitis media. With a history of recurrent infection, she is now admitted for bilateral myringotomy.

REVIEW OF SYSTEMS: Unremarkable. No respiratory, cardiovascular, GI or GU problems.

PAST HISTORY: Operations: None. Allergies: None. Medications: She is finishing up her Ceclor. Illness: No other serious. Family history is unremarkable. No history of bleeding tendencies or anesthetic problems.

PHYSICAL EXAMINATION: Shows a healthy-appearing, young child in no acute distress. Both ears are dull red and retracted with serous fluid. Nose is unremarkable. Mouth shows no oral lesions. Neck is normal and lungs are clear. Heart has a regular sinus rhythm without murmurs.

IMPRESSION: History of recurrent otitis media.
Serous otitis.

RECOMMENDATIONS: Myringotomy and tubes.

Clara Stewart, M.D.

DD: 2-26-20—
DT: 2-26-20—

Source: Delmar/Cengage Learning

FIGURE 3-3
A Short-Stay History

TYPES OF HEALTH INFORMATION SYSTEMS

Patient medical and health information must be maintained and stored for a variety of clinical and legal reasons. There are several record management systems available to physicians and other health care providers. The two most commonly used systems are described in this chapter.

SOURCE-ORIENTED RECORD (SOR)

The **Source-Oriented Record** (SOR) is a traditional way to organize patient records according to the source of the documents involved. Each patient record is subdivided into sections that describe the source of the document or information. In a hospital or large clinic, the record (also called the patient's chart) has dividers labeled "physician," "nursing," "lab and x-ray," "social services," and so forth. As various reports are generated, they are placed behind the appropriate divider. This method is easy to use and requires little training for clerical or support staff. Simply note who signed the report and place it behind the appropriate divider.

For example, behind the *physician divider* you may find the H&P examination, physician orders, physician progress notes, or any other report or document generated or signed by a physician. Following the *nursing divider* would be the nurse's progress notes, nursing assessments, nursing care plans, or other documents that a nurse generated or signed.

Record holders and dividers are available from various record management companies. Commercially prepared divider sets may have dividers that are not necessary in your office or hospital.

PROBLEM-ORIENTED (MEDICAL) RECORD (POR, POMR)

In the 1960s Dr. Lawrence Weed presented a new method for organizing patient medical or health information. The problem oriented record was considered to be a major departure from the traditional source oriented record. The **Problem-Oriented Record** (POR) integrates information from all health care practitioners. The organizing factor of this system is the patient's problems or diagnoses. The patient's record is generated in the same manner that care is delivered. For example, the patient is evaluated, problems or diagnoses are identified, a plan for each problem is developed, and progress or lack of progress is recorded. The patient's record is set up to reflect that process. Each patient's record is divided into four basic sections, described below.

Data Base

The first section of a Problem Oriented Record is the **Data Base**, including a record divider labeled as such. The Data Base would include patient profile, chief complaint, and all patient evaluations, such as the History and Physical Examination, Nursing Assessment, Dietitian Assessment, Social Services Evaluation, and other documents evaluating the patient's state of health.

Problem List

Once the patient has been evaluated, problems or diagnoses are entered on a master **Problem List**. Each problem is given a title and number that stays with that problem during the entire episode of care. Problems can be identified as active or inactive. Active problems are expected to be addressed in the treatment plan.

Plan

The Plan section of the POR must address *each* active problem. All plans for a single problem should be identified by the problem's name and number. Plans can be written on physician order forms, nursing care plans, or other types of patient record forms. Subjective impression, objective clinical evidence, and assessment or diagnosis for each problem are included.

Progress Notes

The **Progress Notes** section of the POR includes both narrative and flow sheet documentation. A narrative progress note can be written by anyone who provides care to the patient. Progress notes are numbered and titled to relate to a specific problem. Whenever possible, the notes address ***s***ubjective information, ***o***bjective results, ***a***ssessment of both the subjective and objective data, and a comment about the need to update or change the treatment ***p***lan. Narrative notes written in this format are often called SOAP notes.

Flow sheets include various documents that carry only a check mark or the initials of the person providing patient care. One example of a flow sheet is the medication record. There is little, if any, narrative documentation on a flow sheet.

The POR requires training for all users, including clerical and support staff. This system is well suited to the physician's office and long-term care settings. Many acute care settings, such as hospitals, have modified the POR to fit the agency's needs. Supplies necessary to set up a POR are readily available from many commercial vendors.

ABBREVIATIONS

The following abbreviations are commonly found in medical H&P examination reports, as well as other patient records. (Note that abbreviations may vary slightly from institution to institution.)

A&P, P&A	auscultation and percussion
AMA	American Medical Association
BP	blood pressure
BUN	blood urea nitrogen
CBC	complete blood count
CC	Chief Complaint
diff	differential white blood cell count
DX, Dx	diagnosis
ECG, EKG	electrocardiogram
ESR	erythrocyte sedimentation rate
FH	family history
GI	gastrointestinal
GU	genitourinary
H&P	history and physical
Hct	hematocrit
HDL	high-density lipoprotein
HEENT	head, eyes, ears, nose, throat
Hgb	hemoglobin
HMO	health maintenance organization
HPI	History of Present Illness
LDL	low-density lipoprotein
MCH	mean corpuscular hemoglobin
MCHC	mean corpuscular hemoglobin concentration
MCV	mean corpuscular volume
PERRLA	pupils are equal, round, react to light and accommodation
PH	Past History
PI	Present Illness
PMH	Past Medical History
POR (POMR)	Problem-Oriented (Medical) Record
Pt	patient

continues

PX, PE	Physical Examination
RBC	red blood cell count
ROS	Review of Systems
RX, Rx	treatment, prescription
SH	Social History
SOAP	subjective, objective, assessment, plan
SOR	Source-Oriented Record
TPR	temperature, pulse, respirations
UA	urinalysis
UTI	urinary tract infection
W/D	well developed
W/N	well nourished
WBC	white blood cell count

ABBREVIATIONS USED WITH LAB RESULTS

cm	centimeters
gm%	grams percent
HPF	high-power field
IU/L	international units per liter
L	liter
LPF	low-power field
mEq	milliequivalent
mEq/L	milliequivalent per liter
mg	milligram
mg%	milligrams percent
mm/Hg	millimeters of mercury
mm^3	millimeters cubed

INTERNET ASSIGNMENT

The American Health Information Management Association (AHIMA) is the professional association that represents specially educated health information management professionals who work to manage, analyze, and use data vital for patient care. Their goal is to make this information accessible to health care providers when it is needed to enhance individual care. They also work to safeguard the confidentiality and privacy of an individual's medical records.

ACTIVITY

Visit the AHIMA's site at **www.ahima.org** and click on About AHIMA in the heading banner to acquaint yourself with this organization. Check its history, mission, and code of ethics. Then provide your instructor with a written response to this question: What role has the AHIMA played in safeguarding the confidentiality of information in the medical record?

Review The Medical History and Physical Examination

- The Medical History and Physical Examination includes the Chief Complaint, Present Illness, Past History, Family History, Social History, Review of Systems, and Diagnostic Impressions and Treatment Plans.
- The Medical History and Physical Examination can be completed by a physician, nurse practitioner, or physician assistant and must satisfy clinical, legal, and regulatory requirements.
- The report may include the names of various diagnostic tests related to blood count, blood chemistry, and lipid profiles; x-rays and other tests may be ordered as patient need indicates.
- There are specific situations when an abbreviated medical history and physical examination format may be used, such as a Short-Stay History and Physical, Interval History and Physical, Consultation, or physician Progress Notes.
- The two most commonly used health information systems are the Problem-Oriented Record (POR), which uses the patient's problems as the organizing factor, and the Source-Oriented Record (SOR), which is organized by the source of the report or document.

Key Terminology Review

In each chapter beginning with this one, words printed in boldface in the text are considered important to your learning process. These words are summarized in the Key Terminology Review for easy reference and use in the practice exercises that follow.

Word	Meaning
atherosclerosis	hardening of arterial walls due to deposits of cholesterol or fats
auscultation	act of listening for sounds within the body
basic biometrics	patient's height, weight, and pain intensity statistics as recorded during a physical examination
blood chemistry profile	analysis of chemical components of the patient's blood
carotid	principal artery in the neck
chief complaint (CC)	subjective description of the symptoms that caused the patient to seek medical attention
cholesterol	fat-soluble, crystalline, steroid alcohol found in animal fat
clinical diagnosis	diagnosis made on the basis of knowledge obtained from the medical history and physical examination
coagulation prothrombin time	measurement of the effectiveness of several blood-clotting factors to adjust prothrombin time

continues

Word	Meaning
consultation	report written by consulting physician on the request of a patient's primary physician
data base	first section of a problem oriented record, including all patient evaluations such as the History and Physical Examination, Nursing Assessment, Dietitian Assessment, Social Services Evaluation, and other documents that evaluate the patient's state of health
diagnosis	identification of a disease or condition by a scientific evaluation of physical signs, symptoms, laboratory tests, and procedures
differential diagnosis	distinguishing between two or more diseases with similar symptoms by comparing their signs and symptoms
diplopia	perception of two images of a single object; double vision
edema	abnormal accumulation of fluid in intercellular spaces; swelling
erythrocyte sedimentation rate (ESR)	rate at which red blood cells settle in a tube within a given amount of time to determine the degree of inflammation in the body
extraocular	outside of the eye
family history (FH)	relevant medical information about the patient's family members
femoral (pulse)	pulse of the femoral artery felt in the groin
fundus, (*pl.*) fundi	back portion of the interior of the eyeball
hemoptysis	spitting up of blood or blood-tinged sputum
hepatosplenomegaly	enlargement of liver and spleen
history	section of the physical and history that contains information to document patient care, justify physician's actions, and secure payment for services rendered
impressions/diagnoses	section of the report in which the physician indicates diagnostic conclusions
interval history and physical examination	abbreviated format sometimes used when a patient is repeatedly hospitalized for the same condition
laboratory diagnosis	diagnosis arrived at after the study of laboratory findings
lacrimation	secretion and discharge of tears
legal health record	documentation of healthcare services provided to an individual, in any aspect of healthcare delivery by a healthcare provider organization
lipid	fat or fatlike substance
lipoprotein	combination of a lipid and a protein having the general properties of proteins
malaise	vague feeling of bodily discomfort
murmur	auscultatory sound, particularly a periodic, short-duration sound of cardiac or vascular origin
palpation	feeling with fingers or hands to determine the physical characteristics of organs or tissues
past history (PH)	information that includes any childhood or adult diseases, surgical procedures, accidents, pregnancies, deliveries, and allergies to medications or other items
percussion	using fingertips to tap the surface area of the body in order to produce sound

continues

Word	Meaning
physical diagnosis	diagnosis supported by both the clinical diagnosis and the laboratory diagnosis
physical examination (PX, PE)	physician's objective assessment of the patient, using auscultation, palpation, percussion, and visualization
plan	section of the report that includes specific laboratory and diagnostic tests, referrals to specialists, specific instructions to the patient, and/or follow-up appointments as needed
present illness (PI)	information provided by patient as to when the symptoms were first noticed, the extent and intensity, and the patient's opinion about what caused the symptoms
primary symptoms	symptoms directly related to a disease
problem list	section of the problem oriented patient record that identifies each problem of a patient (active and inactive)
problem-oriented record (POR)	organizes information in a patient's record by problems or diagnoses
prognosis	physician's conclusions as to the probable outcome of the disease of injury and the prospect of recovery
progress notes	brief notes from a physician documenting a patient's progress
review of systems (ROS)	exchange between doctor and patient to determine presence or absence of signs and symptoms
rubs	scraping or grating noise
secondary symptoms	symptoms that are the result of a disease process
septal	pertaining to a septum
short-stay history and physical examination	abbreviated form of a history and physical often used for ambulatory, same-day, physical examination or short-stay surgical interventions
sign	objective, observable, or measurable manifestation of a disease
social history (SH)	information summarizing the patient's lifestyle and environment to determine whether something about these factors is contributing to the problem
source-oriented record (SOR)	record organized according to the source of the documents included
sputum	matter ejected from the trachea, bronchi, and lungs via the mouth
symptom	subjective indication of disease as reported by the patient
thrills	vibrations felt by way of palpation
trachea	windpipe
triglyceride	neutral fat that is the usual storage form of lipids
tympanic membrane	eardrum
vertigo	sensation as if the patient or the environment is revolving; dizziness
visualization	observation and inspection to assess various body parts by simple use of sight
vital signs	measurement of pulse rate, respiration rate, and body temperature; can also include blood pressure

Key Terminology Practice Exercises

DEFINITIONS

Give the medical term for the following.

1. Listening to sounds in the body ____________
2. Feeling with fingers or hands to determine the physical characteristics of organs or tissues ____________
3. Observation and inspection by the use of sight ____________
4. Tapping surface area of body with fingertips ____________
5. Measurement of temperature, pulse, and respiration ____________
6. Scraping or grating noises ____________
7. A vibration felt by way of palpation ____________
8. Abnormal accumulation of fluid ____________
9. Enlargement of liver and spleen ____________
10. Eardrum ____________
11. First section of the history and physical ____________
12. Analysis of chemical components of the patient's blood ____________
13. First section of a problem oriented record ____________
14. Rate at which red blood cells settle in a tube ____________
15. Measurement of the effectiveness of blood-clotting factors to adjust prothrombin time ____________

SHORT ANSWER

From the Key Terminology Review, identify and define the terms that relate to the eye.

1. ____________
2. ____________
3. ____________
4. ____________

SIGN, SYMPTOM, OR DIAGNOSIS

Identify each of the following terms as a sign, symptom, or diagnosis. (Review the definition of sign, symptom, and diagnosis.)

1. atherosclerosis ____________
2. edema ____________
3. malaise ____________
4. thrills ____________
5. diplopia ____________
6. hemoptysis ____________
7. rubs ____________
8. hepatosplenomegaly ____________

SPELLING

Rewrite the misspelled words.

1. coratid ______________________
2. lipid ______________________
3. femural ______________________
4. vertigo ______________________
5. triglyceride ______________________
6. sputum ______________________
7. trachia ______________________
8. lipoprotein ______________________
9. cholesterol ______________________
10. murmer ______________________
11. septol ______________________

MATCHING

Match the type of diagnosis with its definition.

1. ________ supported by both the clinical and laboratory diagnosis
2. ________ identification of diseases by scientific evaluation
3. ________ distinguishing between two or more diseases
4. ________ diagnosis based on the medical history and physical exam
5. ________ diagnosis arrived at after study of lab results

a. diagnosis
b. clinical diagnosis
c. physical diagnosis
d. laboratory diagnosis
e. differential diagnosis

IDENTIFICATIONS/ABBREVIATIONS

List the headings of a Medical History and Physical Examination in the order in which they appear in a report. Then provide the abbreviation (if any) for each heading.

	Heading	Abbreviation
1.	______________________	__________
2.	______________________	__________
3.	______________________	__________
4.	______________________	__________
5.	______________________	__________
6.	______________________	__________
7.	______________________	__________
8.	______________________	__________
9.	______________________	__________

IDENTIFICATIONS

Write out the words for the following abbreviations. Identify the section of the Medical History and Physical Examination in which each would most likely be found.

1. BP ______________________
2. DX ______________________
3. PERRLA ______________________

4. RX ______________________
5. TPR ______________________
6. W/D ______________________
7. W/N ______________________
8. A&P ______________________
9. UTI ______________________
10. HEENT ______________________

Write out the words for the following abbreviations of laboratory and diagnostic tests.

11. BUN ______________________
12. ECG ______________________
13. UA ______________________
14. HDL ______________________
15. LDL ______________________

Write out the words for the following abbreviations.

16. POR (POMR) ______________________
17. SOR ______________________
18. SOAP ______________________
19. Pt ______________________
20. H&P ______________________

ABBREVIATIONS/IDENTIFICATIONS

Identify the tests included in a complete blood count (CBC). Give the abbreviation and write out the test name.

	Abbreviation	Name of Test
1.	____________	______________________
2.	____________	______________________
3.	____________	______________________
4.	____________	______________________
5.	____________	______________________
6.	____________	______________________
7.	____________	______________________
8.	____________	______________________

MATCHING

Match the laboratory result abbreviations to their meanings.

1. ________ millimeters cubed		a. cm
2. ________ milligram		b. L
3. ________ grams percent		c. HPF
4. ________ low-power field		d. mm^3
5. ________ milliequivalent		e. gm%

continues

6.	__________ millimeters of mercury	f.	mg
7.	__________ milligrams percent	g.	IU/L
8.	__________ centimeters	h.	mEq
9.	__________ international units per liter	i.	mEq/L
10.	__________ high-power field	j.	mm/Hg
11.	__________ liter	k.	LPF
12.	__________ milliequivalent per liter	l.	mg%

ABBREVIATIONS

Provide the abbreviations for these terms.

1. calcium __________
2. cholesterol __________
3. creatinine __________
4. glucose __________
5. phosphorus __________
6. total bilirubin __________
7. genitourinary __________
8. albumin __________
9. Review of Symptoms __________
10. alkaline phosphatase __________
11. hemoglobin __________
12. auscultation and percussion __________
13. Social History __________
14. History of Present Illness __________
15. erythrocyte sedimentation rate __________

SHORT ANSWER

1. Name the four components of the Problem Oriented (Medical) Record.

   ____

   ____

   ____

2. How is the Source Oriented Record organized?

   ____

   ____

3. Differentiate between symptom, sign, and diagnosis.

   ____

   ____

4. Briefly describe the following terms:

   a. Interval History and Physical Examination

   ____

   ____

b. Short-Stay History and Physical Examination

____

____

c. Consultation

____

____

d. Progress Notes

____

____

DISCUSSION

Discuss the need for confidentiality in a medical office.

____

____

____

____

____

____

Word Element Review

Root	Meaning	Example	Definition
path/o	disease	**pathology** (pă-thŏl'ō-jē)	study of disease
Prefix	**Meaning**	**Example**	**Definition**
dys-	bad, labored	**dyspnea** (dĭsp'nē-ah)	labored breathing
ect-	out, outside	**ectopic** (ĕk-tŏp'ĭk)	situated outside of the usual location
epi-	above, upon	**epigastric** (ĕp"ĭ-gă-s'trĭk)	above the stomach
hemi-	half	**hemiplegia** (hĕm"ē'plē'jē-ah)	paralysis of one side of the body
in-	not, into	**incurable** (ĭn-kū'rah-b'l)	not able to cure
infra-	beneath	**infra-axillary** (ĭn"frah-ak'sĭ-lār-ē)	below the axilla
para-	beside	**paraneural** (păr"ah-nū'răl)	alongside a nerve

continues

Prefix	Meaning	Example	Definition
super-	above, in the upper part of	**superior** (soo-pē'rē-or)	situated above
supra-	above, over	**suprapelvic** (soo"prah-pĕl'vĭk)	above the pelvis

Suffix	Meaning	Example	Definition
-algia	pain	**arthralgia** (ar-thrăl'jē-ah)	pain in a joint
-dynia	pain	**cardiodynia** (kăr"dē-ō-dĭn'ē-ă)	pain in the region of the heart
-emesis	vomiting	**hematemesis** (hēm"ah-tĕm'ĕ-sĭs)	vomiting of blood
-ia, -iasis	condition, formation	**lithiasis** (lĭ-thī'ah-sĭs)	condition marked by the formation of stones
-itis	inflammation	**gastritis** (găs-trī'tĭs)	inflammation of the stomach
-malacia	softening	**cardiomalacia** (kăr"dē-ō-mah-lā'shē-ah)	softening of the muscular tissue of the heart
-osis	condition	**fibrosis** (fī-brō'sĭs)	condition of forming fibrous tissue
-pathy	disease	**cardiopathy** (kăr"dē-ŏp'ă-thē)	any disease of the heart
-ptosis	prolapse, downward	**nephroptosis** (nĕf"rŏp-tō'sĭs)	displacement of the downward kidney
-rrhage, -rrhagia	bursting forth, excessive flow	**hemorrhage** (hĕm'ōr-ĭj)	excessive flow of blood
-trophy	development, growth	**atrophy** (ăt'rō-fē)	wasting away, without growth

Word Element Practice Exercises

MATCHING

Match the word elements to their meanings.

1. __________ above, over
2. __________ beside
3. __________ above, in the upper part of
4. __________ out, outside
5. __________ above, upon
6. __________ half

a. ect-
b. epi-
c. hemi-
d. infra-
e. para-
f. super-

7. __________ prolapse, downward
8. __________ beneath
9. __________ not, into

g. supra-
h. ptosis-
i. in-

MEANINGS

In the underlined words below, circle the word element presented in this chapter. Provide the meaning of the word.

1. The patient complains of dyspnea.
   ____
2. The condition, unfortunately, is incurable at the present time.
   ____
3. Pathology was listed as of undetermined origin.
   ____
4. The patient presented with arthralgia.
   ____
5. As a result of the wound, the patient began to hemorrhage.
   ____
6. Her deteriorating condition was marked by cardiomalacia.
   ____
7. Gastritis can be caused by any number of factors.
   ____
8. Her last pregnancy was an ectopic pregnancy.
   ____
9. His aches and pains were attributed to fibrosis.
   ____
10. Epigastric discomfort led her physician to order a series of GI tests.
    ____
11. Hematemesis is a sign of a critical illness.
    ____
12. Gallstones and kidney stones are evidence of lithiasis.
    ____
13. The urologist was concerned about the patient's nephroptosis.
    ____
14. The infra-axillary area was tender to palpation.
    ____
15. Disuse atrophy can be caused by long periods of inactivity.
    ____

WORD ELEMENT MEANINGS

Give the meaning of each word element. Then use your dictionary to find a new word that contains each of the word elements. Specify whether the new word is a noun or an adjective by placing N or A in the last column.

Word Element	Meaning	Word	N or A
1. -algia	______	______	______
2. dys-	______	______	______
3. ect-	______	______	______
4. -emesis	______	______	______
5. dermat/o	______	______	______
6. hemi-	______	______	______
7. -ia, -iasis	______	______	______
8. in-	______	______	______
9. infra-	______	______	______
10. -itis	______	______	______
11. -malacia	______	______	______
12. -osis	______	______	______
13. para-	______	______	______
14. path/o	______	______	______
15. -ptosis	______	______	______
16. -rrhage, -rrhagia	______	______	______
17. super-	______	______	______
18. supra-	______	______	______
19. -trophy	______	______	______

Dictionary Exercises

DICTIONARY EXERCISE 1

Use your dictionary to find the pronunciation and definition of the following words.

	Word	Pronunciation	Definition
1.	adnexa	____________	____________
2.	afebrile	____________	____________
3.	atresia	____________	____________
4.	bruit	____________	____________
5.	cachexia	____________	____________
6.	emaciation	____________	____________
7.	hypertrophy	____________	____________
8.	lesion	____________	____________
9.	rebound pain	____________	____________
10.	rupture	____________	____________

DICTIONARY EXERCISE 2

Pronunciation of the words below is provided. Using your dictionary, find the correct spelling and definition of each word.

	Word	Pronunciation	Definition
1.	____________	ā-tĭp'ĭ-kal	____________
2.	____________	bī-lăt'er-al	____________
3.	____________	kŏn-jĕst'shŭn	____________
4.	____________	dē"hī-drā'shŭn	____________
5.	____________	ĭn"flah-mā'shŭn	____________
6.	____________	ĭn-sŏm'nē-ah	____________
7.	____________	mī'grān	____________
8.	____________	ŏb-strŭk'shŭn	____________
9.	____________	sŭp'l	____________
10.	____________	ū"nĭ-lăt'er-al	____________
11.	____________	ă-rĭth'mē-ă	____________
12.	____________	sēr'ŭs	____________
13.	____________	ă-kŏm"ō-elā'shŭn	____________
14.	____________	văr"ĭ-kŏs'ĭ-tē	____________
15.	____________	tō'sĭs	____________

DICTIONARY EXERCISE 3

Look up the meaning of each italicized word. Place the pronunciation in the space provided. Then rewrite the sentence in your own words.

1. Even though the child was *asymptomatic* (____________________), she had an ear infection.
2. Abdominal *distention* (____________________) hampered the physical examination.
3. Once the nerve was severed, *flaccid* (____________________) paralysis resulted.
4. *Gait* (____________________) disturbances can be caused by many different factors.
5. A *gallop* (____________________) rhythm may signal the need for further cardiac assessment.
6. *Pallor* (____________________) is a symptom and does not identify a specific disease.
7. Dry and moist *rales* (____________________) must be identified by location.
8. The *residual* (____________________) effects of a stroke can be as devastating as the disease itself.
9. On physical examination, a strident *rhonchus* (____________________) was identified.
10. No *cardiomegaly* (____________________), no murmurs, rubs, or gallops were identified.
11. The patient was in *ketoacidosis* (____________________) at the time of admission to the hospital.
12. With a history of recurrent infection, the patient is admitted for bilateral *myringotomy* (____________________).
13. The little girl had a history of recurrent *otitis media* (____________________).
14. The patient reported *palpitations* (____________________) prior to her visit to the cardiac clinic.
15. Patient was transferred to the ICU with multiple injuries and pleural *effusion* (____________________).

StudyWARE™ Connection

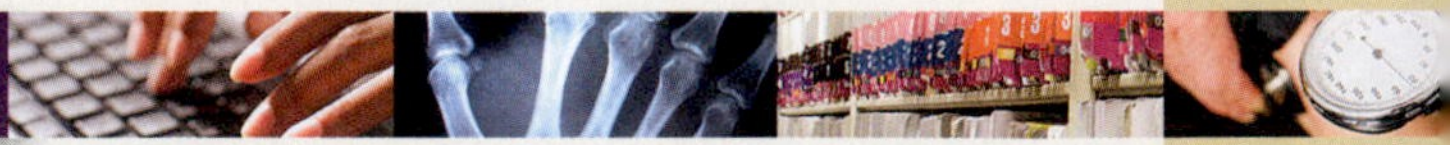

To take a practice quiz or play interactive games that reinforce the content in this chapter, go to your StudyWARE™ CD-ROM.

Listening Exercise

INSTRUCTIONS

All the listening activities in this text are actual medical documents. The words provided in the preview section should be reviewed and practiced before listening to the tape. The words appear in the preview in the same order in which they are used to fill in the blanks in the listening activity.

1. Review the spelling, pronunciation, and meaning of the words provided in the preview.
2. Go to your StudyWARE™ CD-ROM and listen to **Listening Exercise 3-1**. Fill in the blank in the report as the word is dictated.
3. At the end of the activity, check your spelling against the preview words. They appear in the preview in the order in which they are encountered in the activity.
4. Review and practice the words you missed.
5. Look up words that are not familiar.

PREVIEW OF WORDS FOR LISTENING EXERCISE 3-1

Word	Pronunciation	Definition
hemicolectomy	hĕm"ē-kō-lĕk'tō-mē	excision of approximately half of the colon
hematuria	hē"māh-tū'rē-ă	presence of blood in the urine
cataract	kăt'ă-răkt	clouding of the lenses of the eye
ptosis	tō'sĭs	drooping or downward placement
varicosities	văr"ĭ-kŏs'ĭ-tees	enlarged veins
hepatosplenomegaly	hĕp"ă-tō-splē"nō-mĕg'ă-lē	enlargement of liver and spleen

Listening Exercise 3-1

*Study*WARE™ Connection

Listen to the following report being read on your StudyWARE™ CD-ROM. Fill in each blank as the word is dictated.

History and Physical

HISTORY

This 63-year-old man is admitted for a planned right ________________ for a recently discovered cecal carcinoma. The patient denies any history of rectal bleeding, __________________, change in bowel habits, bloating, cramping, or any history of colorectal disorder.

No family history of colon cancer.

PAST MEDICAL HISTORY

No previous medical or surgical hospitalization. Had outpatient removal of a __________________________ with lens implant. Hemorrhoidectomy recently accomplished.

PHYSICAL EXAMINATION

Blood pressure is 145/100. Pulse is 88 and regular. Respirations are 16. Temperature is 98.6°F. The patient is sedated, pleasant, and in no acute distress.

HEENT: Wears glasses. Has ___________ of right upper eyelid. Teeth are in good repair. Tympanic membranes are clear.

Neck is supple. No evidence of thyroid enlargement or cervical lymphadenopathy.

EXTREMITIES: Femoral and popliteal pulses intact. Minor ____________________________ in the right lower leg.

NEUROMUSCULAR: Within normal limits.

ABDOMEN: Soft and nontender; no rebound tenderness. No masses are palpable. Blower sounds are present. There is no _________________or inguinal hernia. Femoral pulsations are equal.

Rectal not done at this time.

IMPRESSION

1. Cecal carcinoma in a mildly hypertensive man.

PLAN: As noted above.

CHAPTER 4

Pharmacology

"There are no really 'safe' biologically active drugs. There are only 'safe' physicians."

—Harold Kaminetzky

OBJECTIVES

When you have completed this chapter on pharmacology, you should be able to

1. Identify significant legislation designed to protect consumers.
2. Distinguish among types of drug names.
3. Name and define drug classifications.
4. Explain various effects of medications.
5. Identify and define methods of drug administration.
6. Identify commonly used drug references.
7. Identify commonly used abbreviations.
8. Identify the meanings of related word elements.

INTRODUCTION

A natural or synthetic chemical substance that affects body function is referred to as a **drug**. These substances may come from plants, minerals, or animals, or they may be synthetic sources manufactured in laboratories (Figure 4-1). **Pharmacology** (fahr"mah-kŏl'ō-jē), the study of drugs, their origins, and how they affect the body, is an important specialty area addressing the following topics:

1. The production of new drugs
2. The use of drugs in treating disease
3. How drugs exert their effects on the body and interact with cells
4. The absorption, distribution, elimination, and duration of effectiveness of drugs
5. The study of drugs as they interact with other drugs or foods

6. The study of drugs as they interact with enzyme systems
7. The study of drugs and their harmful effects, including contraindications

The registered **pharmacist** (R.Ph. or Pharm.D.) dispenses medications ordered by the physician and is the professional who has the ultimate responsibility for the accuracy and appropriateness of those medications. The right patient should get the right medication, in the right amount, at the right time, by the right route of administration, and have the right documentation recorded in the patient's record. These *rights of medication administration* are illustrated in Figure 4-2.

Recognizing these rights, recent federal requirements mandate that a pharmacist shall provide patient counseling concerning drug effects, dosage and form, medication and food compatibility, and dose scheduling. This is very important to the patient because the interaction a medication has with other drugs or foods may determine the potential for an adverse reaction and may alter its effectiveness. This is where the work of a **toxicologist** (tŏk"sĭ-kŏl'ō-jĭst) becomes significant. This pharmacology specialist studies harmful chemicals and their effects on the body and seeks antidotes for drugs that have toxic effects.

Pharmacy and toxicology are but two of the many specialties within the field of pharmacology. Others include medicinal chemistry, nuclear pharmacology, pharmacodynamics, pharmacokinetics, and molecular pharmacology. As modern medicine evolves, new areas continue to open.

CONSUMER SAFETY

In the early 1900s, the first of three laws was passed regulating the dispensing of drugs. The Pure Food and Drug Act, enacted in 1906, required all drugs marketed in the United States to meet minimal standards of strength, purity,

Source	Example	Drug name	Classification
Plants 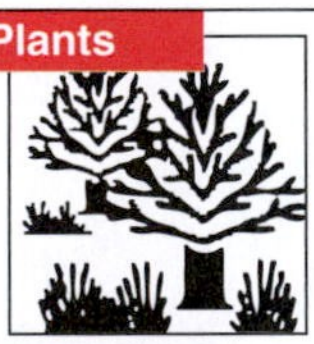	cinchona bark purple foxglove	quinidine digitalis	antiarrhythmic cardiotonic
Minerals 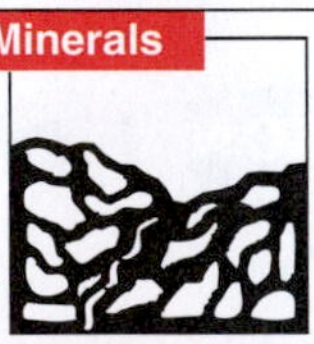	magnesium gold	Milk of Magnesia Solganal; auranofin	antacid, laxative anti-inflammatory used to treat rheumatoid arthritis
Animals 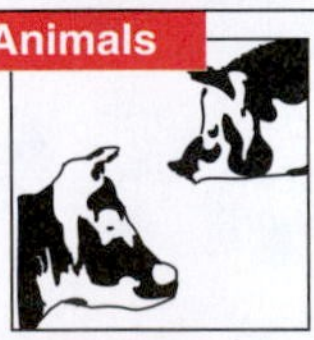	pancreas of cow, hog thyroid gland of animals	insulin thyroid, USP	antidiabetic hormone hormone
Synthetic 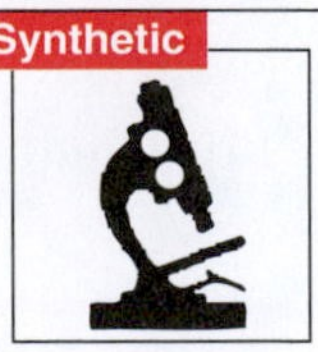	meperidine diphenoxylate	Demerol Lomotil	analgesic antidiarrheal

Source: Delmar/Cengage Learning

FIGURE 4-1
Sources of Drugs

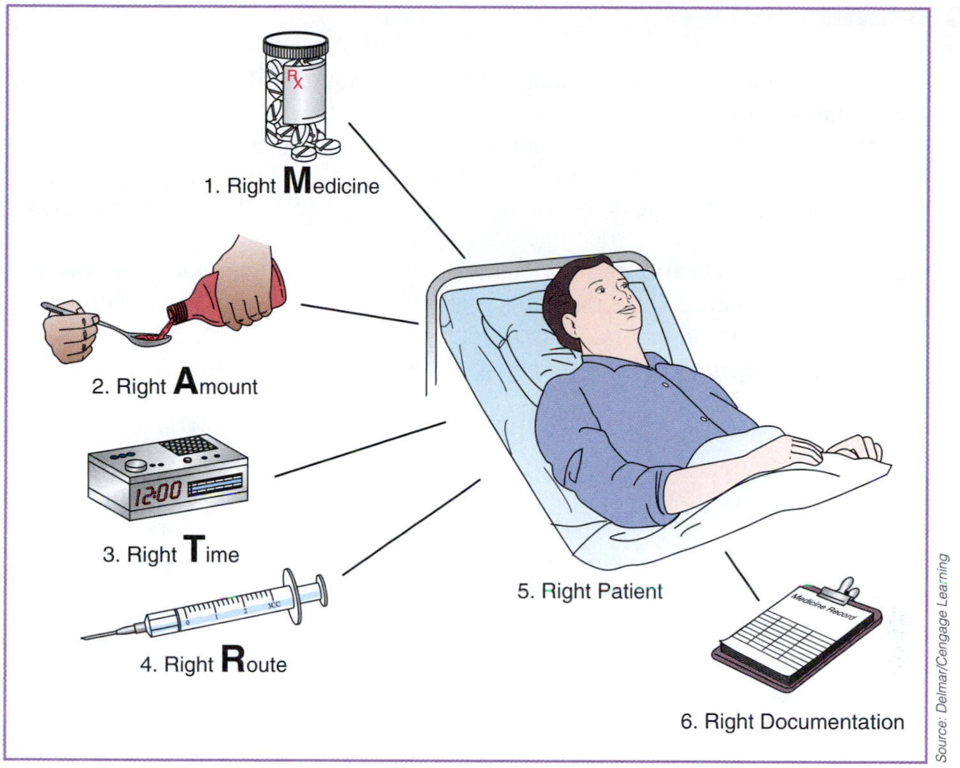

FIGURE 4-2 Six Rights of Medication Administration: (1) Right Medication, (2) Right Amount, (3) Right Time, (4) Right Route, (5) Right Patient, (6) Right Documentation.

and quality. It also established the two references of officially approved drugs: the *United States Pharmacopoeia* (USP) and the *National Formulary* (NF). These two books were later combined into one book, referred to as the USP/NF.

The second law, passed in 1938, was the federal Food, Drug, and Cosmetic Act (with amendments in 1951 and 1965). This legislation provided for more specific regulation of the industry and established the Food and Drug Administration (FDA) as the enforcement agency.

The third law, the Controlled Substances Act, which passed in 1970, established the Drug Enforcement Administration (DEA). The law set much tighter controls on drugs that are depressants, stimulants, psychedelics, and narcotics. One significant part of this act established five levels or schedules into which all drugs are classified. As shown below, the levels—C-I through C-V—are determined by the degree of danger the drug presents. The first three levels all lead to some form of addiction or dependency.

As a result of these three laws, health care workers often are required to keep records according to specific regulations. For example, because prescription pads have the physician's DEA registration number, all pads should be in a secure location.

Class	Description of the Drug	Examples
I	not considered for legitimate use; high risk for addiction	LSD, heroin
II	accepted medical use; high risk for addiction	morphine, codeine, Demerol
III	strict limitation on quantity and length of time; moderate potential for addiction	Butisol
IV	strict limitation on quantity and length of time; less potential for addiction than Class III	Librium, Valium, Darvon, Equanil
V	no limits on prescription; low potential for addiction	Robitussin A-C, Lomotil

DRUG NAMES

Drugs can have four names—a generic name (which any drug manufacturer may use); an official name; a trade, private, or brand name; and a chemical name.

The **generic name** is the common or nonproprietary name by which a medication is known and assigned by the United States Adopted Names (USAN) Council. The name can be used by any manufacturer.

The **official name** is the name of the medication as it appears in the official reference, the USP/NF. Generally, it is the same as the generic name.

The **trade**, **private**, or **brand name** indicates ownership by a manufacturer and usually bears a superscript ® or ™ to the right of the name. The ® indicates registry with the United States Patent and Trademark Office, and ™ indicates a trademark but no federal registration.

The **chemical name** indicates the chemical content of the medication. The chemical name is not commonly used in a physician's practice.

The following is an example of one drug's brand, chemical, and generic names: Sinemet, (-)-3-(3,4-dihydroxyphenyl)-L-alanine, levodopa.

Sometimes a number is a part of the trade name. The purpose of this number is to differentiate it from a product that is almost identical. The number often refers to the *amount* of one of the components of the medication (e.g., 650 mg), but may simply indicate a difference in delivery medium (e.g., liquid vs. tablet) or dosage level (e.g., Tylenol #1, #2, #3, #4). The referenced component of the medication may also be a controlled substance. As a rule, the higher the number, the more of a given substance is present.

A physician may order medications using either the trade or generic name. A list of the 50 most prescribed medications and their generic names follows.

COMMONLY PRESCRIBED MEDICATIONS*

Brand Name	Generic Name
Ambien	zolpidem tartrate
Amoxil	amoxicillin
Ativan	lorazepam
Celebrex	celecoxib
Celexa	citalopram
Cipro	ciprofloxacin
Cymbalta	duloxetine
Darvocet	propoxyphene napsylate
Deltasone	prednisone
Desyrel	trazodone
Diovan	valsartan
Effexor	venlafaxine
Fastin	phentermine
Flexeril	cyclobenzaprine
Glucophage	metformin
Klonopin	clonazepam
Lasix	furosemide
Levaquin	levofloxacin
Lexapro	escitalopram oxalate
Lipitor	atorvastatin calcium

continues

COMMONLY PRESCRIBED MEDICATIONS* *(continued)*	
Brand Name	Generic Name
Lopressor	metoprolol
Lyrica	pregabalin
Naprosyn	naproxen
Neurontin	gabapentin
Nexium	esomeprazole magnesium
Norvasc	amlodipine besylate
Vicodin	hydrocodone bitartrate and acetaminophen
Paxil	paroxetine
Percocet	oxycodone and acetaminophen
Plavix	clopidogrel bisulfate
Prevacid	lansoprazole
Prinivil	lisinopril
Protonix	pantoprazole
Proventil	albuterol
Prozac	fluoxetine
Roxanol	morphine
Seroquel	quetiapine fumarate
Soma	carisoprodol
Synthroid	levothyroxine sodium, evothyroxine
Tenormin	atenolol
Toprol XL	metoprolol succinate
Tramadol	ramadol
Ultram	tramadol
Valium	diazepam
Viagra	sildenafil citrate
Vytorin	ezetimibe
Wellbutrin	bupropion hydrochloride
Xanax	alprazolam
Zocor	simvastatin
Zoloft	sertraline
Zyban	bupropion hydrochloride
Zyrtec	cetirizine

*For the most recent list of frequently dispensed medications, see **www.rxlist.com** or **www.drugtopics.com.**

Check Appendix D for a more comprehensive list of trade and generic medications.

In addition to the terms identified previously, medications may be referred to as OTC drugs, prescription drugs, or controlled substances. OTC is an abbreviation for **over-the-counter drugs**, which are safe to use or self-administer without a physician's prescription. Examples are aspirin and certain ointments. **Prescription drugs** are licensed medications requiring a prescription from a qualified healthcare professional and requiring physician supervision to ensure drug safety and efficacy. Examples are antibiotics and birth control pills. **Controlled substances** are medications that may have a high potential for abuse if taken without supervision, such as codeine and morphine.

CLASSIFICATIONS OF MEDICATIONS

Medications also can be grouped by subcategories called classifications. Within these classifications, medications are grouped by how they affect the body. A few of the more common classifications are presented in the following chart.

For a review of the terms in this list, see the Drug-Related Words and the Dictionary Exercises later in this chapter.

Classification	Effect on Body	Example
analgesics	relieves pain	Aleve (naproxen), aspirin, morphine
antibiotics	treats infection caused by bacteria, fungi, or parasites	erythromycin, Omnipen (ampicillin), Azulfidine (sulfasalazine), Ceclor (cefaclor)
anticoagulants	prevents clotting of blood	heparin, Coumadin (sodium warfarin)
anticonvulsants	treats seizure disorders	Dilantin (phenytoin), phenobarbital, Tegretol (carbamazepine)
antidepressants	mood-lifting medications; includes tricyclics, selective serotonin reuptake inhibitors (SSRIs), and monoamine oxidate inhibitors (MAOIs)	Prozac (fluoxetine), Elavil (amitriptyline), Paxil (paroxetine), Zoloft (sertraline)
antidiabetics	treats diabetes mellitus	insulins, Orinase (tolbutamide), Micronase (glyburide), Glucovance (glyburide and metformin)
anti-inflammatories	reduces inflammation	Motrin, Advil
antihistamines	treats allergies, asthma, nausea, motion sickness, coughing, and itching	Dramamine (dimenhydrinate), Seldane (terfenadine), Claritin (loratadine), Allegra (fexofenadine), Benadryl (diphenhydramine), Hismanal (astemizole)
cardiovascular medications	medications that act on the heart or blood vessels	
• *antianginals*	prevents angina	nitroglycerin, Lopressor (metoprolol)
• *antiarrhythmics*	medications that reduce blood pressure (beta blockers and calcium channel blockers)	Tenormin (atenolol), Procardia (nifedipine)

continues

Classification	Effect on Body	Example
• *antihypertensives*	medications generally used to treat hypertension and congestive heart failure; medications that stimulate heart arteries to enlarge	Inderal (propranolol hydrochloride), Cardizem (diltiazem), Catapres (clonidine)
• *cholesterol-reducing agents*	decreases the production of cholesterol by binding with acids and increasing fecal loss of cholesterol	Questran (cholestyramine), Mevacor (lovastatin), Lipitor (atorvastatin calcium)
• *diuretics*	lowers blood pressure by promoting kidneys to excrete urine	Lasix (furosemide)
• *vasodilators*	relaxes blood vessels and increases blood flow	Apresoline (hydralazine), Nitrostate (nitroglycerine)
gastrointestinal medications	treats gastrointestinal diseases	
• *antacids*	neutralizes acid in stomach	Rolaids (calcium carbonate and magnesia)
• *antiulcer*	blocks secretion of acid in the stomach	Tagamet (cimetidine), Zantac (ranitidine)
• *cathartics*	treats constipation	Peri-Colace (casanthranol and docusate sodium)
• *antinauseants/ antiemetics*	treats nausea and vomiting	Antivert (meclizine), Compazine (prochlorperazine maleate), Zofran (ondansetron hydrochloride), Reglan (metoclopramide)
• *antidiarrheal*	decreases rapid movement of walls of colon	Lomotil (diphenoxylate and atropine), Imodium (loperamide)
• *proton pump inhibitors*	inhibits acid secretion	Prilosec (omeprazole), Prevacid (lansoprazole), Protonix (pantoprazole)
hormones	acts in the same manner as naturally occurring hormones	
• *androgens*	hormones that stimulate the production of male sexual characteristics	Halotestin (fluoxymesterone), Virilon (methyltestosterone)
• *estrogens*	hormones used to treat menopause, prevent osteoporosis, used in oral contraceptives, and to treat some types of cancer	Premarin, estradiol, Nolvadex (tamoxifen)
• *progestin*	medications that treat uterine bleeding	Provera (medroxyabnormal progesterone acetate), Megace (megestrol acetate)
respiratory medications	treats emphysema, asthma, and respiratory infections	Proventil (albuterol), Theo-Dur (theophylline), Vanceril (beclomethasone)

continues

Classification	Effect on Body	Example
sedatives–hypnotics	induce a state of drowsiness to relax and calm nervousness	Halcion (triazolam), Butisol (butabarbital)
steroids	effect development and growth of sex organs; synthetic steroids are used to relieve swelling and inflammation	
• *anabolic*	promotes growth of skeletal muscle and development of male sexual characteristics (androgenic effects) in both men and women	Oxandrin (oxandrolone), Deca Duraboli (nandrolone)
• *mineralocorticoid*	influences salt and water balance	Florinef (fludrocortisone)
• *glucocorticoid*	affects the metabolism of carbohydrates and, to a lesser extent, fats and proteins	Deltasone (prednisone), Decadron (dexamethasone)
• *testosterone*	grows muscle mass and strength; increases bone density	Testoderm (testosterone), Delatestryl (testosterone enanthate)
stimulants	act on the brain to speed up vital processes	caffeine, Dexedrine (dextroamphetamine sulfate)
tranquilizers	treat stress and anxiety	Xanax (alprazolam), Thorazine (chlorpromazine)

EFFECTS OF MEDICATIONS

Effects of medications are categorized as being either systemic or local. Any substance that has the ability to be absorbed and distributed throughout the body has a **systemic effect.** However, when the effect is limited to the area of the body where it is administered, it has a **local effect**. Once a medication is in the body, it is absorbed, distributed, metabolized and, finally, excreted.

Absorption is the process of getting a medication into the body. In most cases it refers to *oral* medications that must disintegrate or dissolve prior to crossing the mucosal membrane and entering the bloodstream. This process is affected by such factors as a medication's formulation, degree of acidity, and particle size, as well as whether there is food in the stomach. That is why some prescriptions instruct one to "take before meals" or "take with food." Another factor that may either impair or enhance the absorption process is whether other prescription drugs might be present in the system. Only when the physician is aware of all medications being taken by the patient can the proper prescription be written.

Distribution is the process by which drugs enter body fluids and tissues following absorption. A medication's specific composition will determine its distribution characteristics. Some are attracted to specific organs or cells, whereas others may or may not be able to cross certain membranes. It depends on organ blood flow, physicochemical properties of the drug (such as lipid solubility), and protein binding.

Metabolism relates to the fate of a medication following its absorption and distribution. The process—which generally takes place in the liver—alters, or *metabolizes*, a medication both physically and chemically into more water-soluble compounds which are then excreted by the kidneys. They may also be eliminated through feces, breast milk, lungs, perspiration, plasma, gastric mucosa, and the lungs or other organs.

Excretion is the process of eliminating from the body substances such as the waste products of drug metabolism—primarily in urine or bile. If not excreted properly, some chemicals may accumulate in the body and may cause **toxicity**. This occurs often during renal insufficiency and creates a poisonous and potentially dangerous situation for the patient. These possible toxic effects must be monitored carefully when certain medications are prescribed.

Toxic and other unintended effects that may occur with some medications are called **side effects** and can lead to a harmful situation for an individual patient. A **contraindication**, on the other hand, refers to a specific situation in which a drug should *not* be used because it may result in an adverse drug reaction, worsening of a medical condition, or cause an interaction with another drug. There are two types of contraindications: relative and absolute. A *relative* contraindication does allow for drug administration but only under close medical supervision. An *absolute* contraindication prohibits the administration of a drug which would result in a life threatening situation.

Additional factors that affect the pharmacologic response to drugs include age, weight, gender, psychological state, other medications and food interacting with one another, dosage, drug resistance or tolerance, genetic factors, allergies, and method of administration.

Other substances have an effect on the body or disease processes and actually predate modern pharmacology. The use of a plant's seeds, berries, roots, leaves, bark, or flowers can be traced back centuries to the people of Egypt, Greece, India, and Asia. Despite the fact that no organization or government body regulates their manufacture or certifies the labeling of herbal preparations, more than 100 million Americans have tried remedies from plants and spend more than $12 billion on *natural* supplements. According to the National Center for Complementary and Alternative Medicine (National Institutes of Health), "natural" doesn't mean safe or without any harmful effects. Unfortunately, individuals taking these substances often do not tell their physicians of their use. This omission can lead to unwanted or unexpected results should a physician prescribe a medication or suggest an OTC product that reacts adversely with the chemical combinations found in herbal medicines.

Because there is little clinical evidence associated with specific herbal agents, claims of effectiveness or safety may not be adequately substantiated. Drug interactions can be significant and may lead to morbidity. Some herbal products can cause allergic reactions, and others can act like a diuretic or a hormone. Still others can affect heart rate, blood pressure, or clotting factors. For example, patients facing surgery are advised to stop taking St. John's wort and ginkgo biloba to avoid bleeding problems or other complications associated with anesthesia. Coumadin's blood-thinning effect is enhanced by Dong Quai root, a popular menopause remedy. Feverfew, sometimes used to prevent migraines, should not be used with nonsteroidal anti-inflammatories such as Advil, Motrin, and Aleve; anticlotting drugs such as warfarin; or blood thinners such as aspirin.

Herbs come in different forms: teas, syrups, oils, liquid extracts, tincture, and dry extracts (pills and capsules). Because of the lack of industry regulation, there is no guarantee that the herb content of any given bottle or package or even from dose to dose is the same. Published analysis of herbal analysis have found differences between what is listed on the label and what is in the bottle. Some have been contaminated with metals, unlabeled prescription drugs, microorganisms, or other substances. Therefore, it is essential that the physician is consulted before herbal medicines are added to one's diet. In addition, infants and pregnant women should not take any herbal remedies.

A list of some of the herbs and their medicinal claims include those in the following chart.

REPRESENTATIVE HERBAL MEDICINES AND THEIR MEDICINAL CLAIMS

Herbal Medicine	Medicinal Claim
aloe	heals
astragalus	enhances energy reserves
barberry	treats bad breath
bilberry leaf	increases night vision
black cohosh	relieves menstrual cramps
burdock leaf, root	treats severe skin problems, cases of arthritis
calendula flower	mends cuts
celery leaf, seed	treats incontinence
chamomile flower	relieves nervous stomach
cranberry	treats, prevents bladder, kidney infections
dandelion leaf	detoxifies poison in liver

continues

REPRESENTATIVE HERBAL MEDICINES AND THEIR MEDICINAL CLAIMS *(continued)*	
Herbal Medicine	**Medicinal Claim**
Don Quai root	prevents, treats menstrual problems
Echinacea root	treats strep throat, lymph glands
feverfew herb	treats migraines
garlic capsules	"nature's antibiotic"
ginger root	treats sore throat
ginkgo biloba	improves blood flow to brain; memory enhancer
ginseng root	slows aging; relieves stress
goldenseal	treats bladder infection, cancers, mouth sores, ulcers
gata kola	improves memory, "memory herb"
hawthorn	strengthens, regulates heart
horsetail	develops strong fingernails, hair
kava kava	induces sleep, calms nervousness
licorice	treats constipation
marshmallow leaf	treats inflammation
pau d'arco	protects immune system
St. John's wort	treats mood disorders
skullcap	sedates nerves
uva-ursi leaf	stimulates digestion
wild yam	helps expel gas
yarrow root	treats flu, fever

Vitamins are not commonly regarded as drugs, but actually are because their administration is associated with a pharmacologic response. They are natural or synthetic substances that have a positive or negative effect on the body. Water-soluble vitamins (vitamins B and C) must be replaced on a regular basis. However, vitamins A, D, E, and K are fat-soluble vitamins whose effects are cumulative. Therefore, if excessive amounts of vitamin A, D, and K are consumed, whether in foods or in natural or synthetic forms, they may increase the risk of toxicity. Vitamin E, however, is not toxic in adults and older children except in extremely rare cases.

DRUG ACTIONS

Drug action has several meanings. For example, drug action can refer to the action the drug has on specific cells, tissues, organs, or systems. Drug action can also refer to the effect the drug has on a disease or disease symptoms. The following words refer to the latter usage of the term *drug action.*

PALLIATIVE

A drug is said to have a **palliative** (păl'ē-ă"tĭv) effect when it relieves the symptoms of the disease but does not cure the disease. A common example is the use of Tylenol to reduce a fever: The medication relieves the symptom (fever) but does not cure or combat the underlying cause of the fever.

PLACEBO

A **placebo** (plah-sē'bō) contains an inert substance lacking any pharmacologic effect. The layman's term for a placebo is sugar pill. Currently, placebos are most commonly used in controlled studies to help determine how well a tested medication works. In the past, however, patients who insisted on medication they did not need were given a placebo—an inactive substance or preparation to satisfy their psychological need.

PROPHYLACTIC

Medications can have a **prophylactic** (prō"fĭ-lăk'tĭk) effect when used to ward off or prevent disease. Immunizations using vaccines are prime examples of prophylactic medications. Antibiotics are often given prophylactically to prevent infection.

THERAPEUTIC

A medication used to cure or treat the disease or disease process is defined as **therapeutic** (ther"-ah-pū'tĭk). Many of the antibiotics are therapeutic medications in that they actually produce a cure.

ADMINISTRATION OF MEDICATIONS

GASTROINTESTINAL (GI) TRACT ROUTES

Medications can be administered in a variety of ways to achieve a desired pharmacologic effect. The most common route of administration is via the **gastrointestinal** (găs"trō-ĭn-tĕs'tĭ-năl) **tract** (GIT). The gastrointestinal tract includes oral (p.o.), nasogastric (NG), and the rectal route of administration.

The oral route of administration is the most frequent route used, but the effects of the medications are delayed 30–60 minutes as adequate absorption must occur from the GIT. These medications may be represented by tablets, capsules, or various forms of liquids (solutions, suspensions, or elixirs). Oral medications may also be administered through a nasogastric tube (NGT) as shown in Figure 4-3. The NGT is generally not inserted for the sole purpose of administering these types of medications, but it may be used when the tube is placed for other reasons.

When drugs are administered rectally, they may be in the form of suppositories or enemas. Actual absorption of a drug given this way may vary depending on its characteristics and therefore influence the therapeutic effect.

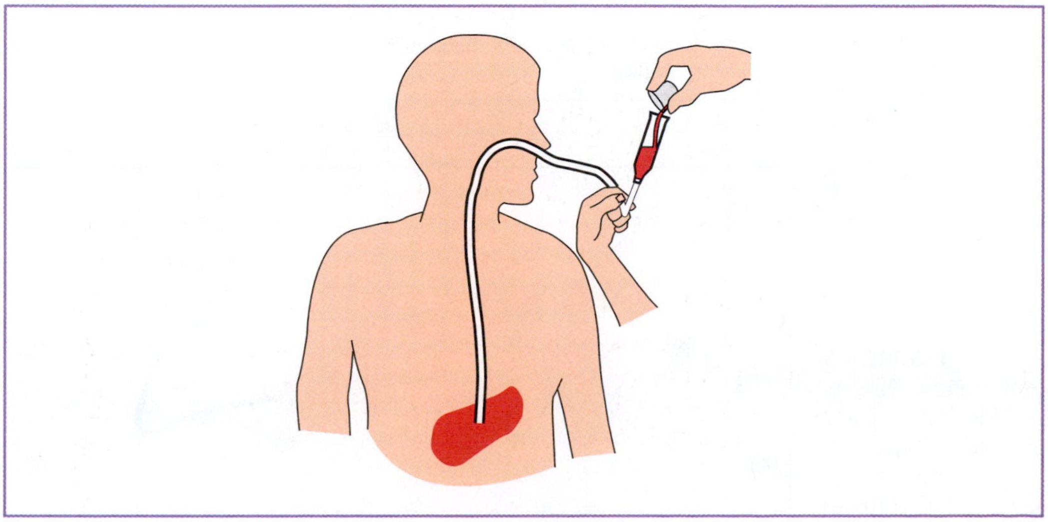

FIGURE 4-3 Medication Delivered Through a Nasogastric Tube

Source: Delmar/Cengage Learning

PARENTERAL ROUTES

Administration of medications by other than the gastrointestinal tract is referred to as **parenteral** (păr-ĕn'tĕr-ăl). Most frequently they are introduced into the system by *intramuscular* (IM), *subcutaneous* (SC), *intravenous* (IV), or *intradermal* (ID) routes (each illustrated in Figure 4-4). Infusion of medications through an IV may be done continuously or by injection with a syringe as shown in Figure 4-5. This method, which generally requires previous placement of an indwelling catheter, provides an almost immediate effect from the drug because it is being introduced directly into the bloodstream.

Medications may also be administered several other ways, one of which is into the ear for direct absorption. Some additional methods are

intra-articular (into a joint space)
epidural (into the epidural space)
intra-ocular (into the eye)
intracardiac (into the heart)
buccal (between the gum and cheek)
sublingual (under the tongue)

Topical administration of a drug refers to the application of a cream, ointment, lotion, or solution where its active ingredient is absorbed through the skin. These medications include vaginal creams, hemorrhoidal preparations, suppositories, oral analgesic creams, and topical steroids. Another example of the topical route is the use of a **transdermal** (trăns-dĕr'măl) **patch**, which provides a sustained delivery of a drug, shown in Figure 4-6. Examples include a synthetic narcotic (fentanyl) and an antimotion sickness medication (transdermal scopolamine).

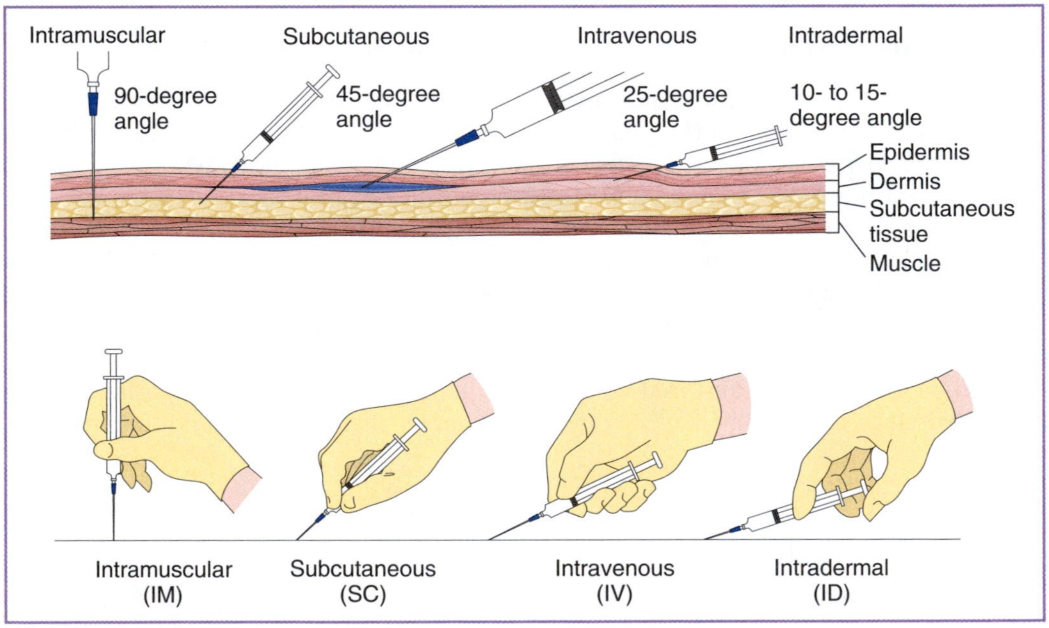

FIGURE 4-4 Administration of Medications by Parenteral Routes

Source: Delmar/Cengage Learning

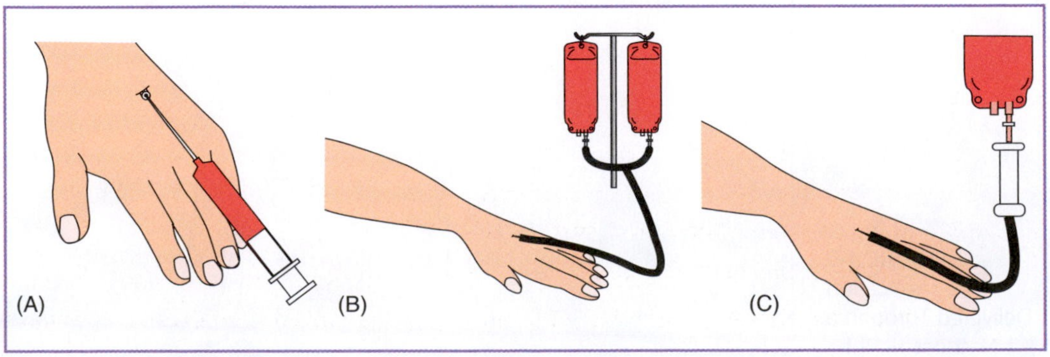

FIGURE 4-5 Intravenous Delivery of Medication: (A) IV push; (B) IV piggyback (intermittent); (C) infusion (continuous)

Source: Delmar/Cengage Learning

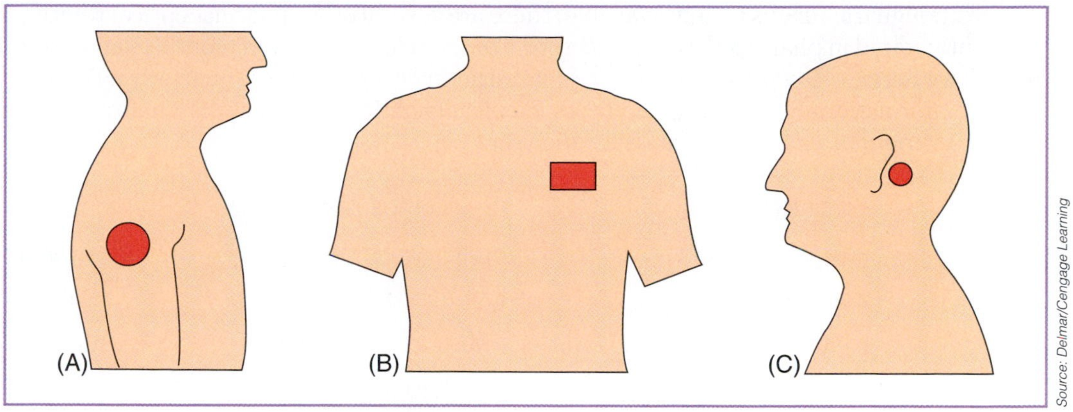

FIGURE 4-6
Transdermal Drug Delivery System: (A, B) for prevention of angina pectoris; (C) for prevention of motion sickness

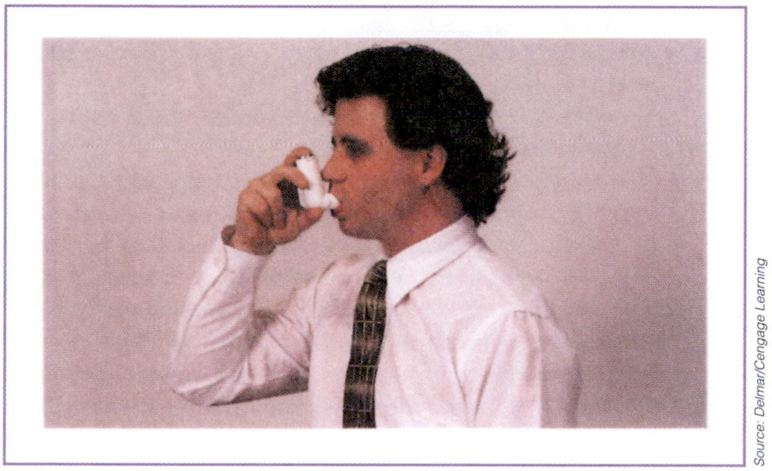

FIGURE 4-7
Nebulizer: Medication by Inhalation

The **inhalation** route includes the administration of drugs from an especially designed device through the nose or mouth. The device may contain a spray, mist, gas, powder that is delivered through a special apparatus such as an inhaler, vaporizer, nebulizer (Figure 4-7), respirator, atomizer, or intermittent positive pressure machine. Examples include medications for asthma, osteoporosis, allergic rhinitis, chronic obstructive pulmonary disease (COPD), cystic fibrosis, and acquired immunodeficiency syndrome (AIDS).

REFERENCE BOOKS

Yearly publications with regular updates are available to physicians seeking information about medications, such as their actions, interactions, and side effects. There are several of these drug references published and they vary in content. The most widely used reference is the *Physicians' Desk Reference* (PDR).

The PDR, published yearly, provides a great deal of information about medications and their manufacturers. The PDR is divided into eight color-coded, alphabetized sections, which provide the following information.

1. Name, address, and phone number of most drug manufacturers in the United States
2. Alphabetical index of drugs produced by each manufacturer
3. Classification of drugs by broad categories such as laxatives
4. Generic or chemical names according to principal ingredients
5. Drug identification by means of color pictures of medications
6. List of drugs with use, dosage, composition, action, and side effects
7. An index of diagnostic products
8. A guide to management of drug overdose

The PDR is distributed to practicing physicians in a single hardcover volume; several supplements are published throughout the year.

Although the PDR is widely available, there are several other pharmaceutical reference guides. The two most frequently found in pharmacies are *Facts and Comparisons* (updated monthly) and, from The American Hospital Formulary Service, *Drug Information* (released annually and updated quarterly). Both serve as excellent sources of drug information. Pharmacies and other medical facilities often maintain many other drug-related books containing a variety of material about drugs including:

administration	drug comparisons	pharmacology
adverse reactions	drug interactions	precautions
available products	indications	relative costs
cautions	investigational drugs	stability
chemistry	overdosage	uses
contraindications	patient information	
dosage	pharmacokinetics	

Depending on the medical environment, you may find one or more of these references available. Examine the introductory section and learn to use its features.

ABBREVIATIONS

According to the Association for Healthcare Documentation Integrity (AHDI) guidelines, periods are not used with short forms of words, such as caps for capsule, or with metric abbreviations. However, time and frequency abbreviations should have periods, as listed in the following tables. The AHDI guide also states that periods for English units of measure should be used as convention dictates and to avoid confusion.

MEDICATION FORMS

Medication	Forms
cap	capsule
inj	injection
sol, soln	solution
supp	suppository
susp	suspension
syr	syrup
tabs	tablets
tinc, tr	tincture
ung	ointment

TIME AND FREQUENCY OF ADMINISTRATION

Abbreviation	Latin Phrase	Meaning
a.c.	*ante cibum*	before meals
ad lib	*ad libitum*	at pleasure
b.i.d.	*bis in die*	twice a day
h.s.	*hora somni*	at bedtime

continues

TIME AND FREQUENCY OF ADMINISTRATION *(continued)*		
Abbreviation	**Latin Phrase**	**Meaning**
p.c.	*post cibum*	after meals
p.r.n., PRN	*pro re nata*	as required, as necessary
q.d.	*quaque die*	every day
q.h.	*quaque hora*	every hour
q.4h.	*quaque quarta hora*	every 4 hours
q.i.d.	*quater in die*	4 times/day
q.o.d.		every other day
stat., STAT	*statim*	immediately
t.i.d.	*ter in die*	3 times/day

DOSAGES AND MEASUREMENTS	
Abbreviation	**Meaning**
cc	cubic centimeter
dr.	dram
fl. dr.	fluid dram
fl. oz.	fluid ounce
gr.	grain
g, gm	gram
gtt.	gutta (drop), guttae (drops)
mEq	milliequivalent
mg	milligram
ml, mL	milliliter
mMol, mMole, mM	millimole
oz.	ounce

SITE OF ADMINISTRATION		
Abbreviation	**Latin Phrase**	**Meaning**
AD	*auris dextra*	right ear
AS	*auris sinistra*	left ear
AU	*aures unitas*	both ears
ID		intradermal
IM		intramuscularly
IV		intravenously
OD	*oculus dexter*	right eye
OS	*oculus sinister*	left eye
OU	*oculus unitas*	both eyes

continues

SITE OF ADMINISTRATION *(continued)*		
Abbreviation	**Latin Phrase**	**Meaning**
p.o., PO	*per os*	orally
PR	*per rectum*	rectally
SL	*sublingual*	sublingually
SQ, SC, subq, subQ		subcutaneously
vag.		vaginally

OTHER ABBREVIATIONS	
Abbreviation	**Meaning**
c	with
disp	dispense
FDA	Food and Drug Administration
NPO	nothing by mouth
OTC	over-the-counter
pt.	patient
s̄	without
sig., Sig.	let it be labeled
×	times, multiplied by

See Appendix D for additional abbreviations.

INTERNET ASSIGNMENT

The U.S. Food and Drug Administration (FDA) is an agency within the U.S. Department of Health and Human Services. Its mission is to review clinical research and take action on the marketing of regulated products and to protect the public health by ensuring product safety and effectiveness. The Center for Drug Evaluation and Research (CDER) is part of the U.S. Food and Drug Administration. One of its best-known activities is the evaluation of new drugs prior to their being made available to the public. Its web site is located at **www.fda.gov/cder**. Clicking the Drug Information button will bring up a list of general and specific drug topics that include:

New Prescription Drug Approvals
Prescription Drug Information
Drug Information Pathfinder
Major Drug Information Pages
Consumer Drug Information
Over-the-Counter Drug Information
Drug Safety and Side Effects
Drug Preparedness and Bioterrorism Response
Clinical Trials Information
Public Health Alerts and Warning Letters
Reports and Publications
Special Projects and Programs

Selecting any of these topics will lead you to detailed articles and lists concerning drugs. For example, in New Prescription Drug Approvals, select Drugs@FDA and you can search for information about FDA approval of various brand names and generic drugs and therapeutic biological products. It includes prescriptive and over-the-counter drugs, as well as discontinued drugs. It does not include dietary supplements or animal drugs.

ACTIVITY

Visit the CDER site and select an article of interest from the Consumer Drug Information selection. Summarize what you have read in a brief memo to your instructor.

Review *Pharmacology*

- Any chemical substance that affects body function is a drug.
- Three major legislative acts standardize the strength, purity, and quality of drugs, and control dangerous, addictive drugs.
- Drugs have four different names: generic, trade, chemical, and official.
- Drugs have either a local or systemic effect and are absorbed, distributed, metabolized, and excreted by the body and/or organ systems.
- The four drug actions are palliative, placebo, prophylactic, and therapeutic.
- Drugs may be administered through the GI tract or parenterally.
- The most widely used drug reference is the *Physicians' Desk Reference (PDR)*.

Key Terminology Review

Word	Definition
absorption	process of getting a drug into the bloodstream
chemical name	name that indicates chemical content of a drug
contraindication	specific situation in which a drug should *not* be used because it may result in an adverse drug reaction, worsening of a medical condition, or cause an interaction with another drug
controlled substances	medications or drugs that may become addictive
distribution	process by which drugs enter body fluids and tissues following absorption
drug	chemical substance that affects body function
excretion	process of eliminating from the body substances such as the waste products of drug metabolism—primarily in urine or bile
gastrointestinal tract (GIT)	most common drug administration route; includes oral, nasogastric, intramuscular, subcutaneous, and rectal routes
generic name	common or nonproprietary name by which a drug is known
inhalation	administration of a drug from an especially designed apparatus through the nose or mouth into the lungs

continues

Word	Definition
local effect	effect limited to the area of the body to which a drug is administered
metabolism	process which alters, or *metabolizes*, a medication—generally in the liver—both physically and chemically into more water-soluble compounds which are then excreted by the kidneys
official name	drug name as it appears in the official reference (USP/NF)
over-the-counter drugs	drugs that do not require a prescription; abbreviated as OTC
palliative	drug that relieves the symptoms of but does not cure the disease
parenteral	any route other than the gastrointestinal tract for administering drugs; examples are *intramuscular* (IM), *subcutaneous* (SC), *intradermal*, and *intravenous* (IV)
pharmacist	one who is licensed to dispense medications ordered by a physician and provide mandated counseling about the drug to the patient
pharmacology	study of drugs, their origins, and how they affect the body
placebo	inactive substance that has no direct pharmacologic effect; sugar pill
prescription drugs	drugs considered unsafe for OTC dispensing; must be prescribed by a physician
prophylactic	drug that prevents or wards off disease
side effects	toxic and other unintended effects that may occur with the use of a drug
systemic effect	effect of a drug that is absorbed and distributed throughout the body
therapeutic	pertaining to medication used treat or to cure a disease
topical administration	external application of a drug to the skin using a cream, ointment, spray, or transdermal patch
toxicity	poisonous and potentially dangerous effect of a drug
toxicologist	one who studies harmful chemicals and their effects on the body
trade, private, or brand name	name by which a manufacturer identifies its product
transdermal patch	provides a sustained delivery of a drug through the skin

Key Terminology Practice Exercises

SHORT ANSWER

Answer the following questions.

1. Distinguish among over-the-counter drugs, prescription drugs, and controlled substances.

2. Name the most widely used drug reference book. List the types of information found in this book.

____

____

____

____

3. Distinguish between systemic effect and local effect.

____

____

____

____

4. Define absorption, distribution, metabolism, and excretion as they refer to the effect of drugs.

____

____

____

____

5. What is the difference between drugs administered sublingually and buccally?

____

____

____

____

6. What is the relationship between contraindications and side effects?

____

____

____

____

FILL IN THE BLANK

Complete the following statements.

1. The common name by which a drug is known, assigned by the United States Adopted Names Council, is the ____________________ name.
2. The name that indicates the chemical content of the drug is ____________________.
3. The study of chemical substances is called ____________________.
4. The pharmacology specialist who studies the effect of harmful chemicals in the body is a ____________________.
5. LSD and heroin are considered class ____________________ drugs.
6. ____________________ is the cumulative effect of drugs that may be harmful.
7. ____________________ is the external application of a drug using a cream, ointment, spray, or transdermal patch.
8. The two main categories for administering drugs are ____________________ and ____________________.
9. Drugs that are not safe to take without a doctor's guidance are ____________________ drugs.
10. A chemical substance that affects body function is a ____________________.

11. The most common route of medication administration is via the ______________________.
12. A drug that relieves the symptoms, but does not cure the disease, is a ______________________ medication.
13. The medical term for a sugar pill is ______________________.
14. Medications that ward off or prevent disease are ______________________ medications.
15. A medication used to treat and cure a disease process is ______________________.
16. A nebulizer is used when the route of administration is ______________________.
17. A topical route that provides a sustained delivery of a drug through the skin is a/n ______________________ patch.
18. The name by which a manufacturer identifies its product is a ______________________, private, or brand name.

MATCHING

Match the abbreviations to their meanings.

1. __________ three times a day
2. __________ ointment
3. __________ capsule
4. __________ intravenously
5. __________ syrup
6. __________ four times a day
7. __________ when requested
8. __________ suspension
9. __________ sublingual
10. __________ orally
11. __________ tablets
12. __________ with

a. c
b. cap
c. IV
d. p.o.
e. p.r.n.
f. q.i.d.
g. ung
h. SL
i. susp
j. syr
k. tab
l. t.i.d.

Root	Meaning	Example	Definition
bucc/o	cheek	**buccal** (bŭk'al)	pertaining to or directed toward the cheek
chem/o	chemical	**chemoreceptor** (kē"mō-rē-sĕp'tor)	receptor sensitive to stimulation by chemical substances
cutane/o, cut/o	skin	**cutaneous** (kū-tā'nē-us)	pertaining to the skin
derm/o	skin	**dermatologic** (der"mah-tō-lŏj'ik)	pertaining to or affecting the skin
hypn/o	sleep	**hypnotic** (hĭp-not'ik)	inducing sleep
lingu/o	tongue	**lingual** (lĭng'gwal)	pertaining to the tongue
narc/o	stupor	**narcosis** (nar-kō'sĭs)	stuporous state induced by a drug
pharmac/o	drug	**pharmaceutical** (fahr"mah-sū'tĭ-kal)	pertaining to pharmacy or drugs
tox/o	poison	**toxic** (tŏk'sik)	poisonous
toxic/o	poison	**toxicant** (tŏk'sĭ-kănt)	poison, poisonous

continues

Prefix	Meaning	Example	Definition
anti-	against	**antispasmodic** (ăn"tĭ-spăz-mŏd'ĭk)	prevents or relieves spasms
contra-	against, opposite	**contraindication** (kon"tră-ĭn"dĭ-kā'shun)	any condition that renders a particular line of treatment improper or undesirable
intra-	within	**intravenous** (ĭn"tră-vē'nŭs)	within a vein
par-	other than	**parenteral** (pah-ren'tĕr-al)	not through the alimentary canal, but by another route
sub-	under, below	**subliminal** (sŭb-lĭm'ĭ-nal)	below the threshold of sensation or conscious awareness
syn-	together, with	**synergy** (sĭn'er-jē)	cooperation of two drugs
trans-	through, across	**transdermal** (trăns-dĕr'măl)	through the skin

Word Element Practice Exercises

CIRCLE AND DEFINE

Circle and define the combining form in the following words.

1. pharmaceutical ______________________________
2. toxicant ______________________________
3. cutaneous ______________________________
4. narcosis ______________________________
5. buccal ______________________________
6. chemoreceptor ______________________________
7. dermatologic ______________________________
8. hypnotic ______________________________
9. toxic ______________________________
10. lingual ______________________________

Circle and define the prefix in the following words.

1. transdermal ______________________________
2. synergy ______________________________
3. parenteral ______________________________
4. intravenous ______________________________
5. subliminal ______________________________
6. antispasmodic ______________________________
7. contraindication ______________________________

COMPLETION

Provide the correct word element to complete the following words.

1. receptor sensitive to stimulation by chemical substances ____________ receptor
2. stuporous state induced by a drug ____________ sis
3. any condition that renders a particular line of treatment improper ____________ indication
4. poison ____________ ant
5. prevents or relieves spasms ____________ spasmodic
6. below the threshold of sensation or conscious awareness ____________ liminal
7. pertaining to or directed toward the cheek ____________ al
8. poisonous ____________ ic
9. other than ____________ -enteral
10. tongue ____________ -al
11. together, with ____________ -ergy
12. within ____________ -venous

MATCHING

Match the terms to their meanings.

1. ________ not through the alimentary canal, but by another route		a. cutaneous
2. ________ poisonous		b. dermatologic
3. ________ pertaining to the skin		c. hypnotic
4. ________ affecting the skin		d. intravenous
5. ________ inducing sleep		e. lingual
6. ________ poison		f. parnetneral
7. ________ cooperation of two drugs		g. syngery
8. ________ pertaining to the tongue		h. toxic
9. ________ injected into the vein		i. toxicant
10. ________ through the skin		j. transdermal

WORD ELEMENT MEANINGS

Give the meaning of each word element. Then use your dictionary to find a new word that contains each of the word elements. Specify whether the new word is a noun or an adjective by placing N or A in the last column.

Word Element	Meaning	Word	N or A
1. anti-	________	________	________
2. bucc/o	________	________	________
3. chem/o	________	________	________

Word Element Practice Exercises continued

Word Element	Meaning	Word	N or A
4. contra-	______	______	______
5. cutane/o, cut/o	______	______	______
6. derm/o	______	______	______
7. hypn/o	______	______	______
8. intra-	______	______	______
9. lingu/o	______	______	______
10. narc/o	______	______	______
11. par-	______	______	______
12. pharmac/o	______	______	______
13. sub-	______	______	______
14. syn-	______	______	______
15. tox/o	______	______	______
16. toxic/o	______	______	______
17. trans-	______	______	______

Dictionary Exercises

Below are drug-related words that have particular meanings for pharmacists and other allied health specialists. After reviewing them, complete the dictionary exercises that follow.

Word	Pronunciation	Definition
allergy		adverse response to a foreign chemical resulting from a previous exposure to that substance
amphetamine	ăm-fĕt'ă-mēn	stimulant for the central nervous system
analgesic	ăn"ăl-jē'zĭk	drug that relieves pain
anaphylactic reaction	ăn"ăh-fĭ-lăk'tĭk	severe allergic response (possibly fatal)
antagonism		interaction created when drugs work against each other
anesthetic	ăn"ĕs-thĕt'ĭk	drug agent that reduces or eliminates sensation
anthelmintic	ănt"hĕl-mĭn'tĭk	antiparasitic drug that destroys worms
antiasthmatic	ănt"ăz-măt'ĭk	agent that prevents or relieves an asthma attack
antibiotic		drug that slows down or stops the growth of bacteria, fungi, or parasites
anticoagulant	ăn"tĭ-kō-ăg'ŭ-lănt	drug that prevents clotting or coagulation of blood
anticonvulsant	ăn"tĭ-kŏn-vŭl'sănt	drug that prevents or reduces the severity of seizure disorders
antidepressant	ăn"tĭ-dē-prĕs'ănt	drug that elevates moods and treats symptoms of depression

continues

Word	Pronunciation	Definition
antidiabetic	ăn"tĭ-dī"ah-bĕt'ĭk	drug that treats Type I and Type II diabetes mellitus
antiemetic	ăn'tĭ-ĕ-mĕt'ĭk	agent that prevents or relieves nausea or vomiting
antihistamine	ăn"tĭ-hĭs'tah-mēn	drug that blocks the action of histamine, a substance that causes allergic reactions
anti-inflammatory	ăn"tĭ-ĭn-flăm'ă-tō-rē	agent that counteracts inflammation
barbiturate	băr-bĭch'oo-rĭt	drug with sedative properties
beta-blockers		drugs that block beta adrenergic receptors used as antiarrhythmics, antianginals, and antihypertensives
cardiovascular drug	kăr"dē-ō-văs'kū-lăr	drug that acts on the heart and/or blood vessels
dependence		situation in which removal or withholding of a drug may cause psychological and/or physical symptoms
diuretic	dī"ū-rĕt'ĭk	drug that increases volume of urine excreted
emetic	ĕ-mĕt'ĭk	drug that induces vomiting
endocrine drug	ĕn'dō-krīn	drug that simulates naturally occurring hormones such as androgens, estrogens, progestins, thyroid, or glucocorticoids
gastrointestinal drug	găs"trō-ĭn-tĕs'tĭ-năl	drug, such as an antacid, antiulcer, antidiarrheal, antinauseant, cathartic, or laxative, which acts on various areas of the gastrointestinal tract
hypersensitivity	hī"pĕr-sĕn"sĭ-tĭv'ĭ-tē	immune response (allergy to a drug)
idiosyncrasy	ĭd"ē-ō-sĭn'krah-sē	unusual response to a drug that is peculiar to the individual
isotonic	ī"sō-tŏn'ĭk	pertaining to solutions that possess the same osmotic pressure
lipid		family of compounds soluble in organic solvents but not in water (e.g., triglycerides, phospholipids, and steroids)
narcotic		drug having both an analgesic and a sedative action; can include substances with morphine-like activity (e.g., meperidine, hydrocodone codeine)
OTC		over-the-counter
placebo	plă-sē'bō	substance that resembles a medication but lacks pharmacologic effect
placebo effect		perceived pharmacologic effect from the administration of a placebo
potentiation	pō-tĕn"shē-ā'shŭn	interaction of two drugs such that one prolongs or multiplies the effect of the other
resistance		decrease in the response to a drug by various factors (e.g., bacteria) or other drugs
sedative		drug that quiets the central nervous system
stimulant		drug that excites or arouses vital processes such as heart rate, respiration, central nervous system activity, or blood flow

continues

Word	Pronunciation	Definition
synergism	sĭn'ĕr-jĭzm	combining of two or more drugs that work together to produce a greater effect than either produces separately
teratogenic effect	tĕr"ah-tō-jĕn'ĭk	effect of a drug taken by a pregnant woman that may cause physical defects in a fetus
tincture	tĭnk'tūr	alcoholic or hydroalcoholic solution
tolerance		decrease in the response to a drug due to its continued use
tranquilizer		drug used to control anxiety
uricosuric agent	ū"rĭ-kō-sū'rĭk	drug that increases the excretion of uric acid in the urine

DICTIONARY EXERCISE 1

Select the correct meaning of each word.

1. Potentiation is
   a. an unusual response to a drug.
   b. interaction of two drugs so that one prolongs or multiplies the effect of the other.
   c. a drug that promotes vomiting.
2. Synergism is
   a repeated doses that decrease the response to the drug.
   b. an unusual response to a drug.
   c. when drugs work together.
3. A beta-blocker is
   a. a drug that blocks beta adrenergic receptors.
   b. a drug that speeds up vital processes such as heart and respiration.
   c. a drug that reduces or eliminates sensation.
4. An amphetamine is
   a. a drug that sedates a person.
   b. a drug used to control anxiety.
   c. a stimulant for the central nervous system.
5. Drugs that mimic naturally occurring hormones such as androgens, estrogens, progestins, and thyroid are
   a. endocrine drugs.
   b. anticonvulsant drugs.
   c. antidiabetic drugs.
6. Drugs such as antacids, antiulcer, anti-diarrheal, antinauseants, cathartics, or laxatives are
   a. endocrine drugs.
   b. gastrointestinal drugs.
   c. antihistamines.

7. An interaction created when one drug cancels or decreases the effect of another is referred to as
   a. synergism.
   b. antagonism.
   c. potentiation.
8. A drug agent that reduces or eliminates sensation is
   a. an anticonvulsant.
   b. an analgesic.
   c. an anesthetic.
9. Drugs that block the action of histamine, a substance that causes allergic reactions, are
   a. anticonvulsants.
   b. antidepressants.
   c. antihistamines.
10. A reduced pharmacologic response to a drug after multiple doses is known as
   a. tolerance.
   b. antagonism.
   c. synergism.
11. Drugs used to control anxiety are
   a. stimulants.
   b. analgesics.
   c. tranquilizers.
12. Drugs that relax an individual by depressing the central nervous system are referred to as
   a. sedatives.
   b. stimulants.
   c. anticonvulsants.
13. Drugs that arouse or excite vital processes such as heart rate and respiration are
   a. sedatives.
   b. stimulants.
   c. amphetamines.
14. An unusual response to a drug is referred to as
   a. an idiosyncrasy.
   b. a teratogenic effect.
   c. an anaphylactic reaction.
15. If a drug produces symptoms of withdrawal, the patient is experiencing
   a. drug dependence.
   b. placebo effect.
   c. anaphylactic reaction.

16. If solutions have the same osmotic pressure, they are referred to as
    a. isotonic.
    b. teratogenic.
    c. anaphylactic.
17. An adverse reaction to a substance is
    a. an antidepressant.
    b. an allergy.
    c. a placebo effect.
18. A drug that treats Types 1 and 2 diabetes mellitus is an
    a. antibiotic.
    b. amphetamine.
    c. antidiabetic.
19. Drugs that increase the volume of urine excreted are
    a. diuretics.
    b. emetics.
    c. analgesics.
20. Drugs that relieve pain are
    a. adjuvant medications.
    b. analgesics.
    c. mentholated rubs.

DICTIONARY EXERCISE 2

Rewrite the following sentences in your own words. Provide the spelling for the underlined pronunciation in the space provided.

1. In the emergency department, the physician ordered an <u>ĕ-mĕt'ĭk</u> (____________________) for the child.

   ____

2. The control group took a <u>plah-sē'bō</u> (____________________) for the entire year.

   ____

3. The patient has been taking an <u>ăn"tĭ-kō-ag'ū-lănt</u> (____________________).

   ____

4. The infant exhibited <u>hī"pĕr-sĕn"sĭ-tĭv'ĭ-tē</u> (____________________) to penicillin.

   ____

5. It was apparent the patient was having an <u>ăn"ah-fĭ-lăk'tĭk</u> (____________________) reaction.

   ____

6. The drug was identified as having a <u>tĕr"ah-tō-jĕn'ĭk</u> (____________________) effect.

   ____

7. She was taking a <u>bar-bĭch'oo-rĭt</u> (____________________).

____

8. The results may be explained by the <u>plah-sē'bō</u> (____________________) effect.

____

9. He asked the physician to prescribe an <u>ăn"ăl-jē'zĭk</u> (____________________).

____

10. Her recovery was assisted by the <u>ăn"tĭ-bī-ŏt'ĭk</u> (____________________) prescribed.

____

11. The <u>ah-lĕr'jĭk</u> (____________________) reaction to the drug was severe.

____

12. The drug was classified as <u>ănt"hĕl-mĭn'tĭk</u> (____________________).

____

13. Because the drug was a <u>dī"ū-rĕt'ĭk</u> (____________________), she experienced some minor inconvenience.

____

14. The substance was classified as a <u>lĭp'ĭd</u> (____________________).

____

15. The physician indicated that use of <u>năr-kŏt'ĭks</u> (____________________) was a primary factor in this situation.

____

16. The pneumonia demonstrated <u>rē-zĭs'tăns</u> (____________________) to antibiotic therapy.

____

17. The physician prescribed <u>tĭnk'tūr</u> (____________________) of opium.

____

18. The physician prescribed a <u>ū"rĭ-kō-sū'rĭk</u> (____________________) agent.

____

19. The physician prescribed an <u>ăn"tĭ-kŏn-vŭl'sănt</u> (____________________).

____

20. An <u>ăn"tĭ-dē-prĕs'sănt</u> (____________________) was prescribed for several weeks.

____

21. Tina was immediately scheduled for a drug <u>dē-tŏk"sĭ-fĭ-kā'shŭn</u> (____________________) program.

____

22. That substance is classified as a <u>hă-loo'sĭ-nō-jĕn</u> (____________________).

____

23. Misuse of <u>ăn"ă-bŏl'ĭk</u> (____________________) steroids in some sports has raised questions about content results.

____

24. Mrs. Weitman experienced an ī-ă"trō-jĕn'ĭk (__________________) disorder from the last drug her doctor prescribed.

____

25. Her grandmother took a bĭs-fŏs'fō-nāt (__________________) once a month.

____

26. At the ER, the doctor prescribed an ĕ-mĕt'ĭk (__________________) for their son.

____

27. A frequently prescribed dī"ū-rĕt'ĭk (__________________) is Diuril.

____

28. After discussing his situation, the psychiatrist prescribed a bĕn"zō-dī-ăz'ĕ-pēn (__________________).

____

29. The pharmacist told Peng that Inderal was a bā'tă-blŏk'ĕr (__________________).

____

30. The physician's assistant explained the difference between băk-tē-rē-ō-stăt'ĭk (__________________) and băk"tĕr-ĭ-sī'dăl (__________________).

____

StudyWARE™ Connection

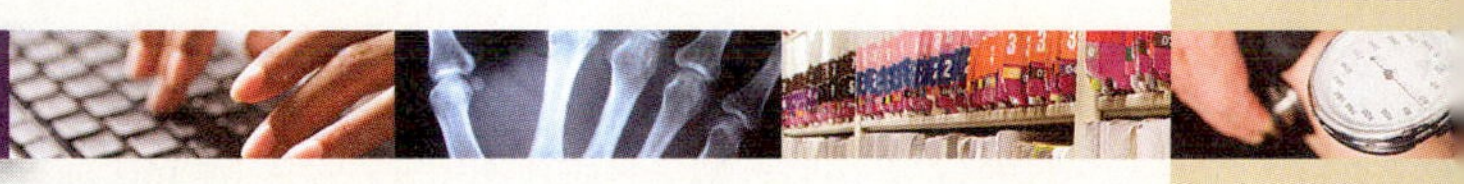

To take a practice quiz or play interactive games that reinforce the content in this chapter, go to your StudyWARE™ CD-ROM.

Listening Exercise

INSTRUCTIONS

1. Review the spelling, pronunciation, and meaning of the words provided in the preview.
2. Go to your StudyWARE™ CD-ROM and listen to **Listening Exercise 4-1**. Fill in the blank in the report as the word is dictated.
3. At the end of the activity, check your spelling against the preview words. They appear in the preview in the order in which they are encountered in the activity.
4. Review and practice the words you missed.
5. Look up words that are not familiar.

PREVIEW OF WORDS FOR LISTENING EXERCISE 4-1

Word	Pronunciation	Definition
Elavil		an antidepressant
pharmaceutical	fahr"mah-sū'tĭ-kal	a medicinal drug
Isordil		coronary vasodilator
h.s.		at bedtime (hour of sleep)
conjunctiva	kŏn"jŭnk-tī'vă	delicate membrane lining the eyelid and covering the eyeball
antidepressant	ăn"tĭ-dē-prĕs'sănt	drugs that prevent or relieve depression

Listening Exercise 4-1

StudyWARE™ Connection

Listen to this report being read on your StudyWARE™ CD-ROM. Fill in each blank as the word is dictated.

History and Physical

History

CHIEF COMPLAINT: This 53-year-old woman presents with vague symptoms of dizziness and nausea.

PRESENT ILLNESS: The patient felt quite well until last Wednesday when she experienced a gradual onset of the abovementioned symptoms. She had been started on ____________________ and it was felt that the symptoms could be related to a reaction to her medication. The patient was seen in the office today to assess her ____________________ regimen.

PAST MEDICAL HISTORY: Past medical history is significant as the patient takes a wide variety of prescription medications. They include Synthroid 0.25 mg per day, ____________________ 20 mg b.i.d., Capoten 50 mg t.i.d., Zantac 150 mg b.i.d., Reglan 10 mg, ____________________ prednisone 25 mg q.i.d., Lopid 600 mg daily in divided doses. The patient denies the use of any OTC drugs.

SOCIAL AND FAMILY HISTORY: Noncontributory.

REVIEW OF SYSTEMS: No significant change from recent examination done on Wednesday, with the exception of the symptoms described above.

Physical Examination

GENERAL: The patient is a well-developed, well-nourished female who expresses concern over the recent onset of nausea and dizziness.

VITAL SIGNS: Wt. 178 lb., BP 150/88. P is 72 and regular; T 98.6°F. RR 20 and labored.

HEENT: Pupils are equal and reactive, and ____________________ are clear. Neck pulses are clear. No bruit.

HEART: No evidence of enlargement or murmurs.

LUNGS: Although respirations are labored, lungs are clear and resonant.

ABDOMEN: No tenderness or guarding. Bowel sounds are present and normal.

GENITALIA: External genitalia is normal female. Vaginal exam not done.

NEUROLOGICAL: Cranial nerves are intact. No evidence of pathology. Remainder of the examination is noncontributory.

IMPRESSION: Current symptoms appear to be related to a reaction to the recently prescribed ____________________.

PLAN: The patient was advised to discontinue Elavil for two days; and if symptoms subside, we will try another antidepressant.

CHAPTER 5

The Integumentary System

"A mole on the neck
You shall have money by the peck."

—Old English Rhyme

OBJECTIVES

When you have completed this study of the integumentary system, you should be able to

1. Spell and define major system components and explain how they operate.
2. Identify the meanings of related word elements.
3. Spell and define diagnostic procedures, diagnoses, treatment procedures, and abbreviations.
4. Spell the names of commonly used medications.
5. Use a dictionary as a tool in processing medical documents.
6. Hear how medical terminology is used in actual medical reports.

INTRODUCTION

The average adult has approximately 7 pounds of skin, which amounts to approximately 20 square feet of tissue—literally all the general public ever sees. As an organ system of the body, the skin, or **integument** (ĭn-tĕg'ū-mĕnt), is considered to be one of the most important systems. The integumentary system includes not only the skin but the hair, nails, and sweat and oil glands. Although the breast is considered an appendage of the skin, its discussion has been deferred to Chapter 16, The Female Reproductive System.

In each chapter that pertains to an organ system of the body or to oncology, the roots, prefixes, and suffixes that pertain to a particular part of the system are identified and defined. Thus beginning in this chapter, the relevant word elements are provided in the Word Element Review section.

SKIN

Dermatology (děr"mă-tŏl'ō-gē) is the branch of medicine concerned with the diagnosis, interpretation, and treatment of diseases of the skin. The physician who specializes in the study of the skin is called a **dermatologist** (děr"mă-tŏl'ō-jĭst).

FUNCTIONS OF THE SKIN

The skin is an organ containing millions of cells and other biological components that protect the inner vital organs. This remarkable organ, the body's first line of defense, serves many functions, but the most important of these are as follows:

1. To protect deeper tissues against drying and being invaded by organisms and many chemicals.
2. To regulate body temperature. Blood vessels in the skin contract when we are cold but dilate when we are warm to dissipate heat. When we are very warm, we perspire and are cooled by the evaporation of the sweat.
3. To sense information about the environment and our position in it.
4. To lubricate the body surface to keep it soft and pliable.

In addition, because of the skin's visibility, it provides valuable information about an individual's general health.

STRUCTURE OF THE SKIN

adip/o	fat
dermat/o, derm/o	skin
cutane/o, cut/o	skin

The surface of the body is covered by three layers of tissue, each different in structure and function. As shown in Figure 5-1, the **epidermis** (ĕp"ĭ-dĕr'mĭs) (6) is the outermost layer. The **dermis** (dĕr'mĭs) (5) is the second layer and contains a framework of connective tissue. These first two layers are referred to as the skin. The third layer is called the **subcutaneous** (sŭb"kū-tā'nē-ŭs) tissue (4) and is composed of deposits of fat in modified connective tissue (**adipose** [ăd'ĭ-pōs] tissue). This layer of fat is sometimes referred to as the panniculus adiposus.

Epidermis

corne/o	horny	melan/o	black
kerat/o	horny	squam/o	scaly

The epidermis is avascular (contains no blood vessels), and is nourished by diffusion from the dermis. It consists of several layers and differs in thickness over the body surface, varying from the eyelids (the thinnest) to the palms and soles (the thickest). When unbroken, the epidermis can prevent most disease germs from entering the body.

The outermost epidermal layer, the **stratum corneum** (strā'tŭm kor'nē-ŭm) (7), is primarily composed of flat, horny cells called squamous cells. The deepest layer, the **stratum basale** (strā'tŭm bā'săl), has cells that are shaped like columns. It is in this layer that cells divide and push already-formed cells into higher layers. During the process, cells flatten, eventually die, and fill with **keratin** (kĕr'ă-tĭn), a dense, fibrous protein material which provides structural strength to skin, hair, and nails. These cells are constantly being shed and replaced by new ones.

The stratum basale also contains melanocytes that produce **melanin** (mĕl'ă-nĭn), the pigment granules which give the skin its color. This coloration also protects the body from injurious ultraviolet light rays.

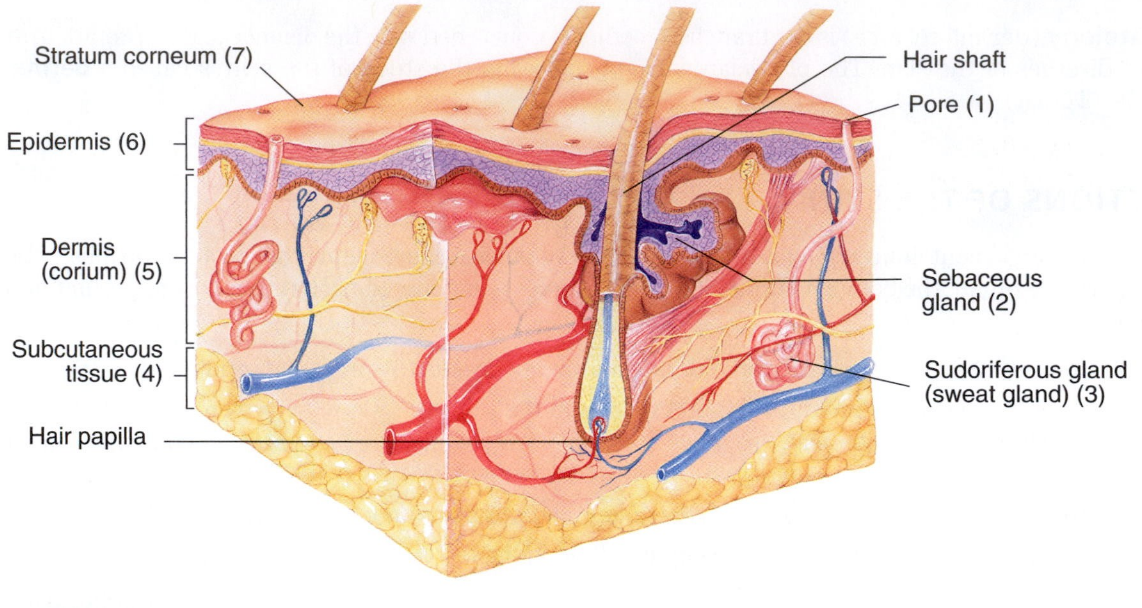

FIGURE 5-1 Structures of the Skin

Dermis (Corium)

hidr/o	sweat
sud/o, sudor/o	sweat
seb/o	sebum

The second layer, the dermis, is also called the **corium** (kō'rē-ŭm) (5). It has a framework of elastic, fibrous connective tissues and contains blood vessels and lymphatics, as well as sweat glands, sebaceous glands, and nerves. Involuntary muscle fibers are also found in the dermis, especially near hairs. Some areas of the dermis are thicker than others, for example, the soles of the feet compared with the eyelids.

There are primarily two types of glands located in the dermis—sweat or **sudoriferous** (sū"dō-rĭf'ĕr-ŭs) glands (2) and oil or **sebaceous** (sĕ-bā'shŭs) **glands** (2). The oily secretion of the sebaceous gland is called **sebum** (sē'bŭm).

The body has some 2 million sweat glands. There are two kinds of sweat glands. The **apocrine** (ăp'ō-krĭn) glands, which are found in the pubic, anal, and mammary regions, open into hair follicles. **Eccrine** (ĕk'rĭn) glands are present almost everywhere and help the body to dissipate excessive heat. These coiled, tube-like structures have an excretory tube that leads to the surface and to a pore (1). Sweat glands can produce two quarts or more of sweat per day under extreme conditions.

There are about as many oil-secreting glands as there are sweat glands. The sebaceous glands have ducts around the hair follicles. Oil secretions prevent the hair from becoming brittle, thus helping the hair remain vital. A certain amount of natural skin oil is also necessary to keep the skin soft and pliable. The largest number of these glands are found in regions of the scalp, face, neck, and upper trunk, which are the areas commonly involved with acne.

A pilosebaceous unit consists of a sebaceous gland opening into the hair canal, the hair apparatus, the arrector pili (smooth muscle attached to the hair follicle wall), and the apocrine gland (in areas where there are apocrine sweat glands). The smooth muscle may contract when the body is chilled, causing piloerection or visible "gooseflesh."

Subcutaneous Layer (Hypodermis)

fasci/o	sheet, band

The dermis is connected to the underlying fascia of the muscles by the subcutaneous layer, also called the hypodermis. The hypodermis is made up of connective tissue, which specializes in the formation of fat. This subcutaneous layer protects deeper tissues and acts as a heat insulator. Some areas of the body, such as the abdomen and buttocks, have characteristically larger accumulations of fat.

StudyWARE™ Connection

Go to your StudyWARE™ CD-ROM to view an animation of the **Skin**. You can also play an interactive game to label structures of the skin.

HAIR AND NAILS

onych/o	nail
pil/o	hair
trich/o	hair

Although the epidermis, dermis, and subcutaneous layers are associated with the skin, one does not normally think of the hair and nails as skin. In fact, hair, fingernails, and toenails are simply modified forms of skin cells.

The major structural material of the hair and nails is keratin. Keratin is produced by the same process that changes living cells into dead, horny cells in the epidermis. A **papilla** (pah-pĭl'ah) is a tiny, cone-shaped structure located at the bottom of a hair follicle, as shown in Figure 5-2. It is here that the root cells grow. Most hair tips project from the skin at a slant.

Oil from the sebaceous gland provides gloss. The hair follicle itself gets its nourishment through tiny capillaries that bring it minerals, proteins, vitamins, fats, and carbohydrates. Like the skin, scalp hair can provide protection and is a visible indicator of age and sometimes general health.

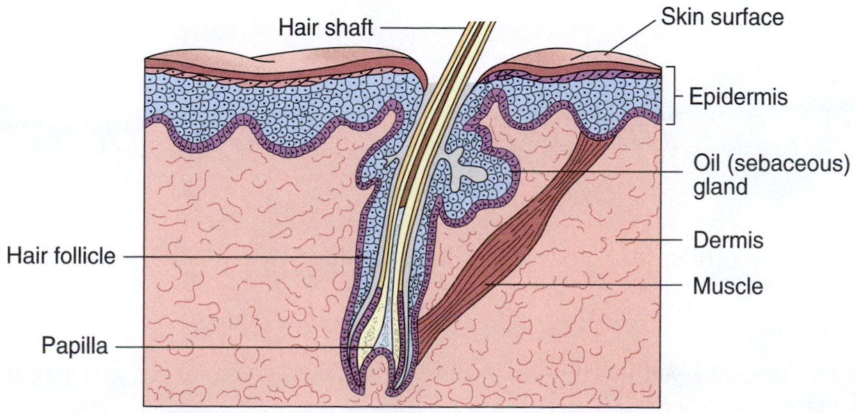

FIGURE 5-2 Structure of a Hair Follicle

Source: Delmar/Cengage Learning

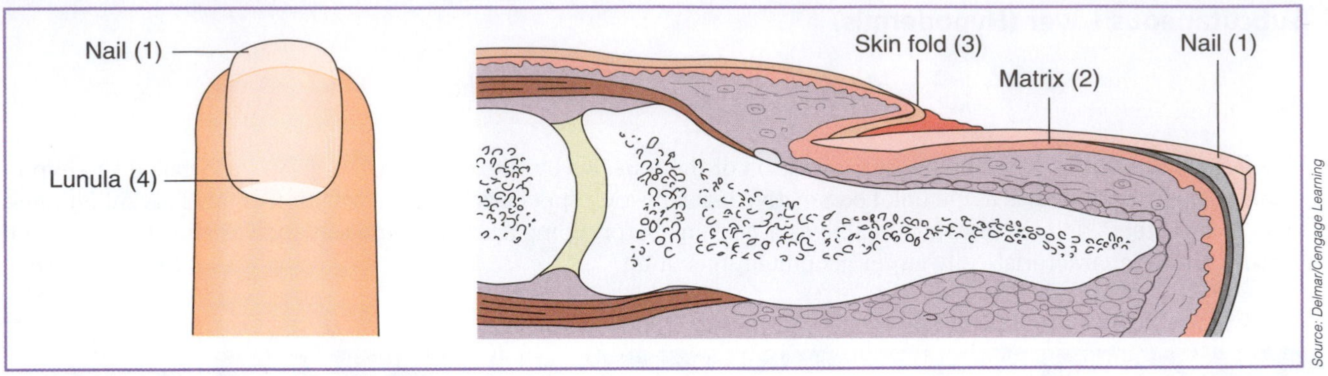

FIGURE 5-3 Structure of the Fingernail

Nails have essentially the same structure as hair, except that nails are flat, hard plates. The living part of a nail (1) lies in the matrix (2), shown in Figure 5-3, which is comprised of modified epidermal cells that produce the hard keratin of the nail.

The matrix lies under the skin fold (3) nearest to the nail and is partially evident under the base of the nail. This is referred to as the **lunula** (loo'nū-lah) (4) or white crescent. As long as the matrix remains intact, new nail will grow. Changes in the appearance of your nails can be a first signal of illness.

INTERNET ASSIGNMENT

The United States National Library of Medicine **(www.nlm.nih.gov)**, the world's largest medical library, provides information through several venues. Its goal is to offer reference and customer service to those in need of biomedical information. The site is divided into 13 sections.

Each of these sections offers a wide range of topics that can be accessed by clicking the name of the listed sections or through the site index in the page header. To illustrate, Health Information leads you to MEDLINEplus, MEDLINE/PubMed, DIRLINE, LOCATORplus, NLM Gateway, TOXNET, and several other sites. MEDLINEplus provides links to dictionaries, drug information, and more.

ACTIVITY

Sign on to the U.S. National Library of Medicine site and go to Search NLM Web Site window. Enter "skin" and get information about skin conditions, skin aging, skin cancer, and other hyperlinks. Click Skin Conditions. Scroll to Related Topics and select one of the several hyperlinks. Summarize your findings for your instructor.

Review *The Integumentary System*

- The skin protects the body, regulates body temperature, and secretes oil to maintain its softness and pliability.
- The first layer of skin, the epidermis, protects the body from injurious light rays or pathogens.
- The second layer, the dermis, contains a network of blood vessels, lymphatics, connective tissue, glands, and nerves.
- The third or subcutaneous layer acts as a heat insulator and protects deeper tissue.
- Hair and nails are modified forms of skin cells and can be indicators of general health.

Key Terminology Review

Word	Meaning
adipose tissue	fat
apocrine glands	sweat glands found in the pubic, anal, and mammary regions and which open into hair follicles
corium	dermis
dermatologist	physician who specializes in the study of the skin
dermatology	branch of medicine concerned with the diagnosis, interpretation, and treatment of diseases of the skin
dermis	second layer of skin; also called the corium
eccrine glands	sweat glands that help dissipate excessive heat
epidermis	outermost layer of skin
integument	skin
keratin	major structural material of hair, fingernails, and toenails; a dense, fibrous protein material
lunula	portion of the nail-forming matrix evident at the base of the nail as a white crescent
melanin	pigment granules that give color to the skin and protect the body from injurious ultraviolet light rays
papilla	small cone-shaped prominence located at the bottom of a hair follicle
sebaceous glands	oil glands located in the dermis
sebum	oily secretion of the sebaceous gland
stratum basale	the deepest layer of the epidermis
stratum corneum	outermost layer of the epidermis
subcutaneous tissue	third layer of tissue covering the body; also called the hypodermis
sudoriferous glands	sweat glands

Terminology Review Practice Exercises

DEFINITIONS

Define the following terms.

1. adipose tissue ______________________________
2. sebaceous glands ______________________________
3. stratum corneum ______________________________
4. corium ______________________________
5. lunula ______________________________

6. sudoriferous glands ______________________________
7. sebum ______________________________

COMPLETION

Complete the following statements.

1. Color pigmentation in the skin is created by ____________________.
2. There are approximately ____________________ sweat glands in the body.
3. Sweat glands are of two types; they are the ____________________ and ____________________.
4. A tiny, cone-shaped structure at the bottom of the hair follicle is called a ____________________.
5. A physician who specializes in the study of the skin is called a ____________________.
6. The three layers of tissue covering the body are the ____________________, ____________________, and ____________________.
7. The major structural material of hair and nails is ____________________.
8. Integument means ____________________.
9. Outermost layer of the epidermis is the ____________________.
10. The subcutaneous layer of skin is composed of deposits of ____________________.

SHORT ANSWERS

Supply a short answer to the following.

1. Why are hair and nails considered part of the skin system?

____

____

____

2. List the four functions of the skin.

____

____

____

____

____

World Element Review

Root	Meaning	Example	Definition
adip/o	fat	**adipocele** (ăd′ĭ-pō-sēl″)	hernia that contains fat or fatty tissue
corne/o	horny	**corneous** (kor′nē-ŭs)	hornlike

continues

World Element Review continued

Root	Meaning	Example	Definition
cutane/o, cut/o	skin	**cutaneous** (kū-tā'nē-ŭs)	pertaining to the skin
dermat/o, derm/o	skin	**dermatitis** (dĕr"mah-tī'tĭs)	inflammation of the skin
fasci/o	sheet, band	**fascicular** (fah-sĭk'ū-lăr)	banding together
hidr/o	sweat	**acrohyperhidrosis** (ăk"rō-hī"per-hī-drō'sĭs)	sweaty hands or feet
kerat/o	horny	**keratosis** (kĕr"ah-tō'sĭs)	horny growth
macul/o	spot	**macula** (măk'ū-lah)	discolored spot on the skin
melan/o	black	**melanoderma** (mĕl"ah-nō-der'mah)	abnormally increased amount of melanin in the skin
myc/o	fungus	**mycosis** (mĭ-kō'sĭs)	any disease caused by fungi
onych/o	nail	**onychitis** (ŏn"ĭ-kī'tĭs)	inflammation of the nail bed
pil/o	hair	**pilose** (pī'lōs)	hairy
seb/o	sebum	**sebum** (sē'bŭm)	oily, fatty matter secreted by the sebaceous glands
squam/o	scale	**squamous** (skwā'mŭs)	scaly
sud/o, sudor/o	sweat	**sudoriferous** (sū"dō-rĭf'er-ŭs)	producing sweat
trich/o	hair	**trichiasis** (trĭ-kī'ah-sĭs)	ingrowing hairs, such as near the eye

Word Element Practice Exercises

COMPLETION

Complete the following statements.

1. Three word elements that mean sweat are ____________________, ____________________, and ____________________.
2. Two word elements that mean skin are ____________________ and ____________________.
3. Two word elements that refer to the hair are ____________________ and ____________________.

IDENTIFY

Provide the word that fits the following definitions.

1. banding together ______
2. hornlike ______
3. pertaining to the skin ______
4. scaly ______
5. sweaty hands or feet ______
6. oily, fatty matter secreted by sebaceous glands ______
7. discolored spot on the skin ______
8. inflammation of the nail bed ______
9. horny growth ______
10. inflammation of the skin ______
11. producing sweat ______
12. hairy ______
13. ingrowing hairs ______
14. any disease caused by fungi ______
15. hernia containing fat or fat tissue ______
16. abnormal amount of melanin in the skin ______

REWRITE

Rewrite the misspelled words.

1. cornious ______
2. melinoderma ______
3. triciasis ______
4. fasicular ______
5. miycosis ______
6. pillose ______
7. suderiferous ______
8. adiposele ______

WORD ELEMENT MEANINGS

Give the meaning of each word element. Then use your dictionary to find a new word that contains each of the word elements. Specify whether the new word is a noun or an adjective by placing N or A in the last column.

Word Element	Meaning	Word	N or A
1. adip/o	______	______	______
2. corne/o	______	______	______
3. cutane/o	______	______	______
4. cut/o	______	______	______

5. dermat/o			
6. derm/o			
7. fasci/o			
8. hidr/o			
9. kerat/o			
10. macul/o			
11. melan/o			
12. myc/o			
13. onych/o			
14. pil/o			
15. seb/o			
16. squam/o			
17. sud/o			
18. sudor/o			
19. trich/o			

Working Practice

The information pertaining to each of the body systems about the type of work done in that specialty is entitled "Working Practice." These sections will vary considerably among specialties. For example, some practices include a great deal of surgery, whereas others have very little or none.

The diagnostic procedures may include radiologic procedures, laboratory tests of blood and other body products, and examinations with instruments. Treatment procedures are indicated for the specific practices they apply to. However, there will be some overlap because certain procedures are pertinent to more than one body system. Common diagnoses for the practices are included, as are abbreviations used and drugs prescribed.

The information presented with each body system is considered sufficient for job-entry qualification. By no means is it intended to be a comprehensive summary of the entire specialty dealing with that body system. You will continue to learn as you begin your career in the allied health field.

DIAGNOSTIC PROCEDURES

Word	Pronunciation	Definition
General		
fungal, bacterial, viral cultures	fŭn'găl	tissue scrapings, purulent (pus-filled) material, exudate viral cultures (accumulated) fluid, or normal body fluids sent to a lab for identification of pathogenic organisms present
immunofluorescent studies for epidermal autoantibodies	ĭm"ū-nō-floo"ō-rĕs'ĕnt ĕp"ĭ-der'măl ăw"tō-ăn'tĭ-bŏd"ēz	fluorescent studies of skin or blood serum under a microscope to identify the specific, abnormal antibody proteins of some cutaneous diseases

continues

DIAGNOSTIC PROCEDURES		
Word	**Pronunciation**	**Definition**
General *(continued)*		
KOH smears		skin scrapings from suspect fungal lesions immersed in 20% aqueous potassium hydroxide and examined under the microscope for hyphae (fungus filaments or threads) or spores
skin biopsy	bī'ŏp-sē	removal of lesions for pathological examination, usually microscopic; a *punch* or *incisional* biopsy is done when it is not possible to remove the entire section of tissue involved
skin tests for allergy or disease		three types of test procedures where the site becomes red disease and swollen when the results are positive after the indicated period of time
• *patch test*		small piece of gauze or filter paper treated with a suspected allergy-causing substance is placed on the skin; reaction occurs after 48 hours
• *scratch test*		small scratches are made in the skin and minute amounts of suspected material are applied; results are examined after 20–60 minutes and again after 24 hours
• *intradermal test*		reactive substances are injected between the dermis and epidermis; results are examined after 20–60 minutes and again after 24 hours
Tzanck smear	tsănk	test of fluid from base of a vesicle; fluid is applied to a glass slide, stained, and examined under microscope; tests reveal multinucleated giant cells in the presence of herpes virus infection
Wood's light examination		detect fluorescent characteristic of examination certain skin infections (usually fungal) in which skin is viewed in a darkened room under ultraviolet light filtered through Wood's glass
Blood		
antibody titer for viral, bacterial, fungal illness	tī'tĕr	blood test used to determine whether the patient has or has had an infection
antinuclear antibody titer (ANA)	ăn"tī-nū'klē-ăr	blood test used to screen for cutaneous lupus erythematosus and similar diseases of the connective tissues
enzyme-linked immunosorbent assay (ELISA)		blood-screening test for antigens of infectious agents (bacteria, viruses, fungi, and Mycoplasma) and antibodies; one of the primary tests for several infectious diseases, in particular HIV
T3, T4, T7, TSH		blood tests to determine thyroid function
Infectious Diseases Caused by Viruses, Bacteria, Fungi, and Parasites		
abscess, furuncle, carbuncle	fū'rŭng-k'l, kăr'bŭng"k'l	localized collection of pus occurring in any body tissue including the skin; a *furuncle* generally occurs around a hair follicle; *carbuncles* are larger abscesses and involve several interconnected furuncles

continues

DIAGNOSES		
Word	**Pronunciation**	**Definition**
Infectious Diseases Caused by Viruses, Bacteria, Fungi, and Parasites *(continued)*		
candidiasis	kăn"dĭ-dī'ă-sĭs	yeast-type fungal infection caused by the yeast *Candida*, often affecting individuals with chronic diseases
cellulitis	sĕl-ū-lī'tĭs	diffuse or spreading inflammation of the skin usually caused by streptococci
cheilitis	kī-lī'tĭs	lip inflammation
exanthem	ĕg-zăn'thĕm	measles-like eruption or rash that may be due to a virus, bacterial toxin, or allergic reaction to a drug
herpes	hĕr'pēz	family of viruses characterized by skin inflammation and the eruption of groups of small vesicles along the course of affected cutaneous nerves; associated with neuralgic pain, especially in the elderly
• *simplex type 1*		commonly called fever blisters and cold sores; usually around lips and nose
• *genitalis (simplex type 2)*	gĕn-ĭ-tăl'ĭs	commonly called genital herpes; highly contagious disease that may be sexually transmitted, but not exclusively so
• *varicella*	văr'ĭ-sĕl'ah	highly contagious childhood disease, commonly called chickenpox; virus becomes dormant after the infection clears
• *zoster*	zŏs'tĕr	reactivation of the varicella virus in adults; appears as blisters grouped along cutaneous nerves; commonly called shingles
impetigo	ĭm-pĕ-tī'gō	bacterial, inflammatory skin disease caused by *Staphylococci* and *Streptococci* characterized by vesicles, pustules, and crusted lesions (See Figure 5-4)

continues

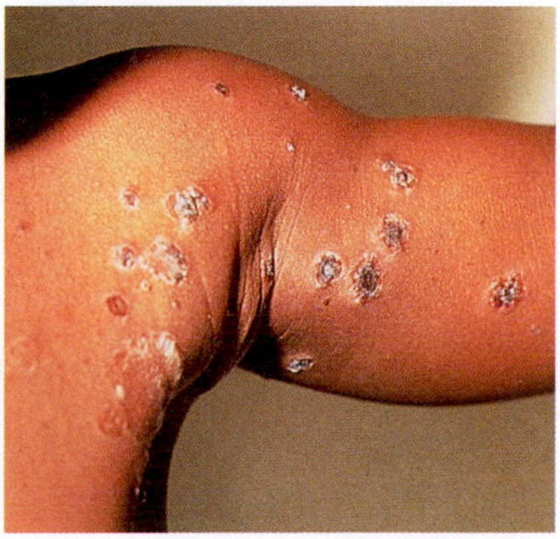

FIGURE 5-4
Impetigo

Source: Courtesy of Robert A. Silverman, M.D., Pediatric Dermatology, Georgetown University

DIAGNOSES		
Word	**Pronunciation**	**Definition**
Infectious Diseases Caused by Viruses, Bacteria, Fungi, and Parasites *(continued)*		
Lyme disease	līm	multisystem infection caused by the lyme spirochetes or Brorrelia burgdorferi, a bacterium; transmitted to humans by the bite of a deer tick
measles		highly communicable disease caused by the rubeola virus, marked by fever and rash; also known as rubeola
pediculosis	pĕ-dĭk"ū-lō'sĭs	condition of being infested with lice, either in the head, body, or pubic area (crabs)
pityriasis rosea	pĭt"ĭ-rī'ă-sĭs	benign rash characterized by scaling, rose-colored spots
scabies	skă'bēz	contagious, parasitic infection of the skin causing intense itching
tinea	tĭn'ē-ă	skin disease caused by fungus; ringworm; the term usually includes the name of the body part affected: may be *corporis* (body), *pedis* (foot), *unguium* (nails), *cruris* (genital area), *faciei* (face), or *capitis* (scalp) (See Figure 5-5)
tinea versicolor	tĭn'ē-ă vĕr'sĭ-kŏl"or	type of superficial fungal infection on the trunk and arms caused by the overgrowth of a saprophytic yeast normally present (*pityrosporum*)
verruca	vĕ-roo'kah	wart; type of common viral skin infection (See Figure 5-6)
Metabolic, Hypersensitivity, Immune, or Idiopathic Disease		
acne vulgaris	ăk'nē vŭl-ga'rĭs	inflammatory disease characterized by oil plugs and inflammation in and around the sebaceous glands; characterized by formation of *comedones*, either white-heads or blackheads, pustules and in severe cases deep, inflammatory nodules
contact dermatitis	dĕr"mă-tī'tĭs	acute or chronic allergic reaction affecting the skin

continues

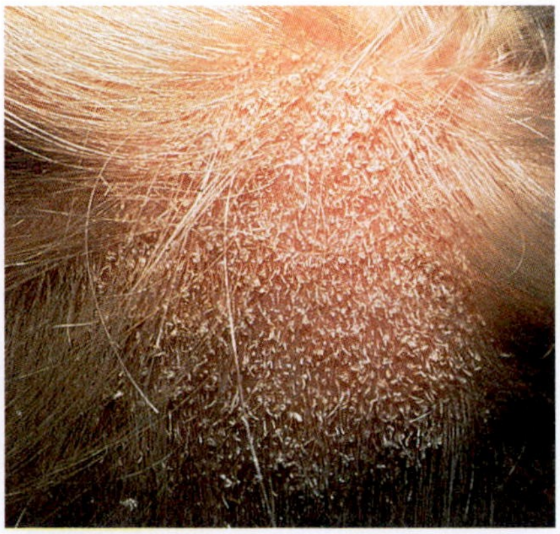

FIGURE 5-5
Tinea Capitis

Source: Courtesy of Robert A. Silverman, M.D., Pediatric Dermatology, Georgetown University

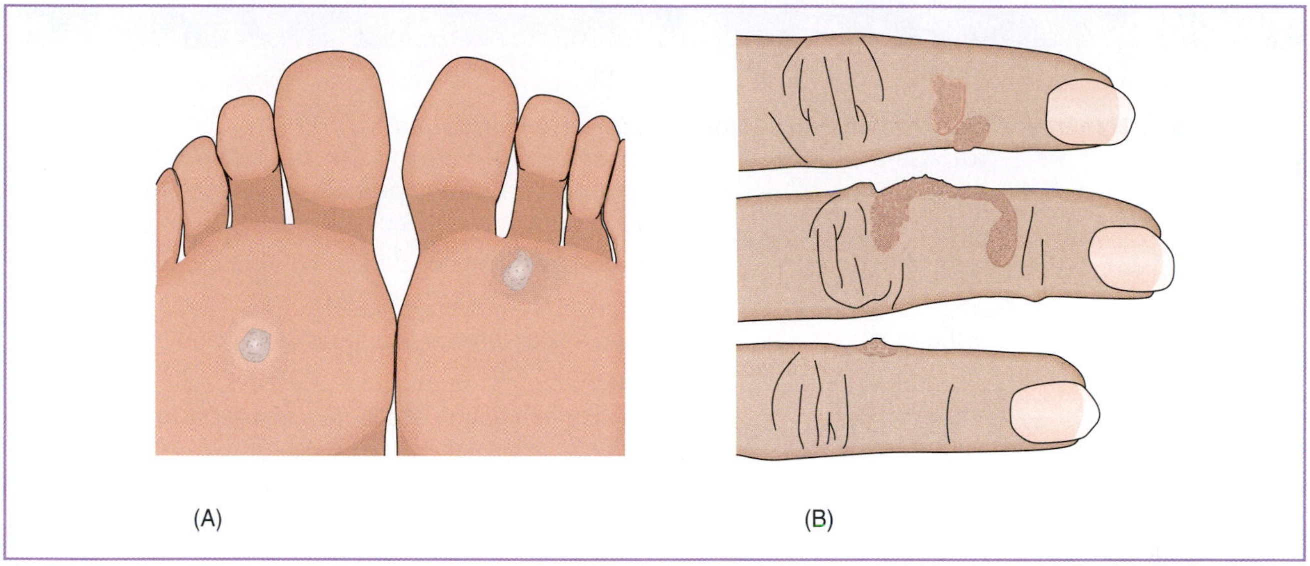

FIGURE 5-6 Warts: (A) Plantar and (B) Verruca

DIAGNOSES		
Word	**Pronunciation**	**Definition**
Metabolic, Hypersensitivity, Immune, or Idiopathic Disease *(continued)*		
eczema	ĕk'zĕ-mă	inflammation of the skin characterized by itching, redness, and vesicles; causes skin thickening in acute stages or dry lichenifications in chronic stages; *atopic dermatitis* is a chronic type of eczema often in families with a history of allergies and asthma; onset is usually two months after birth
lichen planus	lī'kĕn plā'nŭs	recurrent, itchy, inflammatory skin eruption often accompanied by oral lesions
psoriasis	sō-rī'ah-sĭs	chronic skin disease of unknown cause characterized by red, raised plaques with distinct borders and silvery scales (see Figure 5-7)

continues

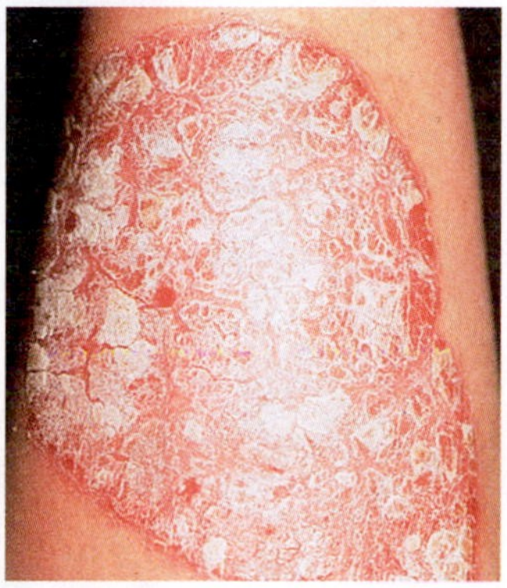

FIGURE 5-7
Psoriasis

DIAGNOSES		
Word	**Pronunciation**	**Definition**
Metabolic, Hypersensitivity, Immune, or Idiopathic Disease *(continued)*		
rosacea	rō-zā'sē-ă	common chronic skin eruption in the central part of the face in which papules and pustules appear on a flushed or red background in middle-aged persons
scleroderma	sklĕr"ă-dĕr'mah	chronic disease caused by thickening of fibrous tissue resulting in "hard skin"
sebaceous cyst	sē-bā'shŭs	cyst that develops when a sebaceous or oil gland becomes blocked
seborrheic dermatitis	sĕb"ō-rē'ĭk dĕr"mă-tī'tĭs	superficial inflammation of the skin associated with heavy production of sebum or oil that is overgrown with oil-bearing yeasts (See Figure 5-8)
systemic lupus erythematosus (SLE)	sĭs-tĕm'ĭk lū'pŭs ĕr"ĭ-thē-mah-tō'sŭs	chronic, inflammatory disease of connective tissue that that may affect the skin, joints, kidneys, and potentially any organ of the body; milder form is chronic discoid lupus erythematous (DLE) that affects skin only
urticaria	ŭr-tĭ-kā'rē-ă	skin condition that may be a reaction to internal or external allergens and often remains of unknown cause; characterized by wheals or hives and local skin swelling; often itchy due to fluids leaking from blood vessels; individual lesions clear within 24 hours but other appear; hives
Benign, Premalignant, and Malignant Tumors and Abnormal Pigmented Lesions		
actinic keratosis	ăk-tĭn'ĭk kĕr-ă-tō'sēs	premalignant condition characterized by growth of scaly, wart-like lesions on sun-exposed areas of skin
albinism	ăl'bĭn-ĭzm	genetic total or partial absence of pigment in skin, eyes, and hair
basal cell carcinoma	bā'săl kăr"sĭ-nō'mah	malignant tumor of the basal cell layer of the epidermis; the most common skin cancer; slowly enlarges but rarely metastasizes

continues

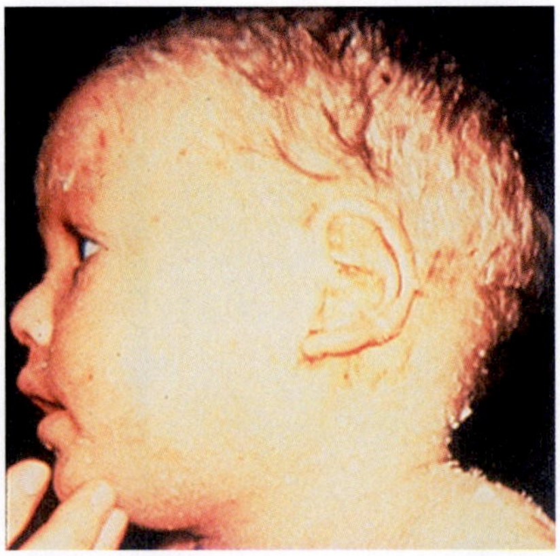

Source: Courtesy of Robert A. Silverman, M.D., Pediatric Dermatology, Georgetown University

FIGURE 5-8
Seborrheic Dermatitis

DIAGNOSES		
Word	**Pronunciation**	**Definition**
Benign, Premalignant, and Malignant Tumors and Abnormal Pigmented Lesions *(continued)*		
ephelis, *pl.* ephelides	ĕf-ē'lĭs, ĕf-ĕl-ī'dēs	freckle
fissure	fĭsh'ūr	crack-like sore in the skin or mucous membrane
hemangioma	hĕ-măn"jē-ō'mah	benign tumor comprising masses of blood vessels (See Figure 5-9)
Kaposi sarcoma	kăp'ō-sē săr-kō'mah	malignant vascular skin tumor; usually not highly malignant except in the case of AIDS
keloid	kē'loid	abnormally large, thickened scar
keratosis	kĕr-ă-tō'sĭs	skin condition characterized by a scaly growth or excessive development of the stratum corneum
lentigo, *pl.* lentigines	lĕn-tī'gō, lĕn-tĭj"ĭ-nēz"	larger, brown patches in the skin
leukoplakia	loo"kō-plā'kō-ah	white, thickened patches on the mucous membrane tissue of the tongue, cheek, or female external genitalia
malignant melanoma	mĕl"ah-nō'mah	malignant, pigmented mole or tumor of the melanocytes that may metastasize (spread) aggressively; tumor malignancy is identified by using the mnemonic aid ABCD (*asymmetry in shape, border irregularity, color variation, and diameter of more than 6mm*)
melasma	mĕl-ăz'mah	condition characterized by dark patches of skin on the face; commonly called mask of pregnancy
metastasis	mĕ-tăs'tă-sis	movement of cancerous cells from one part of the body to another via lymph drainage, bloodstream, or local extension into the skin
nevus, *pl.* nevi	nē'vŭs, nē'vī	mole, birthmark (See Figure 5-10); composed of clusters of pigment-producing cells, or melanocytes, called nevus cells in this circumstance
polyp	pŏl'ĭp	small growth extending on a stalk from a skin or mucous membrane surface
seborrheic keratosis	sĕb"ō-rē'ĭk kĕr-ă-tō'sĭs	benign overgrowth of epithelial cells into brown warty lumps in older individuals

continues

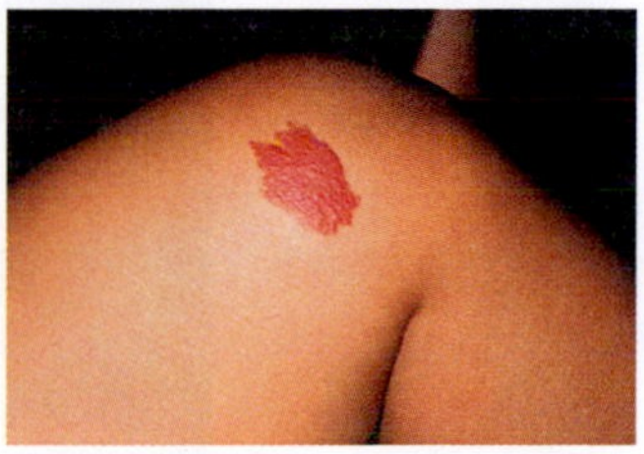

FIGURE 5-9
Hemangioma

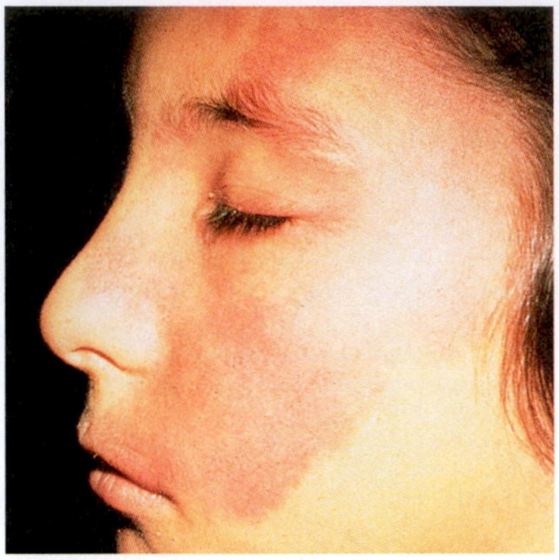

FIGURE 5-10
Nevus Flammeus

Source: Courtesy of Robert A. Silverman, M.D., Pediatric Dermatology, Georgetown University

DIAGNOSES

Word	Pronunciation	Definition
Benign, Premalignant, and Malignant Tumors and Abnormal Pigmented Lesions *(continued)*		
squamous cell carcinoma	skwā'mŭs kăr"sĭ-nō'mah	malignant tumor of the squamous epithelial cells of the epidermis; second most common skin cancer; can metastasize
vitiligo	vĭt-ĭl-ī'gō	condition characterized by destruction of melanocytes in patches of skin that are seen as abnormally white patches in the skin
Diseases of Nail and Hair		
alopecia	ăl"ō-pē'shē-ah	partial or complete hair loss (See Figure 5-11)
folliculitis	fō-lĭk"ū-lī'tĭs	inflammation and infection of the hair follicle
hirsutism	hŭr'sūt-ĭzm	excessive growth of hair
paronychia	păr-ō-nĭk'ē-ah	infection of the skin around the nail (See Figure 5-12)

continues

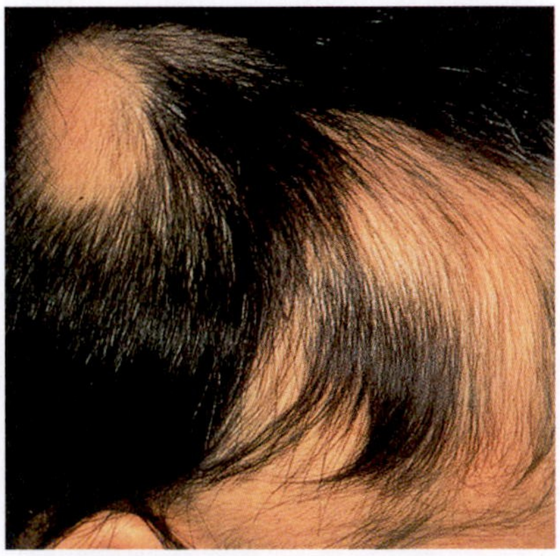

FIGURE 5-11
Alopecia Areata

Source: Courtesy of Robert A. Silverman, M.D., Pediatric Dermatology, Georgetown University

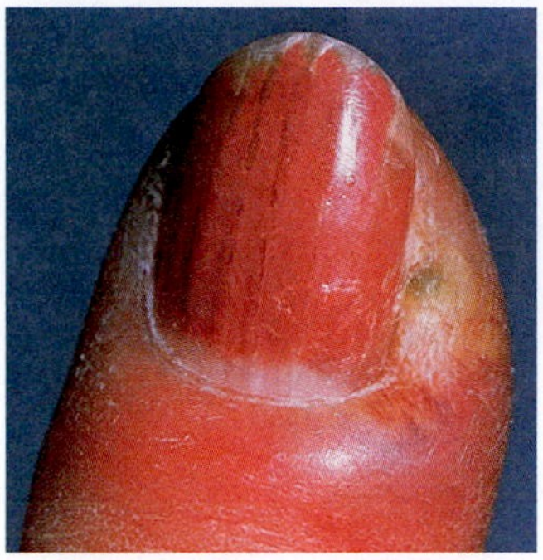

Source: Delmar/Cengage Learning

FIGURE 5-12
Paronychia

DIAGNOSES		
Word	**Pronunciation**	**Definition**
Trauma, Mechanical, Thermal, Electrical, Radiation, and Pressure		
abrasion	ă-brā'zhŭn	scrape; commonly called friction burns or rug burns
avulsion	ă-vŭl'shŭn	trauma caused when a portion of skin or appendage is pulled or torn away
burns		damage to the skin by fire, sun, chemicals, heated objects or fluids, electricity, or other means ranging from minor incidents to life-threatening emergencies; burns are described using four classifications: (1) superficial, or first-degree burns, which affect only the epidermis; (2) partial thickness, or second-degree burns, which affect the epidermis and dermis; (3) full thickness, or third-degree burns, which affect all dermal structures; and (4) deep full thickness, or fourth-degree burns, which extend to the underlying fat, muscles, and bones (See Figure 5-13)
callus	kăl'ŭs	localized thickening of the horny layer of the epidermis due to pressure or friction; usually on the palms of the hands or on the soles of the feet
Cicatrix	sĭk'ă-trĭks	normal scar left by a healed wound
contusion	kŏn-too'zhŭn	bruise
corns		local thickening of tissue, usually on the feet, often painful to pressure and walking
decubitus ulcer	dē-kū'bĭ-tŭs	pressure sore resulting from tissue compression from prolonged confinement in a bed or chair
ecchymosis, *pl.* ecchymoses	ĕk-ĭ-mō'sĭs	bruise or black and blue mark
excoriation	ĕks-kō"rē-ā'shŭn	scratch
frostbite		freezing of tissue, usually on the face, fingers, toes, and ears
hematoma	hē"mah-tō'mah	blood accumulation in the skin or other tissues resulting from bleeding
hyperthermia	hī"pĕr-thĕr'mē-ah	occurs when the body is overheated due to excessive exposure to the sun or a hot environment

continues

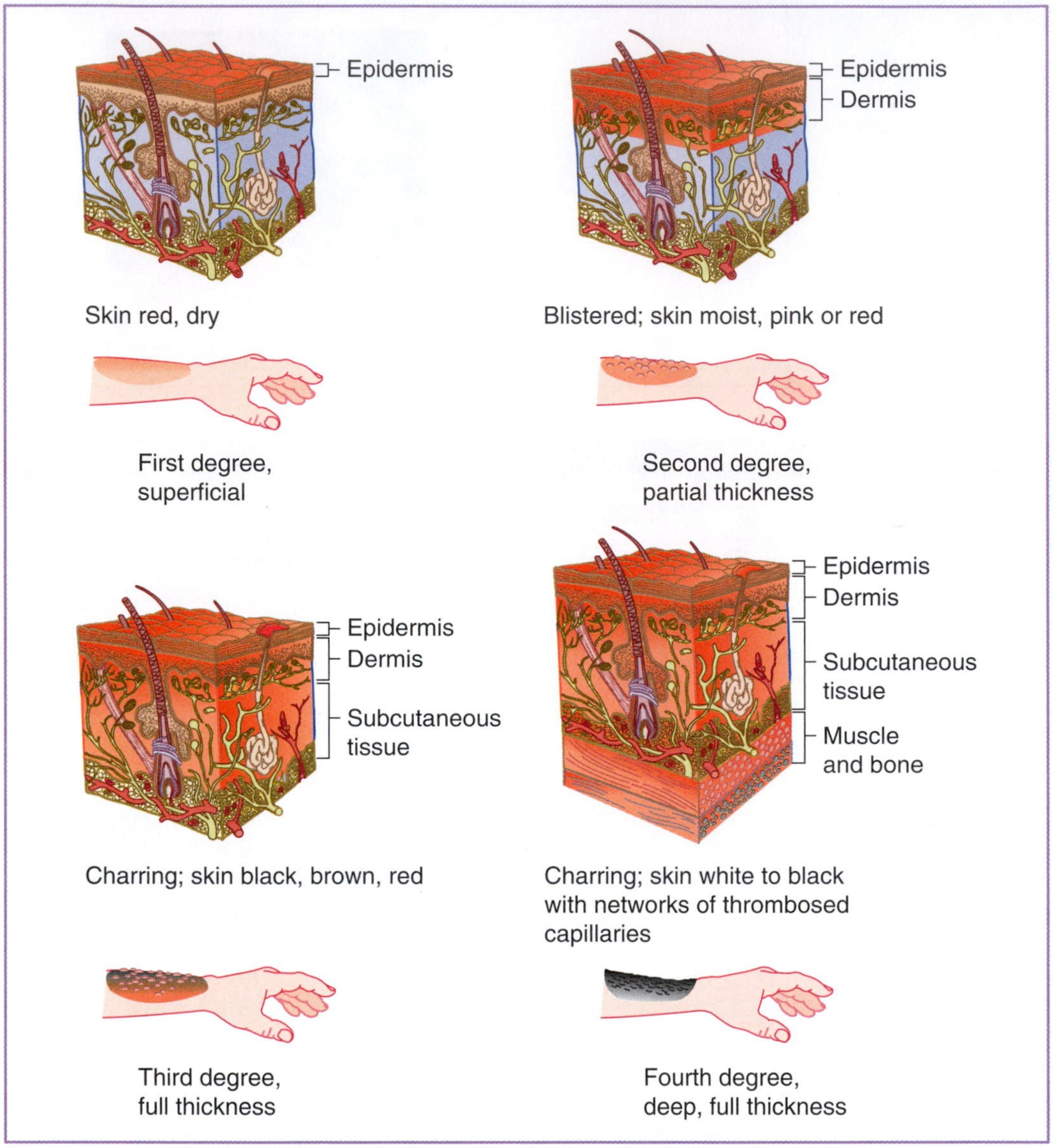

FIGURE 5-13
Four Stages of Burns

DIAGNOSES

Word	Pronunciation	Definition
Trauma, Mechanical, Thermal, Electrical, Radiation, and Pressure *(continued)*		
hypothermia	hī"pō-thĕr'mē-ah	cold thermal injury resulting when the body's core temperature falls to less than 95°F
keloid	kē'lŏyd	abnormal, thick scar left by a healed wound
laceration	lăs"ĕr-ā'shŭn	cut in the skin caused by a sharp object
purpura	pŭr'pū-rah	large bruises in the skin
Other Problems		
comedo, *pl.* comedones or comedos	kŏm'ē-dō	typical small skin lesion of acne vulgaris and seborrheic dermatitis originating from the opening of a hair follicle; may be closed (whitehead) or open (blackhead)

continues

DIAGNOSES

Word	Pronunciation	Definition
Other Problems *(continued)*		
diaphoresis	dī"ă-fō-rē'sĭs	condition marked by profuse perspiration
exfoliative dermatitis or erythroderm	eks-fō'lē-ă-tĭv dĕr"mă-tī 'tĭs, ĕrĭth"rō-dĕr'mah	generalized scaling eruption of the skin; many causes are possible
hyperhidrosis	hī"pĕr-hī-drō'sĭs	excessive perspiration
pemphigoid	pĕm'fĭ-goid	specific blistering disease of the skin
pemphigus	pĕm'fĭ-gŭs	blistering disease of the skin and mucous membrane
petechia, *pl.* petechiae	pĕ-tē'kē-ah, pĕ-tē'kē-ē	fine bleeding points in the skin
primary lesions		basic irregularities in skin disease identified as follows (See Figure 5-14)
• *bulla*		large, fluid-filled accumulation in skin; blister
• *macule*		small, flat discoloration in the skin
• *nodule*		larger, rounded lump in the skin
• *papule*		small, elevated lump in the skin
• *patch*		larger, flat discoloration in the skin
• *plaque*		wider elevation in the skin
• *pustule*		pus-filled swelling in the skin
• *vesicle*		small, clear, liquid accumulation in the skin
• *wheal*		hive; transient swelling in the skin
pruritus	proo-rī'tĭs	itch
secondary lesions		lesions that arise from primary lesions; scales, crusts (scabs), erosions, ulcers, scars, atrophy, excoriations, and lichenification (thickening of skin)
xanthoma	zăn-thō'mah	distinct yellow growth caused by deposits of fat in the skin; usually reflects increased fatty materials in the bloodstream

TREATMENT PROCEDURES

Word	Pronunciation	Definition
allergy immunotherapy		treatment of an allergy by using hyposensitizing injections of allergy serum for specific allergens
cryosurgery	krī"ō-sŭr'jer-ē	use of extreme cold in a localized part of the body to freeze and destroy unwanted tissues
curettage	kū"rĕ-tahzh'	destruction and removal of the surface of the skin or the covering of an organ by scraping with a spoonshaped, sharp instrument
débridement	dā-brēd-mŏn'	removal of debris, foreign objects, or damaged tissue from a wound to prevent infection and encourage healing

continues

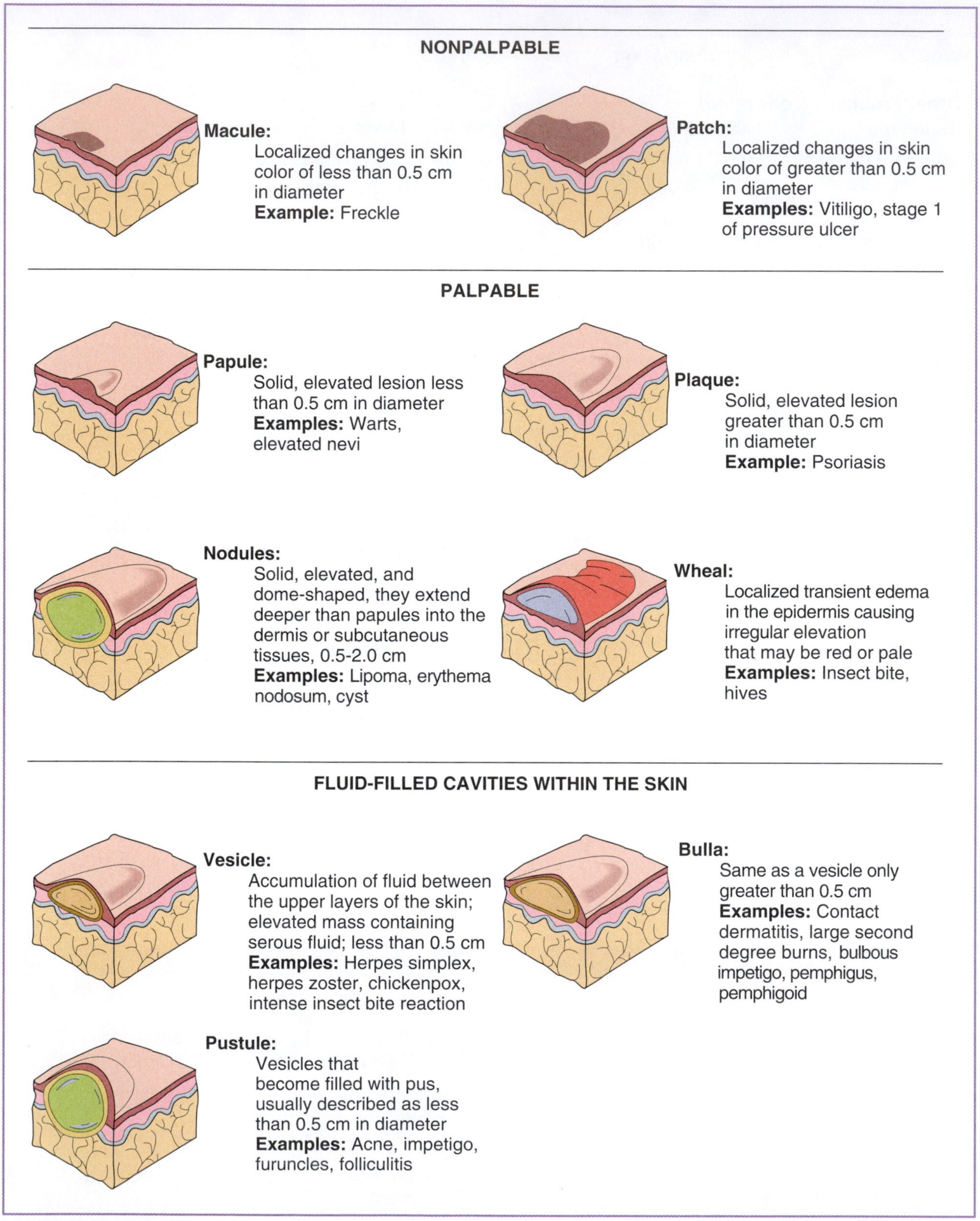

Source: Delmar/Cengage Learning

FIGURE 5-14 Primary Lesions

TREATMENT PROCEDURES		
Word	**Pronunciation**	**Definition**
dermabrasion	dĕr"mah-brā'shun	removal of facial scars and keratose by the use of mechanical or chemical abrasives
electrocoagulation	ē-lĕk"trō-kō-ăg"-ū-lā'shŭn	destruction of tissue by means of a high-frequency electric current concentrated at one point as it passes through tissue (See Figure 5-15)
electrodesiccation	ēlĕk"trō-dĕs"ĭ-kā'shŭn	destruction of warts, growths, or unwanted areas of tissue with a diathermy (electric current) instrument by drying tissue with a hot, electric spark using two electrodes (one positive, one negative) (See Figure 5-15)
escharotomy	ĕs-kăr-ŏt'ō-mē	removal of necrotic tissue resulting from a severe burn
fulguration	fŭl"gū-rā'shŭn	destruction of tissue by electric sparks; uses the same electrode tip as desiccation, but the needle tip is not inserted into the tissue (See Figure 5-15)
laser therapy		destruction of various skin lesions with the use of certain types of lasers, intense monochromatic light that is known to be absorbed by certain skin lesions
Mohs' chemosurgery technique	mōz kēm"ō-sŭr'jĕr-ē	technique for removal of a malignant growth in progressive mapped layers with rapid microscopic evaluation of frozen sections of each layer
photochemotherapy		use of oral or topical psoralen medications followed by exposure to light bulbs emitting light in the long wavelength, ultraviolet light spectrum for treatment of psoriasis and other skin conditions
skin graft		procedure to cover a burn wound to promote healing; may be autograft (from patient), homograft (from another individual), heterograft (from an animal), or synthetic substitutes; also done with patient's own skin to cover sites of skin cancer removal
UVB-phototherapy		exposure to ultraviolet B light (sunburn spectrum) for treatment of psoriasis or other skin conditions

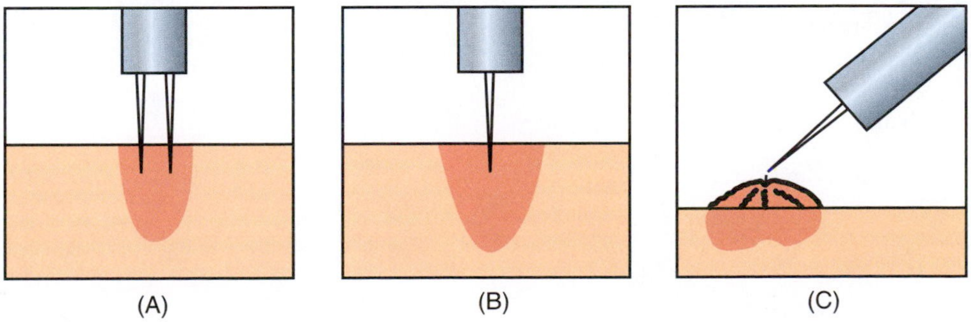

FIGURE 5-15
(A) Electrocoagulation; (B) Electrodesiccation; (C) Fulguration

Source: Delmar/Cengage Learning

MEDICATIONS PRESCRIBED	
Trade Name	Generic Name
Anti-acnes	
Accutane	isotretinoin
Azelex	azelek acid
Cleocin	clindamycin
Differin	adapalene
Emgel, T-Stat, A/T/S	topical erythromycin
Retin A, Avita, Renova	tretinoin
Antifungals	
Diflucan	fluconazole
Exelderm	sulconazole nitrate
Fulvicin P/C, Grifulvin V, Grisactin	griseofulvin
Lamisil	terbinfine
Loprox	ciclopirox topical
Lotrimin, Mycelex	clotrimazole topical
Lotrisone	betamethasone and clotrimazole
Monistat, Mitrazol, Monistat-Derm	miconazole
Naftin	naftifine topical
Nizoral	ketoconazole
Oxistat	oxiconazole topical
Spectazole	econazole topical
Sporanox	itraconazole
Antihistamines	
Atarax, Rezine, Vistaril	hydroxyzine
Benadryl, Banophen	diphenhydramine
Anti-infectives	
Bactroban	mupirocin topical
Bio-Statin, Nilstat, Mycostatin	nystatin
E-Mycin, E.E.S., Robimycin	erythromycin
Keflex	cephalexin
Antivirals	
Famvir	famciclovir
Valtrex	valacyclovir
Zovirax	acyclovir

continues

MEDICATIONS PRESCRIBED	
Trade Name	Generic Name
Bath Dermatologics	
Alpha Keri	
Aveeno Bath	
Balnetar oil	
Lubath	
Zetar	
Burn Treatments	
Baciguent	bacitracin
Betadine	povidone-iodine
Garamycin	gentamicin sulfate
Myciguent	neomycin sulfate
Silvadene	silver sulfadiazine
Sulfamylon	mafenide acetate
Psoriasis Medications	
Dovonex	calcipotriene
Mexate	methotrexate
Oxsoralen	methoxsalen
Tegison	etretinate
Scabicides	
Elamite, Acticin	permethrin
Eurax, Kwell	crotimaton
—	lindane
Topical Steroids	
Aristocort, Kenalog	triamcinolone acetonide
Cordran	flurandrenolide topical
Cort-Dome, Hytone, Nutracort, Cortaid, A-Hydrocort, Westcort, Locoid	hydrocortisone topical
Cutivate	fluticasone propionate
Dermatop	prednicarbate topical
Lidex, Dermacin, Fluex, Flurosyn	fluocinonide topical
Medrol	methylprednisolone
Synalar, Fluonid	fluocinolone acetonide
Temovate, Ciobrevate, Cormax	clobetasol topical
Topicort	desoximetasone topical

continues

MEDICATIONS PRESCRIBED	
Trade Name	**Generic Name**
Topical Steroids *(continued)*	
Ultravate	halobetasol propionate
Valisone, Diprosone, Maxivate, Betaderm, Diprolene	betamethasone

ABBREVIATIONS*	
ANA	antinuclear antibody
bx	biopsy
decub	decubitus ulcer (bed sore)
derm	dermatology
DLE	discoid lupus erythematosus
EIA	enzyme immunoassay
FANA	fluorescent antinuclear antibody
I&D	incision and drainage
ID	intradermal
KOH	potassium hydroxide
PUVA	psorafen psoralen ultraviolet A-range
SLE	systemic lupus erythematosus
subcu, subq, SC, SQ, subcut	subcutaneous
TENS	transcutaneous electrical nerve stimulation
ung	ointment, unguent
UV	ultraviolet

Working Practice Review Exercises

IDENTIFICATION

Identify the following diagnostic procedures.

1. skin test where test materials are applied to small scratches in the skin ____________________

*See Appendix C for additional abbreviations.

2. technique for partial excision of material for pathologic study when total excision is not possible ____________________
3. blood test to screen for cutaneous lupus erythematosus ____________________
4. test of fluid from the base of a vesicle ____________________
5. skin scrapings from lesions immersed in solution and examined for hyphae or spores ____________________
6. skin examination done in a darkened room under light filtered through glass ____________________
7. blood test to see if patient has or has had an infection ____________________
8. one of primary tests for several infections diseases, including HIV ____________________
9. reactive substances are injected between the dermis and epidermis ____________________
10. removal of lesions for pathological examination ____________________

COMPLETION

Fill in the correct treatment procedure.

1. Use of extreme cold in a localized part of the body to freeze and destroy unwanted tissue is ____________________.
2. Destruction and removal of the covering of an organ with a scraping tool is called ____________________.
3. Removal of facial scars and keratose by chemical or mechanical abrasives is known as ____________________.
4. Destruction of warts, growths, or unwanted tissue with a diathermy instrument is known as ____________________.
5. Removal of debris or foreign objects from a wound to prevent infection and encourage healing is ____________________.
6. Removal of necrotic tissue resulting from a severe burn is ____________________.
7. Destruction of tissue by electric spark but without inserting the needle tip into the tissue is ____________________.
8. Technique for removal of a malignant growth, layer by layer is ____________________.
9. Exposure to ultraviolet B light to treat psoriasis or other skin conditions is ____________________.
10. Procedure to cover a burn wound or skin cancer removal to promote healing is known as a ____________________.

MATCHING

Provide the correct diagnosis for the following statements.

1. __________ lip inflammation
2. __________ condition marked by profuse perspiration
3. __________ fire or chemical injury that affects all layers of skin
4. __________ condition marked by excessive hair growth
5. __________ varicella

a. abrasion
b. albinism
c. cheilitis
d. chickenpox
e. contusion

6.	_________ wart	f.	diaphoresis
7.	_________ hard skin	g.	hirsutism
8.	_________ total or partial absence of pigment in skin, eyes, hair	h.	Kaposi sarcoma
9.	_________ keloid	i.	laceration
10.	_________ mask of pregnancy	j.	lentigo
11.	_________ scrape	k.	measles
12.	_________ bruise	l.	melasma
13.	_________ excoriation	m.	petechia
14.	_________ decubitus ulcer	n.	pressure sore
15.	_________ cut in skin	o.	scar
16.	_________ fine bleeding points	p.	scleroderma
17.	_________ abnormally white patches of skin	q.	scratch
18.	_________ large, brown patches of skin	r.	third-degree burn
19.	_________ malignant vascular skin tumor	s.	verruca
20.	_________ rubeola	t.	vitiligo

IDENTIFICATION

Identify the following diagnoses.

1. chronic skin disease displaying silvery scales and red, raised plaques _______________
2. blistering disease of the skin and mucous membranes _______________
3. skin disease caused by fungus _______________
4. condition of infestation with lice _______________
5. pressure sore _______________
6. mole, birthmark _______________
7. hair loss _______________
8. freckle _______________
9. excessive perspiration _______________
10. small, flat discoloration in the skin _______________
11. large bruises in the skin _______________
12. hive _______________
13. pus-filled swelling in the skin _______________
14. small, elevated lump in the skin _______________
15. chronic skin eruption in the central part of the face in which papules and pustules appear on a flushed or red background _______________

Dictionary Exercises

Additional words commonly used by physicians specializing in the system are included at the end of each chapter. They are presented in the form of exercises that will assist you in learning how to use the medical dictionary.

DICTIONARY EXERCISE 1

Use your dictionary to find the pronunciation and definition of the following words.

	Word	Pronunciation	Definition
1.	acrochordon	________	________
2.	bulla	________	________
3.	melanoderma	________	________
4.	collagen	________	________
5.	balanitis xerotica obliterans	________	________
6.	strawberry hemangioma	________	________
7.	dermatitis herpetiformis	________	________
8.	Candida	________	________
9.	dermographism	________	________
10.	photosensitivity	________	________
11.	neurodermatitis	________	________
12.	mycosis fungoides	________	________
13.	xanthelasma	________	________
14.	steatoma	________	________

DICTIONARY EXERCISE 2

Pronunciation of the words below is provided. Using your dictionary, find the correct spelling and definition for each word.

	Word	Pronunciation	Definition
1.	________	sĭk'ā-trĭks	________
2.	________	ĕks-kō-"rē-ā'shŭn	________
3.	________	pū'roo-lĕnt	________
4.	________	tĭn'ē-ă pĕd'ĭs	________
5.	________	kŏn"dĭ-lō'mah	________
6.	________	kŏm'ē-dō	________
7.	________	sĭl'ē-ah	________
8.	________	mŏ-lŭs'kŭm	________
9.	________	stē"ah-tō'mah	________
10.	________	tĕl'ō-jĕn ĕf-loo'vē-ŭm	________
11.	________	pĭt"ĭ-rī'ă-sĭs rō'zē-ah	________

DICTIONARY EXERCISE 3

Rewrite the following sentences in your own words. Provide pronunciation marks for each italicized word.

1. The baby's past medical history included urticaria and *varicella* (________________).

   ____

2. The skin of the feet was characterized by *xerosis* (________________), *pruritus* (________________), and *melasma* (________________), with a *clavus* (________________) on the left toe.

   ____

3. The rash was diagnosed as *erysipelas* (________________).

   ____

4. There was no evidence of *dermatosis* (________________).

   ____

5. The *eruption* (________________) looked like *pityriasis rosea* (________________).

   ____

6. The baby was born with a strawberry *hemangioma* (________________) near the knee.

   ____

7. The final diagnosis was *elephantiasis* (________________).

   ____

8. The *verrucous* (________________) area is located near the *dermatofibroma* (________________).

   ____

9. Psoriasis is an *idiopathic* (________________) disease.

   ____

10. The doctor was concerned about the possibility of *gangrene* (________________).

    ____

11. Naomi learned that *keratoses* (________________) are caused by excessive light.

    ____

12. His diagnoses included *xeroderma* (________________).

    ____

13. After the accident, Jacob experienced *epidermalysis* (________________).

    ____

14. *Causalgia* (________________) is an unpleasant symptom.

    ____

15. One of the characteristics of a melanoma is *asymmetry* (________________).

    ____

StudyWARE™ Connection

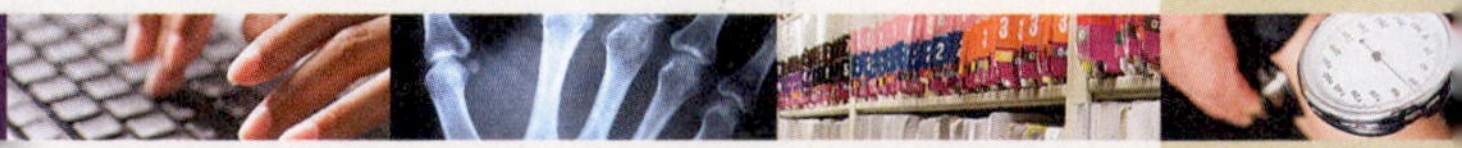

To take a practice quiz or play interactive games that reinforce the content in this chapter, go to your StudyWARE™ CD-ROM.

Listening Exercise

INSTRUCTIONS

1. Review the spelling, pronunciation, and meaning of the words provided in the preview.
2. Go to your StudyWARE™ CD-ROM and listen to **Listening Exercise 5-1**. Fill in the blank in the report as the word is dictated.
3. At the end of the activity, check your spelling against the preview words. They appear in the preview in the order in which they are encountered in the activity.
4. Review and practice the words you missed.
5. Look up words that are not familiar.

PREVIEW OF WORDS FOR LISTENING EXERCISE 5-1

Word	Pronunciation	Definition
malar	mā'lăr	relating to the cheekbone or the cheek; cheekbone
dermatoses	dĕr"mă-tō'sēs	skin disorders not characterized by inflammation
verrucous	vĕr-roŏ'kŭs	pertaining to wartlike elevations
papules	păp'ūlz	small, superficial, solid elevations of the skin
actinic	ăk-tĭn'ĭk	producing chemical action
keratoses	kĕr-ă-tō'sēs	horny growths such as warts or callosities

Listening Exercise 5-1

*Study*WARE™ Connection

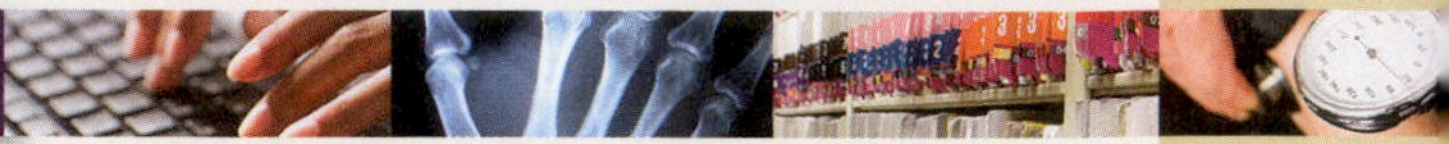

Listen to this report being read on your StudyWARE™ CD-ROM. Fill in each blank as the word is dicted

Letter of Consultation

Dear Dr. Ober:

I examined our mutual patient, Brian Westerhoff, on 8/7/20—. Thank you for sending your clinic notes. As you mentioned, he has had an irregularity on his lip present for several months. This has somewhat diminished since he began using Chapstick with an SPF of 30. In addition, he had a patch on his right ____________________ area that was treated in the last six months with applications of Aclovate cream, that did not clear. The patient is an outdoors person and has had much sun exposure over the years. There is no family history of ____________________ or allergies.

On examination, he exhibited a fine 6 mm irregular scaling patch on his right lower lip centrally. There was also a fine scaling patch on his right malar area. There were tan ____________________ ____________________ on his upper chest, and there were several on his back.

It was my impression he exhibited several ____________________ ____________________, as well as multiple
seborrheic keratoses. I discussed these with him and proceeded to treat the two actinic keratoses with application of liquid nitrogen.

I did suggest he return for follow-up in several months.

Thank you for this consultation.

Sincerely yours,

George Quackenbush, MD

CHAPTER

6

The Musculoskeletal System

"Those who think they have no time for bodily exercise will sooner or later have to find time for illness."

—Edward Stanley

OBJECTIVES

When you have completed this study of the musculoskeletal system, you should be able to

1. Spell and define major system components and explain how they operate.
2. Identify the meanings of related word elements.
3. Spell and define diagnostic procedures, diagnoses, treatment procedures, and abbreviations.
4. Spell the names of commonly used medications.
5. Use a dictionary as a tool in processing medical documents.
6. Hear how medical terminology is used in actual medical reports.

INTRODUCTION

The musculoskeletal system is composed of bones, muscles, tendons, ligaments, and joints. This system involves the specialties of orthopedic surgery, physical medicine, rheumatology, and sports medicine. **Orthopedic** (or"thō-pē'dĭk) **surgery** is the surgical correction of deformities, traumas, and chronic diseases of bones and joints. **Physical medicine** is the treatment of illnesses by clinical use of physical agents such as heat, water, electricity, ultraviolet radiation, massage, and exercise. **Rheumatology** (roo"mă-tŏl'ō-jē) is the study of diseases of the joints. **Sports medicine** and **exercise science** are committed to the diagnosis, treatment, and prevention of sports-related injuries. Basic to all of these specialties are the various components of the musculoskeletal system: bones, joints, and muscles.

BONES

oste/o	bone

There are 206 bones in the human body. Each bone is an organ with its own system of blood and lymphatic vessels and nerves. Bones are divided into four classes according to their shape—long, short, flat, and irregular.

COMPOSITION OF BONES

Bones are living **osseous** (ŏs'ē-ŭs) tissue, one of the hardest materials in the body. Note in Figure 6-1 that almost all bones are covered on the outside by a membrane called **periosteum** (pĕr"ē-ŏs'tē-ŭm) (1), which contains many nerve fibers and lymphatics. The hard material forming the exterior of the bone is called compact or **cortical** (kor'tĭ-kăl) **bone** (2). **Cancellous** or **spongy bone** (3) is found in the interior. Spaces within the cancellous bone contain two kinds of marrow, red and yellow bone marrow (4). **Red bone marrow** is found in certain parts of all bones and manufactures most of the blood cells. **Yellow bone marrow** is found primarily in the central cavities of the long bones and is composed chiefly of fat cells.

PROCESSES AND DEPRESSIONS

The contour of bones has many projections. Often there are places for muscle attachments. To identify these areas the term **process** is used. Some of the common bony processes are as follows.

Process	Pronunciation	Meaning
condyle	kŏn'dīl	rounded portion of bone that joins with another
epicondyle	ēp"ĭ-kŏn'dīl	small projection located on or above a condyle
head		end of a long bone, often set off from the shaft of the bone by a neck

continues

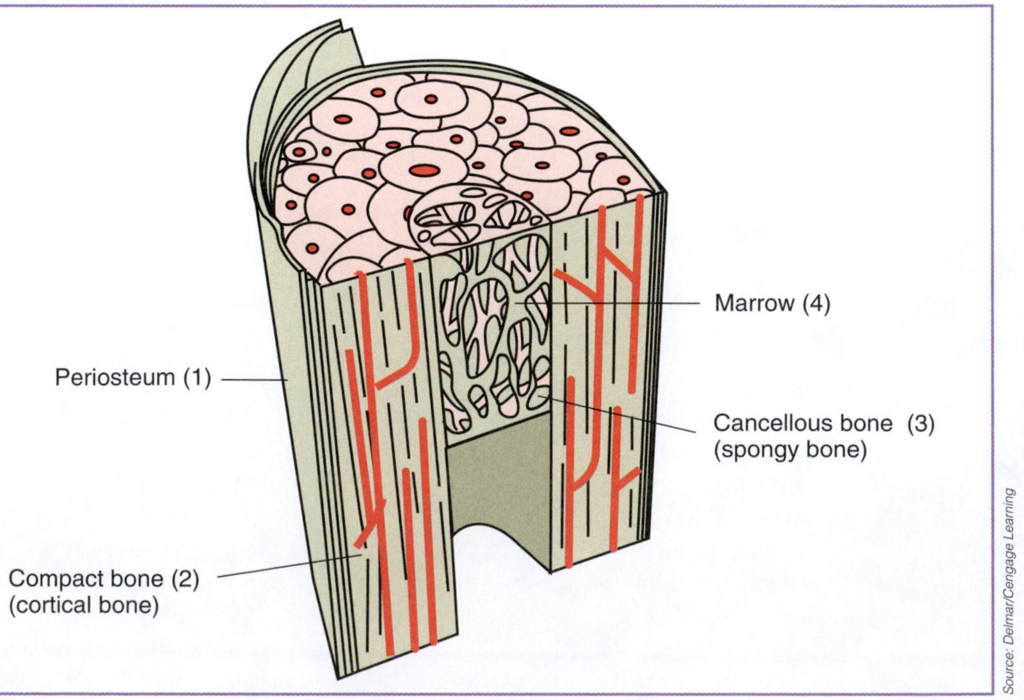

FIGURE 6-1
Interior Bone Structure

Process	Pronunciation	Meaning
trochanter	trō-kăn'ter	large, somewhat blunt process on the femur that serves as a site for attachment
tubercle	too'ber-k'l	nodule or small, rounded process that serves as the site for tendon or muscle attachment
tuberosity	too"-bĕ-rŏs'ĭ-tē	broad process, larger than a tubercle

Openings or hollow regions that help to join one bone to another are **depressions**. The following are some of the common bony depressions.

Depression	Pronunciation	Meaning
fissure	fĭs'sur	narrow, deep, slit-like opening
foramen	fō-rā'mĕn	hole for blood vessels and nerves
fossa	fŏs'ah	depression or cavity in a bone, for articulation or muscle attachment
sinus	sī'nŭs	air cavity within a bone
sulcus	sŭl'kŭs	groove

Other descriptive structural terms include the following:

Term	Pronunciation	Meaning
crest		sharp, prominent, bony ridge
facet	făs'ĕt	small, flat-surfaced area on a bone
fovea	fō'vē-ah	pit generally used for attachment
line		slight, bony ridge
meatus	mē-ā'tŭs	canal; passage; opening

THE SKELETON

The complete bony framework of the body is known as the skeleton. It is divided into two main groups of bones—the axial (ăk'sē-ăl) skeleton and the appendicular (ăp"ĕn-dĭk'ŭ-lar) skeleton.

Axial Skeleton

caud/o	tail	lumb/o	loin, lower back
cephal/o	head	maxill/o	upper jaw bone
cervic/o	neck	sacr/o	sacrum
cleid/o	clavicle	spondyl/o	vertebra
cost/o	rib	vertebr/o	vertebra
crani/o	skull, head		

The **axial skeleton** includes the bony framework of the head and trunk.

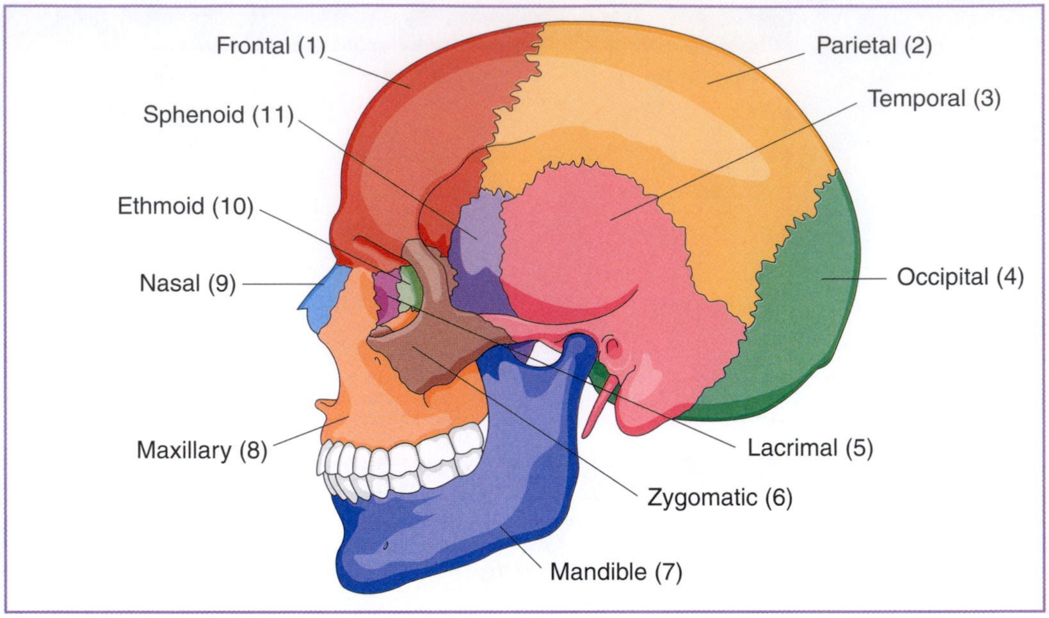

FIGURE 6-2 The Skull

Source: Delmar/Cengage Learning

Head. The framework of the head is called the **skull**; it is subdivided into two parts, called the cranium and the facial bones. Figure 6-2 illustrates the cranium bones: frontal (1), parietal (pah-rī'ĕ-tăl) (2), temporal (3), ethmoid (ĕth'moid) (10), sphenoid (sfē'noid) (11), and occipital (ŏk-sĭp'ĭ-tăl) (4). The facial bones shown in Figure 6-2 are the mandible (măn'dĭ-bl) (7), maxillary (măk'sĭ-lĕr"ē) (8), zygomatic (zī"gō-măt'ĭk) (6), and smaller bones, including the nasal (9) and lacrimal (lăk'rĭ-măl) (5).

Trunk. The framework of the trunk includes the vertebral column and rib cage. The **spinal column** is divided into five regions, shown in Figure 6-3. These spinal column regions are the cervical (1), thoracic (2), lumbar (3), sacral (să'krăl) (4), and coccygeal (kŏk-sĭj'ē-ăl) (5). These bones protect the spinal cord and enable a human to stand in an upright position. A physician records or identifies each by indicating region and number; for example, the twelfth thoracic vertebra is T12.

The **rib cage** has twelve pairs of ribs attached to the vertebral column at the back. Ten of these pairs are also attached directly or indirectly to the breastbone or **sternum** (ster'nŭm) in the front. The remaining two pairs, referred to as floating ribs, are attached only to the vertebral column. The rib cage serves to support the chest and protect the heart, lungs, and other organs.

StudyWARE™ Connection

Play an interactive game labeling structures of the **Skull** on your StudyWARE™ CD-ROM.

Appendicular Skeleton

carp/o	wrist	ili/o	ilium
cheir/o, chir/o	hand	ischi/o	hip
dactyl/o	finger, toe	ped/o, pod/o	foot
digit/o	finger, toe	tars/o	of or pertaining to the edge of the foot

The **appendicular skeleton** is usually referred to as the extremities and includes both upper and lower extremities.

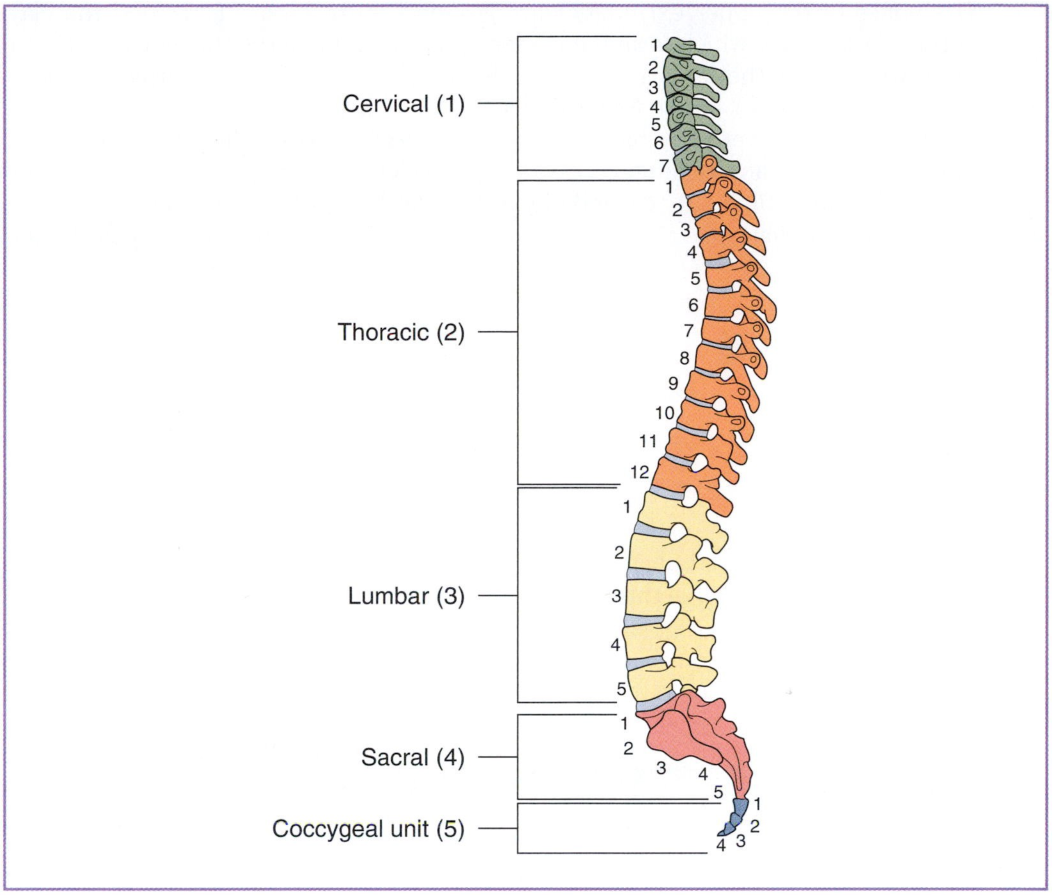

FIGURE 6-3
Regions of the Spinal Column

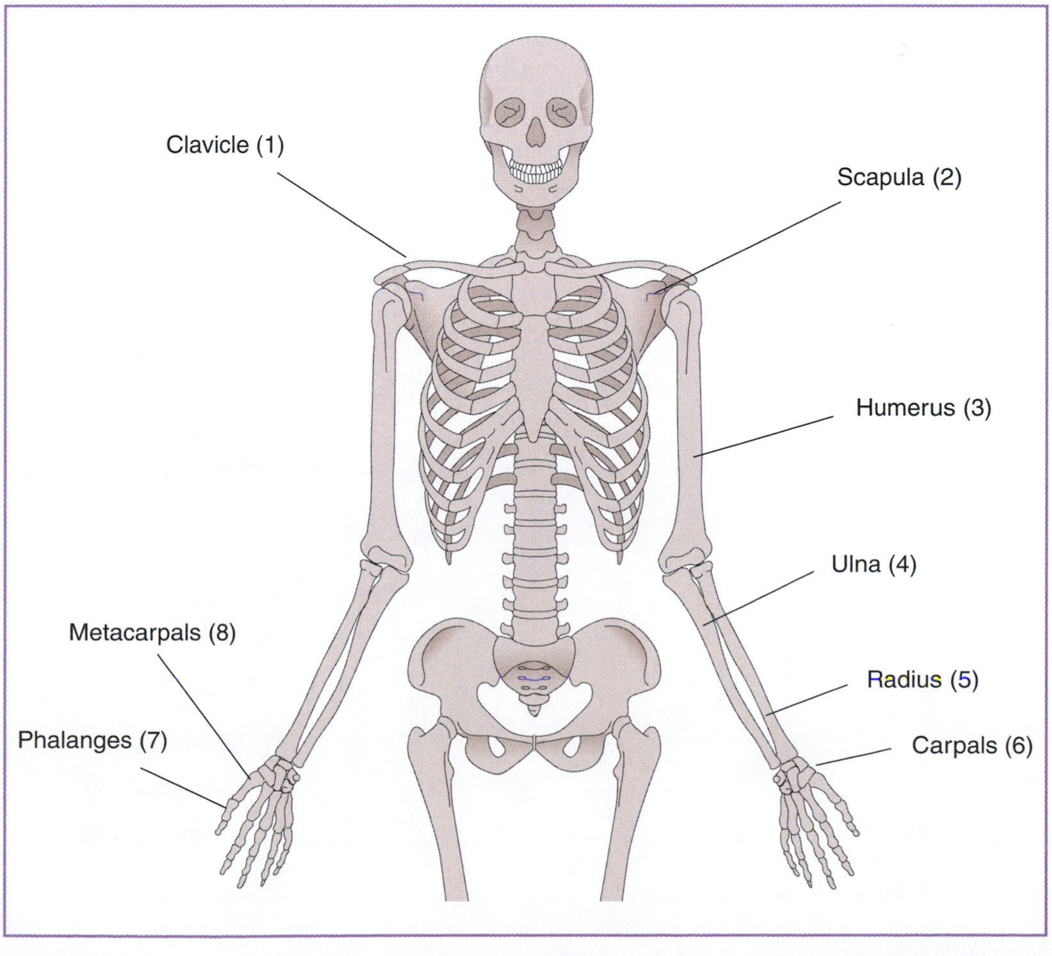

FIGURE 6-4
Bones of the Upper Extremities

The bones of the upper extremities are grouped as shown in Figure 6-4: the clavicle (klăv'ĭ-kl) (1) and scapula (skăp'ū-lah) (2), which form the pectoral girdle; the humerus (hū'mer-ŭs) (3); the ulna (ul'nah) (4) and radius (5), which form the forearm; the carpals (kăr'păls) (6), the metacarpals (mĕt"ah-kăr'păls) (8), and the phalanges (fah-lăn'jēz) (7), which form the hand.

The bones of the lower extremities (Figure 6-5) are grouped in a similar fashion, as follows: the ilium (ĭl'ē-ŭm) (1), pubis (pū'bĭs) (2), and ischium (ĭs'kē-ŭm) (3), which form the pelvic girdle; the femur (fē'mur) (4), patella (pah-tĕl'ah) (5), tibia (tĭb'ē-ah) (6), and fibula (fĭb'ū-lah) (7), which form the leg; the tarsals (tahr'săls) (8), the metatarsals (9), and phalanges (10), which form the foot. The femur is the strongest bone in the body.

Joints

arthr/o	joint	ligament/o	ligament
articu/o	joint	synov/o	synovial membrane
burs/o	sac		

A region in which two or more bones meet is called a **joint** or an articulation (see Figure 6-6). Most are classified as freely movable joints, called **diarthroses** (dī"ăr-thrō'sēz), and are lined with a **synovial** (sĭ-nō'vē-ăl) **membrane** (1) that secretes lubricating synovial fluid (2). The shoulder is an example of this type of joint. Others are classified as slightly movable or **fixed joints**, which occasionally allow slight motion, but these do not have a distinct cavity containing fluid. The suture joints of the skull are considered examples of a fixed joint.

StudyWARE™ Connection

View an animation of different types of **Diarthroses (synovial joints)** on your StudyWARE™ CD-ROM.

Stability is added to joints by connective tissue bands called **ligaments**. Certain joints have a saclike structure called a **bursa** (bĕr'sah) surrounding them that prevents friction between the moving parts, such as tendons and bones. Common bursal locations are at the elbow, knee, and shoulder joints.

The chief function of the freely movable joints is to allow changes of position and to provide for motion. Some of these movements are identified and illustrated in Figure 6-7.

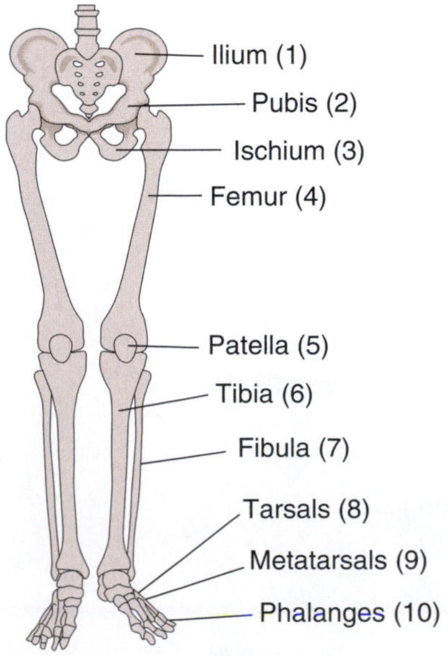

FIGURE 6-5 Bones of the Lower Extremities

Source: Delmar/Cengage Learning

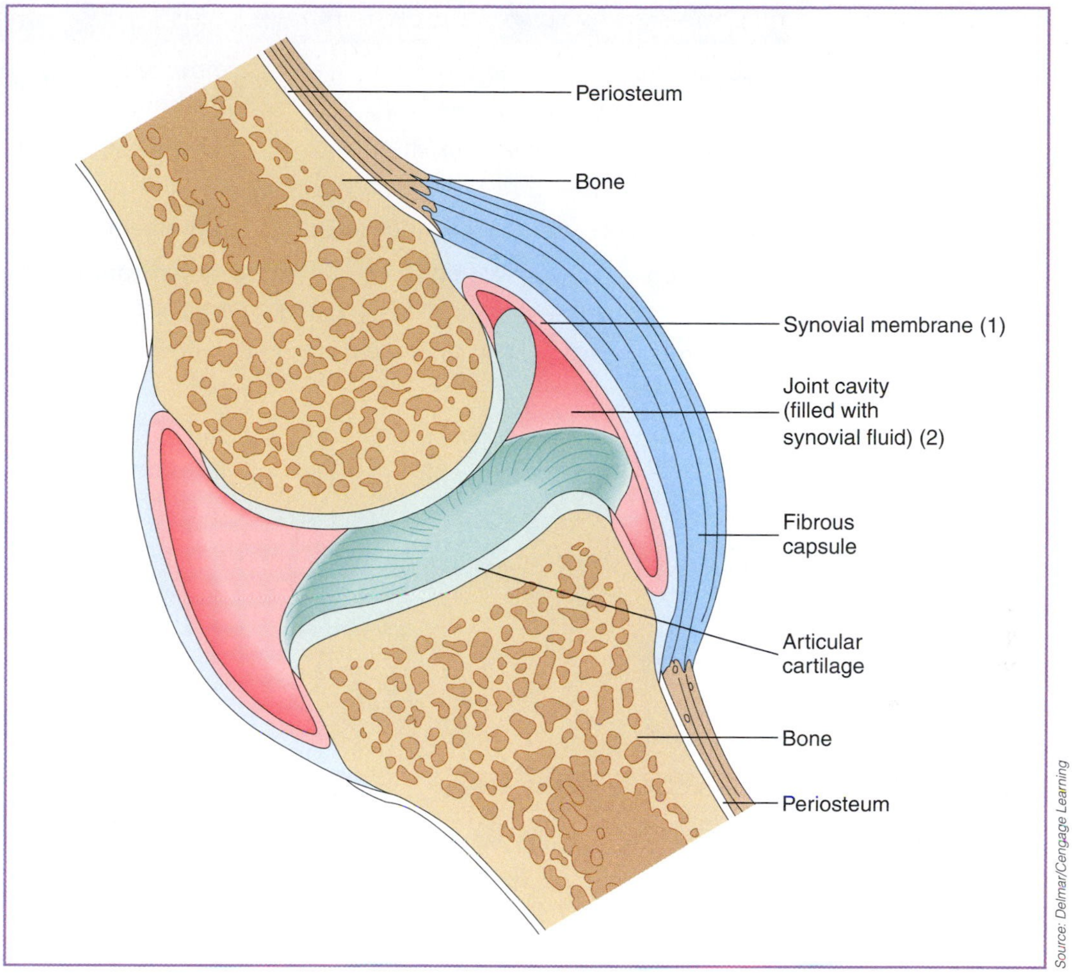

FIGURE 6-6
The Structure of a Synovial Joint

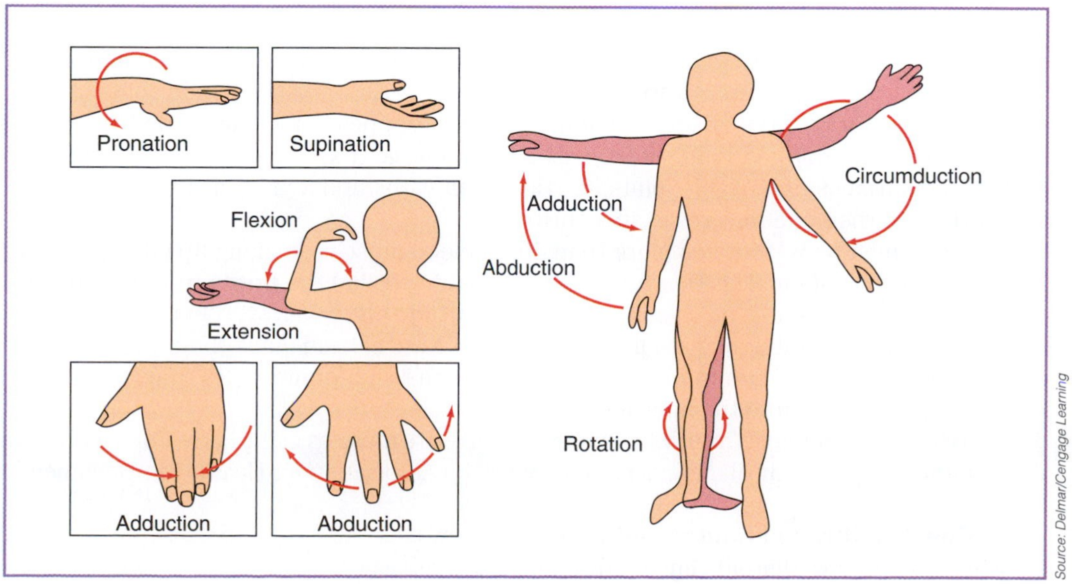

FIGURE 6-7
Movement of Joints

Movement	Pronunciation	Meaning
abduction	ăb-dŭk'shŭn	movement away from the midline of the body
adduction	ah-dŭk'shŭn	movement toward the midline of the body
circumduction	ser'kŭm-dŭk'shŭn	movement in a circular direction
extension	ĕk-stĕn'shŭn	movement that brings the members of a limb into or toward a straight condition
flexion	flĕk'shŭn	act of bending or condition of being bent
pronation	prō-nā'shŭn	turning the hand so that the palm faces downward or backward
rotation	rō-tā'shŭn	motion around a central axis
supination	soo"pĭ-nā'shŭn	turning of the palm or foot upward

MUSCLES

chondr/o	cartilage	spas/o	draw, pull
muscul/o	muscle	tend/o, ten/o, tendin/o	tendon
my/o	muscle	tens/o	stretch
phren/o	diaphragm		

There are three kinds of basic muscle tissue—skeletal, smooth, and cardiac. Skeletal (or striated) muscles may be regarded as organs because they are made of a combination of muscle and connective tissue. These muscles give form and shape to the body and are referred to as **voluntary muscles** because they operate at will. Enveloping and separating the skeletal muscles is a fibrous tissue called **fascia** (făsh'ē-ah). It contains the blood, nerves, and other supplies for muscles. Smooth and cardiac muscles are considered **involuntary muscles** because they generally function without direction from an individual. Examples of involuntary muscles are the muscles that control the digestive tract, blood vessels, and heart (see Figures 6-8A and 6-8B).

Most muscles have two or more attachments to the skeleton. The method of attachment varies. In some cases, the connective tissue within the muscle is attached directly to the periosteum of the bone. These attachments are called **tendons**. If these connective tissues are broad and sheetlike and attached to bone or to other tissue, they are referred to as **aponeurosis** (ăp"ō-nū-rō'sĭs). Muscle may in some instances attach to **cartilage**. Cartilage, a specialized type of dense connective tissue, appears in the adult body in several regions, including the nasal septum, external ear, lining of the eustachian tube, larynx, trachea, bronchi, between bodies of the vertebrae, and on the surfaces of movable joints. Cartilage can withstand a great deal of stress; however, interference with this surface of the bone may result in arthritis.

The human body contains more than 400 skeletal muscles, making up about 40 to 50% of body weight. The one muscle or set of muscles that initiates movement is called the **prime mover**. When an opposite movement is to be made, another set of muscles known as the **antagonist** takes over. In this way, body movements are coordinated, and a large number of complicated movements are carried out without the necessity of planning in advance how to perform them. All muscular activity occurs as a result of messages transmitted from the brain through the central nervous system to the muscles.

To follow are some of the most commonly referred to muscles in the body. For a more comprehensive list, consult *Gray's Anatomy,* a medical dictionary, or contact the Association for Healthcare Documentation Integrity (AHDI).

Muscles of the shoulder and upper extremities
biceps, triceps, deltoid (injection site), pectoralis major

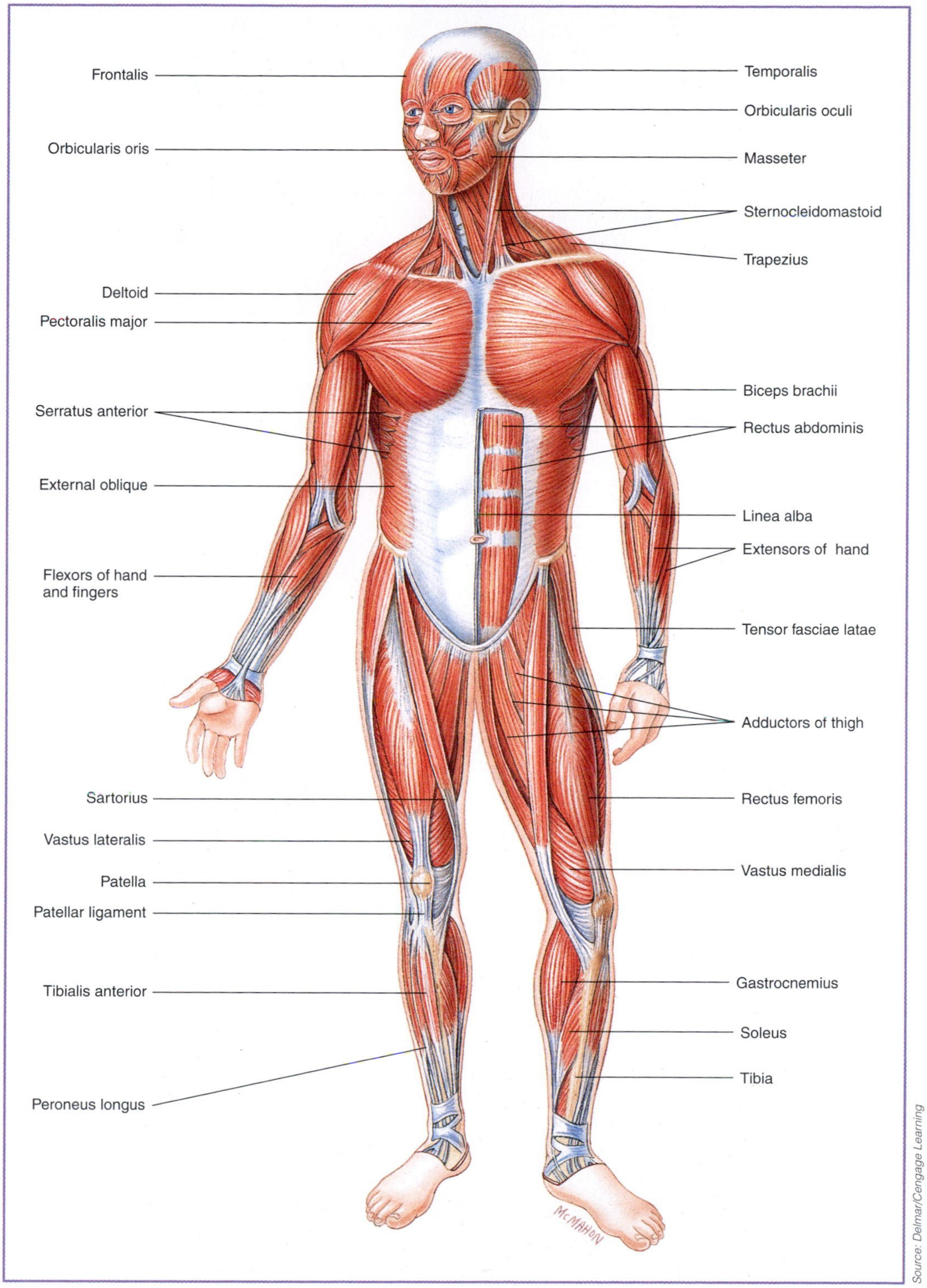

FIGURE 6-8A The Superficial Muscles of the Body (Anterior View)

Muscles of the chest and back
pectoralis major and minor, serratus anterior, intercostal muscles, latissimus dorsi

Muscles of the lower extremities
gluteus maximus (injection site), gluteus medius and minimus, iliopsoas, quadriceps femoris, hamstring group, gastrocnemius, soleus, tibialis anterior and posterior, peroneus brevis and longus

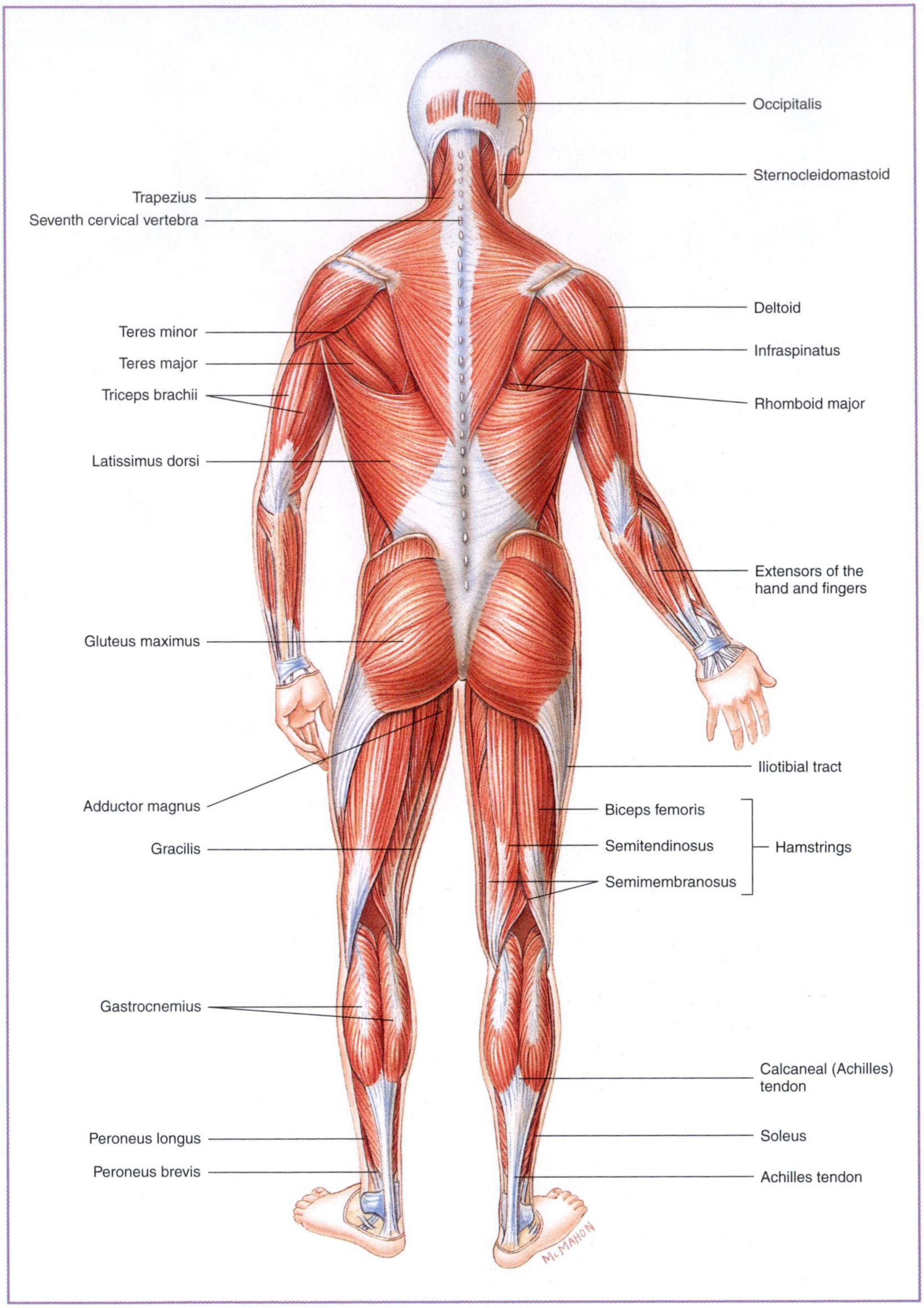

FIGURE 6-8B The Superficial Muscles of the Body (Posterior View)

Source: Delmar/Cengage Learning

Muscles of the abdomen
external and internal oblique, transversus and rectus abdominis

Diaphragm
The diaphragm is an important muscle that divides the thoracic cavity from the abdominal cavity. It has three major openings for the esophagus, aorta, and inferior vena cava, as well as several smaller structures.

When muscles do not function as they should, a disability occurs and a physiatrist may become involved.

THE ROLE OF PHYSICAL MEDICINE

dynam/o	power	therm/o	heat
-plegia	paralysis	traumat/o	wound, injury
therap/o	treatment, therapy		

A **physiatrist** (fĭz"ē-ăt'rĭst) is a physician who specializes in physical medicine and rehabilitation. Skill in applying physical agents is combined with evaluating the patient's mental, social, and vocational problems. Rehabilitation helps a person reach maximum potential for normal living. This practice recognizes that diagnosing the problem is not enough. The critical issue is finding a solution that best benefits the patient.

Disabilities occur because of trauma, such as an accident, a birth defect, a disease, or a cerebrovascular or cerebrocardiovascular accident. Three sources account for most cerebrovascular accidents: thrombosis, embolism, and hemorrhage. Diseases may be of the connective tissue or the nervous system. Trauma may affect the brain or spinal cord, as do several congenital diseases. Sports medicine, a field that deals with injuries related to sports, has evolved from the treatment of trauma and accidents.

Regardless of the type of trauma, a variety of evaluative methods are used to diagnose the nature and degree of disability. Taking the patient's history and examining him or her physically are the first steps.

HISTORY

The physiatrist takes a patient's history using a format similar to that identified in Chapter 3; however, the focus is somewhat different. The first step involves determining the chief complaint. The diseases most likely to produce the complaints a physiatrist addresses usually involve the musculoskeletal, neurological, or cardiovascular system.

Present illness will specify what effect the illness has on self-care activities. The physiatrist wants to know how much the patient depends on others to perform activities of daily living, such as walking, transfer activities, dressing activities, eating skills, and personal hygiene.

Social and vocational history evaluates the patient's environment and provides insight into the patient's psychological makeup.

Review of systems and past medical history contribute to the assessment of residual capacity. Essentially, the physician is looking for the following cardinal signs in each of these systems.

Past medical history attempts to identify residual effects of prior disease or trauma.

System	Pronunciation	Cardinal Signs
cardiovascular	kăr"dē-ō-văs'kū-lăr	dyspnea (dĭsp'nē-ah) or orthopnea (or"thŏp-nē'ă) (types of labored breathing), chest pain, limb claudication (klaw"dĭ-kā'shŭn) (pain from exercise resulting in limping), palpitations
musculoskeletal	mŭs"kū-lō-skĕl'ĕ-tăl	pain, deformity, weakness, limitation of movement, stiffness
nervous		numbness, weakness, fainting, loss of consciousness, dizziness, pain, headache, defective memory or thinking
respiratory	rĕ-spī'rah-tō"rē	cough, sputum, hemoptysis (hē-mŏp'tĭ-sĭs) (spitting up blood), chest pain, dyspnea

PHYSICAL EXAMINATION

A physical examination serves three functions: It searches for deviations from normal, tries to identify secondary problems, and attempts to assess residual strengths. All areas of a traditional examination are covered, with emphasis on the neurological and musculoskeletal areas.

An essential step in the evaluation of function in a patient is measuring joint angle movement or motion, or **goniometry** (gō-"nē-ŏm'ĕ-trē). Methods for recording measurements vary. In addition to the planes and directions indicated in Chapter 2 and the movements illustrated in Figure 6-6, the following directions are used.

Direction	Pronunciation	Meaning
dorsiflexion	dor"sĭ-flĕk'shŭn	backward bending of the hand or foot
opposition		moving the thumb into contact with the pads of the other digits
plantar flexion	plăn'tăr flĕk'shŭn	bending the foot toward the ground

The rehabilitative process includes assessment of speech and language disorders, psychological assessment and management, psychosocial diagnoses, vocational assessment and management, and electrodiagnosis. All help determine realistic goals and the types of therapeutic techniques necessary to achieve those goals. Therapeutic techniques include heat and cold treatment (local), **diathermy** (dī'ah-ther"mē) (deep heating), hydrotherapy, ultraviolet therapy, electrical stimulation, **iontophoresis** (ī-ŏn"tō-fō-rē'sĭs), and exercise.

Physical medicine is a creative practice that utilizes the expertise of people trained in occupational therapy, physical therapy, and speech therapy. A team approach is most effective in providing the various types of therapeutic treatments that will enable an individual to regain as much normalcy as possible.

MASSAGE THERAPY

Massage therapy—the systematic manual treatment of disease—and physical exercise are techniques that have a curative effect on the human condition. The modern day version of these techniques was first used as far back as 3000 B.C. by the Chinese, Hindu, Egyptian, Japanese, Persian, and Turkish cultures. They claim massage therapy can relieve stress and anxiety, increase the blood supply to tissues, hasten the elimination of waste stored in muscles, improve energy level, aid recovery from damaged muscles and ligaments, and relieve certain repetitive motion injuries related to job activities. In the broad perspective, it may provide anything from soothing relaxation to deeper therapy for specific physical problems as well as compensate for the lack of physical activity when an individual must remain sedentary.

The medical profession views massage therapy as an addition or possible alternative to regular medical treatment. Research confirms its benefits. Recent publications such as the *International Journal of Neuroscience* and the *Professional Nurse* have reported the use of compression to treat lymphedema in breast cancer patients and the enhancement of the immune system's cytotoxic capacity in treating cancer or human immunodeficiency virus (HIV)-positive patients.

Integrated approaches such as prenatal therapy, infant therapy, and geriatric therapy have become part of certain practices. But perhaps one of the most widely accepted and used approaches is in sports massage.

Sports massage is based on **osteology** (ŏs-tē-ŏl'ō-jē), the study of the skeleton, and **myology** (mī-ŏl'ō-jē), the study of muscles, their attachments, and the actions they perform. Deep and repetitive compressions of fiber-spreading techniques produce a hyperemia (dilation of the total range of blood vessels). These treatments bring blood and oxygen to the muscles and result in an increase in free motion.

The American Massage Therapy Association has spearheaded a national certification process, and some states have already begun to license massage therapists. Some of the techniques used are listed below.

Technique	Pronunciation	Meaning
compression		use of pressure on the body to spread tissue against underlying structures; may be pinpoint compression (direct pressure) or ischemic pressure (applied at acupressure points)
effleurage	ĕf-loor-ăzh'	use of gliding strokes applied horizontally in relation to tissue masses
friction		use of small deep movements, either circular or transverse, performed on a local area; movements focus directly on underlying tissue
pètrissage	pā"trē-săzh'	use of kneading-like action where soft tissue is lifted, rolled, wrung, and squeezed
rocking		use of rhythmic motion applied with a deliberate full-body movement
shaking		use of quick, loose movements to a body area to relax muscle groups or an entire limb
tapotement	tă-pōt-mŏn'	use of springy blows to the body at a (percussion) fast rate to create rhythmical compression
vibration		use of compression first and then a trembling action; transmits to surrounding tissue to create reflexive response

Other professions that use manipulation techniques described above are chiropractic and osteopathy.

Chiropractic treats disease by manipulating the vertebral column based on the assumption that all diseases are caused by pressure on the nerves. This pressure is the result of faulty alignment of the bones.

Osteopathy is founded on the theory that the body is a single organism made up of interrelated systems dependent upon one another for good health. Practitioners are called Doctors of Osteopathic Medicine (D.O.s) or osteopaths. They treat specific illnesses in the context of the whole person by using generally accepted physical, medicinal, and surgical methods of diagnosis and therapy. The emphasis of this treatment is on the importance of normal body mechanics and manipulative methods to detect and correct faulty structure.

Massage therapy, chiropractic, and osteopathy practitioners each use their knowledge of the musculoskeletal system to help their patients remain healthy and pain free.

INTERNET ASSIGNMENT

The American Academy of Orthopaedic Surgeons (AAOS) is a not-for-profit organization that advocates for improved patient care and informs the public about the science of orthopedics. Members of the Academy are concerned with the diagnosis, care, and treatment of musculoskeletal disorders. The orthopedist's scope of practice includes disorders of the body's bones, joints, ligaments, muscles, and tendons. AAOS's web site is **www.aaos.org**.

On the home page clicking the Patient Information button brings up a picture representation of each component of the musculoskeletal system. A list of links to fact sheets about each system component is presented by clicking on the appropriate picture. For more information, make a selection from the list. The patient information has been reviewed by surgeons to ensure accuracy.

ACTIVITY

Access the AAOS at **www.aaos.org**. On the home page, click Patient Information and then one of the pictures. From the hyperlinks provided, select one that interests you. Summarize your findings in a short report for your instructor, focusing on new information that you learned.

Review *The Musculoskeletal System*

- Bones are made up of one of the hardest materials in the body. They are long, short, flat, or irregular in shape; covered by periosteum; and filled with red and/or yellow marrow.
- The skeleton consists of the axial skeleton (head and trunk) and appendicular skeleton (upper and lower extremities).
- Contours on the bones, called processes and depressions, provide places for muscle attachments that join one bone to another.
- A joint, or articulation, is where two or more bones join. Some joints are movable; others are not.
- Skeletal muscles are voluntary muscles. They give shape to the body and are regarded as organs.
- Smooth and cardiac muscles are involuntary muscles and function without direction from the individual.
- Muscles are attached to the bone with tendons or connective tissue called aponeurosis.
- The physiatrist, a physician specializing in physical medicine, diagnoses problems with special attention to the residual effects on the mental, social, and vocational aspects of a patient's life.
- Massage therapists, chiropractors, and osteopaths are some of the professionals who use knowledge of the musculoskeletal system in helping individuals to be healthy and pain free.

Key Terminology Review

Word	Definition
antagonist	muscle that opposes movement initiated by a prime mover muscle
aponeurosis	broad, sheetlike connective tissue that attaches muscles to bone or other tissue
appendicular	skeleton bony framework of the extremities
axial skeleton	bony framework of the head and trunk
bursa	saclike structure surrounding certain bony processes to prevent friction
cancellous (spongy) bone	soft, spongy material found in the interior of bone
cartilage	specialized type of dense connective tissue
chiropractic	system of treating disease by manipulating the vertebral column
compact (cortical) bone	hard material forming the exterior of bone
depressions	openings or hollow regions that help to join one bone to another

continues

Word	Definition
diarthrosis *pl.* diarthroses	freely movable joint lined with synovial membrane that secretes synovial fluid
diathermy	deep heating
fascia	fibrous tissue separating and enveloping muscles
fixed joints	joints that have little or no movement
goniometry	measurement of joint movement or angle
involuntary muscles	smooth and cardiac muscles that move without conscious thought
iontophoresis	process of transferring ions of the body by an electromotive force
joint	region where two or more bones join
ligaments	connective tissue bands that add stability to joints
massage therapy	systematic, therapeutic manual treatment of disease
myology	study of the muscles and their parts
orthopedic surgery	surgical correction of deformities, traumas, and chronic diseases of bones and joints
osseous	referring to bone; bony
osteology	study of the structure and function of bones
osteopathy	treatment based on the importance of normal body mechanics and manipulative methods to detect and correct faulty structure; *literally means* any bone disease
periosteum	membrane covering the outside of most bones
physiatrist	physician specializing in physical medicine and rehabilitation
physical medicine	treatment of illnesses by clinical use of physical agents such as heat and water
prime mover	muscle that initiates a movement
process	projection on bones for muscle attachments
red bone marrow	soft, organic material found in spaces within the spongy bone; source of red blood cells
rheumatology	study of diseases of the joints
rib cage	24 bones attached to the vertebral column and sternum; supports chest and protects heart, lungs, and other organs
skull	framework of the head
spinal column	structure that protects the spinal cord and allows humans to stand upright
sports medicine and exercise science	diagnosis, treatment, and prevention of sports-related injuries
sternum	breastbone
synovial membrane	inner layer of a movable joint that secretes lubricating synovial fluid
tendons	connective tissues within muscles that attach directly to the periosteum of bones
voluntary muscles	skeletal (or striated) muscles; operate at will
yellow bone marrow	soft organic material found in central cavities of long bones; composed chiefly of fat cells

Key Terminology Practice Exercises

COMPLETION

Complete the following statements.

1. The systematic therapeutic manual treatment of disease is referred to as ______________________.
2. Projections of the bones that often serve as places for muscle attachment are called ______________________.
3. Bones are made of tissue ______________________.
4. The two kinds of bone are ______________________ and ______________________.
5. Most bones are covered by a membrane called ______________________.
6. A physician would identify the fifth lumbar vertebra as ______________________.
7. A physician who specializes in physical rehabilitation is a ______________________.
8. The five regions of the spinal column are the ______________________, ______________________, ______________________, ______________________, and ______________________.
9. Muscles make up from ______________________ to ______________________ percent of body weight.
10. The measurement of joint angle or movement is ______________________.
11. Hollow regions that help to join one bone to another are called ______________________.
12. The bone framework of the head and trunk is the ______________________ skeleton; the upper and lower extremities are known as the ______________________ skeleton.
13. The framework of the head is called the ______________________; the framework of the trunk includes the ______________________ and the ______________________.
14. Ribs are attached to ______________________ or breastbone in front
15. The region where two or more bones join is a ______________________ or articulation.
16. Freely movable joints are called ________________; they are lined with ______________________ membrane.
17. Connective tissue bands that give joints stability are ______________________; some of these have a sac-like structure surrounding them, called ______________________.
18. ______________________ muscles, operating at will, are covered with fibrous tissue called ______________________.
19. Attachment of connective tissue within a muscle directly to periosteum of bone are called ________________; broad sheets attaching to bone or other tissue are called ______________________.
20. A dense, specialized type of connective tissue, found in nasal septum, is called ______________________.

CHOICES

Circle the correct answer in each statement.

1. (Red marrow/yellow marrow) is composed chiefly of fat cells.
2. The (axial skeleton/appendicular skeleton) is composed of the extremities.
3. A (joint/bursa) is the region where two or more bones come together.
4. A (tendon/ligament) is connective tissue within a muscle that attaches directly to the periosteum of the bone.
5. (Synovial membrane/bursa) is the lining that secretes lubrication for movable joints.
6. (Cartilage/ligaments) are connective tissue bands that add stability to joints.

MATCHING

Match the terms to their meanings.

1.	________ motion around a central axis	a.	abduction
2.	________ motion away from the body	b.	adduction
3.	________ motion toward the body	c.	antagonist
4.	________ straightening or stretching	d.	diathermy
5.	________ bending motion	e.	dorsiflexion
6.	________ backward bending of the hand or foot	f.	extension
7.	________ moving the thumb toward the digit pads	g.	flexion
8.	________ bending the foot toward the ground	h.	iontophoresis
9.	________ muscle that initiates a movement	i.	myology
10.	________ muscle that opposes an initiated movement	j.	opposition
11.	________ deep heating	k.	osteology
12.	________ transferring ions of body by electromotive force	l.	plantar flexion
13.	________ study of structure and function of bones	m.	prime mover
14.	________ study of muscles and their parts	n.	rotation

Word Element Review

Root	Meaning	Example	Definition
arthr/o	joint	**arthrocentesis** (ăr"thrō-sĕn-tē'sĭs)	puncture of a joint with a needle to remove fluid
articul/o	joint	**articular** (ăr-tĭk'ū-lăr)	pertaining to a joint
burs/o	sac	**bursitis** (bĕr-sī'tĭs)	inflammation of a bursa (fluid-filled sac)
carp/o	wrist	**carpal** (kăr'păl)	pertaining to the wrist
caud/o	tail	**caudal** (kaw'dăl)	pertaining to a tail-like structure; inferior position
cephal/o	head	**cephalic** (sĕ-făl'ĭk)	pertaining to the head
cervic/o	neck	**cervical** (sĕr'vĭ-kĭl)	pertaining to the neck

continues

Root	Meaning	Example	Definition
cheir/o, chir/o	hand	**cheirospasm** (kī'rō-spăsm) **chirospasm** (kī'rō-spăzm)	spasm of the muscles of the hand; writer's cramp (Note the similar pronunciation and meaning of these two terms but the different spellings.)
chondr/o	cartilage	**chondrocostal** (kŏn'drō-kŏs'tăl)	pertaining to the ribs and costal cartilages
cleid/o	clavicle	**sternocleidomastoid** (ster"nō-klī"dō-măs'toid)	one of two muscles arising from the sternum and inner part of the clavicle
cost/o	rib	**intercostal** (ĭn"ter-kŏs'tăl)	between the ribs
crani/o	skull, head	**cranial** (krā'nē-ăl)	pertaining to the skull and head
dactyl/o	finger, toe	**dactylitis** (dăk"tĭ-lī'tis)	inflammation of a finger or toe in very young children
digit/o	finger, toe	**digital** (dĭj'ĭ-tăl)	pertaining to or resembling a finger or toe
ili/o	ilium	**iliac** (ĭl'ē-ăk)	referring to the ilium
ischi/o	hip	**ischium** (ĭs'kē-ŭm)	lower portion of the hip bone
ligament/o	ligament	**ligamentous** (lĭg"-ah-men'tăs)	pertaining to or of the nature of a ligament
lumb/o	loin, lower back	**lumbago** (lŭm-bā'gō)	nonspecific term for a dull, aching pain in the lumbar region of the back
maxill/o	upper jaw bone	**maxilla** (măk-sĭl'ah)	upper jaw bone
muscul/o	muscle	**musculoskeletal** (mŭs'kū-lō-skĕl'ĕ-tăl)	pertaining to the muscles and skeleton
my/o		**myocarditis** (mī"ō-kăr-dī'tĭs)	muscle inflammation of the middle layer of the heart wall
oste/o	bone	**osteoarthritis** (ŏs"tē-ō-ăr-thrī'tĭs)	chronic disease involving the joints
ped/o, pod/o	foot	**podiatry** (pŏ-dī'ah-trē)	specialized field dealing with the study and care of the foot
phren/o	diaphragm	**phrenic nerve** (frĕn'ik)	nerve to the diaphragm
sacr/o	sacrum	**sacroiliac** (sā"krō-ĭl'ē-ăk)	pertaining to the sacrum and ilium
spas/o	draw, pull	**spasticity** (spăs-tĭs'ĭ-tē)	state of increased muscle tone over the normal

continues

Root	Meaning	Example	Definition
spondyl/o	vertebra	**spondylolysis** (spŏn"dĭ-lŏl'ĭ-sĭs)	degenerative changes in the spine
synov/o	synovial membrane	**synovitis** (sĭn-ō-vī'tĭs)	inflammation of the synovial membrane, especially that of a joint
tars/o	foot	**tarsus** (tahr'sŭs)	ankle
tend/o, ten/o, tendin/o	tendon	**tendinitis** (tĕn"dĭ-nī'tŭs) (preferred spelling) **tendonitis** (tĕn"dō-nī'tĭs)	inflammation of a tendon
		tenorrhaphy (tĕn-or'ah-fē)	suturing of a tendon
tens/o	stretch	**tensor** (tĕn'sor)	any muscle that makes a body part tense
vertebr/o	vertebra	**vertebral column** (vĕr'tē-brăl)	spinal column
Physical Medicine			
dynam/o	power	**dynamometer** (dī"nah-mŏm'ĕ-ter)	an instrument for measuring muscular strength
therap/o	treatment,	**physical therapist** (thĕr'a-pĭst)	a person skilled in the treatment of diseases or disorders using physical agents such as massage, heat, hydrotherapy (water), radiation, electricity, and exercise
therm/o	heat	**thermotherapy** (ther"mō-thĕr'ah-pē)	therapeutic application of heat
traumat/o	wound, injury	**traumatic** (traw-măt'ĭk)	pertaining to or resulting from a wound or an injury (trauma)
-paresis	partial paralysis	**hemiparesis** (hĕm"ē-păr'ĕ-sĭs)	paralysis of one arm and one leg on either side of the body
-plegia	paralysis	**paraplegia** (păr"ah-plē'jē-ah)	paralysis of the lower part of the body
		quadriplegia (kwŏd"rĭ-plē'jē-ah)	paralysis of all four limbs
-spasm	twitching, contraction of muscles	**cheirospasm** (kī'rō-spăsm)	writer's cramp; spasm of the muscles of the hand

Word Element Practice Exercises

WORD ELEMENTS

Name the word elements that refer to the following parts.

1. head ______________________
2. hand ______________________
3. foot ______________________
4. back ______________________

MATCHING

Match the word elements to their meanings.

1. ________ clavicle		a. arthr/o
2. ________ muscle		b. burs/o
3. ________ sac		c. cleid/o
4. ________ ilium		d. cost/o
5. ________ diaphragm		e. ili/o
6. ________ bone		f. ischi/o
7. ________ rib		g. maxill/o
8. ________ joint		h. muscul/o, my/o
9. ________ hip		i. oste/o
10. ________ upper jawbone		j. phren/o

PRONUNCIATION AND DEFINITION

Provide the pronunciation and definition for the following terms.

1. intercostal ______________________

____

2. arthrocentesis ______________________

____

3. bursitis ______________________

____

4. myocarditis ______________________

____

5. osteoarthritis ______________________

____

6. spondylolysis ______________________

____

7. tensor ______________________

____

MATCHING

Match the terms to their meanings.

1. __________	paralysis of the lower limbs	a. articular
2. __________	person skilled in the treatment of diseases and disorders either with or using physical agents	b. carpal
3. __________	instrument for measuring muscular strength	c. caudal
4. __________	pertaining to the wrist	d. cervical
5. __________	upper jaw bone	e. chirospasm
6. __________	pertaining to or resulting from a wound or injury	f. chondrocostal
7. __________	any muscle that makes a body part tense	g. dynamometer
8. __________	specialized field studying the foot	h. ischium
9. __________	pertaining to a ligament	i. ligamentous
10. __________	pertaining to a joint	j. maxilla
11. __________	pertaining to the neck	k. paraplegia
12. __________	state of increased muscle tone over the normal	l. phrenic
13. __________	therapeutic application of heat	m. physical therapist
14. __________	writer's cramp	n. podiatry
15. __________	pertaining to ribs and costal cartilages	o. spasticity
16. __________	ankle	p. tarsus
17. __________	nerve to diaphragm	q. tendonitis
18. __________	pertaining to tail-like structure	r. tensor
19. __________	lower portion of hip bone	s. thermotherapy
20. __________	inflammation of a tendon	t. traumatic

WORD ELEMENT MEANINGS

Give the meaning of each word element. Then use your dictionary to find a new word that contains each of the word elements. Specify whether the new word is a noun or an adjective by placing N or A in the last column.

Word Element	Meaning	Word	N or A
1. arthr/o	__________	__________	______
2. articul/o	__________	__________	______
3. burs/o	__________	__________	______
4. carp/o	__________	__________	______
5. caud/o	__________	__________	______
6. cephal/o	__________	__________	______
7. cervic/o	__________	__________	______
8. cheir/o	__________	__________	______
9. chir/o	__________	__________	______
10. chondr/o	__________	__________	______
11. cleid/o	__________	__________	______

Word Element	Meaning	Word	N or A
12. cost/o			
13. crani/o			
14. dactyl/o			
15. digit/o			
16. dynam/o			
17. ili/o			
18. ischi/o			
19. ligament/o			
20. lumb/o			
21. maxill/o			
22. muscul/o			
23. my/o			
24. oste/o			
25. -paresis			
26. ped/o			
27. phren/o			
28. -plegia			
29. pod/o			
30. sacr/o			
31. -spasm			
32. spas/o			
33. spondyl/o			
34. synov/o			
35. tars/o			
36. tend/o			
37. ten/o			
38. tendin/o			
39. tens/o			
40. therap/o			
41. therm/o			
42. traumat/o			
43. vertebr/o			

DIAGNOSTIC PROCEDURES		
Word	**Pronunciation**	**Definition**
General Tests		
arthrocentesis (synovial fluid space for analysis studies)	ăr"thrō-sĕn-tē'sĭs	synovial fluid is removed with a needle from a joint
arthroscopy	ăr-thrŏs'kō-pē	examination of the interior of a joint by entering the joint with an arthroscope (a fiber-optic camera) (See Figure 6-9)
Bone marrow aspiration	ăs-pĭ-rā'shŭn	use of a needle to remove a small sample of bone marrow for examination
electromyography	ē-lĕk"trō-mī-ŏg'rah-fē	recording and studying the strength of a muscle contraction as a result of electrical stimulation
muscle biopsy	bī'ŏp-sē	removal of muscle tissue for pathological examination
Nuclear Medicine		
bone scan		scan that measures uptake of a radioactive phosphate substance that is injected intravenously
Dual photon absorptiometry	ăb-sŏrp"shē-ŏm'ĕ-trē	noninvasive procedure that beams a minimal amount of radiation through the bones
indium 111WBC scan (^{111}indium)	ĭn'dē-ŭm	scan for infection or abscess by tagging white blood cells
gallium scan	găl'ē-ŭm	scan that tracks white cells (infection)
Radiology		
arthrography	ăr-thrŏg'rah-fē	study of the joints after injection of an opaque contrast material
computerized axial tomography (CAT, CT)	tō-mŏg'rah-fē	computer-assisted x-ray technique used to distinguish pathological conditions such as tumors and fractures
diskography	dĭs-kŏg'rah-fē	x-ray of the spine to study the intervertebral disks

continues

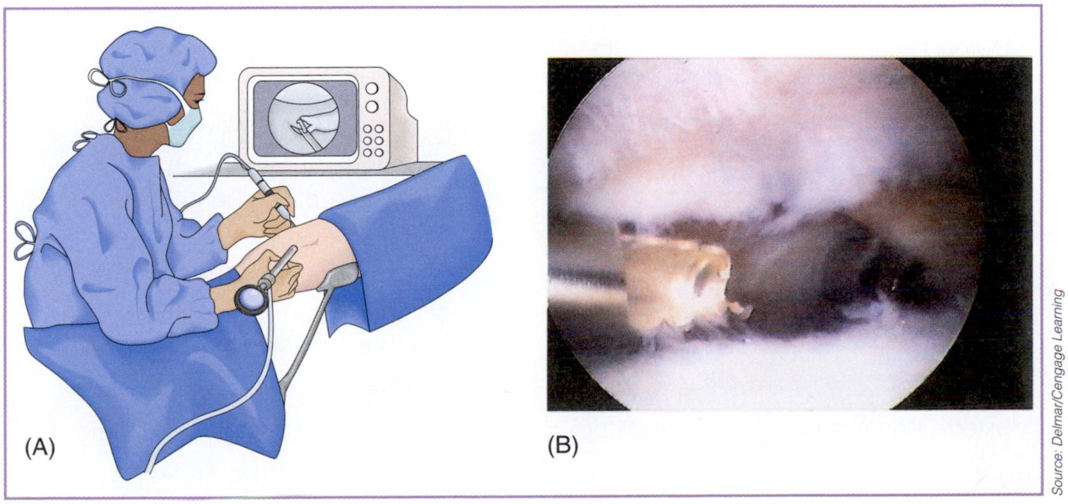

FIGURE 6-9 Arthroscopy of the Knee: (A) arthroscope in use; (B) internal view of the knee during arthroscopy

DIAGNOSTIC PROCEDURES		
Word	**Pronunciation**	**Definition**
Radiology *(continued)*		
dual energy x-ray absorptiometry (DEXA)	ăb-zorp"shē-ŏm'ĕ-trē	noninvasive procedure that measures bone density by generating energy protons that pass through the bones
magnetic resonance imaging (MRI)		production of detailed pictures of internal structures, using combination of computers and magnetism, for diagnostic purposes without invasive surgical procedures
myelography	mī"ĕ-lŏg'rah-fē	study of the spinal column after injection of opaque contrast material
skeletal survey		x-ray overview of the entire skeleton
Blood Tests		
antinuclear antibody (ANA)	ăn"tĭ-nū'klē-ăr ăn'tĭ-bŏd"ē	test for autoimmune disorders such as lupus erythematosus (LE) which can cause inflammatory arthritis
C-reactive protein	prō'tēn	test that indicates an inflammatory process in the body
erythrocyte sedimentation rate	ĕ-rĭth'rō-sīt	measurement of the rate that erythrocytes settle out of solution when an anticoagulant is added; elevation indicates an inflammatory process
lupus erythematosus	loo'pŭs ĕr"ĭ-thĕm" ah-tō'sŭs	test for lupus erythematosus, a cutaneous or cell test connective tissue disease
rheumatoid factor	roo'mă-toyd	blood test that measures the presence of antibodies that develop in a number of connective tissue diseases
serum calcium s (Ca)	sērŭm kăl'sē-ŭm	measurement of the amount of calcium in the blood
serum creatine kinase (CK)	sērŭm krē-ah-tĭn kī'nās	measurement of the amount of creatine kinase present in the blood
serum phosphorus (P)	sērŭm fŏs'fŏ-rŭs	measurement of the amount of phosphorus in the blood
uric acid	ū'rĭk	measurement of the amount of uric acid in the blood
Diseases of Bone		
bunion	bŭn'yŭn	inflammation and thickening of first metatarsal joint of the great toe associated with metatarsal joint deformity; sometimes called hallux valgus
Ewing sarcoma	ū'ĭng săr-kō'mah	second most common malignant bone tumor in patients 5-30 years old
exotosis	ēk"sō-tō'sĭs	benign new growth projecting from a bone surface
kyphosis	kī-fō'sĭs	improper posture characterized by shoulders that roll forward (See Figure 6-10B)
lordosis	lŏr-dō'sĭs	improper posture characterized by forward curvature of the lumbar spine; swayback (See Figure 6-10C)
multiple myeloma	mī-ĕ-lō'mah	malignant disease characterized by infiltration of the bone and bone marrow by neoplastic plasma cells
myeloma	mī-ĕ-lō'mah	tumor originating in the bone marrow
osteochondroma	ŏs"tē-ō-kŏn-drō'mă	common benign bone tumor

continues

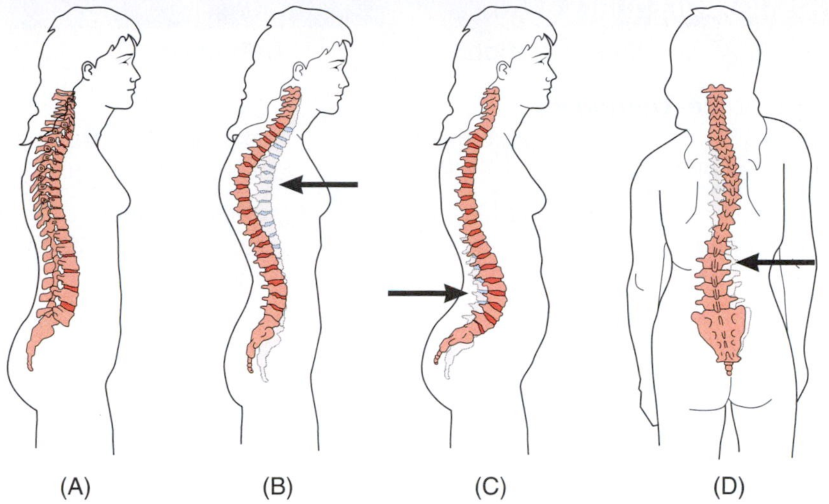

FIGURE 6-10
Common Forms of Improper Posture: (A) normal; (B) kyphosis, in which shoulder rolls forward; (C) lordosis, swaybacked posture; (D) scoliosis, a sideways curvature of the spine

DIAGNOSTIC PROCEDURES		
Word	Pronunciation	Definition
Diseases of Bone *(continued)*		
osteomalacia	ŏs"tē-ō-mah-lā'shē-ah	condition marked by softening of the bones as a result of calcium loss from the bones
osteomyelitis	ŏs"tē-ō-mī"ĕ-lī'tĭs	inflammation of bone and bone marrow due to infection
osteoporosis	ŏs"tē-ō-pō-rō'sĭs	condition caused by decrease in bone mass resulting in thinning and weakening of bone (See Figure 6-11)

continues

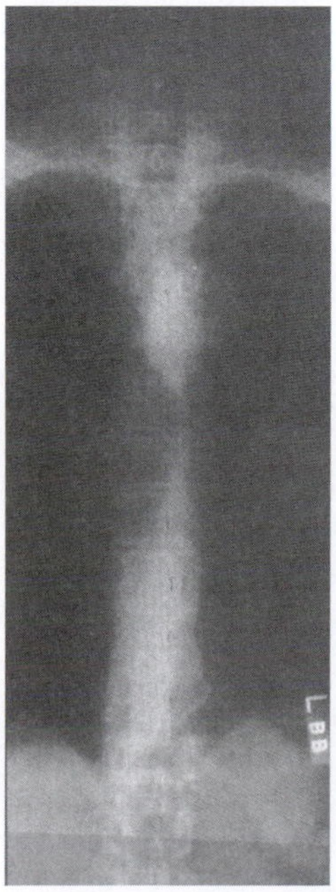

FIGURE 6-11
Fracture of the Thoracic Spine caused by Osteoporosis

DIAGNOSTIC PROCEDURES		
Word	**Pronunciation**	**Definition**
Diseases of Bone *(continued)*		
osteosarcoma (osteogenic sarcoma)	ŏs"tē-ō-săr-kō'mah (ŏs"tē-ō-jĕn'ĭk)	malignant cancer of the bone; typically afflicts adolescents
Paget's disease (osteitis deformans)	păj'ĕt (ŏs-tē-ī'tĭs dĕ-fŏr'mănz)	chronic metabolic bone disease in older persons that affects bone formation because of increased bone turnover
scoliosis	skō"lē-ō'sĭs	abnormal rotational and lateral curvature of the spine (See Figure 6-10D)
spondylosis	spŏn"dĭ-lō'sĭs	disorder in which the spine becomes stiff and loses flexibility over time
talipes	tăl'ĭ-pēz	congenital deformity of the foot; clubfoot
Diseases of Joints, Muscles, and Connective Tissue		
Arthritis	ăr-thrī'tĭs	inflammation of bone joints; may be ankylosing spondylitis, gout, osteoarthritis, and rheumatoid arthritis
• *ankylosing* • *spondylitis*		affects the vertebral column and causes deformities of the spine
• *gout*		inflammation of joints caused by excessive uric acid in the body
• *osteoarthritis (degenerative arthritis)*		chronic, non-inflammatory, degenerative disease of bone and joints due to degenerative changes in cartilage (See Figure 6-12A)
• *rheumatoid arthritis*		condition marked by the inflammation of a joint, as well as stiffness (See Figure 6-12B)

continues

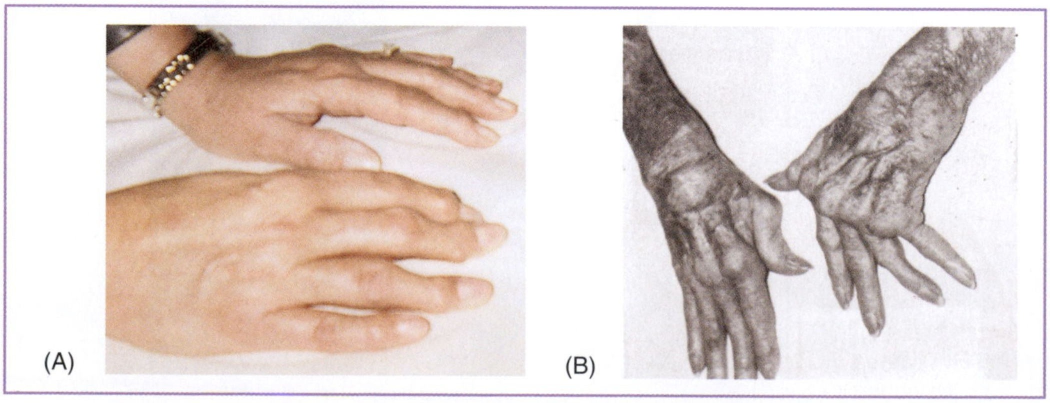

FIGURE 6-12 Comparison (A) Osteoarthritis; (B) Rheumatoid Arthritis: hands and joints

DIAGNOSTIC PROCEDURES		
Word	**Pronunciation**	**Definition**
Diseases of Joints, Muscles, and Connective Tissue *(continued)*		
Dupuytren's contracture	dū-pwē-trănz' kōn-trăk'chūr	disorder characterized by a hardening of the lining of tissue beneath skin of the palm of the hand
fibromyalgia	fī"brō-mī-ă'jē-ah	chronic disorder characterized by aches, pain, and stiffness in joints and muscles
ganglion cyst	găng'glē-ŏn	cystic lump on the wrist and other areas (See Figure 6-13)
hallux valgus	hăl'ŭks văl'gŭs	deformation of the great toe metatarsophalangeal (MTP) joint with abduction of the phalanges; often referred to as a bunion (See Figure 6-14)
Lyme disease	līm	acute, recurrent inflammatory infection transmitted by the bite of an infected deer tick
muscular dystrophy (MD)	dĭs'trō-fē	inherited disease characterized by a progressive weakness of muscle fibers
myasthenia gravis	mī"ăs-thē'nē-ah grăv'ĭs	disorder marked by lack of muscle strength or even paralysis
polymyositis	pŏl"ē-mī"ō-sī'tĭs	chronic progressive disease of muscles characterized by muscle weakness and atrophy; relatively uncommon
systemic lupus erythematosus (SLE)	sĭstĕm'ĭk lū'pŭs ĕr"ĭ-thĕm"ah-tō'sŭs	chronic, autoimmune, inflammatory disease involving the joints, skin, kidneys, nervous system, heart, and lungs
temporomandibular joint (TMJ) syndrome	tĕm"pō-rō-măn-dĭb'ū-lăr	condition characterized by severe headaches and pain in the jaw joint with decreased ability to open the mouth
tetanus	tĕt'ă-nŭs	acute infectious, life-threatening disease characterized by painful, uncontrolled contractions of skeletal muscle; lockjaw
Trauma		
bursitis	bĕr-sī'tĭs	inflammation of the bursa, often caused by repetitive motions

continues

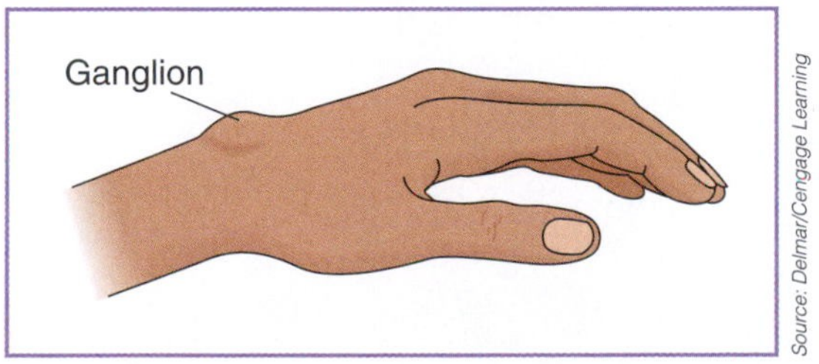

FIGURE 6-13 Ganglion

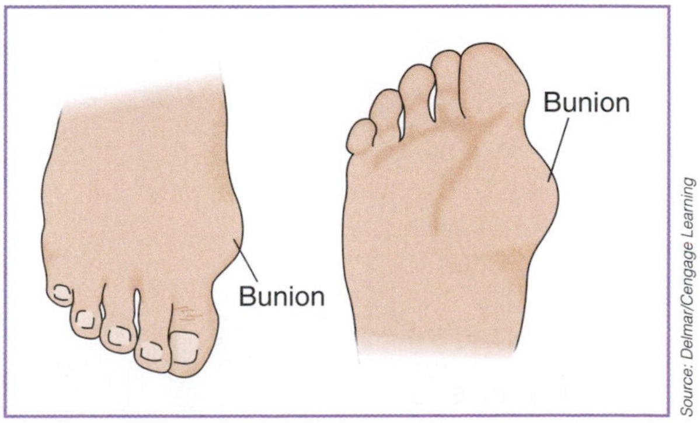

FIGURE 6-14 Bunion or hallux valgus

DIAGNOSTIC PROCEDURES		
Word	Pronunciation	Definition
Trauma *(continued)*		
carpal tunnel syndrome	kăr'păl	compression of the nerve as it passes between the bones and tendons of the wrist, often caused by repetitive motions
cruciate ligament tear	kroo'shē-āt	torn ligament, most commonly in the knee; usually associated with athletic injury (see Figure 6-16)
dislocation		disruption of ligaments allowing joints to separate (see Figure 6-15)
fractures		sudden breaking of a bone; terms describing fractures and related injuries
• *closed (simple)*		bone is broken, but there is no open wound in the skin (See Figure 6-17B)
• *Colles' fracture*		fracture that is at the lower end of the radius, within 1 inch of the wrist bones (See Figure 6-18)
• *comminuted*		bone is broken into more than two pieces (See Figure 6-17E)
• *compression fracture*		caused by bone surfaces being forced against each other with loss of height (See Figure 6-19)
• *greenstick (incomplete)*		bone is partially bent and broken (See Figure 6-17A)
• *hairline*		stress fracture; appears as a very thin hairline between two segments of bone
• *impacted*		bone is broken and one end is wedged into the fracture surface of the other (See Figure 6-17D)
• *open (compound)*		bone is broken with an open wound in the skin (See Figure 6-17C)
• *pathological*		bone break because of a preexisting weakness or defect
herniated nucleus pulposus (HNP)	hĕr-nē-ā'tĕd nŭ'klē-ŭs pŭl-pō'sŭs	herniated disc; ruptured disc (See Figure 6-20)

continues

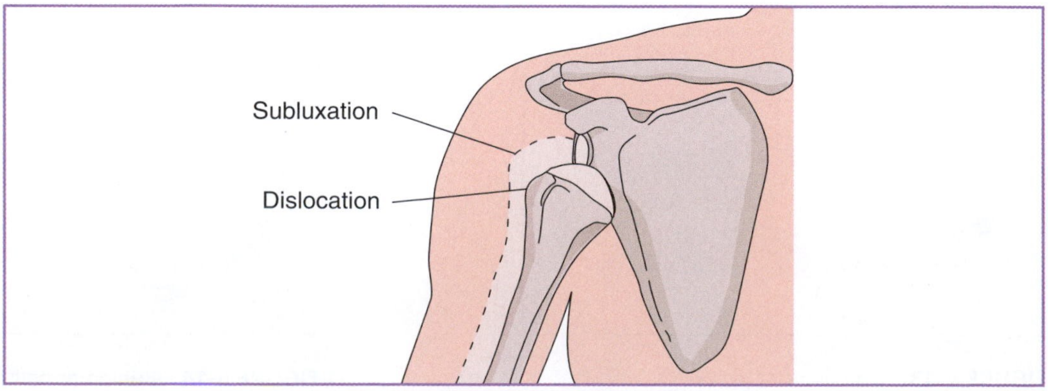

FIGURE 6-15
Dislocation and Subluxation

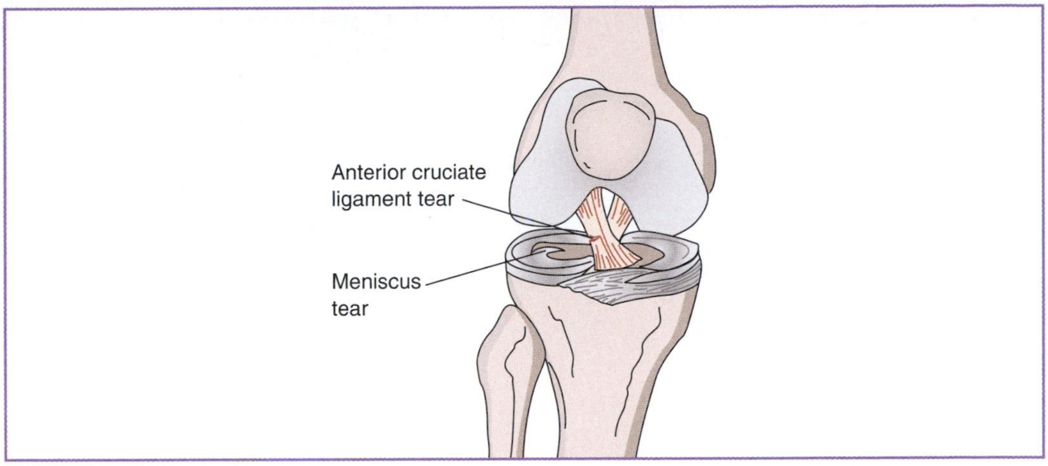

FIGURE 6-16 Meniscus and Anterior Cruciate Ligament Tear

DIAGNOSTIC PROCEDURES		
Word	Pronunciation	Definition
Trauma *(continued)*		
low back pain		common disorder of the lumbar area of the spine that may be acute or chronic
plantar fasciitis	plăn'tăr făs"ē-ī'tĭs	inflammation of the thick connective tissue and the sole of the foot
shin splint		overuse injury to the periosteum and extensor muscle attachments to the lower leg
sprain		traumatic injury to a joint with partial or complete tearing of ligaments
strain		overstretching injury of a muscle leading to tenderness, soreness, and pain
subluxation	sŭb"lŭks-ā'shŭn	a partial separation of a bone from its normal position in a joint (See Figure 6-15)
tendonitis	tĕn"dah-nī'tĭs	inflammation of a tendon, often in the shoulder

continues

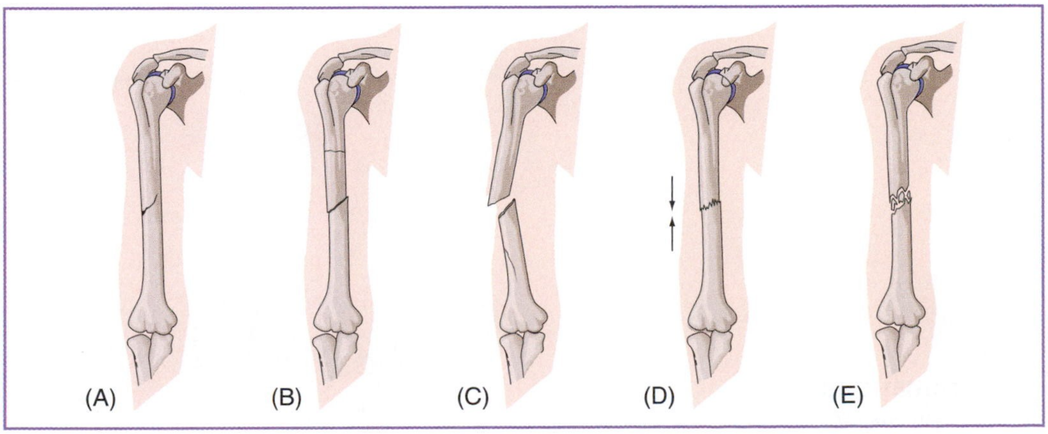

FIGURE 6-17 Types of Fractures: (A) greenstick (incomplete); (B) closed (simple, complete); (C) open (compound); (D) impacted; (E) comminuted

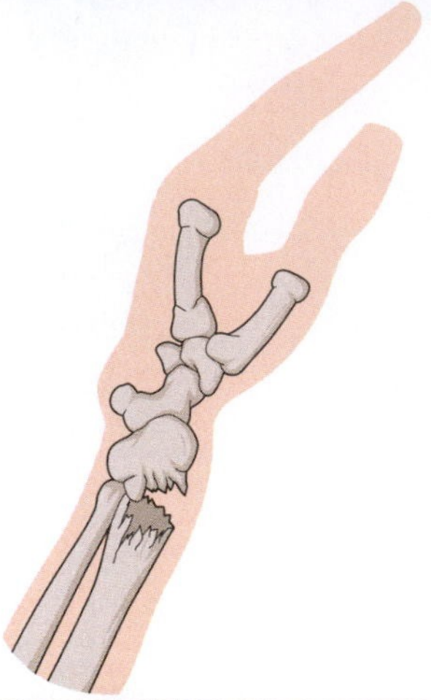

FIGURE 6-18
Colles' Fracture

DIAGNOSTIC PROCEDURES

Word	Pronunciation	Definition
Trauma *(continued)*		
torn rotator cuff		injury to the tendinous portion of a group of muscles that hold the head of the humerus in the shoulder socket area
torn meniscus	mĕn-ĭs'kŭs	injury to cartilage pads that are in the knee

TREATMENT PROCEDURES

Word	Pronunciation	Definition
anterior cruciate ligament (ACL) reconstruction	ăn-tēr'ē-or kroo'shē-āt	replacement of a torn ACL with a biological graft; usually done by arthroscopic surgery
arthrodesis	ăr"thrō-dē'sĭs	fusion of a joint with loss of motion to provide stability; sometimes done for pain from arthritis
arthroplasty	ăr'thrō-plăs"tē	surgical reconstruction of a joint
arthroscopy	ăr'thrŏ-skō"pē	surgical procedures performed on joints with an arthroscope (a fiber-optic camera) (See Figure 6-9)
arthrotomy	ăr"thrŏt'ō-mē	surgical opening of a joint

continues

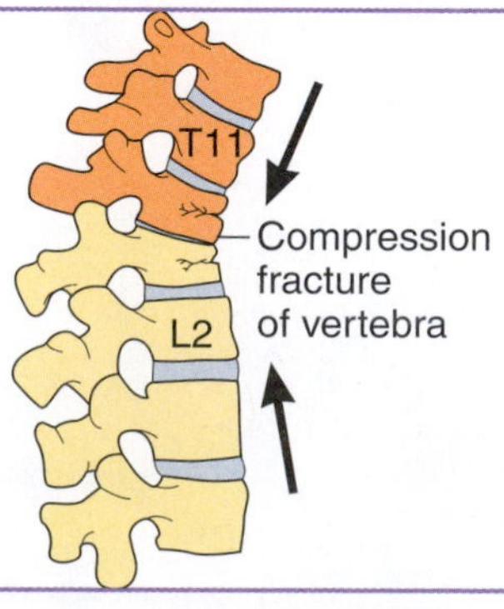

FIGURE 6-19
Compression Fracture

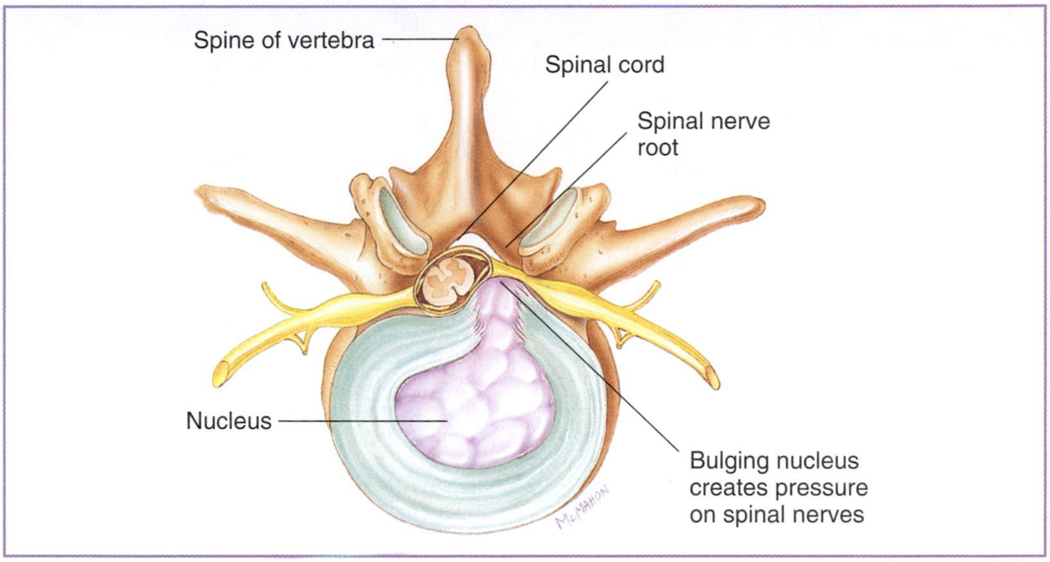

FIGURE 6-20
Herniated Nucleus Pulposus

TREATMENT PROCEDURES

Word	Pronunciation	Definition
bunionectomy	bŭn-yŭn-ĕk'tō-mē	removal of the bursa and bone deformity of the great toe
capsulorrhaphy	kăp"sū-lor'ah-fē	suture of a tear in any joint capsule
carpal tunnel release	kăr'păl	cutting the wrist ligament to relieve nerve pressure (See Figure 6-21)
chondroplasty	kŏn'drō-plăs"tē	shaving or smoothing of rough or fragmented articular cartilage; done by arthroscopic surgery

continues

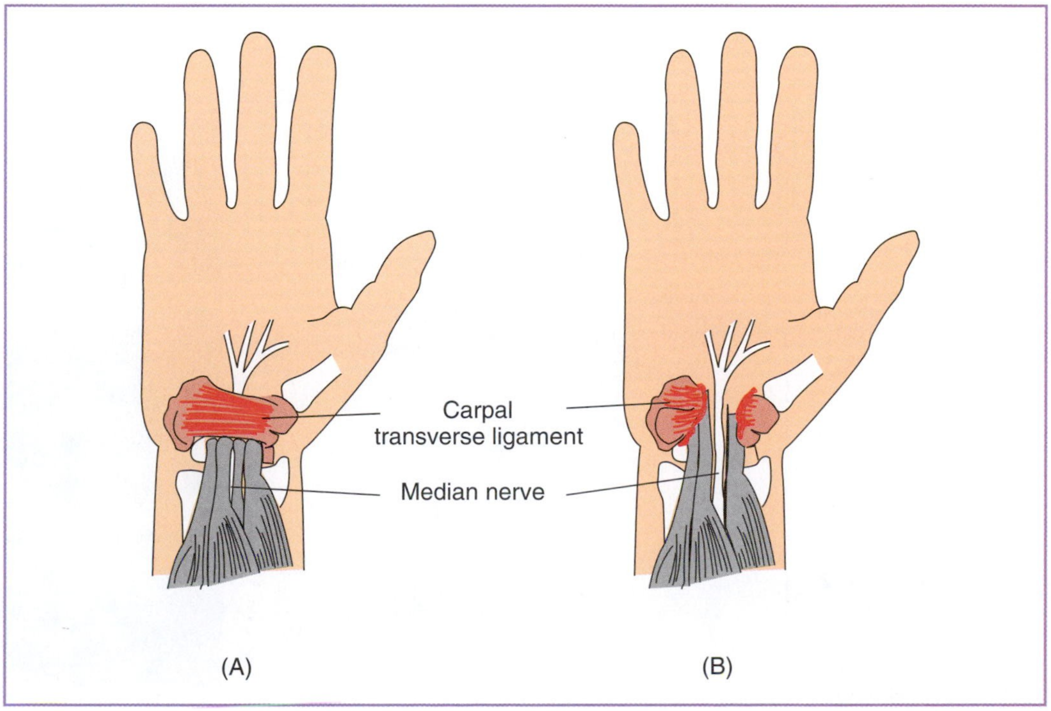

FIGURE 6-21
Carpal Tunnel Release: (A) before; (B) after procedure

TREATMENT PROCEDURES		
Word	Pronunciation	Definition
fasciectomy	făs"ē-ĕk'tō-mē	surgical removal of fascia
laminectomy	lăm"ĭ-nĕk'tō-mē	removal of a portion of a vertebra in order to remove disc tissue
meniscectomy	mĕn"ĭ-sĕk'tŏ-mē	removal of knee cartilage (meniscus)
microdiskectomy	mī"krō-dĭs-kĕk'tŏ-mē	removal of ruptured disc or disc fragments using small incisions and minimal approach
microvascular anastomosis	mī"krō-văs'kū-lăr ah-năs"tō-mō'sĭs	use of an operating microscope to repair minute blood vessels and nerves
neurolysis	nū-rōl'ĭ-sĭs	freeing the nerve of surrounding scar tissue; may be median, ulnar, or radial
osteotomy	ŏs-tē-ŏt'ō-mē	correction of a bone deformity by cutting and repositioning the bone
reduction		restoration of a fracture to normal position; *closed reduction* is manipulation without an incision; *open reduction* is when an incision is made into the fracture site
resection		removal of all or part of a bone
revision arthroplasty	ăr'thrō-plăs"tē	redoing total hip arthroplasty or total knee arthroplasty after failure or loosening of originally placed components
spinal fusion		bony union of two or more vertebrae; spinal fusion with bone graft and internal fixatives such as plates, rods, and cables
synovectomy	sĭn"ō-vĕk'tō-mē	removal of the synovium or tissues lining the joints
total hip replacement (arthroplasty)	(ăr'thrō-plăs"tē)	surgical reconstruction by implanting a prosthetic hip joint (See Figure 6-22)

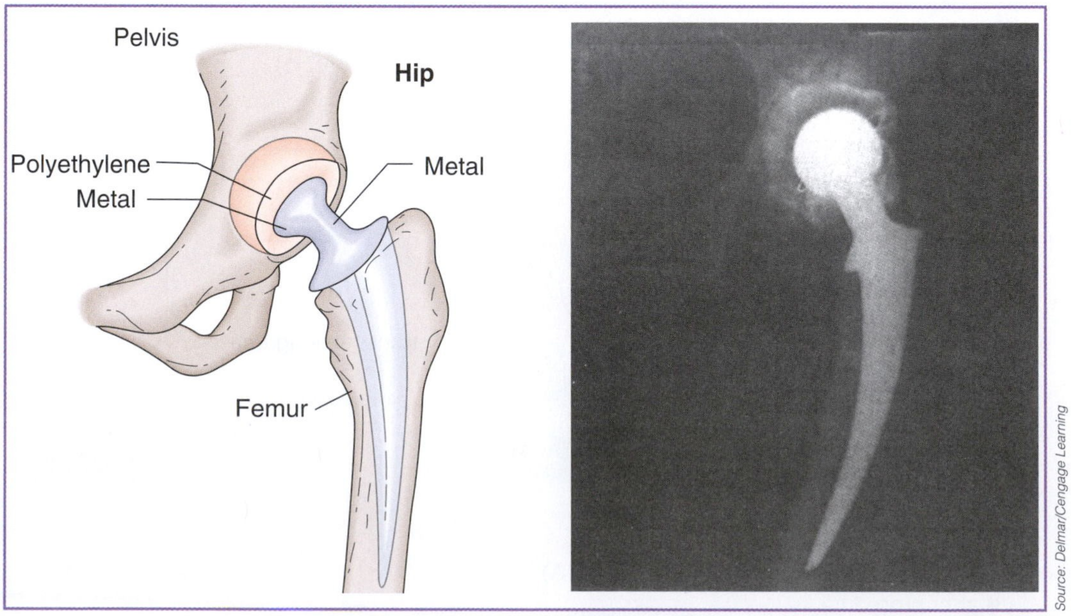

FIGURE 6-22 Total Hip Replacement: implanted artificial joint

MEDICATIONS PRESCRIBED	
Trade Name	Generic Name
Analgesics	
Darvon	propoxyphene
Flexeril, Cycloflex	cyclobenzaprine HCl
Fioricet	caffeine, butalbital, and APAP
Fiorinal	caffeine, butalbital, and ASA
Lortab, Lorcet, Vicodin, Dolacet, Hydrocet	hydrocodone and acetaminophen
OxyContin	oxycodone
Robaxin	methocarbamol
Soma	carisoprodol
Tylenol, Panadol, Excedrin, Anacin	acetaminophen and APAP
Ultram	tramadol HCl
Antibiotics	
Cipro	ciprofloxacin
Keflex	cephalexin
Mandol	cefamandole
Muscle Relaxants	
Flexeril, Cycloflex	cyclobenzaprine HCl
Robaxin	methocarbamol
Soma	carisoprodol
Valium	diazepam
Disease-Modifying Antirheumatic Drugs (DMARDs)	
Azulfidine	sulfasalazine
Cytoxan	cyclophosphamide
Imuran	azathioprine
Minocin	minocycline
Neoral, Sandimmune	cyclosporine
Rheumatrex, Trexall	methotrexate
Osteoporosis Treatment	
Actonel	risedronate sodium
Calcimar, Miacalcin	calcitonin
Didronel	etidronate
Evista	raloxifene hydrochloride
Fosomax	alendronate

continues

MEDICATIONS PRESCRIBED	
Trade Name	Generic Name
Osteoporosis Treatment (*continued*)	
Menest	esterified estrogen
Reclast	zoledronic acid
Rocaltrol	calcitriol
Nonsteroidal Anti-Inflammatory Drugs (NSAIDs)	
Advil, Motrin, Midol, Rufen	ibuprofen
Anaprox, Naprosyn	naproxen sodium
Ansaid	flurbiprofen
Celebrex	celecoxib
Clinoril	sulindac
Daypro	oxaprozin
Feldene	piroxicam
Indocin	indomethacin
Lodine	etodolac
Nalfon	fenoprofen calcium
Orudis, Oruvail	ketoprofen
Relafen	nabumetone
Tolectin	tolmetin sodium
Voltaren	diclofenac sodium ophthalmic
Gout	
—	colchicine
Anturane	sulfinpyrazone
Benemid, Probalan	probenecid
Lopurin, Purinal, Zyloprim	allopurinol
Glucocorticoids/Steroids	
Artisocort	triamcinolone acetonide
Cortone	cortisone
Cortef, Hydrocortone	hydrocortisone
Decadron, Hexadrol	dexamethasone
Deltasone, Orasone	prednisone
Medrol	methylprednisolone
Prelone	prednisolone

continues

MEDICATIONS PRESCRIBED	
Trade Name	Generic Name
Biological Response Modifiers	
Enbrel	etanercept
Remicade	infliximab

ABBREVIATIONS	
ACJT	acromioclavicular joint
ACL	anterior cruciate ligament
ANA	antinuclear antibody
C1, C2, etc.	cervical vertebrae
Ca	calcium
CK	creatine kinase
CPK	creatine phosphokinase
CTS	carpal tunnel syndrome
DEXA	dual-energy x-ray absorptiometry
DIPJ	distal interphalangeal joint
DMARD	disease-modifying antirheumatic drug
DTR	deep tendon reflex
EMG	electromyography
ESR	erythrocyte sedimentation rate
Fx	fracture
Ga	gallium
IM	intramuscular
L1, L2, etc.	lumbar vertebrae
LE	lower extremity
LE cell	lupus erythematosus cell
NSAID	nonsteroidal anti-inflammatory drug
ortho	orthopedics
phos, P	phosphorus
RA	rheumatoid arthritis
RF	rheumatoid factor
RLE	right lower extremity
ROM	range of motion
RUE	right upper extremity

continues

ABBREVIATIONS	
Sed rate	sedimentation rate
SLE	systemic lupus erythematosus
T1, T2, etc.	thoracic vertebrae
THR	total hip replacement
TKR	total knee replacement
TMJ	temporomandibular joint
UE	upper extremity

Working Practice Review Exercises

SPELLING

Rewrite the misspelled words.

1. capsuloraphy ____________________
2. fascectomy ____________________
3. lupis erythematosis ____________________
4. arthrotomy ____________________
5. menisectomy ____________________

DEFINITIONS

Define the following diagnostic procedures.

1. arthroscopy

   ____

2. arthrography

   ____

3. synovial fluid studies

   ____

4. latex fixation or rheumatoid factor

   ____

5. electromyography

   ____

6. skeletal survey

____

7. C-reactive protein

____

8. magnetic resonance imaging

____

9. serum creatine kinase

____

10. erythrocyte sedimentation rate

____

11. gallium scan

____

12. myelography

____

IDENTIFICATION

Name the following treatment procedures.

1. removal of knee cartilage _______________
2. removal of the bursa and bone of the great toe _______________
3. incision made into a fracture site to return bone to its normal position _______________
4. cutting the wrist ligament to relieve nerve pressure _______________
5. surgical opening of a joint _______________
6. surgical implantation of a prosthetic hip joint _______________
7. union of two or more vertebrae _______________
8. surgical procedures performed on joints with an arthroscope _______________
9. surgical reconstruction of a joint _______________
10. restoration of a fracture to normal position _______________

DEFINITIONS

Define the underscored diagnoses.

1. The patient was seen today because of suspected <u>atrophic</u> <u>arthritis</u>.

____

2. The injury to the leg was a <u>greenstick</u> <u>fracture</u>.

____

3. He complained of <u>gout</u> for years.

____

4. The patient has myasthenia gravis.

____

5. The diagnosis in her case is osteomyelitis.

____

6. The dentist was suffering from carpal tunnel syndrome.

____

7. The doctor suspected he suffered from Paget's disease.

____

8. The patient complained of discomfort related to a ganglion cyst.

____

9. The doctor indicated that scoliosis was causing her symptoms.

____

10. James has a torn meniscus as a result of his participation in the football game.

____

Dictionary Exercises

DICTIONARY EXERCISE 1

Use your dictionary to find the pronunciation and definition of the following words.

	Word	Pronunciation	Definition
1.	anomaly	_______	_______
2.	calcific	_______	_______
3.	collateral ligaments	_______	_______
4.	costochondral	_______	_______
5.	coxa	_______	_______
6.	de Quervain's disease	_______	_______
7.	flail joint	_______	_______
8.	genu	_______	_______
9.	Legg-Calvé-Perthes disease	_______	_______
10.	pes planus	_______	_______
11.	osteoplasty	_______	_______
12.	ossification	_______	_______
13.	intertrochanteric	_______	_______
14.	osteoclast	_______	_______

DICTIONARY EXERCISE 2

Select the correct meaning and provide the pronunciation of each term.

1. capitulum (________________)
   a. small, rounded end of a bone
   b. the shaft of a long bone
2. diaphysis (________________)
   a. resembling a pit or socket
   b. the shaft of a long bone
3. giant cell tumor (________________)
   a. bony outgrowth, usually branched in shape
   b. arises from the marrow of a long bone or from a tendon sheath
4. glenoid (________________)
   a. resembling a pit or socket
   b. the bony process of the ulna at the elbow
5. glenoid cavity (________________)
   a. removal of tissue to form a shallow depression
   b. hollow socket in the head of the shoulder blade that receives the head of the humerus
6. hemarthrosis (________________)
   a. passage of blood into the cavity of a bony joint
   b. spotty osteoporosis of bone in posttraumatic states
7. lamina (________________)
   a. bony outgrowth, usually branched in shape
   b. a thin, flat layer
8. metaphysis (________________)
   a. fusing together of two or more toes or fingers
   b. growth zone of a long bone between the epiphysis and diaphysis
9. nucleus pulposus (________________)
   a. semi-fluid cushion in the center of an intervertebral disk
   b. bonelike structure that develops on a bone or occasionally at another site
10. olecranon (________________)
    a. free-floating bone that resembles a grain of sesame in size and shape
    b. bony process of the ulna at the elbow
11. ostectomy (________________)
    a. surgical removal of dead bone
    b. excision or resection of bone
12. osteoma (________________)
    a. arises from the marrow of a long bone or from a tendon sheath
    b. bonelike structure that develops on a bone or occasionally at another site
13. osteophyte (________________)
    a. a bony outgrowth, usually branched in shape
    b. resembling a pit or socket
14. rheumatologist (________________)
    a. physician who treats joint diseases
    b. physician who manipulates the spinal column
15. polymyositis (________________)
    a. inflammatory condition of muscular tissue in which an area of abnormal bone formation occurs
    b. inflammation of uncertain origin of several muscles at once
16. saucerization (________________)
    a. removal of tissue to form a shallow depression
    b. surgical removal of dead bone
17. sequestrectomy (________________)
    a. surgical removal of dead bone
    b. removal of synovial membrane lining a joint capsule
18. sesamoid (________________)
    a. free-floating bone that resembles a grain of sesame in size and shape
    b. resembling a pit or socket
19. Sudeck's atrophy (________________)
    a. complete or incomplete separation of a portion of joint cartilage from underlying bone
    b. spotty osteoporosis of bone in posttraumatic states
20. syndactylism (________________)
    a. hollow back; convexity of spine
    b. fusing together of two or more toes or fingers

DICTIONARY EXERCISE 3

Pronunciation of the words below is provided. Using your dictionary, find the correct spelling and the definition of the word.

	Word	Pronunciation	Definition
1.	____________	ăs"ĕ-tăb'ū-lŭm	____________
2.	____________	mī"ĕ-lō'mah	____________
3.	____________	ōs"tē-ō-kŏn-drī'tĭs dĭs'ĕ-kănz	____________
4.	____________	sŭb"lŭks-ā'shŭn	____________
5.	____________	zĭf'oid prŏs'ĕs	____________
6.	____________	krĕp"ĭ-tā'shŭn	____________
7.	____________	făs"ē-ī'tĭs	____________
8.	____________	dĭs-plā'sē-ah	____________
9.	____________	kŏn"drō-mah-lā'shē-ah	____________
10.	____________	ăng"kĭ-lō'sĭs	____________
11.	____________	ŏs"ĭ-fĭ-kā'shŭn	____________
12.	____________	lah-săgz' sign	____________
13.	____________	mĕ-nĭs'kŭs	____________
14.	____________	mī"ō-sī'tĭs ŏ-sĭf'ĭ-kănz	____________
15.	____________	spŏn"dĭ-lō-lĭs'thē-sĭs	____________
16.	____________	ō-lĕk'răn-ŏn	____________
17.	____________	tor"tĭ-kŏl'ĭs	____________

DICTIONARY EXERCISE 4

Look up the definition of each of the italicized words. Write the pronunciation in the space provided. Then rewrite the sentence in your own words.

1. The patient was placed in a *Denis Browne* splint.

   ____

2. *Ortolani's* (____________) sign was evident.

   ____

3. She was scheduled for a *patellectomy* (____________) on Thursday.

   ____

4. There was evidence of *spondylolysis* (____________), as well as *myositis* (____________).

   ____

5. During the procedure *tenodesis* (____________) was achieved.

   ____

6. A *tenoplasty* (____________) was performed two years ago.

   ____

7. On examination, a *trigger finger* was noted on the right hand.

____

8. Both a *tenosynovectomy* (____________________) and *tenotomy* (____________________) were required.

____

9. The pathology report indicated an *osteochondroma* (____________________).

____

10. On physical examination, the patient presented with a *metatarsus varus* (____________________).

____

11. There was a *contracture* (____________________) present, as well as *lordosis* (____________________).

____

12. The problem was diagnosed as *Baker's cyst*.

____

13. Patient is suffering from *Paget's* (____________________) *disease*.

____

*Study*WARE™ Connection

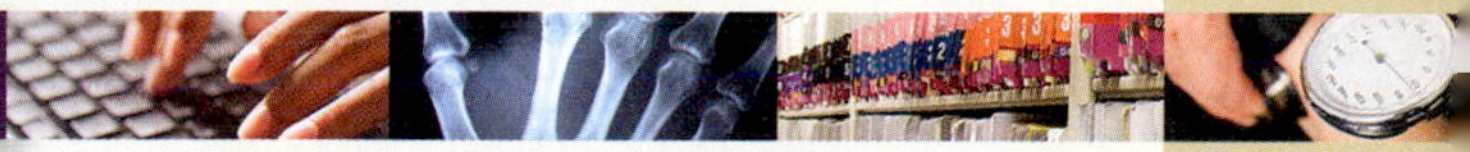

To take a practice quiz or play interactive games that reinforce the content in this chapter, go to your StudyWARE™ CD-ROM.

Listening Exercise

INSTRUCTIONS

1. Review the spelling, pronunciation, and meaning of the words provided in the preview.
2. Go to your StudyWARE™ CD-ROM and listen to **Listening Exercise 6-1**. Fill in the blank in the report as the word is dictated.
3. At the end of the activity, check your spelling against the preview words. They appear in the preview in the order in which they are encountered in the activity.
4. Review and practice the words you missed.
5. Look up words that are not familiar.

PREVIEW OF WORDS FOR LISTENING EXERCISE 6-1

Word	Pronunciation	Definition
crepitus	krĕp'ĭ-tŭs	dry, crackling sound or sensation, as in the grating of the ends of a fractured bone
effusion	ĕ-fū'zhŭn	escape of fluid into a part
varus gait	vārŭs gāt	style of walking characterized by an inward bend toward the midline of the body
medially	mē'dĕ-ăl-lē	toward the midline of the body
patellofemoral	pă-tĕl"ō-fĕm'ō-răl	pertaining to the patella (kneecap) and femur (thigh bone)
arthroplasty	ăr'thrō-plăs"tē	surgical reconstruction of a joint

Listening Exercise 6-1

*Study*WARE™ Connection

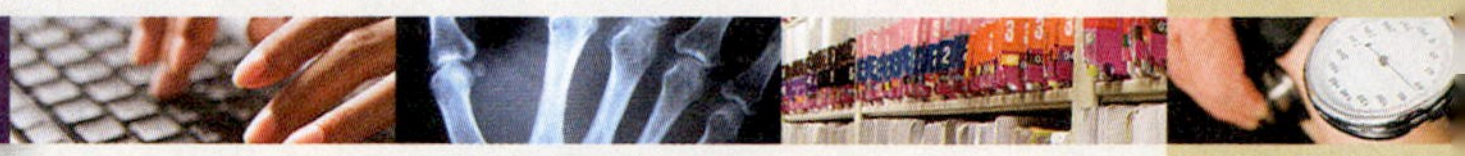

Listen to this report being read on your StudyWARE™ CD-ROM. Fill in each blank as the word is dictated.

Letter of Consultation

Dear Dr. Zemstov:

I had the pleasure of seeing your patient, Mr. Roger Petrov, who is a 75-year-old very active gentleman who has had a long history of increasing pain associated with his right knee. He states his problem began when he sustained trauma to his knee while playing high school football. Although he got better originally, over the last few years he has experienced increasing discomfort within his knee with activities. In addition, he has noted a deformity, specifically a genu varum or bowleggedness, that has gotten worse. He finds that on occasion he will sense catching and locking. He has noted considerable amounts of ______________________ along with periodic episodes of ______________________.

You have maintained him so appropriately over these last few years with anti-inflammatory medication, the use of cold therapy, and some physical therapy with reasonable success. However, his symptoms now have worsened to the point where his daily living activities have become more difficult, including such simple things as walking to the mailbox, cutting the grass and doing minimal manual tasks around his house, or going shopping.

On physical examination he is a healthy appearing, very pleasant man complaining of right knee pain. He walks with a limp with an obvious ______________________. Closer examination reveals no limb-length discrepancy. He does carry about a half inch of atrophy of his thigh. There is relative instability ______________________ with a 2+ effusion. Considerable crepitus is noted throughout his knee. There is discomfort along the medial side during the course of the exam as well. He has no edema, has full pulses, and no other lower extremity joint problems.

We have obtained standing x-rays, in addition to the usual lateral and Merchant views. The films show end-stage degenerative arthritis involving primarily the medial compartment of his knee with lesser involvement of the ______________________ compartment. He is bone on bone medially.

I think this man has exhausted all forms of conservative measures for his condition of degenerative arthritis. He is an excellent candidate for a total knee ______________________ in an effort to improve his pain and reduce his other symptoms, as well as to alter his alignment. He is interested in pursuing a corrective course and arrangements will be made for this to be done sometime within the next few weeks.

Thank you for this referral. I will keep you informed as to his progress, both in the hospital and postoperatively.

Sincerely yours,

Juanita Montoya, MD

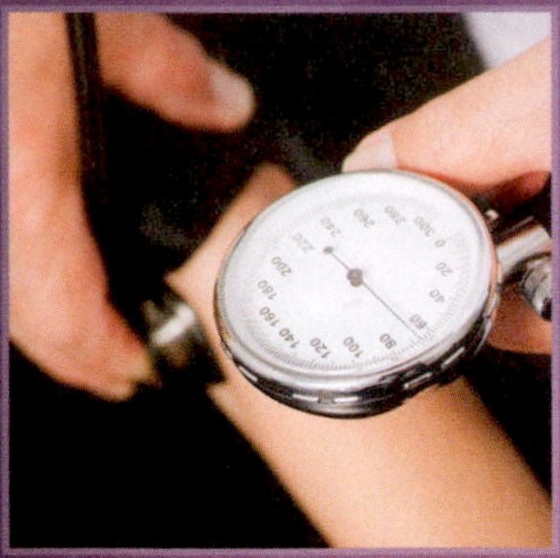
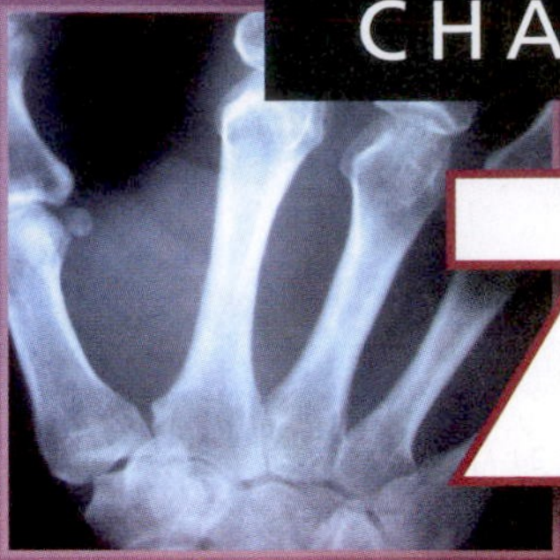
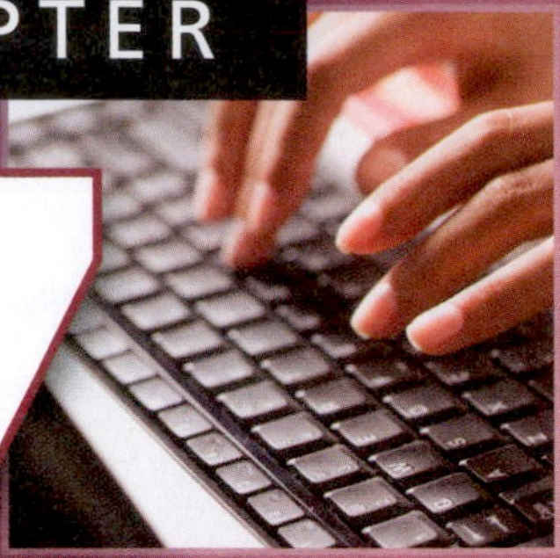
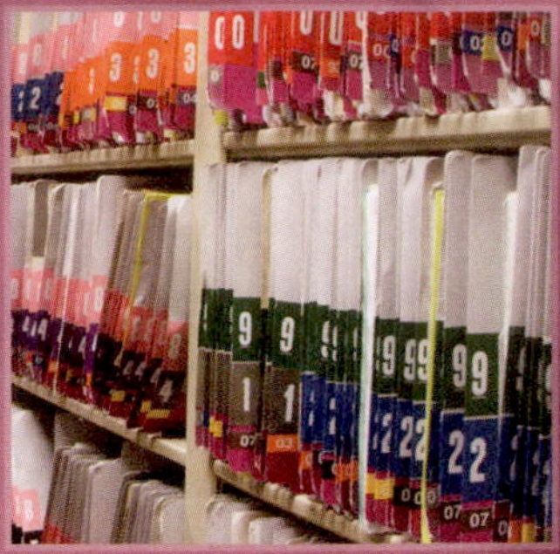

CHAPTER 7

Surgery

"Surgery does the ideal thing—
it separates the patient from his disease."

—Logan Clendening

OBJECTIVES

When you have completed this chapter on surgery, you should be able to

1. Identify the components of an Operative Report.
2. Spell and define commonly used anesthesia terminology.
3. Identify and spell commonly used surgical positions, incisions, and instruments.
4. Explain the difference between suture material and suture technique.
5. Identify the meanings of related word elements.
6. Hear how medical terminology is used in actual medical reports.

INTRODUCTION

Surgical intervention is often required to repair injuries to the body, to correct deformities or defects, and to diagnose, treat, or cure certain disease processes. A surgeon is a physician who has completed five or more years of postgraduate training in one or more of a broad range of surgical specialties. Some of these surgical specialties are listed below.

Specialty	Organs or Systems Involved
General surgery	various organs or systems
Gynecology	external and internal female reproductive organs
Neurosurgery	nervous system and associated structures
Ophthalmology	eyes and associated structures, including ocular muscles, tear ducts, and glands

continues

Specialty	Organs or Systems Involved
Orthopedic	surgery musculoskeletal system
Otorhinolaryngology	ear, nose, and throat and related structures
Plastic surgery	repair and reconstruction of various body structures
Thoracic surgery	thorax (chest) and diseases related to the bronchi, lungs, and mediastinum
Urology	male and female urinary tract, male reproductive organs
Vascular and cardiac	heart, blood vessels, and lymphatic vessels surgery

The terminology associated with surgery and surgical reports is highly specialized as well. Surgical terminology includes terms related to anesthesia; names of surgical positions, instruments, and incisions; and suture techniques and materials. The surgical report contains a detailed technical description of how the procedure was performed.

Although the surgeon is responsible for providing the information for the report, support staff may be responsible for processing or producing it. Therefore, it is important to recognize the required components of the report, know basic information about anesthetics, and become familiar with other surgical terminology.

COMPONENTS OF THE OPERATIVE REPORT

A written report is required for every surgical procedure. The report may be called an operative note, an operative report, a surgical note, or a surgical report. The term **Operative Report** will be used throughout this chapter.

The Operative Report is used to assist in further patient care, to secure payment for services provided, and as a legal document to support the surgeon's actions. There are required components of the Operative Report mandated by various state and federal laws and by other regulatory agencies. Each report must contain a preoperative and postoperative diagnosis, the name of the operation or procedure, indications for the procedure, and a description of findings and techniques.

In addition, the Operative Report will include the patient's name, date of the procedure, and the surgeon's name. These items may be listed at the beginning of the report under appropriate headings. Some agencies include the case number, patient room number, and the names of any assisting surgeons or physicians.

PREOPERATIVE DIAGNOSIS

All regulatory and accrediting agencies require a **Preoperative Diagnosis**, which helps explain why the operation or procedure is necessary. The diagnosis can be stated as a specific disease. When the diagnosis is not clearly evident, the Preoperative Diagnosis is stated as a "rule out" or "suspected" diagnosis, or in other general terms.

EXAMPLES

Patient A has been diagnosed with acute appendicitis. An appendectomy is performed. In this case the Preoperative Diagnosis will be appendicitis.

Patient B may have several symptoms of appendicitis, but the physician cannot make a clear-cut diagnosis. In this case the Preoperative Diagnosis could be suspected appendicitis, rule out appendicitis, or it could be severe abdominal pain with high fever, with an unknown reason or cause.

In any case, the Preoperative Diagnosis *must* be present and *must* be related to the procedure performed.

POSTOPERATIVE DIAGNOSIS

The **Postoperative Diagnosis** is also required by all regulatory and accrediting agencies. It states the diagnosis after the operation or procedure is completed. The Postoperative Diagnosis is a short descriptive title of what was actually found.

As with the Preoperative Diagnosis, the Postoperative Diagnosis can be explicit when a specific disease is identified. There are also situations in which several diagnoses or contributing factors are identified.

EXAMPLES

An appendectomy is performed on patient A. Only the appendix is inflamed with no other complications or contributing factors. The Postoperative Diagnosis would be appendicitis.

Patient B, however, has an appendectomy and the surgeon finds an inflamed appendix and a stenosis between the small and large intestine. The Postoperative Diagnosis would be appendicitis, with localized peritonitis, or inflammation of the peritoneum.

In all cases, the Preoperative and Postoperative Diagnosis should be the same or closely related. If the Postoperative Diagnosis is different or unrelated to the Preoperative Diagnosis, the surgeon must explain why the diagnoses are different in the body of the Operative Report.

The Preoperative and Postoperative Diagnosis should be written in acceptable medical terms, without abbreviations or use of layman's terms. It is poor practice to simply write "SAME" for the Postoperative Diagnosis. The following are examples of correct ways to write Preoperative and Postoperative Diagnoses.

EXAMPLES

Example A	Preoperative Diagnosis:	Appendicitis
	Postoperative Diagnosis:	Appendicitis
Example B	Preoperative Diagnosis:	Severe abdominal pain
	Postoperative Diagnosis:	Appendicitis

OPERATION

The **Operation** section of the report, required by all regulatory agencies, describes the name of the operation or procedure performed. The length of this section, which is sometimes called *Procedure* or *Procedure Performed,* depends on the surgeon's writing style and the complexity of the operation. Below are three examples of how the Operation section could be written using appendicitis as the Preoperative and Postoperative Diagnosis.

EXAMPLES

Operation	**Interpretation**
Appendectomy	Removed the appendix
Laparotomy with appendectomy	Opened the abdomen and removed the appendix
Exploratory laparotomy with appendectomy	Opened the abdomen, looked around, and removed the appendix

INDICATIONS

The **Indications** section gives the reason for the operation or procedure. If the Preoperative Diagnosis is vague, the surgeon uses this section to describe the problems or symptoms that led to the decision to operate.

The indications can be stated as a separate section or included in the main body of the report. Examples of a separate Indications section are shown below.

EXAMPLES

INDICATIONS: This is a 34-year-old woman who gives a history of intermittent right upper quadrant pain that radiates to the right shoulder. It is associated with meals. The pain has been worse for the last several months. It is now associated with a three-day history of nausea, vomiting, fever, and chills. A sonogram done today revealed multiple stones.

INDICATIONS: This is a 21-year-old man with a three-month history of thrombocytopenia and easy bruising. He has been on high doses of steroids.

FINDINGS AND TECHNIQUE

The **Findings and Technique** section usually is the longest and most technical part of the Operative Report. This section may be called *Description of Operation* or *Description of Procedures*, but whatever name used, specific information must be included in this section. The required items are discussed below.

Type of Anesthesia

The type of anesthesia tells how the patient was protected from feeling the pain of the operation. The surgeon must give the type of anesthesia and tell how it was administered. The specific name of the anesthesia is usually included. For example, the surgeon may say, "The patient was injected with a local anesthetic." This means that the patient received a shot of a medication that numbed the area where the procedure was to be performed. More information about anesthesia terms is presented later in this chapter.

Surgical Position

Surgical position describes how the patient was placed on the operating table. A thorough Operative Report includes the name of the surgical position. However, if the surgical position is not given, the report is still considered complete. You must *never* include the name of a surgical position that you *think* is correct. Only the surgeon may provide this information. Certain types of surgical positions are associated with specific operative procedures.

The more commonly used surgical positions are listed and illustrated later in this chapter.

Incision

The **incision** (ĭn-sĭzh'ŭn) is a surgical cut used to access various parts of the body. The surgeon will describe the location, length, direction, and depth of the incision. A complete description of the incision is a requirement of the Operative Report.

Incisions often are named after the individual who perfected the procedure. The name of the incision is also related to the location of the incision or the operation being performed. Commonly used incisions are listed below, with those named for an individual capitalized. Illustrations of some surgical incision locations are presented later in the chapter.

Bergmann	Lempert	Pfannenstiel	subcostal
chevron	midline	Rocky-Davis	superficial
crescent	muscle splitting	semilunar	supraumbilical
endaural	oblique	sharp and blunt	transverse
Kocher	paramedian	skin	vertical
lateral rectus	Perthes	stab	

Description

Most of the Findings and Techniques section is devoted to a detailed description of the entire operative procedure. The surgeon will describe what was done, how and why it was done, and the patient's response. The description paragraphs are filled with the names and sizes of instruments, suture materials and techniques, and the condition of the organs and tissue examined or removed. An example of a brief technical description, with a layman's translation, follows.

EXAMPLES

DESCRIPTION: The patient was brought to the operating room and placed on the operating table in the upright position. Tonsils were injected with 2% Xylocaine. After waiting for the anesthesia to take effect, the tonsils were clamped with a curved Allis clamp and removed using blunt and sharp dissection and the snare technique.

LAYMAN'S INTERPRETATION: The patient was brought to the operating room. The table was raised so he was sitting up. The glands at the back and sides of the throat were given a shot of a medicine to make them numb. When the glands were completely numb, a curved clamp was used to grab them. Two kinds of cutting methods (blunt and sharp) were used. The tonsils were trapped in the clamp and removed.

Closure

The final paragraphs of the Findings and Technique section describe how the incision was closed, state that all surgical tools have been accounted for, and may include information about blood loss, and type or volume of fluid replacement.

Types and locations of catheters and drains should be included, as well as any complications encountered. Any specimens removed during surgery should be listed, as well as any procedures requiring extra effort such as extensive types of adhesions and the time that was required. Include any preventive measures that were taken.

The surgeon describes how each layer of skin and tissue was sutured, the type of suture material and techniques used, and the condition of the incisional wound. There are many types of suture materials and techniques, which are discussed later in this chapter.

An important part of the Findings and Techniques section is the sponge count. Every Operative Report must state that the surgeon can account for all surgical tools. Prior to every procedure, a member of the surgical team counts items like sponges, needles, and instruments. After the procedure, these items are counted again to ensure that nothing was left inside the patient. The Operative Report *must* have a statement that the count was done.

EXAMPLES

The sponge, needle, and instrument counts were correct.

You *must not* include a sponge count statement if the surgeon does not include one. You should, however, alert the surgeon of this omission, because it is the surgeon's responsibility to authorize the inclusion of this information.

If the patient received blood during the procedure, information about blood loss and blood replacement may appear in this section. This information may be included as a separate heading of the Operative Report.

EXAMPLES

Due to excessive blood loss, the patient received 2 units of whole blood.

Patient Condition

The final statement in the Operative Report concerns the condition of the patient and is usually one or two sentences in length.

EXAMPLES

The patient was sent to the recovery room in stable condition.

If there is some question about the patient's ability to survive the operation, the statement could read:

EXAMPLES

The patient was sent to the recovery room in poor condition. Prognosis is poor.

In the case of a poor **prognosis** (prŏg-nō'sĭs) (probable outcome), a reason will be given.

SIGNATURE BLOCK

The surgeon must sign the Operative Report. It is important to *carefully proofread* the completed report before you submit it for signature. A standard signature block format is acceptable. It contains the name of the surgeon followed by the initials of the individual who transcribed or typed the report. If the report was dictated and transcribed, a notation beneath the signature block indicates the date dictated and the date transcribed.

Figure 7-1 is an example of a completed Operative Report.

ANESTHESIA TERMINOLOGY

Anesthesiology (ăn"ĕs-thē"zē-ŏl'ŏ-jē), a specialty that developed as a result of Joseph Priestley's discovery of nitrous oxide in 1772, is the study of anesthesia and anesthetic agents. An **anesthesiologist** (ăn"ēs-thē"zē-ŏl'ŏ-jĭst) is a physician who specializes in anesthesiology. An **anesthetist** (a-nĕs'thĕ-tĭst) is a nurse with additional education and training in anesthesia who administers anesthetic agents.

Anesthesiology is closely related to surgery in that most surgical or operative procedures include some type of anesthesia. To understand and produce Operative and Procedural Reports, it helps to have a basic knowledge of anesthesiology terms. The following basic information covers types of anesthesia, modes of induction, and the names of commonly used anesthetic agents.

TYPES OF ANESTHESIA

Anesthesia (ăn"ĕs-thē'zē-ah), loss of feeling or sensation, is usually identified as being general, regional, local, or topical. The type of surgery or procedure performed determines the type of anesthesia that will be used. Each anesthesia category has unique characteristics.

General Anesthesia

General anesthesia produces a loss of consciousness with an absence of pain sensation over the entire body. This type of anesthesia is given to the patient by two methods: **inhalation** (ĭn"hah-lā'shŭn) (breathing in) and **intravenous** (ĭn"trah-vē'nŭs) (into the vein). Under general anesthesia the patient feels no pain and often has to be placed on respiratory support. The patient's vital signs are closely monitored. Adjustments in the level of unconsciousness can be made throughout the operative procedure.

Regional Anesthesia

Regional anesthesia interrupts nerve conduction from a specific region of the body. The patient remains conscious, but does not feel pain. In this type of anesthesia the anesthetic agent is injected close to the nerve to be blocked. Regional anesthesia is sometimes called **block anesthesia**. A **field block** prevents pain sensations in the area around the operative site. A **nerve block** focuses the anesthetic agent very close to the nerve that supplies the operative area.

Local Anesthesia

Local anesthesia is confined to one part of the body. The patient remains conscious but does not experience pain in the specific area. Local anesthesia involves introducing a nerve-conduction blocking agent into tissues surrounding a nerve that serves only the tissue at the surgical site. A local anesthetic agent may be rubbed directly on the skin or tissue in the area involved—topical application—or injected into the layers of the skin or tissue—**subcutaneous** (sŭb"kŭ-tā'nē-ŭs) application.

Topical Anesthesia

Topical anesthesia is applied directly to the area involved, usually as a solution or gel. The patient is conscious, and only the surface area is pain free. Topical anesthesia is confined to the skin, mucous membranes of the upper digestive tract, urethra, vagina, and rectum.

HILLCREST Medical Center

OPERATIVE REPORT

Patient Name: James Kent
Attending Physician: Roger Clements, MD
Preoperative Diagnosis: Abdominal pain, unknown etiology
Postoperative Diagnosis: Appendicitis

Hospital No.:
Room No.: 456
Date of Surgery: December 1, 20—
Surgeon: Martha Sandburg, MD
Anesthesia: General endotracheal tube

Operative Procedure: Exploratory laparotomy
INDICATIONS: Mr. Kent is a 31-year-old male who had been feeling well until approximately 3 o'clock in the morning prior to his admission. He awoke with sharp periumbilical pain that localized in his right lower quadrant over the next several hours. This pain was associated with nausea, vomiting, chills, and anorexia. Upon inital presentation in the emergency room, it was felt that the patient had appendicitis. The patient had a WBC of approximately 13,000 upon admission. His temperature in the emergency room went from 99.6 to 102.6 F. The patient was felt to have a "hot" appendix with appendicitis and was taken to the operating room.

PROCEDURE: After appropriate permission was obtained and the risks and benefits of the procedure were explained to the patient, he was put to sleep with a general endotracheal anesthetic. The abdomen was prepared and draped in the usual sterile fashion. A Rocky-Davis incision was used with a #10 blade. Hemostasis was obtained with electrocautery. A muscle-splitting incision was used and carried to the peritoneum. The peritoneum was grasped with two small hemostats, lifting it away from the intra-abdominal cavity. A small incision with a #10 scalpel was made, being careful not to injure any intra-abdominal contents. The incision was then carried sharply along the entire length of the incision. The cecum was grasped with a Babcock's forceps and delivered through the wound. The vermiform appendix was identified and appeared to be grossly normal. Upon limited exploration of the abdomen, there were no abnormal abdominal findings with the exception of some of the mesenteric nodes, which appeared to be inflamed. It was elected at that time to complete the appendectomy.

The mesentery attaching to the appendix was divided using hemostat clamps, doubly ligated, and transected. The appendiceal artery was identified and doubly clamped, transected, and ligated. A 2-0 silk pursestring was then passed around the base of the appendix. A straight clamp was then used to rush the base of the appendix. The clamp was placed above a 1-0 chromic tie, tied under the previously placed clamp, and the appendix was excised using a #10 scalpel. The appendix, clamp, and scalpel were passed off the field. Electrocautery was used to cauterize the remaining tip of the appendix. The previously placed clamp was used to invert the appendix as the pursestring was tied. This buried the stump of the appendix. A Z-stitch was then used to oversew the remaining deformity.

The wound was thoroughly irrigated, and the posterior fascia was closed with #1 Prolene in a running fashion. The anterior fascial layer was closed in a similar manner. The wound was thoroughly irrigated. The skin was closed with staples. The sponge, needle, and instrument counts were correct.

The patient was extubated in the operating room and sent to the recovery room in stable condition.

Martha Sandburg, MD/X

DD: 12-1-20—
DT: 12-2--

FIGURE 7-1 Completed Operative Report

ANESTHETIC AGENTS

Although types of anesthesia routinely fall into one of these four categories, there are a multitude of **anesthetic agents**, which are drugs used to induce anesthesia. Various factors are considered when choosing an anesthetic, such as the type of operation or procedure, patient allergies, available anesthetic agent, and the surgeon's or physician's previous experience with a particular anesthetic agent. The following is a list of several of the more commonly used anesthetic agents.

ANESTHETIC AGENTS	
Trade Name	Generic Name
General Anesthetics	
Inhaled	
Ethrane	enflurane
Fluothane	halothane
Forane	isoflurane
Ultane	sevoflurane
Suprane	desflurane
–	nitrous oxide
Intravenous	
Diprivan	propofol
Ketalar	ketamine
Pentothal	thiopental
–	Opioids (fentanyl, sufentanil, alfentanil)
Regional Anesthetics	
Carbocaine, Polocaine	mepivacaine
Nesacaine	chloroprocaine
Xylocaine, Lignocaine	lidocaine
Local Anesthetics	
Novocaine	procaine
Xylocaine, Lignocaine	lidocaine
Pontocaine, Cetacaine	tetracaine
Marcaine, Sensorcaine	bupivacaine
Topical Anesthetics	
Americaine	benzocaine
Xylocaine	lidocaine
Cinchocaine	dibucaine
Pramoxine	pramoxine
Butyl aminobenzoate	butamben
Pontocaine	tetracaine

MODES OF INDUCTION

The ways in which anesthetic agents are introduced into the body are referred to as **modes of induction**. The mode of induction varies depending on the type of anesthesia used. General anesthetics usually are administered by inhalation of a gaseous mixture or injection of an intravenous fluid. Regional anesthetics are most often injected. Local anesthetics can be introduced by injection into a specific region of the body and by subcutaneous or topical methods. Topical anesthetics are placed on the surface of the skin or tissue. The more commonly used modes of induction are identified and defined to follow.

Block

Block is a generic term that means the anesthetic agent is injected near or along a nerve path in order to stop nerve impulses to the area supplied by the nerve. The block method is also called nerve block and can include the name of the nerve or nerve group to be anesthetized. Block modes of induction are associated with regional anesthetics. Some of the more frequently used block methods are presented here.

Epidural (ĕp"ĭ-dū'ral) block
An anesthetic injected into the epidural space of the spinal column to anesthetize the pelvic, abdominal, or genital area.

Intercostal (ĭn"ter-kŏs'tal) block
An anesthetic injected into the intercostal nerves to prevent the conduction of nerve impulses. Intercostal nerves are located near or along the rib cage.

Saddle block
A local anesthetic injected into the area of the spine that affects the buttocks, perineum, and inner aspects of the thighs. The **perineum** (per"ĭ-nē'ŭm) is the area between the anus and genitalia. This type of anesthesia is frequently associated with childbirth.

Spinal block
A local anesthetic injected into the **subarachnoid** (sŭb"ah-răk'noid) **space** around the spinal cord. The area below the injection site is affected.

Endobronchial

The **endobronchial** (ĕn"dō-brong'kē-al) mode of induction is the administration of a gaseous mixture through a tube placed in a large bronchus. The **bronchus** (brŏng'kŭs) is one of two larger air passages to the lung beyond or below the trachea. The endobronchial mode is associated with general anesthesia.

Endotracheal

The **endotracheal** (ĕn"dō-trā'kē-al) method is the administration of a gaseous mixture through a tube placed in the **trachea** (trā'kē-ah), or windpipe. This method produces a general anesthetic condition.

Infiltration

Infiltration is the injection of anesthetic agent into tissues. This is a common way to administer a local anesthetic.

Inhalation

Inhalation is when the patient breathes in or inhales a gaseous anesthetic agent. This method is used most often with general anesthetics.

Insufflation

Insufflation (ĭn"sŭ-flā'shŭn) is the introduction of a gaseous anesthetic agent into the respiratory tract through a slender tube. It is another method of general anesthesia.

Intravenous

The **intravenous** method is the administration of an anesthetic agent into a vein by injection. This method usually indicates a general anesthesia.

Topical

The **topical** mode of induction is the application of an anesthetic agent directly to the surface of the area involved in the procedure. Topical induction does not compromise the integrity of the skin or membrane involved.

OTHER SURGICAL AND OPERATIVE TERMINOLOGY

There are several other categories of specialized surgical and operative terminology. These categories include the names of surgical positions, instruments, and incisions, as well as suture materials and techniques.

POSITION

Surgical position describes how the patient is placed on the operative or examination table. The surgeon chooses the position best suited for the procedure to be performed. The Operative Report includes the surgical position. The names of several surgical positions and when they are used are identified below. The more commonly used surgical positions are illustrated in Figure 7-2.

Position	Description
decubitus (right, left, lateral)	lying on the right or left side; position for urological procedures
dorsal (supine)	flat on back with legs extended; position for abdominal surgery
dorsal recumbent	flat on back with knees drawn up and thighs turned outward; position for vaginal procedures
Fowler	trunk raised to form a 45-degree angle, thighs also raised, pelvis at bottom of "V"
Kraske	prone on abdomen with head and foot of table dropped, buttocks raised; position for rectal surgery
lateral decubitus	on side, body elevator raised under patient, head and foot lower; position for kidney procedure
lithotomy	on back with legs in stirrups; position for obstetrics and gynecology
prone	flat on abdomen; position for back surgery
Sims'	on left side with left arm in back, resting on chest, right knee drawn up; position for rectal procedures
Trendelenburg	on back with table tilted 45 degrees toward head, bent at knees; stirrups may be used; position for pelvic surgery

INSTRUMENTS

A wide variety of instruments are used to perform surgical procedures. They are classified according to their function: cutting, grasping/holding, clamping, retracting, probing, dilating, suturing, or suctioning. Specific examples are shown in the list of Commonly Used Surgical Instruments below. Other instruments that do not fit into these classifications are referred to as accessory instruments.

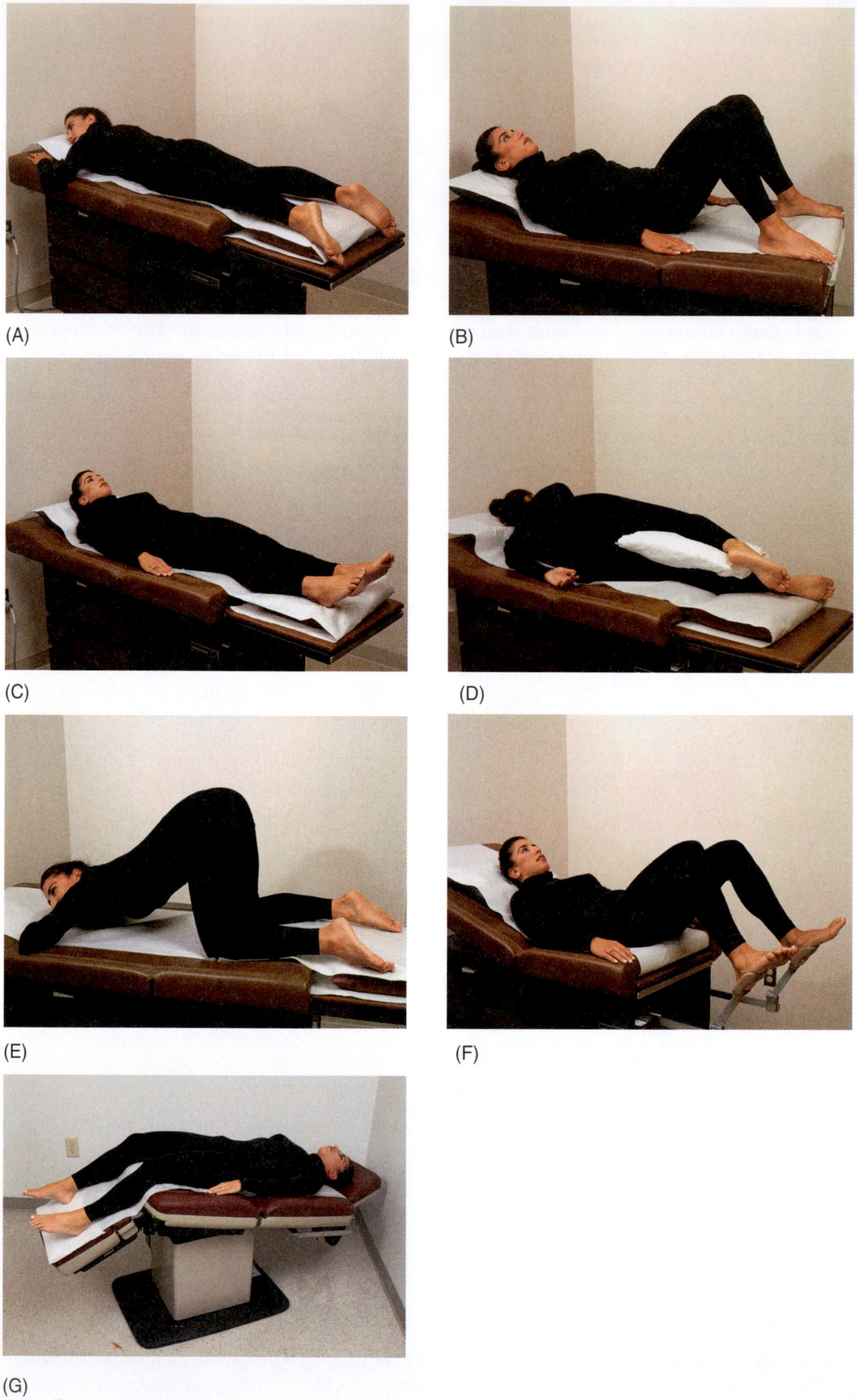

Source: Delmar/Cengage Learning

FIGURE 7-2 Surgical and Examination Positions: (A) prone; (B) dorsal recumbent; (C) supine; (D) Sims'; (E) knee-chest; (F) lithotomy; (G) Trendelenburg

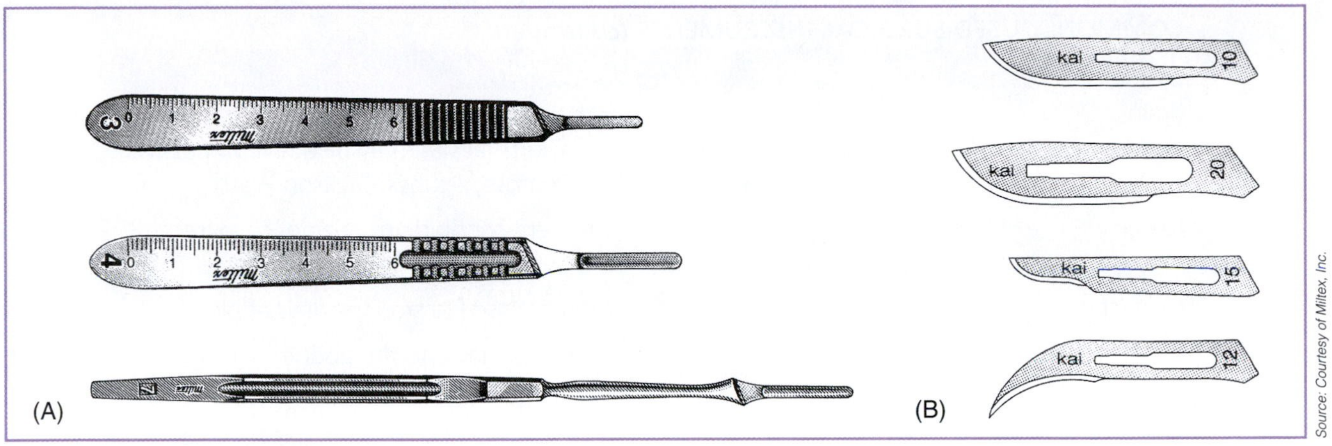

FIGURE 7-3 (A) Scalpel Handles: #3, #4, and #7; (B) Scalpel Blades: #10, #20, #15, and #12

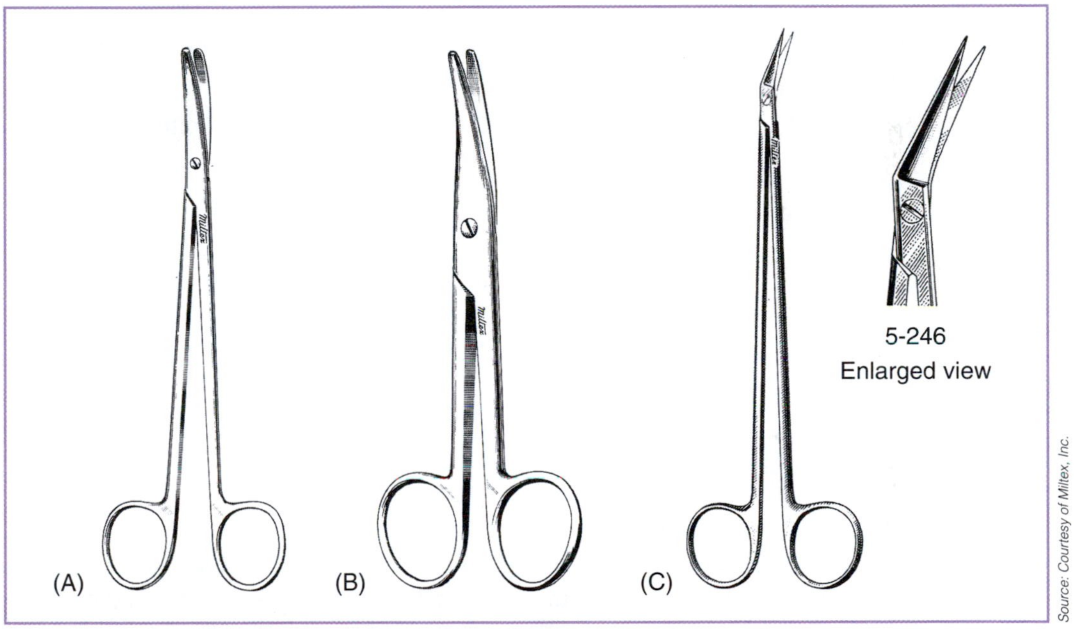

FIGURE 7-4 Scissors: (A) Metzabaum; (B) curved Mayo; (C) Potts-Smith

COMMONLY USED SURGICAL INSTRUMENTS		
Name	**Pronunciation**	**Description**
aspirator	ăs'pĭ-rā'tŏr	instrument that suctions fluid or gas
cannula	kăn'ū-lă	tube fitted with a trocar for insertion into a duct or cavity; the trocar is removed and the fluids are drained
catheter	kăth'ĕ-tĕr	tubular instrument inserted into a vessel or body cavity structure
clamp		instrument for gripping, joining, supporting, or compressing an organ or vessel
curet, curette	kū-rĕt'	spoon-shaped instrument for scraping and removing tissue
dilator	dī-lā'tōr	instrument used to enlarge an opening by stretching

continues

COMMONLY USED SURGICAL INSTRUMENTS *(continued)*		
Name	Pronunciation	Description
drains		tubes used for removal of air and/or fluids from a surgical site; may be active or passive (e.g., Penrose, T-tubes, Jackson Pratt)
forceps	fōr'cĕps	instrument for holding, seizing, or extracting tissue or organs
hemostat	hē'mō-stăt	instrument used to stop the flow of blood
insufflator	ĭn'sŭ-flā"tor	infuses CO_2 gas into the abdominal cavity for laparoscopic procedures
irrigation/aspiration units (I/A)	ăs-pĭ-rā'shŭn	device powered by nitrogen gas used to remove foreign material or tissue from a traumatic or infected wound
retractor	rē-trăk'tōr	instrument for pulling back the edges of a wound or incision
scalpel	skăl'pĕl	small, straight knife
syringes		plastic or glass devices fitted with a needle; used to irrigate wounds, aspirate fluids, or inject medications; vary in capacity from 3–60 mL (most common is 10 mL)
tenaculum	tĕ-năk'ū-lŭm	hook-like instrument for seizing and holding
trocar	trō'căr	sharply pointed instrument with cutting edges inserted in a cannula; used to penetrate a body cavity to permit drainage of the fluid

Cutting instruments are used for incision, sharp dissection, or excision and include knives, scalpels, scissors, and bone-cutting instruments. Scalpel handles come in several sizes (#3, #4, #7, and #9) and are usually not disposable (Figure 7-3A). The blades are disposable and fit a specific handle (Figure 7-3B). The #10 blade is the most frequently used. Scissors are designed for specific cutting purposes: tissue, suture, wire, or bandage/dressings (Figure 7-4).

Grasping and holding instruments are designed to stabilize fractured bone or to facilitate dissection or suturing. They vary in type and length, and the gripping surfaces may have teeth, serrations, or be smooth. Common examples include Adson, Ferris-Smith, DeBakey, Brown, Russian, Geral, Cushing bayonet forceps, Allis, Babcock, and Kocher.

Clamping instruments are designed to constrict tissue. Figure 7-5 shows finger rings and ratchets engineered to lock the instrument in place.

Retracting instruments are used to allow the surgeon to see the operative site (Figure 7-6). Sizes and shapes vary according to the surgical site. For example, wide curved retractors are used to retract abdominal walls.

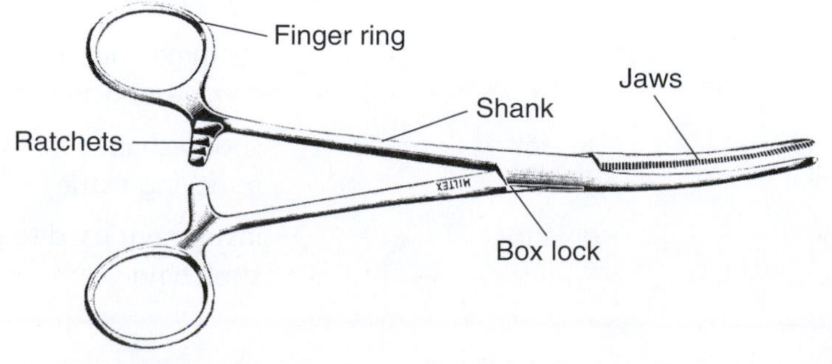

FIGURE 7-5
Clamping Instrument: clamp showing finger rings and ratchets

Source: Courtesy of Miltex, Inc.

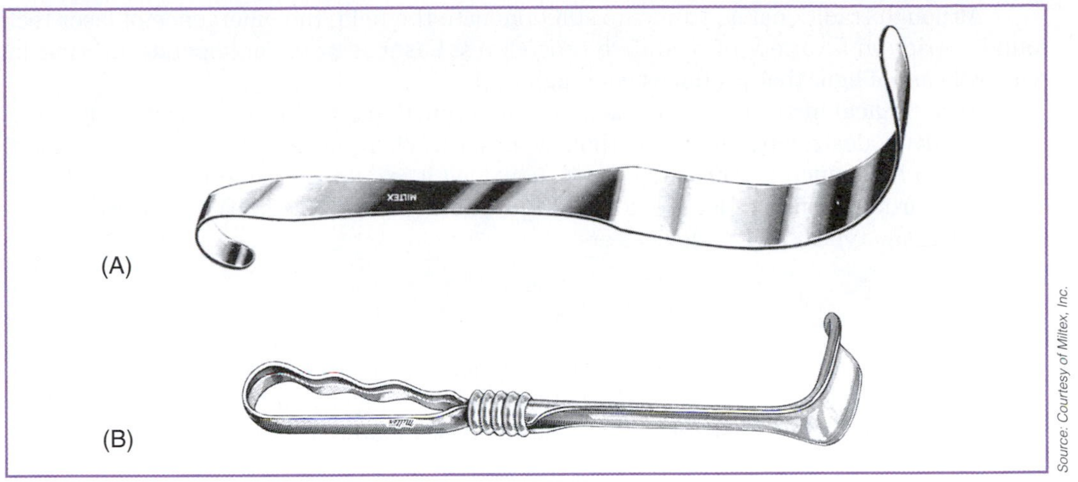

FIGURE 7-6 Retractors: (A) Deaver; (B) Richardson

Suturing instruments called needle holders are used to hold a curved suturing needle (Figure 7-7). Most holders are scissor-like clamps (A) with a ratchet or other locking device to lock the needle within the blades. The blades (B) are usually straight, but may be curved to meet special needs. For the subtle maneuvers needed for microsurgical, ophthalmic, and some vascular procedures, the holder is designed with a spring-action ratchet to protect the delicate suture needles.

Suctioning instruments remove blood and body fluids from the operative site. The suction instruments in Figure 7-8 are representative of the many standard and specialized devices available.

Other specialized equipment includes endoscopes, power tools, and lasers. Flexible endoscopes, for example, may be used before, during, or after a surgical procedure for diagnosis, biopsy, visualization, and/or repair of a structure within a body cavity. Power tools may be driven by compressed air or nitrogen, electricity, or battery and are used to cut, drill, or reshape bones. They may also be used to cut skin (grafting) or grind skin (dermabrasion).

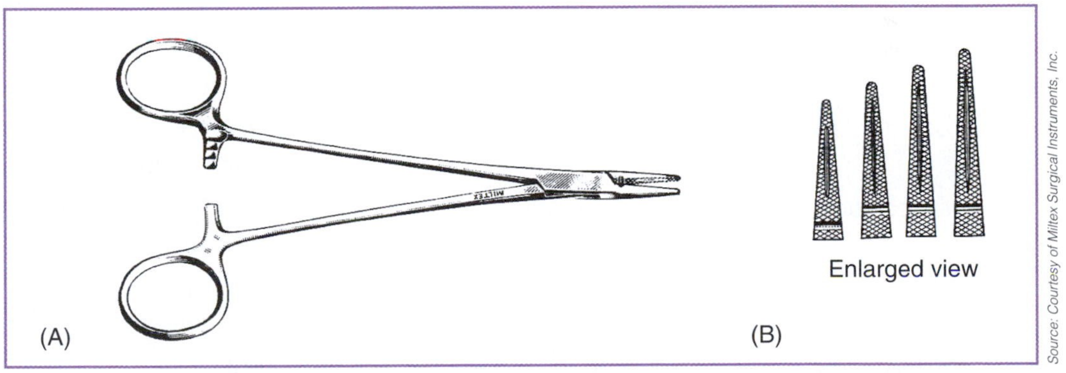

FIGURE 7-7 Needle Holder

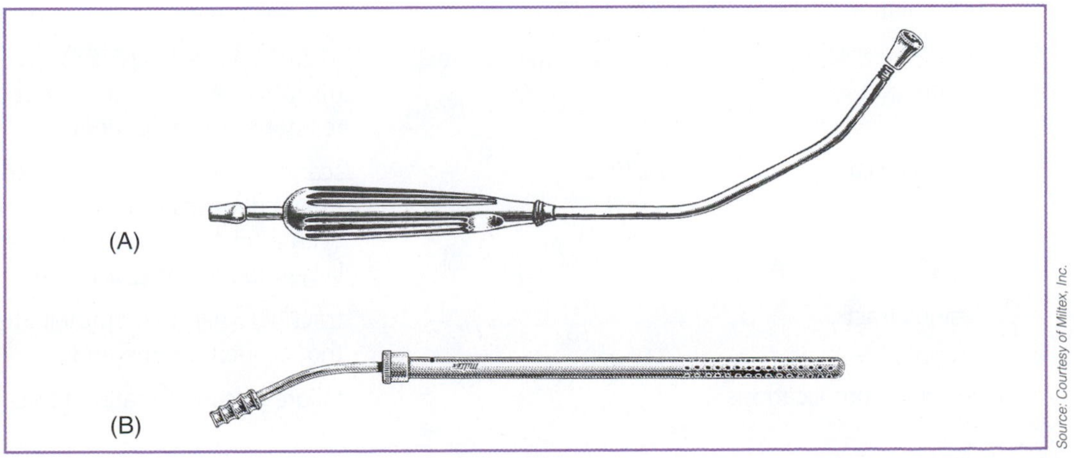

FIGURE 7-8 Suctioning Instruments: (A) Yankauer suction tip; (B) Poole suction tip

Although traditional instruments still dominate the field, the emergence of laser technology has had a profound impact on a variety of operative procedures. **Laser** instruments operate by emitting a powerful and very narrow beam of light that produces very high heat.

As a surgical instrument, the laser is a multifunctional tool that can cut, coagulate, vaporize tissue, weld, and selectively destroy pigmented pathologic tissues. When the laser beam is focused on the tissue, what it does depends on how much power is delivered, how long it is delivered, and the size of the exposed area. It can, for example, harden tissue or clot blood by **coagulation** (kō-ăg'ū-lā'-shŭn) or perform surgical cuts with very little bleeding. Some types of laser devices are

Ho:YAG	CO_2	argon
Nd:YAG	KTP	excimer

Laser technology does, however, present unique safety considerations because laser light can be harmful to skin and eyes. For this reason, both the patient and the surgical team must keep these areas adequately covered. Fire also is a real hazard, and appropriate extinguishing materials must be readily available.

TYPES OF SURGICAL INCISIONS

The surgical procedure determines the type of surgical incision. Location and direction are major considerations. A variety of factors affect the decision: procedure performed, access desired, surgeon's preferences, patient's physical condition, speed of entry required, and sites of previous surgeries. Figure 7-9 describes the location of common abdominal surgical incisions.

When tissue is traumatized by surgery or accident, a patient is vulnerable to infection and other complications. Some of the factors that influence the rate at which a wound heals are age, nutritional status, disease, use of tobacco, radiation exposure, and the condition of the patient's immune system. Other complications are listed below.

Application of the principles of sterile techniques is probably the best defense against keeping microbial counts to a minimum. The sterility of all surfaces, instruments, and personnel must be of prime concern both before and during any surgical procedure.

Complication	Pronunciation	Description
adhesion	ăd-hē'zhŭn	abnormal attachment of two surfaces that normally are separate
dehiscence	dē-hĭs'ĕns	partial or total separation of a layer or layers of tissue after closure
evisceration	ē-vĭs"ĕr-ā'shŭn	exposure of the viscera through the edges of a totally separated wound
fistula	fĭs'tū-lă	tract between two epithelium-lined surfaces that is open on both ends
hemorrhage	hĕm'ĕ-rĭj	uncontrolled bleeding
herniation	hĕr-ne-ā'shŭn	results from wound dehiscence occurring 2–3 months postoperatively
infection		microbial contamination that overrides the resistance of the patient
keloid scar	kē'lŏyd	scar composed of fibroblast (connective tissue) deposits that continue to multiply even after the wound is healed, forming large mounds of scar tissue
sinus tract		tract between two epithelium-lined surfaces that is open on one end
suture complications		failure of suture material to properly absorb

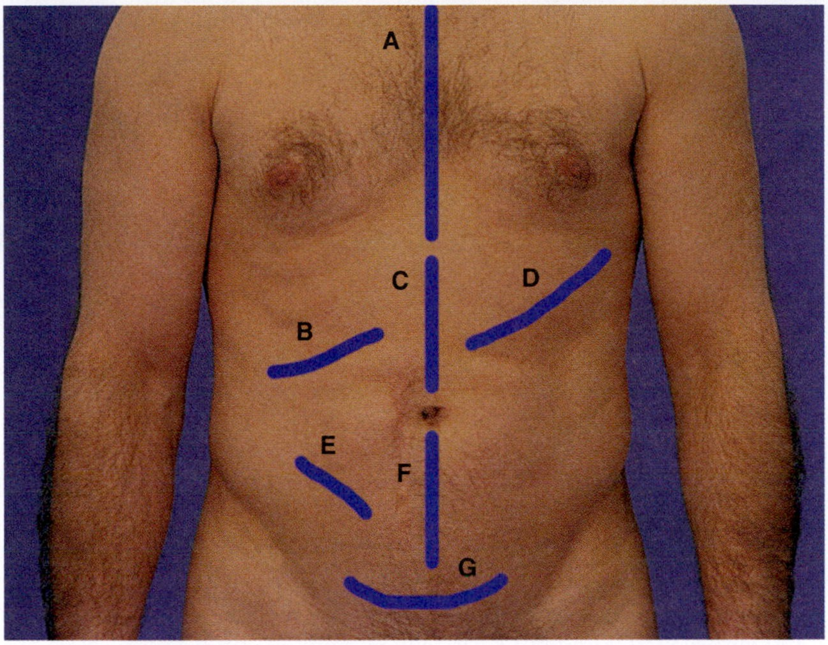

INCISION	LOCATION	ORGAN
A. Sternal Split	Begins at the top of the sternum and extends downward to the sternal notch.	Heart
B. Oblique Subcostal	Begins in the epigastric area and extends laterally and obliquely below the lower costal margin.	Right side: Gallbladder, Biliary Left side: Spleen
C. Upper Vertical Midline	Begins below the sternal notch and distally around the umbilicus.	Stomach, Duodenum, Pancreas
D. Thoracoabdominal	Begins midway between the xiphoid process and the umbilicus and extends across the seventh or eighth intercostal space to the midscapular line.	Thorax, Heart
E. McBurney	Begins below the umbilicus, goes through McBurney's point, and extends toward the right flank.	Appendix
F. Lower Vertical Midline	Begins below the umbilicus, downward toward the symphysis pubis.	Bladder, Uterus
G. Pfannenstiel	Begins 1.5 inches above the symphysis pubis with a curved transverse cut across the lower abdomen.	Uterus, Fallopian tubes, Ovaries

FIGURE 7-9 Location of Common Surgical Incisions

SUTURE MATERIALS

Suture materials are threads, wires, or other materials used to stitch parts of the body together. Some suture materials are absorbable and others are not. Absorbable material will dissolve in the body fluids and then disappear. The rate of absorption depends on the type of material used. Absorbable sutures do not have to be removed by the surgeon or physician. Nonabsorbable suture material remains intact until it is removed. Suture materials are described by size and composition, as follows.

Size

Suture material size has been standardized by governmental regulations. The thickest or largest available size is #5, about the size of commercial string. Sizes progress downward from #5 to #0 and then from #2-0 to #11-0, the smallest. This "n-0" format was chosen as a more convenient way to express the number of zeros in the finer, more delicate suture sizes. For example, suture size 0000 is written as 4-0. Suture material is available in lengths from 13 cm to 150 cm.

Composition

Natural and synthetic materials are used for sutures. Natural materials include plain catgut, surgical cotton and silk, and chromic catgut. Synthetic materials include nylon and polyester. There are many types of natural and synthetic suture materials. The surgeon chooses the type of material best suited to the tissue being sutured.

In many cases surgical staples are used to close incisions. Staples can be made of surgical steel, plastic, or a Teflon-like material. Below are some of the more commonly used suture materials.

catgut	Dexon	Nurolon	surgical cotton
chromatic catgut	Ethilon	nylon	surgical silk
Dacron	Mersilene	PDS II	Tantalum
Dermalene	Monocryl	Prolene	Vicryl
Dermalon	Novafil	stainless steel	

SUTURE TECHNIQUE

Suture technique refers to the method used to unite parts. There are two basic suturing methods: continuous and interrupted. A continuous suture runs from one end of the incision to the other without being snipped or tied between. The interrupted suture is tied and cut with each completed stitch so that each stitch is independent of any other stitch. Figure 7-10 illustrates the continuous and interrupted suture methods.

There are many types of suture techniques. Most are modifications of the continuous or interrupted methods. Suture techniques are often named for the general appearance of the suture or for the person who developed the technique. Below are some of the more interesting names of suture techniques. It is easy to imagine what these sutures look like.

baseball	chain	fish hook	pursestring
blanket	circular	mattress	sliding
button	crown	noose	zipper

Some of the more commonly used suture techniques are illustrated in Figure 7-11.

REFERENCES

This chapter presents the basic information needed to use and understand surgical terminology. For more detailed assistance, the medical secretary and surgical transcriptionist can turn to one of the many surgical word reference books available or the Internet. These sources contain listings of surgical equipment and specific information about surgical specialties.

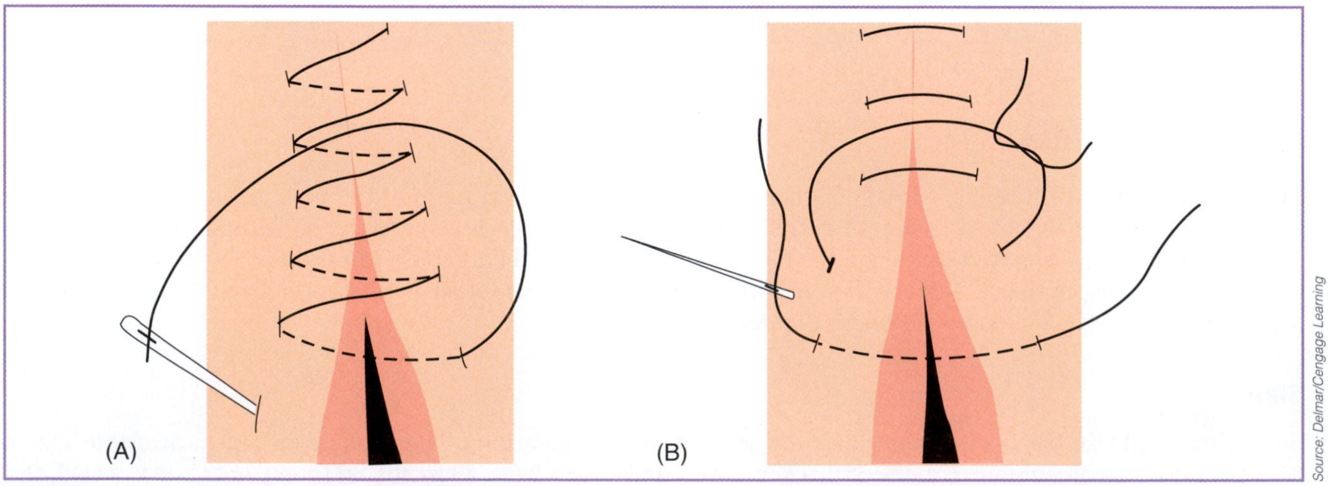

FIGURE 7-10 (A) Continuous Sutures; (B) Interrupted Sutures

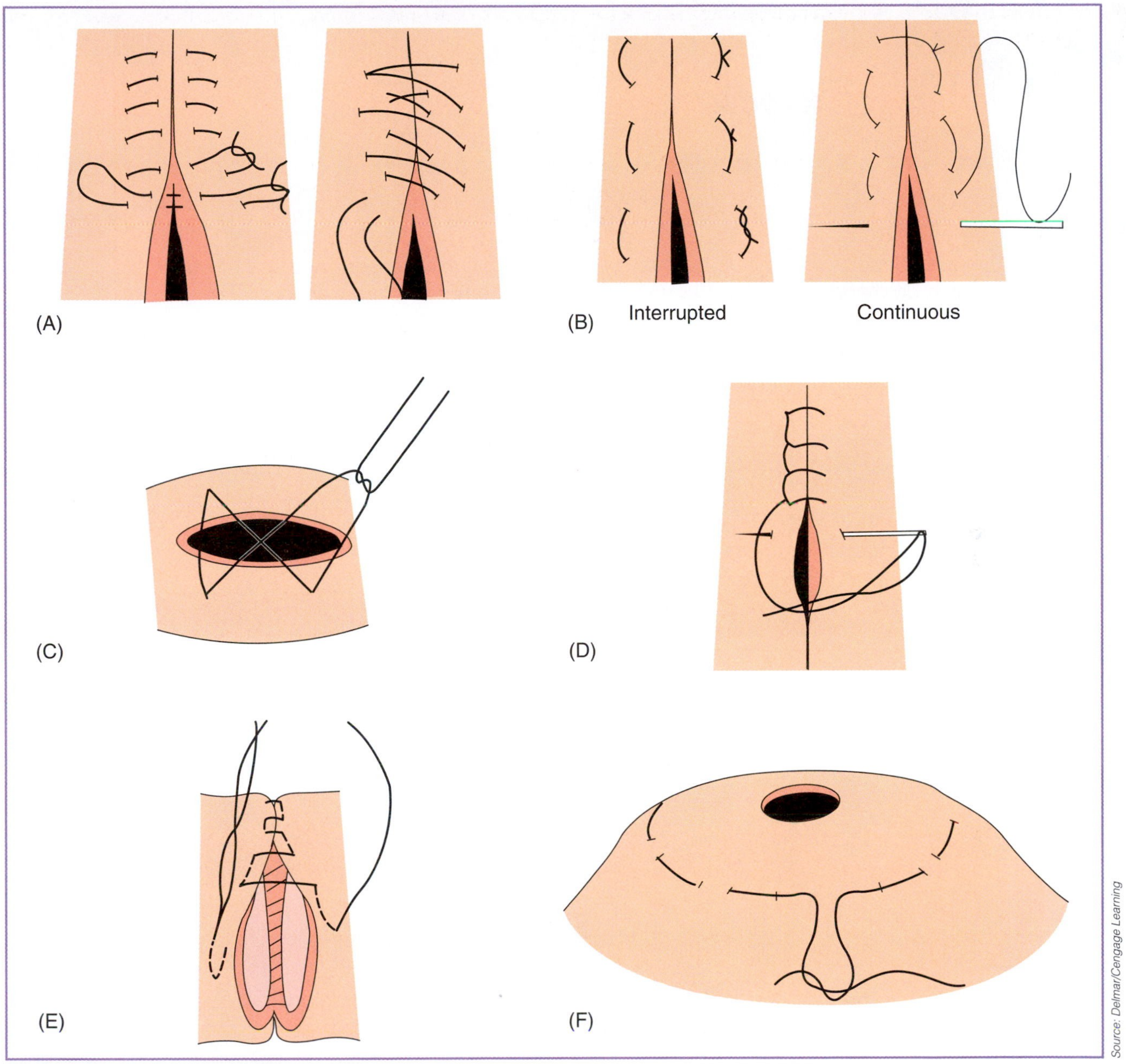

FIGURE 7-11 Commonly Used Suture Techniques: (A) vertical mattress; (B) horizontal mattress (left: interrupted; right: continuous); (C) figure-of-eight; (D) lock-stitch; (E) Connell; (F) pursestring

INTERNET ASSIGNMENT

Labtestsonline.org is a collaborative resource for individuals who want more information about clinical tests. It provides a test description, conditions and diseases for which tests are used, a screening guide including recommendation of a wide range of organizations, and much more. The site is organized by the American Association for Clinical Chemistry (AACC) in an effort to help you to better understand clinical lab tests.

ACTIVITY

Access **labtestsonline.org**. Three choices are provided: Tests, Conditions and Diseases, and Screening. Select one item in each set of choices. Summarize your results for your instructor.

Review *Surgery*

- Surgical intervention may be required to repair, correct, diagnose, or treat problems or disease processes.
- Operative Reports must be written for every surgical procedure performed and must contain information mandated by state and federal laws and other regulatory agencies.
- In addition to identifying information, an Operative Report must include Preoperative and Postoperative Diagnoses, name of the operation and indications for performing it, findings and techniques, patient's condition, and a signature block.
- The patient is usually anesthetized in one of several ways with a specific anesthetic agent.
- The patient is placed in specific positions for various surgical procedures, and the surgeon uses a multitude of instruments, including laser beams, during the procedure.
- The surgeon may select from a variety of incisions, suture techniques, and materials to close an incision appropriately.

Key Terminology Review

Word	Definition
anesthesia	loss of feeling or sensation; may be general, regional, local, or topical
anesthesiologist	physician who specializes in anesthesiology
anesthesiology	branch of medicine that studies anesthesia and anesthetic agents
anesthetic agent	drug used to induce anesthesia
anesthetist nurse	trained in administering anesthetic agents
block anesthesia	anesthetic agent injected near or along a nerve path to stop nerve impulses to the area supplied by that nerve
bronchus	one of the two larger air passages to the lungs below the trachea
coagulation	clotting of blood or hardening of tissue
endobronchial induction	administration of an anesthetic gas through a tube placed in a large bronchus
endotracheal induction	administration of an anesthetic gas through a tube placed in the trachea
epidural block	injection of anesthetic into the epidural space of the spinal column

continues

Word	Definition
field block	anesthesia produced by injecting a local anesthetic along the course of a nerve or nerves to prevent pain sensation in the area around the operative site
Findings and Technique	part of the Operative Report that includes type of anesthesia, surgical position, incision, description, closure, patient condition, and signature block
general anesthesia	anesthesia that produces loss of consciousness with an absence of pain sensation over the entire body
incision	surgical cut
Indications	part of the operative report that describes why the procedure was necessary
infiltration	injection of anesthetic into tissue
inhalation	breathing in of a gaseous anesthetic agent
insufflation	introduction of an anesthetic agent through a slender tube into the respiratory tract
intercostal block	anesthesia produced by injecting the anesthetic agent into the nerves along or near the ribs
intravenous	introduction of anesthetic agent into a vein
laser	instrument used to cut, coagulate, or vaporize tissue by way of an intense, narrow light beam that produces heat
local anesthesia	anesthetic agent confined to one specific part of the body
modes of induction	ways in which anesthetic agents are introduced into the body
nerve block	regional anesthesia that follows a nerve or group of nerves
Operation	part of the Operative Report that describes the procedure(s) performed
Operative Report	written record of a surgical procedure that contains mandated information
perineum	area between the anus and genitalia
Postoperative Diagnosis	part of the Operative Report that states the diagnosis after surgery is completed and gives a short descriptive explanation of what was actually found
Preoperative Diagnosis	part of the Operative Report that describes the diagnosis before surgery is performed
prognosis	probable outcome
regional anesthesia	anesthetic agent that interrupts nerve impulse conduction from a specific region of the body
saddle block	local anesthesia produced by injecting anesthetic into the area of the spine that affects the buttocks, perineum, and inner aspects of the thighs
spinal block	regional anesthesia produced by injecting anesthetic into the subarachnoid space around the spinal cord
subarachnoid space	space between the arachnoid and pia layers of the brain and spinal cord
subcutaneous	beneath the skin
suture materials	threads, wires, and other materials used to stitch parts of the body together
suture technique	method used to unite body parts; may be interrupted or continuous
topical anesthesia	anesthetic agent applied to the surface of the area involved in a procedure
trachea	windpipe

Key Terminology Practice Exercises

SHORT ANSWER

Supply a short answer to the following:

1. Name and define the major components of an Operative Report.

____

____

____

____

____

____

2. Name three modes of induction for general anesthesia.

____

3. Name three modes of induction for regional anesthesia.

____

4. Name two modes of induction for local anesthesia.

____

5. Identify the required items in the Findings and Technique section.

____

COMPLETION

Complete the following statements.

1. The ______________________ section of the Operative Report can be a separate paragraph or included in the main body of the report.
2. ______________________ describes how the patient was placed on the operating table.
3. A surgical cut used to access various parts of the body is called an ______________________.
4. The ______________________ and ______________________ section of the Operative Report includes a detailed and technical narrative of the entire operation.
5. ______________________ ______________________ are threads, wires, or other materials used to stitch parts of the body together.
6. The methods used to unite body parts are called ______________________.
7. A ______________________ suture runs from one end of the incision to the other.
8. An ______________________ suture is tied and cut with each completed stitch.
9. As an instrument, the ______________________ is used to cut, coagulate, or vaporize tissue.
10. The ______________________ ______________________ is an accounting for all surgical tools such as sponges, needles, and instruments.
11. A loss of consciousness and absence of pain sensation in the entire body is ______________________ ______________________.
12. Two modes of induction for general anesthesia are ______________________ and ______________________.
13. Another name for regional anesthesia is ______________________ anesthesia.
14. Anesthesia confined to one part of the body is ______________________.
15. Application of an anesthetic agent directly to the surface of the area involved in a procedure is ______________________ anesthesia.

MATCHING

Match the following definitions with the correct surgical instrument.

1. __________ small, straight knife
2. __________ hook-like instrument for seizing and holding
3. __________ instrument used to penetrate a body cavity to drain fluid
4. __________ instrument used to pull back edges of a wound or incision
5. __________ infuses CO_2 gas into abdominal cavity for laparoscopic a procedure
6. __________ instrument used to stop blood flow
7. __________ instrument used to enlarge an opening
8. __________ tube fitted with a trocar for insertion into a duct or cavity
9. __________ spoon-shaped instrument for scraping and removing tissue
10. __________ instrument for holding, seizing, and extracting tissue or organs

a. cannula
b. curette
c. dilator
d. forceps
e. hemostat
f. insufflator
g. retractor
h. scalpel
i. tenaculum
j. trocar

COMPLETION

Complete the following statements about surgical complications.

1. Exposure of viscera through the edges of a totally separated wound is ______________________.
2. Partial or total separation of layers of tissue after closure is ______________________.
3. Abnormal attachment of two surfaces that normally are separate is ______________________.
4. Open ended tract between two epithelium-lined surfaces is a ______________________.
5. Results from wound dehiscence about 2-3 months postoperative is ______________________.
6. A scar made up of fibroblast deposits that continue to multiply even after the wound is healed is a ______________________ scar.
7. Microbial contamination that overrides resistance of the patient is ______________________.

IDENTIFICATION—MATERIALS AND TECHNIQUES

Identify the following terms as suture material (M) or suture technique (T).

1. mattress ______________________
2. Mersilene ______________________
3. pursestring ______________________
4. Vicryl ______________________
5. Dacron ______________________
6. catgut ______________________
7. Monocryl ______________________
8. sliding ______________________
9. Connell ______________________
10. lock-stitch ______________________

IDENTIFICATION

Identify the following surgical positions.

1. flat on back with legs extended ______________________
2. flat on abdomen; position for back surgery ______________________
3. lying on back with table tilted toward the head, bent at knees ______________________

4. lying on right or left side ______________________
5. lying on back with legs in stirrups ______________________

SPELLING

Rewrite the misspelled words.

1. anestethist ______________________
2. epidural ______________________
3. currete ______________________
4. dialator ______________________
5. hemostat ______________________
6. scalple ______________________
7. insuflation ______________________
8. coagulation ______________________
9. intravenus ______________________
10. perineum ______________________

Word Element Review

Root	Meaning	Example	Definition
esthesi/o	feeling, sensation	**esthesiogenic** (es-thē"zē-ō-jĕn'ik)	producing sensation
Prefix	**Meaning**	**Example**	**Definition**
ant-, anti-	against	**antiemetic** (ăn"tĭ-ē-mĕt'ĭk)	medication that prevents or alleviates vomiting
hyper-	above, more than	**hyperemia** (hī"per-ē'mē-ah)	excess blood in a part
pro-	before, in front of, favoring	**proptosis** (prŏp-tō'sĭs)	forward displacement or bulging
Suffix	**Meaning**	**Example**	**Definition**
-cele	hernia	**cystocele** (sĭs'tō-cēl)	protrusion of the bladder through the vaginal wall
-centesis	puncture and aspiration of	**thoracentesis** (thŏ"rah-sĕn-tē'sĭs)	surgical puncture of chest wall for aspiration of fluids
-desis	binding, fixation	**arthrodesis** (ăr"thrō-dē'sĭs)	surgical fusion of a joint
-ectomy	surgical removal, excision	**gastrectomy** (găs-trĕk'tō-mē)	surgical removal of the stomach or a portion of it

continues

Suffix	Meaning	Example	Definition
-lysis	breakdown, destruction, loosening, setting free	**hemolysis** (hē-mŏl'ĭ-sĭs)	destruction of red blood cells with the setting free of hemoglobin
-oid	like, resembling	**dermoid** (der'moid)	skin-like
-oma	tumor, neoplasm	**carcinoma** (kar"sĭ-nō'mah)	malignant new growth or tumor
-ostomy	creation of a new opening	**colostomy** (kŏ-lŏs'tō-mē)	surgical creation of a new opening between the colon and the body surface
-otomy	incision into	**gastrotomy** (găs-trŏt'tō-mē)	incision into the stomach
-pexy	surgical fixation	**hysteropexy** (hĭs'ter-ō-pĕk"sē)	surgical fixation of a displaced uterus
-plasty	surgical correction or repair	**arthroplasty** (ăr'thrō-plăs"tē)	surgical repair of a joint
-rrhaphy	suture of	**herniorrhaphy** (her"nē-ōr'ah-fē)	surgical repair of a hernia, with suturing
-rrhexis	break, burst forth, rupture	**angiorrhexis** (ăn"jē-ō-rĕk'sĭs)	rupture of a blood vessel
-tripsy	crushing, friction	**lithotripsy** (lĭth'ō-trĭp"sē)	crushing of a stone within the bladder or urethra

Word Element Practice Exercises

MATCHING

Match the terms to their meanings.

1. __________ surgical fixation of a displaced uterus
2. __________ creation of a new opening between the colon and the body surface
3. __________ destruction of red blood cells with the setting free of hemoglobin
4. __________ skin-like
5. __________ forward placement or bulging
6. __________ suture of a hernia
7. __________ excision of the stomach or a portion of it
8. __________ rupture of a blood vessel
9. __________ surgical puncture of the chest wall for aspiration of fluids

a. angiorrhexis
b. antiemetic
c. arthrodesis
d. arthroplasty
e. carcinoma
f. colostomy
g. cystocele
h. dermoid
i. esthesiogenic
j. gastrectomy
k. gastrotomy

10. __________ malignant new growth or tumor
11. __________ excess blood in a part
12. __________ crushing of a stone in the bladder or urethra
13. __________ protrusion of the bladder through the vaginal wall
14. __________ incision into the stomach
15. __________ surgical repair of a joint
16. __________ surgical fusion of a joint
17. __________ medication that prevents or eliminates vomiting
18. __________ producing a feeling or sensation

l. hemolysis
m. herniorrhaphy
n. hyperemia
o. hysteropexy
p. lithotripsy
q. proptosis
r. thoracentesis

WORD ELEMENTS AND DEFINITIONS

In the underlined words below, circle the word element presented in this chapter. Then provide the definition of the word.

1. The patient is scheduled for a <u>gastrotomy</u> tomorrow.

   ____

2. The <u>arthroplasty</u> of her knee allowed her to walk without crutches.

   ____

3. A <u>proptosis</u> of the eye can be corrected by surgery.

   ____

4. We hope the problem will be solved after the patient's scheduled <u>arthrodesis</u>.

   ____

5. <u>Hyperemia</u> was caused by additional swelling around the elastic bandage wrap.

   ____

6. An <u>antiemetic</u> was given after the chemotherapy session.

   ____

7. The surgeon found evidence of a <u>carcinoma</u> in the upper abdomen.

   ____

SPELLING

Rewrite the misspelled words.

1. herniorhaphy ______________________
2. angiorrexis ______________________
3. lithotripsy ______________________
4. cystosele ______________________
5. colostomy ______________________
6. dermoyd ______________________

WORD ELEMENT MEANINGS

Give the meaning of each word element. Then use your dictionary to find a new word that contains each of the word elements. Specify whether the new word is a noun or an adjective by placing N or A in the last column.

Word Element	Meaning	Word	N or A
1. anti-, ant-	________	________	________
2. -cele	________	________	________
3. -centesis	________	________	________
4. -desis	________	________	________
5. -ectomy	________	________	________
6. esthesi/o	________	________	________
7. hyper-	________	________	________
8. -lysis	________	________	________
9. -oid	________	________	________
10. -oma	________	________	________
11. -ostomy	________	________	________
12. -otomy	________	________	________
13. -pexy	________	________	________
14. -plasty	________	________	________
15. pro-	________	________	________
16. -rrhaphy	________	________	________
17. -rrhexis	________	________	________
18. -tripsy	________	________	________

Dictionary Exercises

DICTIONARY EXERCISE 1

Use your dictionary to find the pronunciation and definition of the following words.

Word	Pronunciation	Definition
1. ampulla	________	________
2. anastomosis	________	________
3. aponeurosis	________	________
4. bifurcation	________	________

5. cautery	__________	__________
6. cicatrix	__________	__________
7. cruciate	__________	__________
8. electrocoagulation	__________	__________
9. enucleation	__________	__________
10. exudate	__________	__________
11. fulguration	__________	__________
12. imbricated	__________	__________
13. intubation	__________	__________
14. microinstrumentation	__________	__________
15. peritoneum	__________	__________

DICTIONARY EXERCISE 2

Pronunciation of the words below is provided. Using your dictionary, find the correct spelling and definition of each word.

	Word	Pronunciation	Definition
1.	__________	ā'pĕks	__________
2.	__________	ăs'pĭ-rāt	__________
3.	__________	kah-rī'nah	__________
4.	__________	kŏl'oyd	__________
5.	__________	ĕn-kăp"sū-lā'shŭn	__________
6.	__________	fĭm'brē-āt-ĕd	__________
7.	__________	ĭn-sī'tū	__________
8.	__________	ĭn'dū-rāt"ĕd	__________
9.	__________	lī-gā'shŭn	__________
10.	__________	loo'mĕn	__________
11.	__________	lī'sĭs	__________
12.	__________	rē-flĕk'shŭn	__________
13.	__________	sā'lēn	__________
14.	__________	sē-rō'sah	__________
15.	__________	sē'rŭs	__________

DICTIONARY EXERCISE 3

Look up the meaning of each italicized word. Write the pronunciation in the space provided. Then rewrite the sentence in your own words.

1. The bleeder was *clamped* and *ligated* (____________________).

   ____

2. Several skin conditions can be treated with *cryotherapy* (____________________).

   ____

3. The surgeon was able to remove the growth *en bloc* (____________________).

____

4. A *freely movable mass* was identified during exploratory surgery.

____

5. During the colonoscopy, the lining of the colon was very *friable* (____________________).

____

6. *Hemostasis* (____________________) was secured.

____

7. Adhesions were removed by *blunt* and *sharp dissection* (____________________).

____

8. The *Scultetus bandage* (____________________) was best suited for the wound.

____

9. *Ligatures* (____________________) are used by surgeons and orthodontists.

____

10. Dilation and *curettage* (____________________) are used to remove tumors.

____

11. The tumor cells were *undifferentiated* (____________________).

____

12. There are *tumor markers* for specific proteins, antigens, genes, hormones, or enzymes, but they are not 100% accurate.

____

13. A surgical procedure may be classified as *curative* (____________________).

____

14. Jamming a knee or finger will result in *somatic* pain (____________________).

____

15. Salicylates, acetaminophen, and NSAIDs are *nonopioid* (____________________) drugs.

____

*Study*WARE™ Connection

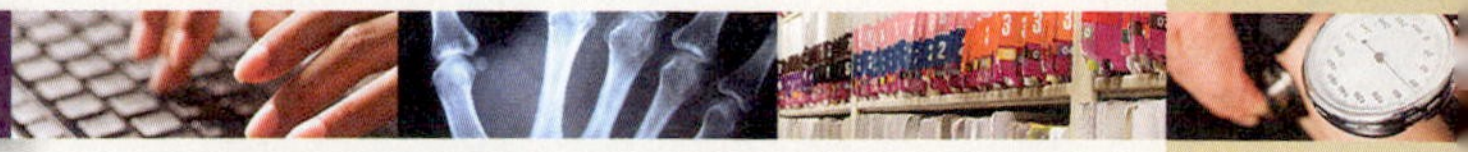

To take a practice quiz or play interactive games that reinforce the content in this chapter, go to your StudyWARE™ CD-ROM.

Listening Exercise

INSTRUCTIONS

1. Review the spelling, pronunciation, and meaning of the words provided in the preview.
2. Go to your StudyWARE™ CD-ROM and listen to **Listening Exercise 7-1**. Fill in the blank in the report as the word is dictated.
3. At the end of the activity, check your spelling against the preview words. They appear in the preview in the order in which they are encountered in the activity.
4. Review and practice the words you missed.
5. Look up words that are not familiar.

PREVIEW OF WORDS FOR LISTENING EXERCISE 7-1

Word	Pronunciation	Meaning
hyperalimentation	hī"pĕr-ăl"ĭ-mĕn-tā'shŭn	intravenous infusion of fluids to augment or substitute for nutritional requirements of patients with severe absorption problems in the GI tract
Xylocaine	zī'lō-kāne	anesthetic agent to sterilize surgical site
Trendelenburg	trĕn-dĕl'ĕn-bŭrg	surgical position in which patient's head is low and the body and legs are on an elevated and inclined plane
fluoroscopic	floŏ"or-ō-skŏp'ĭc	pertaining to the use of an x-ray device that allows the surgeon to visualize on a screen the internal area in which the procedure is being done
clavicle	klăv'ĭ-k'l	collarbone
lumen	lū'mĕn	space within a tube, artery, vein, or intestine. In this case, the catheter has a single entrance.

Listening Exercise 7-1

StudyWARE™ Connection

Listen to this report being read on your StudyWARE™ CD-ROM. Fill in each blank as the word is dictated.

OPERATIVE NOTE

DATE OF PROCEDURE: 8/21/20—

PROCEDURE

1. Placement of Hickman catheter for ____________________ and hydration.

SURGEON: Dr. Sean O'Shancy

ANESTHESIA: Versed 3.5 mg, Demerol 50 mg IV, 1% ____________________ with epinephrine.

INDICATIONS: This is a 65-year-old female with short bowel syndrome who needed intravenous access for IV fluids and hyperalimentation. She had a port removed recently because of persistent infection.

FINDINGS: Normal anatomy, no difficulty in entering the left internal jugular vein.

PROCEDURE: After usual prep and drape, the left internal jugular area was infiltrated with Xylocaine with the patient in ____________________ position. The needle was introduced into the internal jugular vein without difficulty and a J-wire threaded under guidance. A small incision was made by the J-wire entrance site and subsequently a counter incision was made near the left breast medially about 15 cm below the ____________________. A tunnel was developed and a single-Hickman by Bard with Vitacath was advanced through the tunnel. Venous dilator and introducer were placed around the J-wire through the superior vena cava and the catheter, which was cut to an appropriate length, was then threaded under fluoroscopic guidance. After position of the catheter, the neck site was closed with 3-0 nylon vertical mattress suture. The catheter was secured with 3-0 nylon tied in a Chinese fingertrap fashion. Betadine ointment was applied to the exit site and dressing was applied. A chest x-ray was ordered.

Signature ____________________

Sean O'Shancy, MD

CHAPTER 8

The Cardiovascular System

"Everywhere he feels his heart because its vessels run to all limbs."

—Anonymous

OBJECTIVES

When you have completed this study of the cardiovascular system, you should be able to

1. Spell and define major system components and explain how they operate.
2. Identify the meaning of related word elements.
3. Spell and define diagnostic procedures, diagnoses, treatment procedures, and abbreviations.
4. Spell the names of commonly used medications.
5. Use a dictionary as a tool in processing medical documents.
6. Hear how medical terminology is used in actual medical reports.

INTRODUCTION

Blood travels through a closed circular system referred to as the cardiovascular system, which is composed of the heart and blood vessels or vascular network. Blood continuously travels through the heart, into the arteries and their smaller branches, then to the capillaries, into the branches of the vein structure, and back to the heart. The heart serves as the pump that keeps the blood moving. A physician who specializes in the study of the heart is a cardiologist.

HEART

The heart is one of the strongest organs in the human body. It does an incredible amount of work during a person's life span. With an average 70 to 80 beats per minute, the heart will beat more than 2.5 *billion* times in seventy years. An adult heart pumps about 4,000 gallons of blood a day. Most people do not even recognize this activity as a strenuous one.

COMPOSITION

aort/o	aorta	pericardi/o	pericardium
atri/o	atrium	steth/o	chest
brady-	slow	tachy-	fast, rapid
cardi/o	heart	valv/o, valvul/o	valve
coron/o	heart	ventricul/o	ventricle
-megaly	enlargement		

The heart is a muscular organ slightly bigger than a fist. It is located between the lungs, somewhat to the left of the midline of the body.

As shown in Figure 8-1, there are actually three layers in the heart wall. The first is the **endocardium** (ĕn"dō-kăr'dē-ŭm) (1), which is the membrane that lines the interior of the heart. It is also the material that forms the valves of the heart. The second and thickest layer is the **myocardium** (mī"ō-kăr'dē-ŭm) (2), which is the muscle of the heart. The third and outermost layer is the **epicardium** (ĕp"ĭ-kăr'dē-ŭm) (4). The heart itself is surrounded by the **pericardial** (pĕr"ĭ-kăr'dē-ăl) **sac** (3), whose lining is called the **pericardium** (pĕr"ĭ-kăr'dē-ŭm). In the space between the pericardium and the epicardium there is a small amount of lubricating fluid.

Physicians sometimes refer to the left and right heart because the heart is responsible for two specific types of circulation. The left heart is involved in systemic circulation, which is the movement of blood from the heart to all parts of the body and back to the heart. The right heart is involved in pulmonary circulation, which is the movement of blood from the heart to the lungs and back to the heart.

Imagine the left and right sides of the heart as back-to-back pumps that beat or function as one. The two sides are completely separated by a partition called the **septum** (sĕp'tŭm). Note in Figure 8-2 that the upper part of the partition is called the **interatrial** (ĭn"ter-ā'trē-ăl) **septum** (8), and the lower portion is called the **interventricular** (ĭn"ter-vĕn-trĭk'ū-lăr) **septum** (9). The septum prevents the blood in the two sides of the heart from mixing. In fact, to get from one side of the heart to the other, blood must go through the entire body.

Each side of the heart has two chambers or sections. One is a receiving chamber and the other is a pumping chamber. The **left atrium** (ā'trē-ŭm) (4), one of the upper chambers of the heart, receives blood high in oxygen

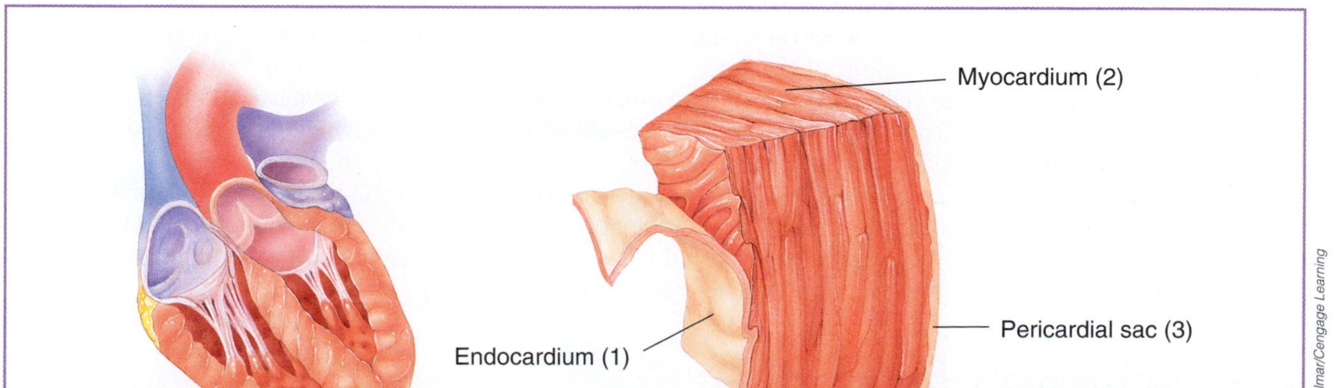

FIGURE 8-1 Layers of the Heart Wall

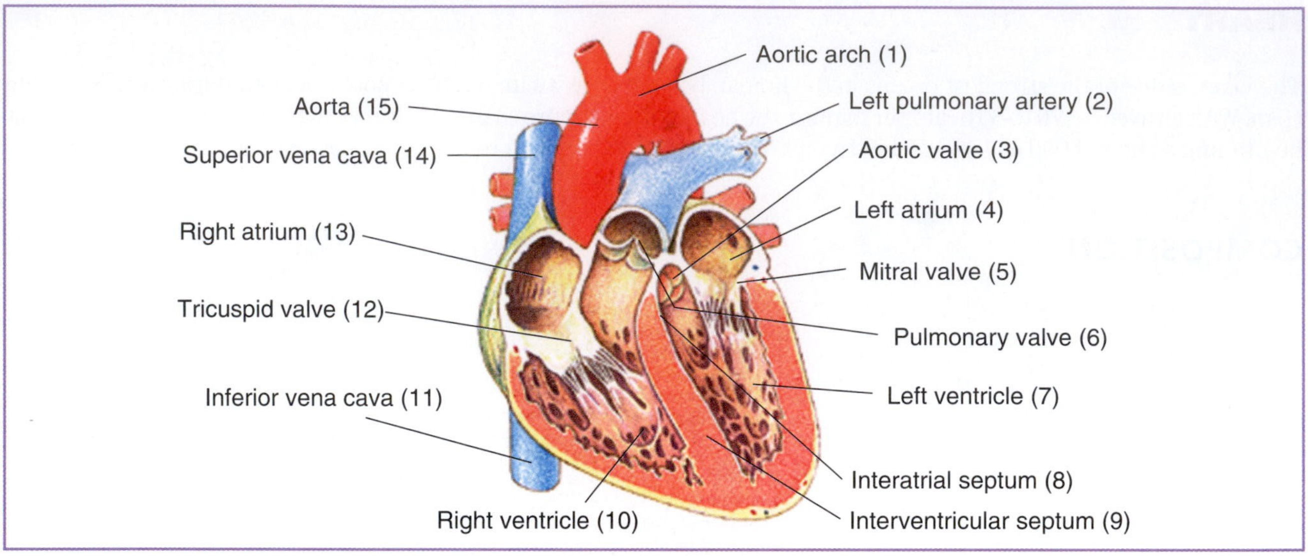

Source: Delmar/Cengage Learning

FIGURE 8-2 A Section of the Heart

content as it returns from the lungs by way of the pulmonary veins. The pulmonary vein is the only vein that carries oxygen-rich blood. The blood then moves to the lower chamber or **left ventricle** (vĕn'trĭ-k'l) (7)—which has the thickest walls of all the chambers—where newly oxygenated blood is pumped to all parts of the body.

Blood leaves the left ventricle and goes through the arteries via the **aorta** (ā-or'tah) (15), called the great artery. The aorta curves in a great aortic arch (1) up from the heart, down the spine, and into the abdomen. From there several smaller arterial systems carry the blood to the head, digestive organs, arms, legs, and other body parts, where it discharges its load of nutrients and oxygen.

The blood then collects carbon dioxide and castoffs from cells and flows into the venules. From there it makes its way back to the heart through the two largest veins of the body called **venae cavae** (vē'nē kā'vē). The **superior vena cava** (vē'nah kā'vah) (14) drains blood from the upper part of the body, and the **inferior vena cava** (11) carries blood from the lower part of the body. Both drain this "used" blood into the upper chamber of the heart or **right atrium** (13). The blood next moves into the lower chamber or **right ventricle** (10), which contracts to send the deoxygenated blood to the **pulmonary** (pul'mō-nĕr"ē) **artery** (2). The pulmonary artery takes the blood back to the lungs, where it absorbs fresh oxygen. This whole process, which takes about one minute, then starts all over.

Each pumping chamber, or ventricle, has two valves, one at the entrance and one at the exit. The purpose of the valves is to seal the chambers tightly so that contracting muscles have something to work against. The valves also prevent a backflow of blood.

The **tricuspid** (trī-kŭs'pĭd) **valve** (12) at the entrance to the right ventricle prevents blood from returning to the right atrium. When the right ventricle has finished emptying, the **pulmonary valve** (6) closes to prevent blood pumped out to the lungs from returning to the right ventricle. On the other side of the heart, muscles of the powerful left ventricle begin their contraction, and the **mitral** (mī'trăl) **valve** (5), made of two heavy flaps, closes the chamber's entrance to keep blood from returning to the left atrium. At the end of the contraction, the **aortic valve** (3) closes to prevent the backflow of the enriched aortic blood.

Abnormal heart sounds are called murmurs. Often **murmurs** are caused by faulty valve action such as failure to close tightly so that blood will not seep back into a chamber. Another condition giving rise to an abnormal sound is the narrowing, or **stenosis** (stĕ-nō'sĭs), of a valve orifice.

Many conditions can cause abnormal heart sounds. These sounds, which can be heard with a stethoscope, might be caused by congenital defects, disease, or physiological variation. An abnormal sound caused by a structural change in the heart or the vessels connected with the heart is called an organic murmur. A functional murmur is one that does not necessarily involve an abnormality in the heart structure.

WORK OF THE HEART

Although the right and left sides of the heart are completely separate, they work together. The blood is squeezed through the chambers by a contraction of heart muscle, first in the thin-walled upper chambers (the atria) and then in the thick muscle of the lower chambers (the ventricles). The right and left atria contract together; then the right and left ventricles contract together.

The active phase of contraction, or pumping, is called **systole** (sĭs'tō-lē), and is followed immediately by a short resting period known as **diastole** (dī-ăs'tō-lē). The contraction of the walls of the atria is completed as the contraction of the ventricles begins. Thus, the resting phase begins in the atria at the same time the contraction begins in the ventricles.

Although the heart muscle is capable of contracting in rhythm independent of outside control, impulses from the nervous system are required to cause a beat rapid enough to maintain circulation effectively. The normal heartbeat range for an adult is usually 60 to 100 beats per minute and is referred to as the **pulse rate**.

StudyWARE™ Connection

Play an interactive game labeling structures of the **Heart** on your StudyWARE™ CD-ROM.

CONDUCTION SYSTEM OF THE HEART

Specialized masses of tissue in the heart wall form the conduction system of the heart to regulate the order of events. Two of these specialized masses are called nodes, and the third is a branching structure called the **atrioventricular bundle**.

Figure 8-3 shows the **sinoatrial** (sĭ"nō-ā'trē-al) **node** (SA) (1) in the upper wall of the right atrium. Its function is to act as a pacemaker. The second node is called the **atrioventricular** (ā"trē-ō-vĕn-trĭk'ū-lar) **node** (AV) (2) and is located at the septum at the junction between the interatrial portion and the interventricular portion.

The atrioventricular bundle, or the **bundle of His** (hĭss) (4), is located in the interventricular septum, with branches extending to all parts of the ventricle walls.

The order in which the impulses travel through the heart is as follows.

1. The beginning of the heartbeat is in the sinoatrial node (1), the pacemaker.
2. The excitation wave travels throughout the muscles of the atria (3 and 7), causing them to contract.

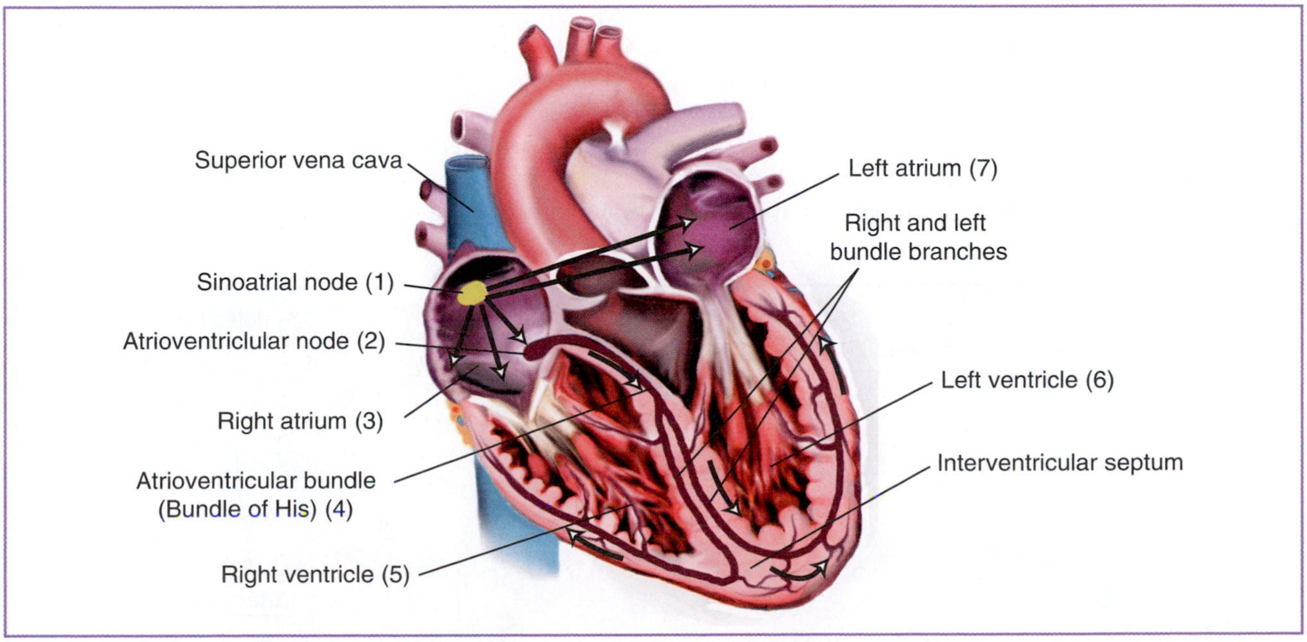

Source: Delmar/Cengage Learning

FIGURE 8-3 Conduction System of the Heart

3. The atrioventricular node (2) is stimulated next and transmits a wave to the bundle of His (4) with a rapid spread to all parts of the ventricle walls (5 and 6).
4. The entire ventricular musculature then contracts—practically all at once.

All of these events happen without conscious thought or action. It is easy to see why the function of the heart is so critical to the effective operation of the cardiovascular system.

StudyWARE™ Connection

Go to your StudyWARE™ CD-ROM to watch an animation of the conduction system of the heart.

VASCULAR SYSTEM

When the blood leaves the heart, it enters the vascular system. This system is composed of a variety of vessels that transport the blood to all parts of the body, provide for the exchange of certain substances between the blood and body fluids, and eventually return the blood to the heart. Physicians who specialize in surgical procedures performed on veins and arteries are called cardiovascular surgeons.

TYPES OF BLOOD VESSELS

angi/o	blood vessel	phleb/o	vein
arter/o, arteri/o	artery	thromb/o	clot, lump
ather/o	yellowish plaque, fatty substance	vascul/o, vas/o	vessel
furc/o	division, fork	ven/o	vein

On the basis of function, blood vessels may be divided into three groups: arteries, capillaries, and veins, as illustrated in Figure 8-4. **Arteries** (2) (with the exception of the pulmonary artery) carry oxygen-rich blood from the pumping chambers of the heart to the organs and other parts of the body. The pulmonary artery carries deoxygenated blood from the right ventricle of the heart to the lungs. The arteries have the thickest walls and are composed of three layers. These are the **intima** (ĭn'tĭ-mah) (or endothelium), the smooth innermost surface; a bulky layer of involuntary muscle called the **media**; and an outer tunic of supporting connective tissue called the **adventitia** (ăd"vĕn-tĭsh'ē-ah).

The arterial system starts with the aorta. It is the largest artery, with a diameter of about one inch, and also has the thickest wall. Arteries branch and rebranch throughout the body and become smaller and smaller. The smallest subdivision, the **arterioles** (ar-tē'rē-ōls) (1), have thinner walls with little connective tissue and more muscle.

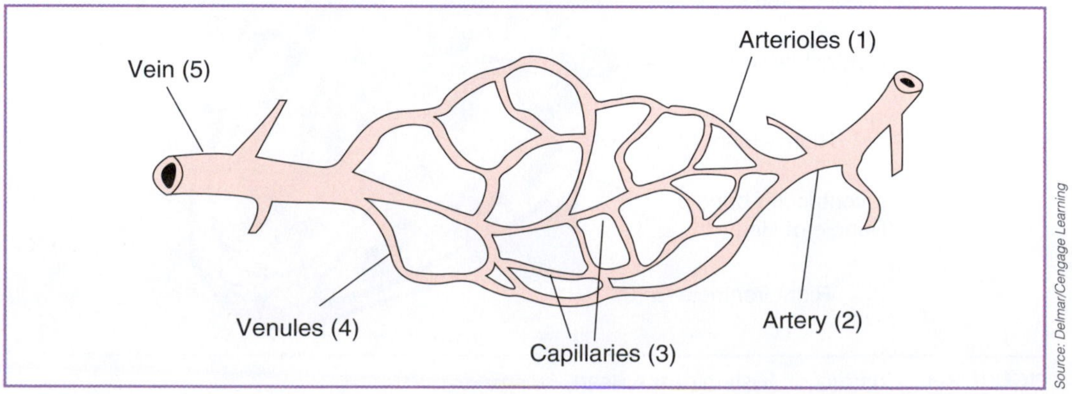

FIGURE 8-4 Types of Blood Vessels

The microscopic branches of these tiny connecting vessels, **capillaries** (3), have the thinnest walls of any vessels—only one cell layer. Because of this thinness, exchanges between the blood and the body cells are possible. During the outbound pass of arterial blood, oxygen leaves the blood and passes freely through these thin capillary walls to enter body cells.

On the return, capillaries drain waste products from tissues into **venules** (vĕn'ūls) (4), the smallest veins. Venules are formed by the union of capillaries; their walls are only slightly thicker than those of the capillaries. Venules then join to form **veins** (5). With the exception of the pulmonary vein, veins carry deoxygenated blood back to the heart. The pulmonary vein carries oxygen-rich blood from the lungs to the left atrium. Like arteries, veins have three layers. They are much thinner than arteries and collapse easily. Therefore, only slight pressure by a tumor or some other mass may interfere with the return blood flow. Essentially arteries and veins are a long, continuous tube, with the capillaries being the smallest portion.

Systemic Arteries

All arteries, carrying oxygen-rich blood, branch from the aorta. In Figure 8-5 is the aortic arch (3), which gives rise to the right innominate (ĭ-nŏm'ĭ-nāt) (brachiocephalic) (19), carotid (kah-rŏt'ĭd) (20 and 1), and left subclavian (sŭb-klā'vē-ăn) (18 and 2) arteries. The next section of the descending aorta is the **thoracic** (thō-răs'ĭk) **aorta** (4), located from the arch to the level of the diaphragm. The thoracic aorta consists of nine or ten pairs of intercostal arteries that reach between the ribs, sending branches to the muscles and other structures of the chest wall.

Below the thoracic section and extending downward to the common iliac is the **abdominal aorta** (15) section. This is the longest aortic section and spans the abdominal cavity. Branches of the abdominal aorta may be unpaired or paired. The unpaired vessels have three important parts: the celiac (sē'lē-ăk) (17) trunk, the superior mesenteric (mĕs"ĕn-tĕr'ĭk) (16) artery, and the inferior mesenteric (6) artery. The paired branches are the phrenic (frĕn'ĭk), suprarenal, renal, ovarian or testicular, and lumbar arteries. (These are smaller arteries and are not shown in the drawing.)

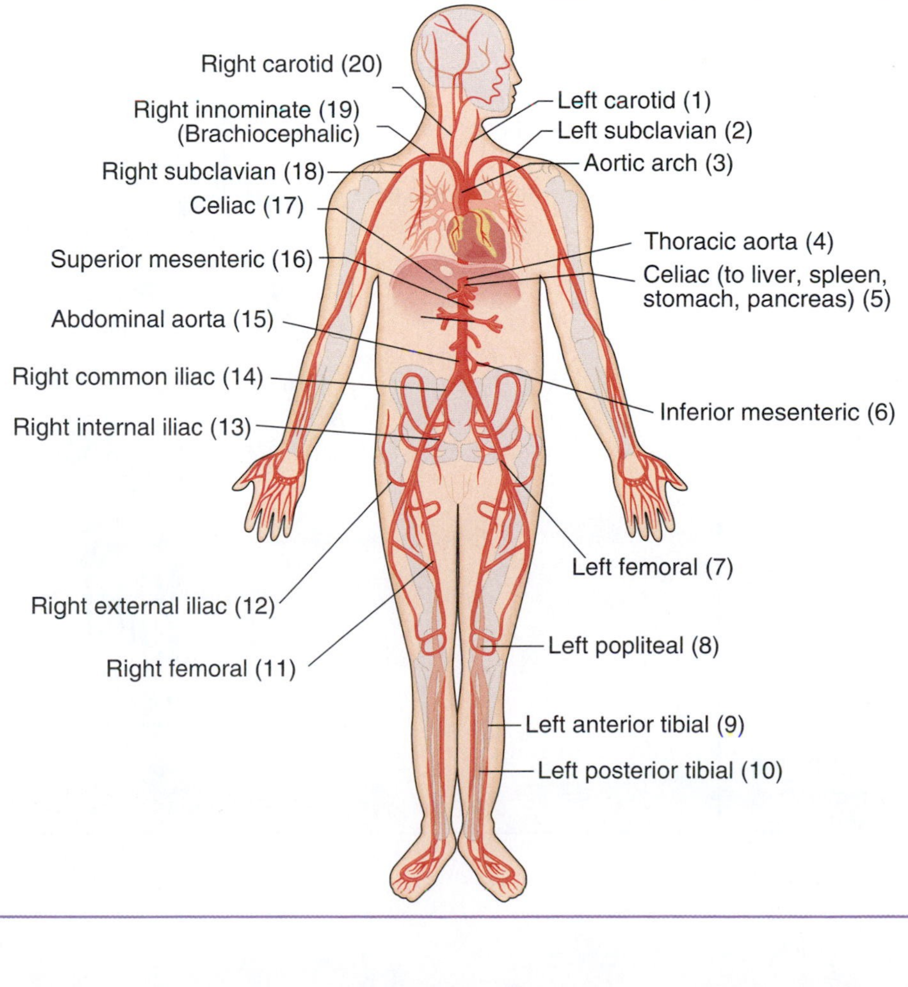

FIGURE 8-5
Major Arteries of the Body

Source: Delmar/Cengage Learning

The abdominal aorta finally divides into two common iliac (14) arteries. Each extends into the pelvis and subdivides into the internal (13) and external (12) iliac arteries. The internal iliac vessels send branches to the pelvic organs, including the urinary bladder, rectum, and some reproductive organs. The external iliac arteries continue into the thigh, where the name of these tubes is changed to femoral (fĕm'or-ăl) arteries (7 and 11). These vessels branch off in the thigh at the level of the knee and become the popliteal (pŏp-lĭt'ē-ăl) (8) arteries. Below the knee they further subdivide into the tibial (tĭb'ē-ăl) (9 and 10) arteries and extend into the ankle and foot.

Systemic Veins

Although most arteries are located and protected in deep areas, the veins are found both in protected areas and near the surface. Those near the surface are called **superficial veins**, because they lie just beneath the skin and return blood from the skin and the subcutaneous regions to the deep veins. The **saphenous** (sah-fē'nŭs) **veins**, the longest veins of the body, are in the lower extremities. (These can be used in heart bypass surgery.) The veins on the back of the hand and at the front of the elbow are superficial veins. They are called cephalic (sĕ-făl'ĭk) (5), basilic (bah-sĭl'ĭk) (4), and median cubital (kū'bĭ-tal) (6) and are illustrated in Figure 8-6.

The deep veins travel alongside an artery and have the same name as the artery, although there are a few exceptions to this pattern. The femoral (7) and iliac (ĭl'ē-ăk) (8) vessels are found in the lower part of the body, and the brachial (brā'kē-ăl) (3), axillary (2), and subclavian (sŭb-klā'vē-ăn) (1) veins are in the

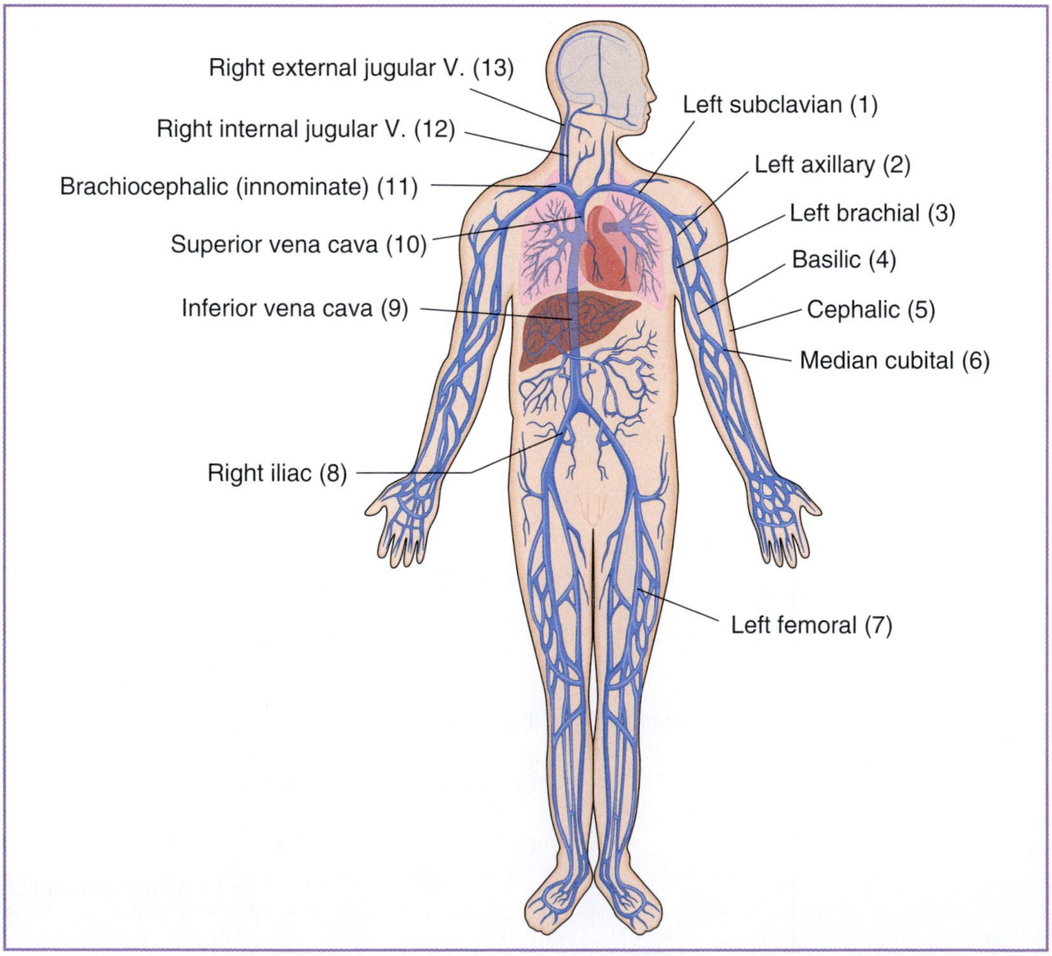

FIGURE 8-6
Major Systemic Veins of the Body

upper extremities. Jugular (jŭg'ū-lăr) (12 and 13) veins drain the areas supplied by the carotid arteries. Two brachiocephalic (innominate) veins (11) are formed, one on each side of the neck, by the union of the subclavian and jugular veins.

All veins finally converge into one of two large trunks: the superior vena cava (10) and the inferior vena cava (9). The superior vena cava drains the veins of the head, neck, upper extremities, and chest, and the **azygos** (ăz'ĭ-gŏs) **vein** drains the veins of the chest wall.

The inferior vena cava is much longer than the superior vena cava and drains blood from parts of the body below the diaphragm. The large veins can be divided into two groups, paired and unpaired. The paired veins, such as the lumbar, renal, suprarenal, and hepatic veins, drain paired parts and organs.

The unpaired veins come from parts of the digestive tract and empty into a special vein called the portal tube. The blood coming from the intestines enters the liver through the portal system. Here, a good portion of the glucose and protein is extracted and stored for future use. From there the blood flows through the hepatic vein and empties into the inferior vena cava.

PULSE AND BLOOD PRESSURE

Both pulse and blood pressure are good indicators of the efficiency of the cardiovascular system.

Pulse

The ventricle pumps blood into arteries at a normal rate ranging from 60 to 100 times per minute. The force of ventricular contraction starts a wave of increased pressure beginning in the heart and traveling through the arteries. This wave is called the pulse. There are several factors that can influence the pulse rate. Here are a few of them.

1. The pulse is somewhat faster in smaller people and usually slightly faster in women than in men.
2. In a newborn infant, the rate may be from 120 to 140 beats per minute.
3. Physical activity influences the pulse rate. The rate can be 100 or higher with strenuous exercise, but may be as slow as 60 beats per minute during sleep.
4. Emotional disturbances can increase the pulse rate.
5. The pulse rate increases with a rise in temperature, such as with infection.

Blood Pressure

Blood pressure is the pressure exerted on the arterial walls by the blood, influenced by the rate of flow and resistance to flow. The instrument used to measure blood pressure is called a **sphygmomanometer** (sfig"mō-mah-nŏm'ĕ-ter) (also called a "cuff"). It records blood pressure at two specific times.

Systolic pressure
The pressure on the arterial walls during the heart muscle contraction. Normal systolic pressure averages around 120 millimeters (mm) of mercury and may vary from 90 to 140 mm of mercury.

Diastolic pressure
The pressure on the arterial walls during relaxation, or the rest period, of the heart muscle. Normal diastolic pressure ranges from 50 to 90 mm of mercury and averages around 80 mm.

Lower-than-normal blood pressure is called **hypotension** (hī"pō-tĕn'shŭn). **Hypertension** (hī"per-tĕn'shŭn) is higher-than-normal blood pressure. The condition of the small arteries may have more effect on the diastolic pressure, thus making it more important than systolic pressure.

INTERNET ASSIGNMENT

The web site healthfinder.gov is a free guide to reliable consumer health and human services information. It was developed by the Office of Disease Prevention and Health Promotion of the U.S. Department of Health and Human Services in collaboration with other Federal agencies. Healthfinder.gov can lead you to more than 1,500 selected online publications, clearinghouses, data bases, carefully reviewed web sites, and support and self-help groups, as well as government agencies and not-for-profit and professional organizations that produce reliable health information for the public.

The home page provides links to a health library, consumer guides and a directory of healthfinder organizations. As an example of topic content, the directory of healthfinder organizations provides a list of related organizations based on a topic you enter. Clicking one of these organizations will bring up a list of organizations concerned about that topic, with links to their home pages. Alternatively, you may click on a letter to browse available topics and then click on a topic of choice and make your specific selection.

ACTIVITY

Access healthfinder at **www.healthfinder.gov**. Click on Health Library to get a list of general categories. You then may either select a category to get a browse list of available topics and choose one, or enter a specific topic in the search field at the top of the page. For this activity, key "how the heart works" into the search window. From the choices presented, select one, cite the source, and summarize the information found for your instructor.

Review *The Cardiovascular System*

- The heart consists of two separate parts that are divided by the septum: The left side receives oxygenated blood and pumps it into the aorta for distribution to the body; the right side receives "used" blood as it returns from the tissues.
- The period of contraction, when the heart is beating, is referred to as systole; the resting phase of the heart is called diastole.
- Beating rate is controlled by the sinoatrial node or the pacemaker, the atrioventricular node, and the bundle of His.
- After blood leaves the heart, a system of arteries, arterioles, capillaries, venules, and veins circulates the blood through the body.
- The aorta is the largest artery, and the superior and inferior venae cavae are the largest veins.
- The rate at which blood is pumped is referred to as the pulse rate.
- Blood pressure readings are a combination of systolic and diastolic pressure readings.

Key Terminology Review

Word	Definition
abdominal aorta	longest aortic section; spans the abdominal cavity
adventitia	outermost layer of an artery wall
aorta	great artery; its main trunk arises from the left ventricle
aortic arch	continuation of the ascending aorta that gives rise to the brachiocephalic, carotid, and subclavian arteries
aortic valve	valve that prevents enriched blood from the aorta from returning to the left ventricle
arteries	vessels that carry blood from the heart to the body
arterioles	smallest divisions of arteries
atrioventricular bundle (bundle of His)	specialized bundle of tissue that spreads impulses to all parts of the ventricle walls
atrioventricular node	specialized mass of tissues in the heart wall that carries impulses generated by the sinoatrial node to the bundle of His and ventricle walls
atrium, left and right (*pl.* atria)	upper chambers of the heart
azygos vein	vessel draining the veins of the chest wall into the superior vena cava
capillaries	tiny vessels that connect arterioles and venules to provide for the exchange between oxygenated and deoxygenated blood
diastole	resting phase of the heart muscle
endocardium	membrane that lines the interior of the heart
epicardium	outermost layer of the heart
hypertension	higher-than-normal blood pressure
hypotension	lower-than-normal blood pressure
intima (endothelium)	innermost structure of an artery wall
media	middle layer of an artery wall
mitral valve	valve that prevents blood from the left ventricle from returning to the left atrium
murmurs	abnormal heart sounds
myocardium	muscle of the heart; middle and thickest layer
pericardial sac	sac surrounding the heart
pericardium	lining of the pericardial sac that surrounds the heart
pulmonary artery	artery that leads deoxygenated blood from the right ventricle to the lungs
pulmonary valve	valve that prevents blood from returning to the right ventricle
pulse rate	number of times per minute that the heart beats
saphenous veins	longest veins of the body located in the lower extremities
septum, interatrial and interventricular	partition that separates the two sides of the heart

continues

Word	Definition
sinoatrial node	natural pacemaker of the heart
sphygmomanometer	instrument used to measure blood pressure; a "cuff"
stenosis	narrowing
superficial veins	veins located near the body surface
systole	pumping or contracting phase of the heart muscle
thoracic aorta	section of the descending aorta from the aortic arch to the level of the diaphragm
tricuspid valve	valve that prevents blood from the right ventricle from returning to the right atrium
veins	vessels that carry blood from the body to the heart
vena cava, superior and inferior (*pl.* venae cavae)	largest veins of the body
ventricle, left and right	lower chambers of the heart
venules	smallest divisions of veins, formed by the union of capillaries

Key Terminology Practice Exercises

SHORT ANSWER

Supply a short answer to the following.

1. Name the four chambers of the heart and specify the function of each.

____

____

____

____

2. Name three types of blood vessels and state their function.

____

____

____

____

3. Explain the difference between diastolic and systolic blood pressure readings.

____

____

____

____

4. Name and define the layers of the heart wall.

____

____

____

____

5. Name and define the layers of the blood vessels.

____

____

____

____

COMPLETION

Complete the following statements.

1. The two sides of the heart are separated by a partition called the ____________.
2. The four valves of the heart are the ____________, ____________, ____________, and ____________.
3. Abnormal heart sounds are called ____________.
4. The active phase of the heart is ____________; the resting period is ____________.
5. Two types of heart murmurs are ____________ and ____________.
6. The pulse rate is ____________ to ____________ beats per minute.
7. The order in which the heart operates is controlled by the ____________ system.
8. The sinoatrial node is often referred to as the ____________ of the heart.
9. The smallest veins are called ____________.
10. The aortic arch sends off three branches; they are the ____________, ____________, and ____________.
11. The instrument used to measure blood pressure is called a ____________.
12. The two major trunks of veins are the ____________ and ____________.
13. The largest artery of the body is the ____________.
14. The origin of all arteries carrying oxygen-rich blood is the ____________.
15. The longest section of the aorta is the ____________.

MATCHING

Match the terms to their meanings.

1. __________ continuation of ascending aorta
2. __________ upper chamber of the heart
3. __________ interior lining of heart
4. __________ middle layer of an artery wall
5. __________ outermost layer of an artery wall
6. __________ muscle of the heart
7. __________ vessel draining chest wall veins into superior vena cava
8. __________ innermost structure of an artery wall
9. __________ vessels that carry blood from heart to body
10. __________ outermost layer of the heart
11. __________ narrowing
12. __________ smallest divisions of arteries
13. __________ connects arterioles and venules for exchange of oxygenated and deoxygenated blood
14. __________ lower chambers of the heart
15. __________ longest veins of body located in the lower extremities

a. adventitia
b. aortic arch
c. arteries
d. arterioles
e. atrium, left and right
f. azygos vein
g. capillaries
h. endocardium
i. epicardium
j. intima
k. media
l. myocardium
m. saphenous veins
n. stenosis
o. ventricles, left and right

Word Element Review

Root	Meaning	Example	Definition
angi/o	blood vessel	**angiitis** (ăn"jē-ī'tĭs)	inflammation of a blood vessel
		angioma (ăn"jē-ō'mah)	tumor made of blood or lymph vessels
aort/o	aorta	**aortorrhaphy** (ā"ŏr-tor'ah-fē)	suture of the aorta
arter/o, arteri/o	artery	**arterioplasty** (ăr-tē"rē-ō-plăs'tē)	surgical repair of an artery
		arteriorrhaphy (ăr-tē"rē-or'ah-fē)	suture of an artery

continues

Root	Meaning	Example	Definition
ather/o	yellowish plaque, fatty substance	**atheroma** (ăth"er-ō'mah)	mass of plaque of degenerated, thickened arterial intima (inner lining of an artery), occurring in atherosclerosis
atri/o	atrium	**atrial** (ā'trē-ăl)	pertaining to an atrium
		atriomegaly (ā"trē-ō-mĕg'ah-lē)	abnormal enlargement of an atrium of the heart
cardi/o disease	heart	**cardiomyopathy** (kăr"dē-ō-mī-ŏp'ah-thē)	diagnostic term designating myocardial
		myocardial infarction (mī"ō-kăr'dē-ăl ĭn-fărk'shŭn)	a "heart attack"
coron/o	heart	**coronary** (kor'ŏ-nā-rē)	applying to arteries of the heart and the pathology of them
furc/o	division, fork	**bifurcation** (bī'fur-kā'shŭn)	division into two parts
		furcal (fur'kăl)	shaped like a fork
pericardi/o	pericardium	**pericardiectomy** (pĕr"ĭ-kăr"dē-ek'tō-mē)	removal of a portion of the pericardium
phleb/o	vein	**phlebitis** (flĕ-bī'tĭs)	inflammation of a vessel
		phlebostenosis (flĕb"ō-stĕ-nō-'sĭs)	narrowing of a vein
steth/o	chest	**stethoscope** (stĕth'ō-skōp)	instrument for listening to body sounds
thromb/o	clot, lump	**thrombosis** (thrŏm-bō'sĭs)	formation of a blood clot in a vessel or an organ
		thrombus (thrŏm'bŭs)	clot in a blood vessel formed by coagulation of the blood (note the similarity in sound, spelling, and meaning of these two words)
valv/o, valvul/o	valve	**valvular** (văl'vū-lăr)	pertaining to a valve
vascul/o, vas/o	vessel	**vascular** (văs'kū-lăr)	pertaining to a blood vessel

continues

Root	Meaning	Example	Definition
		vasodilator (văs"ō-dī-lāt'or)	agent that dilates the blood vessels
ven/o	vein	**venous** (vē'nŭs)	pertaining to a vein
ventricul/o	ventricle	**ventriculotomy** (vĕn-trĭk"ū-lŏt'ō-mē)	incision into the ventricle of the heart
Prefix	**Meaning**	**Example**	**Definition**
brady-	slow	**bradycardia** (brăd"e-kăr'dē-ah)	slow heartbeat
tachy-	fast, rapid	**tachycardia** (tăk"ē-kăr'dē-ah)	fast heart rate
Suffix	**Meaning**	**Example**	**Definition**
-megaly	enlargement	**cardiomegaly** (kăr"dē-ō-mĕg'ah-lē)	condition characterized by an enlarged heart

Word Element Practice Exercises

COMPLETION

Complete the following statements.

1. ________________________ is a rapid heartbeat.
2. ________________________ applies to arteries of the heart and the pathology of them.
3. A ________________________ is commonly known as a "heart attack."
4. A ________________________ is an instrument for listening to the heart and other body sounds.
5. Suture of the aorta is ________________________; suture of an artery is ________________________.
6. ________________________ refers to a valve.
7. The clot in a blood vessel is a ________________________, but the formation of a clot is a________________________.
8. A diagnostic term designating myocardial diseases is ________________________.
9. ________________________ is the abnormal enlargement of an atrium of the heart.
10. Removal of a portion of the pericardium is ________________________.

SPELLINGS AND DEFINITIONS

Mark any spelling errors in these words. Then define each and specify whether it is a noun or an adjective by placing an N or A in the last column.

	Definition	N or A
1. cardiomegaly	______________________	________
2. bradicardia	______________________	________
3. tachicardia	______________________	________
4. ventriclotomy	______________________	________
5. venus	______________________	________

DEFINITIONS

Provide the medical term for the following definitions.

1. surgical repair of an artery ______________________
2. division into two parts ______________________
3. inflammation of a vessel ______________________
4. narrowing of a vein ______________________
5. pertaining to a blood vessel ______________________
6. agent that dilates the blood vessels ______________________
7. shaped like a fork ______________________
8. pertaining to an atrium ______________________
9. mass of plaque ______________________
10. tumor made of blood and lymph vessels ______________________

WORD ELEMENT AND MEANING

In the following terms, circle the word element presented in this chapter. Then provide the definition of the term.

1. cardiomyopathy ______________________
2. atrial ______________________
3. coronary ______________________
4. vasodilator ______________________
5. angioma ______________________
6. atheroma ______________________

WORD ELEMENT MEANINGS

Give the meaning of each word element. Then use your dictionary to find a new word that contains each of the word elements. Specify whether the new word is a noun or an adjective by placing N or A in the last column.

Word Element	Meaning	Word	N or A
1. angi/o	________	________	____
2. aort/o	________	________	____
3. arter/o	________	________	____
4. arteri/o	________	________	____
5. ather/o	________	________	____
6. atri/o	________	________	____
7. brady-	________	________	____
8. cardi/o	________	________	____
9. coron/o	________	________	____
10. furc/o	________	________	____
11. -megaly	________	________	____
12. pericardi/o	________	________	____
13. phleb/o	________	________	____
14. steth/o	________	________	____
15. tachy-	________	________	____
16. thromb/o	________	________	____
17. valv/o	________	________	____
18. valvul/o	________	________	____
19. vas/o	________	________	____
20. vascul/o	________	________	____
21. ven/o	________	________	____
22. ventricul/o	________	________	____

DIAGNOSTIC PROCEDURES		
Word	**Pronunciation**	**Definition**
General		
cardiac catheterization	kăth"ĕ-tĕr-ĭ-zā'shŭn	intensive study of the heart that uses catheters to perform angiocardiography and/or pressure and flow measurement to determine the severity of suspected cardiac disease
Doppler ultrasound flowmeter		procedure using an apparatus that measures sound waves as echoes bounce off red blood cells
echocardiogram	ĕk"ō-kăr'dē-ō-grăm"	graphic record of reflected ultrasound waves from the heart
electrocardiogram (EKG, ECG)	ē-lĕk"trō-kăr'dē-ō-grăm"	electrical record of heart activity monitored by electrodes placed on the chest wall (Figure 8-7 provides an explanation of a normal tracing.)
exercise stress test		screening tool for the detection of significant coronary artery disease
Holter monitor		compact recording device that monitors EKG activity over a long period of time by using electrodes attached to a patient's chest; "24-hour EKG" (See Figure 8-8)
Nuclear Medicine		
angiocardiography	ăn"jē-ō-kăr"dē-ŏg'rah-fē	x-ray of the blood vessels after an injection of radioactive isotope material into the bloodstream
positron emission tomography scan (PET)	tō-mŏg'ră-fē	test that shows blood flow and myocardial function after the uptake of a radioactive substance

continues

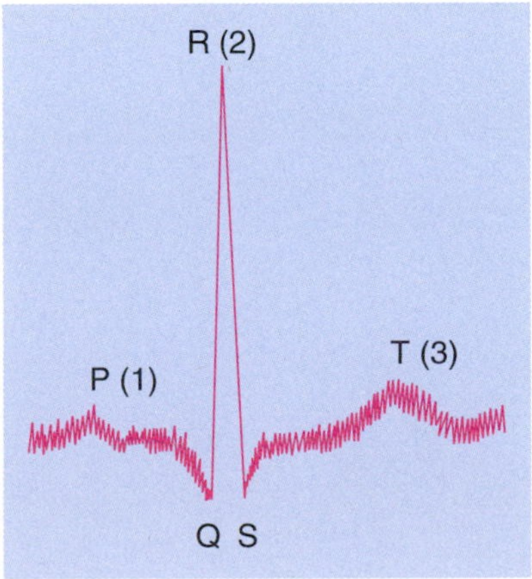

FIGURE 8-7 Electrocardiogram Components (1) P wave denotes the electrical impulse from the sinoatrial node through the atrial sinus; (2) QRS complex denotes ventricle wall contraction; (3) T wave denotes ventricular recovery (rest) phase after contraction

Source: Delmar/Cengage Learning

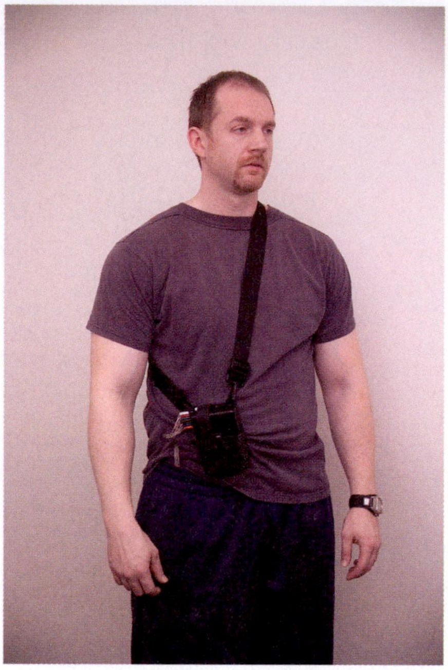

Source: Delmar/Cengage Learning

FIGURE 8-8
Holter Monitor

DIAGNOSTIC PROCEDURES		
Word	Pronunciation	Definition
Nuclear Medicine (*continued*)		
radionuclide angiography (multiple-gated acquisition scan [MUGA scan])	rā"dē-ō-nū'klīd ăn"jē-ŏg'rah-fē	x-ray that uses radioactive isotopes injected into the blood vessels to evaluate the condition heart
thallium stress test (technetium Tc99m sestamibi scan)	thăl'ē-ŭm těk-nē'shē-ŭm	use of thallium imaging during exercise stress testing to detect decreased blood flow to a portion of the heart muscle
Radiology		
arteriography	ăr-tē"rē-ŏg'rah-fē	x-ray of an artery or the artery system after an injection (angiography) of radiopaque material into the bloodstream; See Figure 8-9 for an image from an arteriography
cardiac magnetic resonance imaging (MRI)		test that uses magnetic waves beamed at the heart to produce an image; used to detect detailed information about various heart problems
computed axial tomography (CAT)	ăk'sē-ăl tō-mŏg'ră-fē	diagnostic x-ray technique that uses ionizing radiation to produce a cross-sectional image of the body

continues

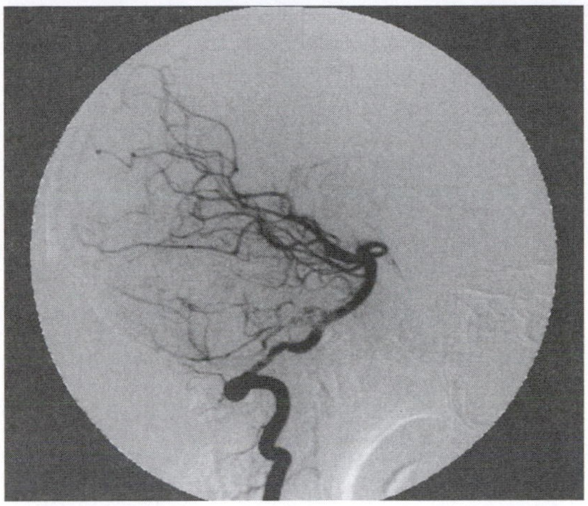

FIGURE 8-9
Arteriogram

Source: Delmar/Cengage Learning

DIAGNOSTIC PROCEDURES		
Word	Pronunciation	Definition
Radiology (*continued*)		
CT angiography	ăn"jē-ŏg'ră-fē	diagnostic x-ray technique that uses ionizing radiation to produce images of the myocardial vasculature, including the coronary arteries
PA (posteroanterior) and lateral of the chest	pŏs"tĕr-ō-an-tēr'ē-or	routine x-ray views of the lung fields and heart
venography	vē-nŏg'rah-fē	x-ray of the veins after an injection of radiopaque material into the bloodstream
Blood Tests		
arterial blood gases (ABGs)	ăr-tē'rē-ăl	measurement of oxygen, carbon dioxide, and metabolic balance from an arterial blood sample
cardiac enzymes	ĕn'zīms	measurement of the blood for the following: • *AST*—aspartate aminotransferase (ăs-păr'tāt ăm'nē'-trănz-fĕr'ās), which is found in its highest concentration in the heart muscle, brain, and liver • *CPK*—creatine phosphokinase (krē'ah-tĭn fŏs"fō-kī'nās), which is released into the blood when the heart or skeletal muscles are injured • *LDH*—lactate dehydrogenase (lăk'tāt dē-hī-drŏj'ĕ-nās), which is an enzyme found primarily in the heart muscles, skeletal muscles, kidneys, liver, and red blood cells • *Troponin I and Troponin T*—cardiac-specific enzyme released from dying heart muscle cells

continues

DIAGNOSTIC PROCEDURES		
Word	Pronunciation	Definition
complete blood count (CBC)		measurement of the blood for the following: hemoglobin, hematocrit, red blood count, white blood count, and differential (the types and number of white blood cells present)
electrolytes	ē-lĕk'trō-līts	measurement of the blood for chloride, sodium, and potassium
serum lipids (lipid profile)		measurement of the blood cholesterol, high- and low-density lipoprotein, very low-density lipoprotein, and triglycerides
prothrombin time (PT)	prō-thrŏm'bĭn	tests the coagulation of blood

DIAGNOSES		
Word	Pronunciation	Definition
Diseases and Disorders of the Heart		
angina pectoris	ăn-jī'nah pĕk'tŏr-ĭs	attacks of severe chest pain caused by insufficient blood reaching the heart muscle
arteriosclerotic (coronary) heart disease (ASHD)	ăr-tē"rē-ō-sklĕ-rŏt'ĭk	heart disease produced by coronary artery disease
cardiomyopathy	kăr"dē-ō-mī-ŏp'ah-thē	weakening of the heart muscle
carditis	kăr-dī'tĭs	inflammation of the heart
congestive heart failure	kŏn-jēs'tĭv	condition caused by the inability of the heart to pump (beat) adequately, resulting in an accumulation of fluid in tissues (edema or swelling) or in the lungs (see Figure 8-10)
endocarditis (bacterial endocarditis)	ĕn"dō-kăr-dī'tĭs	inflammation of inner lining of the heart (bacterial caused by bacteria)
hypertensive heart disease	hī"pĕr-tĕn'sĭv	disease characterized by prolonged high blood pressure with varying degrees of heart failure
hypertrophic obstructive cardiomyopathy	hī"pĕr-trōf'ĭk, kăr"dē-ō-mī-ŏp'ah-thē	abnormal thickening of the heart muscle resulting in a restriction of the flow of blood from the heart
ischemia	ĭs-kē'mē-ah	inadequate flow of blood to a part of the body, caused by constriction or blockage of the blood vessels supplying it (See Figure 8-11)
myocardial infarction (MI)	mi"ō-kăr'dē-ăl ĭn-făr'k'shŭn	heart attack; blood clot blocks the flow in one or more coronary arteries resulting in the death of myocardial tissue
myocarditis	mi"ō-kăr'dī'tĭs	inflammatory disease of the myocardium
pericarditis	per"ĭ-kăr'dī'tĭs	inflammatory disease of the pericardium

continues

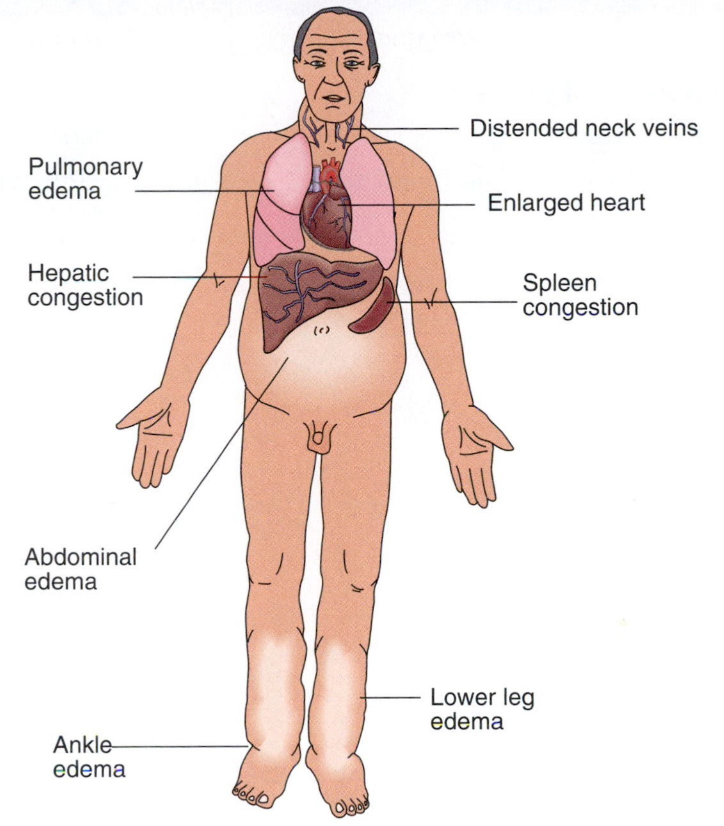

FIGURE 8-10
Signs of Congestive Heart Failure

Source: Delmar/Cengage Learning

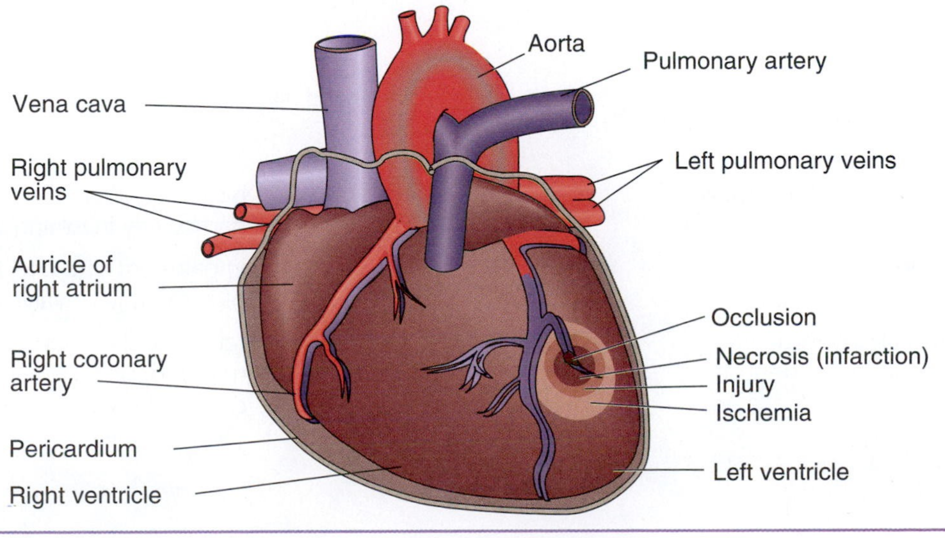

FIGURE 8-11
Areas of Ischemia After Myocardial Infarction

Source: Delmar/Cengage Learning

DIAGNOSES		
Word	Pronunciation	Definition
Congenital Diseases of the Heart		
congenital heart disease		abnormalities of the heart at birth
coarctation of the aorta	kō"ărk-tā'shŭn	localized congenital malformation resulting in narrowing of the aorta, often resulting in hypertension
patent ductus arteriosus (PDA)	păt'ĕnt dŭk'tŭs ăr-tēr-ē-ō'sŭs	small duct between the aorta and pulmonary artery stays open, instead of closing at birth
tetralogy of Fallot	tĕ-trăl'ō-jē of făl-ō'	congenital malformation of the heart that has four defects: 1. pulmonary artery stenosis, restricts blood flow from heart to the lungs 2. ventricular septal defect, allows deoxygenated blood from right ventricle to communicate with oxygenated blood in the left ventricle and from there to the aorta 3. shift of aorta to the right, aorta overrides the interventricular septum 4. hypertrophy of the right ventricle, occurs because the myocardium has to work harder to pump blood through the obstructed pulmonary artery
transposition of the great vessels		two major arteries of heart are reversed and resulting in two non-communicating circulatory systems
Diseases of Heart Valves		
infective endocarditis	ĭn-fec'tĭv ĕn"dō-kăr-dī'tĭs	inflammatory disease of the endocardium
mitral valve prolapse	mī'trăl, prō'lăps	extraneous and floppy mitral valve tissue causing the heart valve to fail to close properly
murmur		abnormal sound in the heart or vascular system
regurgitation	rē-gŭr"jĭ-tā'shŭn	a backward flow through a defective heart valve
rheumatic heart disease	roo-mă'tĭk	disease produced by rheumatic fever, particularly involving the valves
stenosis	stĕn-ō'sĭs	impairment of blood flow due to narrowing of a passage or valve
valvular insufficiency, valvular heart disease	văl'vū-lăr	failure of the heart valves (aortic, mitral, tricuspid, or pulmonic) to close completely, causing leakage

continues

DIAGNOSES

Word	Pronunciation	Definition
Disorders of Heart Rate and Rhythm		
arrhythmia (dysrhythmia)	ah-rĭth'mē-ah (dĭs-rĭth'mē-ah)	irregular heartbeat; cause may be for one of several reasons
• *ectopic*	ĕk-tŏp'ĭk	• small variation in the heartbeat, often called extrasystoles
• *atrial fibrillation*	ā'trē-ăl fĭ'brĭl-ā'shŭn	• uncoordinated muscle contractions in the atria
• *atrial flutter*	ā'trē-ăl	• atria contract too often
• *heart block (atrioventricular block)*	(ā"trē-ō-vĕn-trĭk'ū-lăr)	• interference with the normal condition of electric impulses that control the activity of heart muscle
• *paroxysmal atrial tachycardia*	păr"ŏk-sĭz'măl ā'trē-ăl tăk"ē-kăr'dē-ă	• rapid heart beat
• *ventricular tachycardia and fibrillation*	vĕn-trĭk'ū-lăr tăk"ē-kăr'dē-ă fĭ'brĭl-ā'shŭn	• muscle fibers of ventricles are uncoordinated
bradycardia	brăd"ē-kăr'dē-ah	slow heart beat
sick sinus syndrome		sinus node initiates beats too slowly, pauses too long between beats, or stops producing beats
Disorders of Arteries, Veins, and Circulation		
acrocyanosis	ăk"rō-sī-ă-nō-sĭs	bluish discoloration of the extremities caused by lack of oxygen to these parts
aneurysm	ăn'ū-rĭzm	weakness in the wall of a blood vessel, which causes the vessel to bulge or enlarge abnormally
atherosclerosis	ăth"ĕr-ō-klĕ-rō'sĭs	hardening of the arteries caused by deposits of cholesterol and calcium in the arterial walls (See Figure 8-12)
coronary artery disease		narrowing of arteries that supply blood to the heart muscle
deep venous thrombosis (DVT)	thrŏm-bō'sĭs	clotting occurring in femoral and pelvic veins (see Figure 8-13)
embolism	ĕm'bō-lĭzm	free-moving clot or debris from a buildup of atherosclerotic plaque that may plug an artery
gangrene	găng'grēn	death of tissue resulting from deficient or absent blood supply

continues

StudyWARE™ Connection

To watch an animation on **Congestive Heart Failure,** go to your StudyWARE™ CD-ROM.

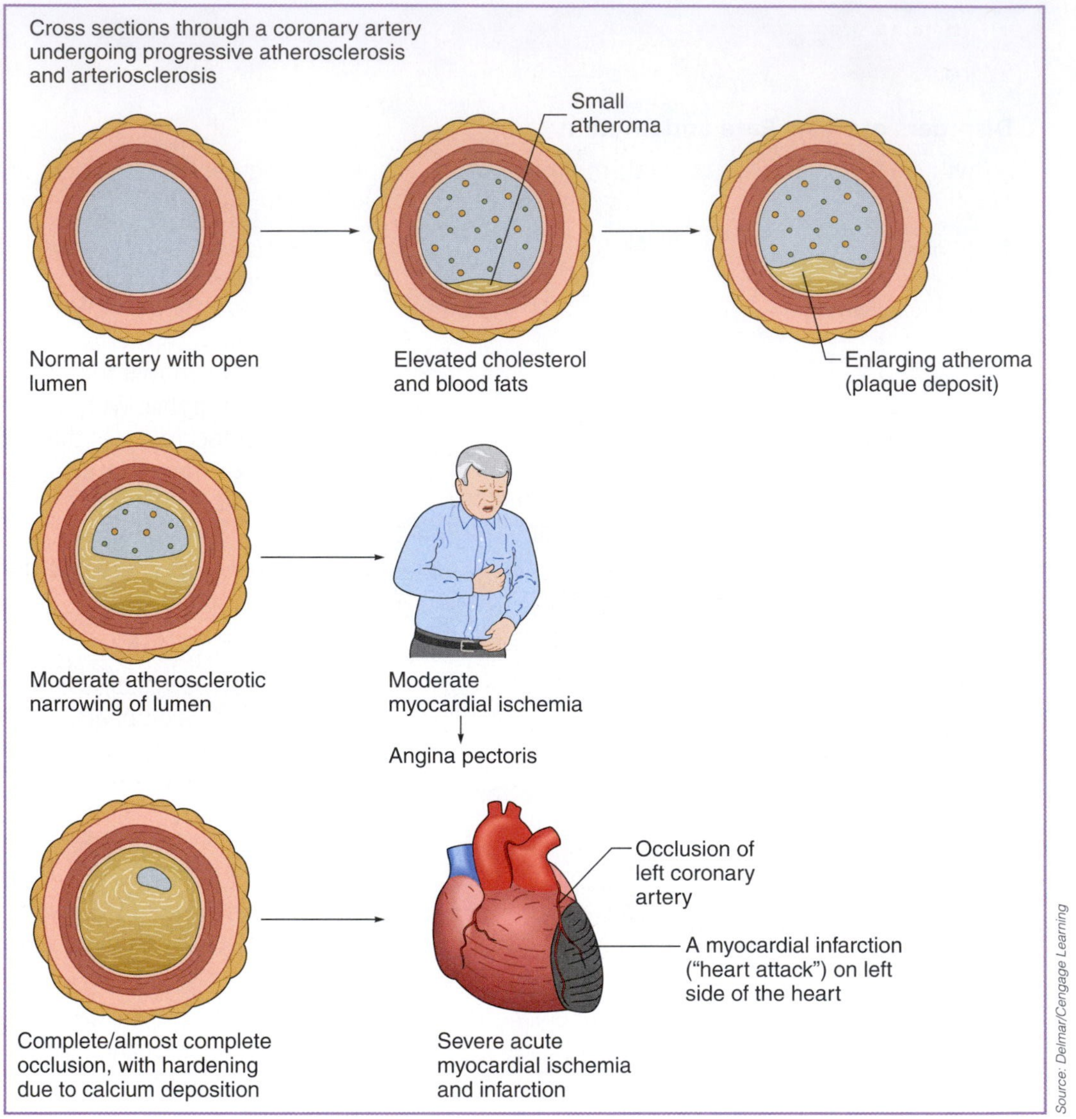

FIGURE 8-12 Atherosclerosis

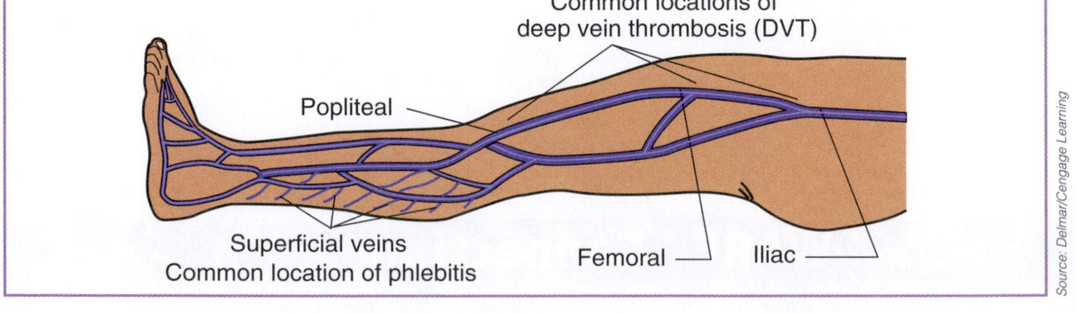

FIGURE 8-13 Superficial vs. Deep Veins in the Development of Phlebitis and Thrombosis

DIAGNOSES		
Word	**Pronunciation**	**Definition**
Disorders of Arteries, Veins, and Circulation (*continued*)		
hypertension	hī"pĕr-tĕn'shŭn	high blood pressure; may be *primary or essential* (idiopathic gradual onset) or *secondary* (due to another problem)
hypotension	hi"pō-tĕn'shŭn	low blood pressure
infarct	ĭn'fărkt	death of tissue resulting from inadequate blood supply
lymphedema	lĭmf-ĕ-dē'mah	abnormal accumulation of tissue fluid, often caused by venous obstruction
peripheral arterial occlusive disease	pĕr-ĭf'ĕr-ăl ăr-tē'rē-ăl ŏ-kloo'sĭv	obstruction of the arteries of the extremities
peripheral (hypertensive) vascular disease (PVD)		persistent high blood pressure caused by one of several diseases of the arteries
phlebitis	flĕ-bī'tĭs	inflammation of a superficial vein
Raynaud's phenomenon	rā-nōz' fĕ-nŏm'ĕ-nŏn	short episodes of pallor and numbness in the fingers and toes due to the temporary constriction of arterioles in the skin (See Figure 8-14)
thrombophlebitis	thrŏm"bō-flĕ-bī'tĭs	development of a clot in an inflamed vessel
thrombus	thrŏm'bŭs	fixed blood clot
varicose veins	văr'ĭ-kōs	abnormally swollen veins, usually occurring in the legs (See Figure 8-15)

TREATMENT PROCEDURES		
Word	**Pronunciation**	**Definition**
aneurysmectomy	ăn"ū-rĭz-mĕk'tō-mē	surgical removal of an aneurysm
angioplasty	ăn'jē-ō-plăs"tē	percutaneous repair of a blood vessel (See Figure 8-16)
artery graft		replacement of a portion of an artery by another open structure (e.g., aortofemoral bypass graft, which is a graft between the abdominal aorta and the femoral artery)

continues

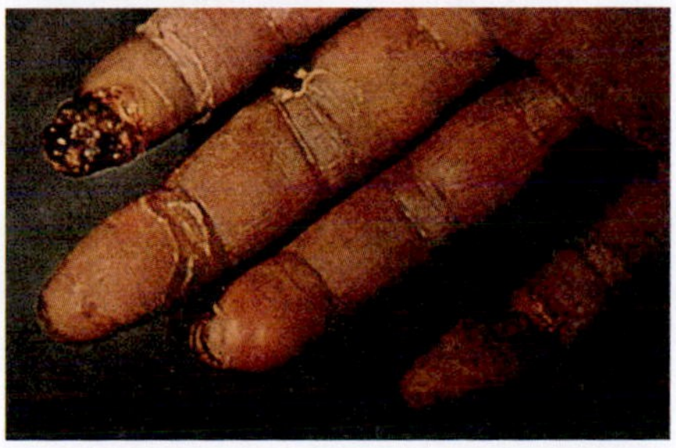

FIGURE 8-14
Arterial Ulcers as a Result of Raynaud's Phenomenon

Courtesy of Marvin Aceman, M.D., Scarsdale, NY

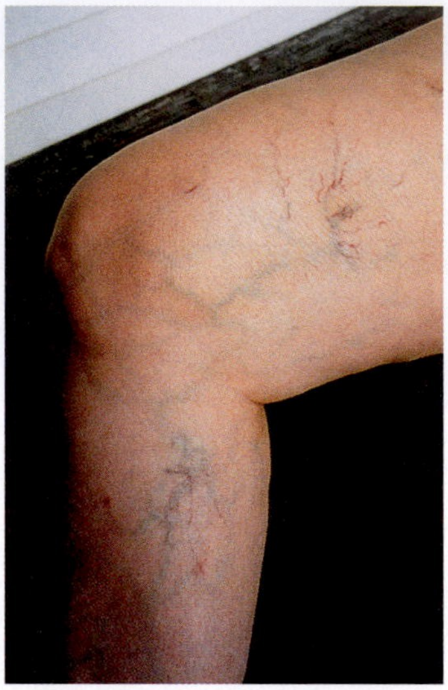

Source: Delmar/Cengage Learning

FIGURE 8-15
Varicose Veins

TREATMENT PROCEDURES		
Word	**Pronunciation**	**Definition**
atherectomy	ăth-ĕr-ĕk'tō-mē	technique using high-speed drills to remove atheromatous plaque from arteries
cardiomyoplasty	kăr"dē-ō-mī'ō-plăs-tē	surgical implantation of skeletal muscle to either supplement or replace myocardial muscle
cardiopulmonary resuscitation (CPR)	kăr"dē-ō-pŭl'mō-nĕr-ē rē-sŭs"ĭ-tā'shŭn	mouth-to-mouth breathing and chest compression
cardiotomy	kăr"dē-ŏt'ŏ-mē	surgical incision or opening of the heart for repair
cardioversion	kar'dē-ō-vĕr"zhŭn	brief charges of electricity applied to the chest to stop cardiac arrhythmia
commissurotomy	kŏm"ĭ-shūr-ŏt'ō-mē	surgical incision of the connecting bands of a commissure; done to correct valvular stenosis (narrowing)
coronary artery bypass	kor'ŏ-nā-rē	open-heart surgery for the purpose of bypassing an obstructed coronary artery (See Figure 8-17)
correction of atrial septal defect	ā'trē-ăl sĕp'tăl	closure of an abnormal opening in the interatrial septum
correction of ventricular septal defect	vĕn-trĭk'ū-lăr	repair of an abnormal opening in the interventricular septum
defibrillation	dē-fĭb"rĭ-lā'shŭn	delivery of electric shock during emergency situation to return heart to normal rhythm
embolectomy	ĕm"bō-lĕk'tō-mē	removal of an embolus (a plug or clot) from a blood vessel
endarterectomy	ĕnd"ăr-ter-ĕk'tō-mē	removal of the interior portion of an artery and occluding fatty deposits
extracorporeal	ĕks"tră-kŏr'ē-ăl	circulation of blood outside of the body for purposes of circulation removing or exchanging substances

continues

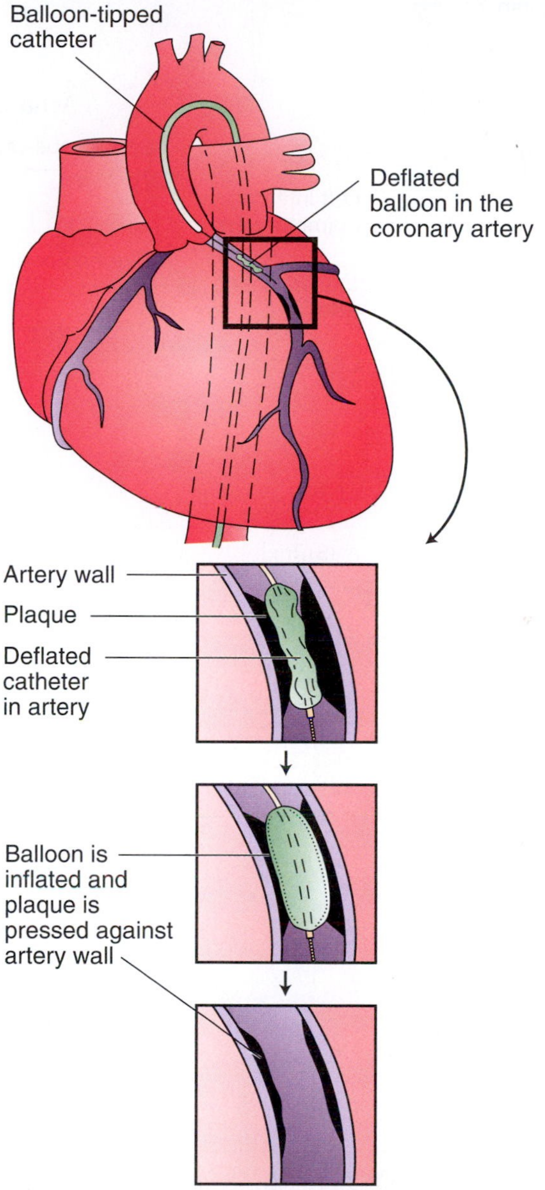

FIGURE 8-16
Coronary Artery Angioplasty

TREATMENT PROCEDURES

Word	Pronunciation	Definition
heart transplantation		replacement of the patient's malfunctioning heart with a donor's heart
heart valve valvuloplasty	văl'ŭ-lō-plăs"tē	insertion of a guidewire (with a balloon on its tip) through an artery to a diseased valve where the balloon is inflated (Figure 8-18 illustrates this procedure.)
internal cardioverter-defibrillator (ICD)	kăr'dē-ō-vĕr"tĕr dē-fĭb"rĭ-lā'tŏr	battery-driven device implanted in the chest to sense abnormal heart rhythm and emit a signal to bring it back to normal

continues

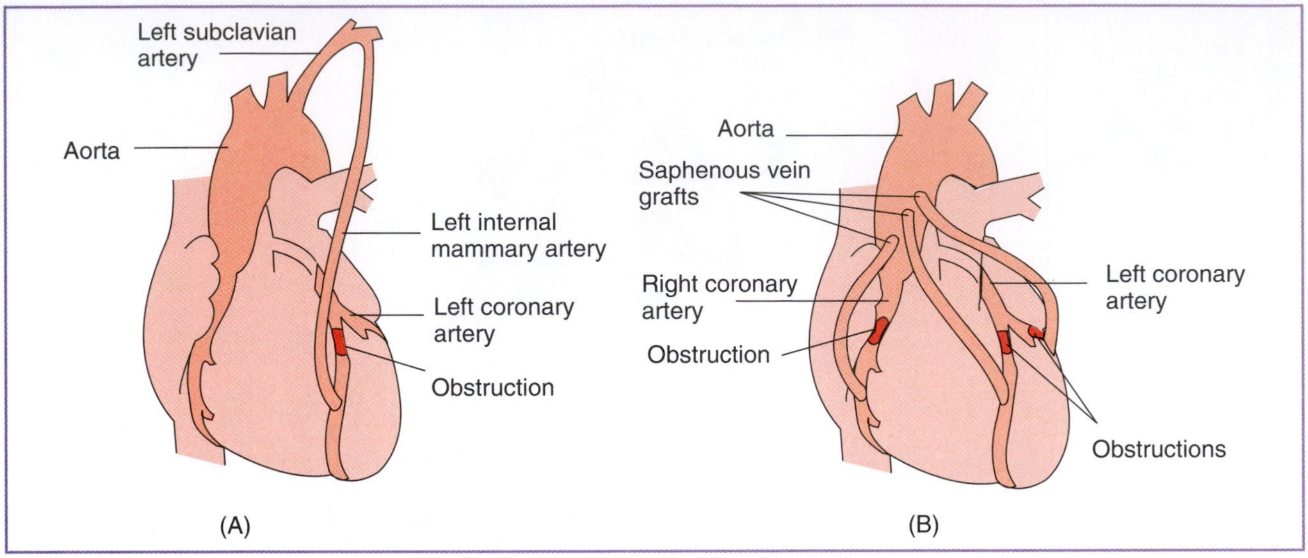

FIGURE 8-17 Coronary Bypass; (A) Single; (B) Triple

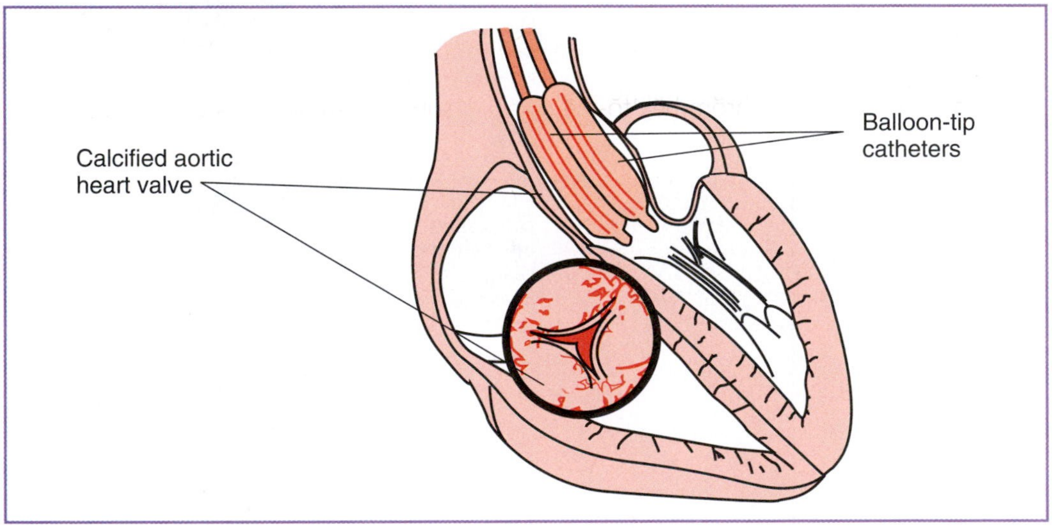

FIGURE 8-18 Heart Valve Valvuloplasty

TREATMENT PROCEDURES		
Word	**Pronunciation**	**Definition**
intra-aortic balloon pump (IABP)	ĭn"tră-ā-or'tĭc	mechanical device to help improve coronary blood flow and systemic circulation in weak hearts
left ventricular assist device (LVAD)	vĕn-trĭk'ū-lăr	external circulatory support device used after bypass surgery to ensure unidirectional blood flow
pacemaker cardiac defibrillator (PCD)	dē-fĭb"rĭ-lă'tŏr	small electronic device consisting of a battery and an electrode implanted in the chest and heart, respectively, that provides an electrical signal to ensure a steady heartbeat and to defibrillate the heart in case of severe arrhythmia

continues

TREATMENT PROCEDURES		
Word	**Pronunciation**	**Definition**
percutaneous transluminal coronary angioplasty (PTCA)	per"kū-tā'nē-ŭs trăns-loo'mĭ-năl kor'ō-nā-rē ăn'jē-ō-plăs"tē	opening an obstructed coronary artery with a balloon catheter (See Figure 8-16)
pericardiectomy	pĕr"ĭ-kăr"dē-ĕk'tō-mē	incision and partial removal of the pericardium to relieve the heart of adhesions
pericardiocentesis	pĕr"ĭ-kăr-dē-ō"sĕn-tē'sĭs	procedure to aspirate excess fluid from the pericardial space
permanent pacemaker (PPM)		small electronic device consisting of a battery and electrode implanted in the chest and heart, respectively, that provides an electrical signal to ensure a steady heartbeat
phlebectomy	flĕ-bĕk'tō-mē	excision or resection of a vein
phlebotomy	flĕ-bŏt'ō-mē	cutting into a vein
sclerotherapy	sklĕr"ō-thĕr'ă-pē	treatment that injects a chemical into a vein to harden, fill, or destroy it
stent	stĕnt	metal sleeve placed in an artery after angioplasty surgery to keep it from narrowing again (See Figure 8-19)
thrombectomy	thrŏm-bĕk'tō-mē	surgical removal of a clot from a blood vessel
thrombolytic therapy	thrŏm-bō-lĭt'-ĭk	procedure where drugs that dissolve clots are injected into bloodstream
valve replacement		excision of a diseased, incompetent valve, which is replaced with a prosthetic (artificial) valvular structure
vein ligation	lī-gā'shŭn	tying off an involved section of vein with a suture
venipuncture	vĕn'ĭ-pŭnk"tūr	surgical puncture of a vein
vein stripping		removal of a diseased portion of a vein

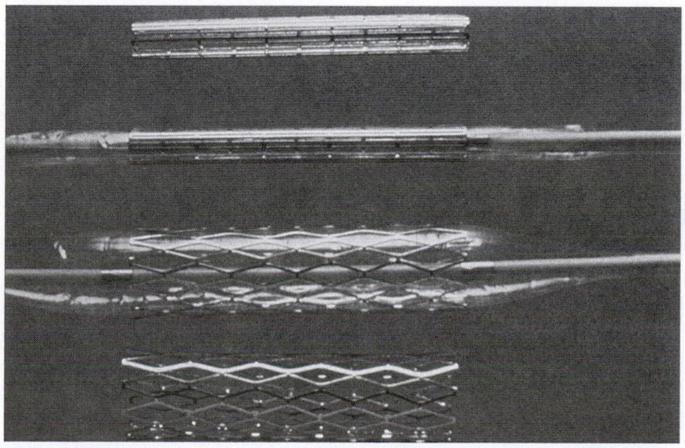

FIGURE 8-19 Four Stages of Stent Replacement (top to bottom): (1) nondeployed stent, (2) stent on delivery balloon, (3) balloon inflated stent expanded, and (4) expanded stent

Source: Courtesy of Cordis, a Johnson & Johnson Company, New Brunswick, NJ

MEDICATIONS PRESCRIBED	
Trade Name	Generic Name
Diuretics	
Aldactazide	spironolactone with HCTz
Aldactone	spironolactone
Bumex	bumetanide
Diuril	chlorothiazide
Dyazide	triamterene/HCTz
Dyrenium	triamterene
Enduron	methyclothiazide
HydroDIURIL, Esidrix	hydrochlorothiazide (HCTz)
Hygroton	chlorthalidone
Lasix	furosemide
Lozol	indapamide
Midamor	amiloride hydrochloride
Zaroxolyn	metolazone
Alpha-adrenergic Blockers	
Aldomet	methyldopa
Cardura	doxazosin mesylate
Catapres	clonidine hydrochloride
Hytrin	terazosin hydrochloride
Minipress	prazosin hydrochloride
Regitine	phentolamine mesylate
ACE Inhibitors	
Vasotec	enalapril maleate
Zestril	lisinopril
Angiotensin II Receptor Blockers (ARBs)	
Atacand	candesartan cilexetil
Cozaar	losartan
Beta-adrenergic Blockers	
Blocadren	timolol
Inderal	propranolol hydrochloride
Lopressor	metoprolol
Tenormin	atenolol
Toprol XL	metoprolol succinate

continues

MEDICATIONS PRESCRIBED	
Trade Name	Generic Name
Calcium Channel Blockers	
Calan, Isoptin	verapamil
Cardene	nicardipine
Cardizem	diltiazem hydrochloride
Norvasc	amlodipine
Procardia	nifedipine
Direct Vasodilators	
Apresoline	hydralazine hydrochloride
Hyperstat	diazoxide
Nipride	nitroprusside sodium
Other Cardiac Medications	
Adrenalin	epinephrine
Cordarone, Pacerone	amiodarone hydrochloride
Lanoxin	digoxin
Mexiletine	mexiletine hydrochloride
Nitrostat	nitroglycerine
Norpace	disopyramide phosphate
Pronestyl	procainamide hydrochloride
Quinidex	quinidine
Rythmol	propafenone hydrochloride
Tambocor	flecainide acetate
Thrombolytic Agents	
Abbokinase	urokinase
Activase	alteplase
Retavase	reteplase
Streptase	streptokinase
Anticoagulants	
—	Heparin
Coumadin	warfarin sodium
Fragmin	dalteparin
Lovenox	enoxaparin

continues

MEDICATIONS PRESCRIBED	
Trade Name	**Generic Name**
Antibiotics	
Amoxil	amoxicillin
Cipro	ciprofloxacin
Garamycin	gentamicin sulfate
Kefzol	cefazolin
Vancocin	vancomycin hydrochloride
V-Cillin K	penicillin V potassium
Other Supplements or Removing Agents	
Colestid	colestipol
K-Lor, Slow-K, Kay Ciel, Klor-Con, K-Tab, Ten-K, Micro-K	potassium chloride
Lipitor	atorvastatin
Mevacor	lovastatin
Questran	cholestyramine
Pravachol	pravastatin sodium
Zocor	simvastatin

ABBREVIATIONS	
ABG, ABGs	arterial blood gas(es)
ACE inhibitors	angiotensin-converting enzyme inhibitors
AI	aortic insufficiency
AMI	acute myocardial infarction
AS	aortic stenosis
ASD	atrial septal defect
ASHD	arteriosclerotic heart disease
AV, A-V	atrioventricular
BBB	bundle branch block
BP blood	pressure
CABG	coronary artery bypass graft
CAD	coronary artery disease
cath	catheterization
CCU	coronary care unit
CHD	coronary heart disease
CHF	congestive heart failure

continues

ABBREVIATIONS	
CoA	coarctation of the aorta
CPR	cardiopulmonary resuscitation
CVD	cardiovascular disease
DSA	digital subtraction angiography
DVT	deep venous thrombosis
ECC	extracorporeal circulation
ECG, EKG	electrocardiogram
ECHO	echocardiography
ETT	exercise tolerance test
HDL	high-density lipoprotein
IABP	intra-aortic balloon pump
ICD	internal cardioverter-defibrillator
LDL	low-density lipoprotein
LVAD	left ventricular assist device
MI	mitral insufficiency, myocardial infarction
MR	mitral regurgitation
MS	mitral stenosis
MUGA	multiple-gated acquisition scan
MVP	mitral valve prolapse
PAC	premature atrial contraction
PAT	paroxysmal atrial tachycardia
PCD	pacemaker cardiac defibrillator
PCI	percutaneous coronary intervention
PDA	patent ductus arteriosus
PPM	permanent pacemaker
PTCA	percutaneous transluminal coronary angioplasty
PVC	premature ventricular contraction
PVD	peripheral vascular disease
SA, S-A	sinoatrial
VSD	ventricular septal defect
VT	ventricular tachycardia

Working Practice Review Exercises

MATCHING

Match the terms to their meanings.

1.	________ recording device attached to the chest to monitor heart activity for a long period of time	a.	angiocardiography
2.	________ bypass of an obstructed coronary artery	b.	arterial blood gases
3.	________ x-ray visualization of the heart and blood vessels after contrast material is injected into the bloodstream	c.	artery graft
4.	________ surgical incision of connecting bands of commissure	d.	commissurotomy
5.	________ measurement of oxygen, carbon dioxide, and metabolic balance from an arterial blood sample	e.	coronary artery bypass
6.	________ screening tool for the detection of significant coronary artery disease	f.	endarterectomy
7.	________ removal of a diseased portion of a vein	g.	exercise stress test
8.	________ surgical removal of a clot from a blood vessel	h.	Holter monitor
9.	________ removal of the interior portion of an artery	i.	phlebectomy
10.	________ excision or restriction of a vein	j.	prothrombin time
11.	________ replacement of a portion of an artery by another open structure	k.	stent
12.	________ tests the coagulation of blood	l.	stress thallium test
13.	________ metal sleeve placed in an artery after angioplasty to keep it from narrowing again	m.	thrombectomy
14.	________ use of a radioactive tracer given during exercise to detect decreased blood flow to a portion of the heart muscle	n.	vein stripping
15.	________ x-ray of veins after injection of radiopaque material into the blood stream	o.	venography

SPELLING

Rewrite the misspelled words.

1. electrolights ________________________
2. enzemes ________________________
3. sodium ________________________
4. trigylcefides ________________________
5. potassium ________________________
6. hematocrit ________________________
7. cholesterol ________________________
8. prothronbin ________________________
9. extracorpeal ________________________
10. stint ________________________
11. translumenal ________________________

IDENTIFICATION

Identify the following diagnoses.

1. irregularity of the heartbeat ____________________
2. disease characterized by prolonged high blood pressure ____________________
3. heart disease produced by coronary artery disease ____________________
4. inflammatory disease of the endocardium ____________________
5. abnormality in the heart at birth ____________________
6. condition caused by a weakened heart resulting in an accumulation of fluid in tissues ____________________
7. low blood pressure ____________________
8. fixed blood clot ____________________
9. clotting and associated inflammation in the vein ____________________
10. fast heart rate ____________________
11. inflammation of a superficial vein ____________________
12. abnormal accumulation of tissue fluid ____________________
13. backward flowing through a defective heart valve ____________________
14. hardening of arteries ____________________
15. inadequate flow of blood to a body part ____________________

ABBREVIATIONS

Give the abbreviation for each of the following.

1. arteriosclerotic heart disease ____________________
2. atrioventricular ____________________
3. mitral insufficiency; myocardial infarction ____________________
4. premature ventricular contraction ____________________
5. sinoatrial ____________________
6. digital subtraction angiography ____________________
7. exercise tolerance test ____________________
8. internal cardioverter-defibrillator ____________________
9. permanent pacemaker ____________________
10. congestive heart failure ____________________

COMPLETION

Complete the following statements.

1. An ______________________ results when inadequate blood supply causes death of tissue.
2. When a blood vessel bulges or enlarges abnormally, an ______________________ results.
3. Disease of an artery, causing high blood pressure, often results in ______________________.
4. A localized malformation in the muscular wall of the aorta that makes it narrow is referred to as ______________________.
5. Abnormally swollen veins are ______________________ veins.
6. The removal of a diseased portion of a vein is ______________________.
7. Failure of a heart valve to close completely is called ______________________.
8. A graphic record of reflected ultrasound waves from the heart is a/an ______________________.
9. A heart attack is a/an ______________________.
10. Clotting occurring in the femoral and pelvic veins is referred to as ______________________.
11. Free-moving clot or debris from a buildup of atherosclerotic plaque is a/an ______________________.
12. A brief charge of electricity applied to the chest to stop cardiac arrhythmia is referred to as a/an ______________________.
13. Delivery of electric shock during an emergency situation to return heart to normal rhythm is referred to as ______________________.
14. Cutting into a vein is a procedure called ______________________.
15. Surgical puncture of a vein is referred to as ______________________.

CLASSIFICATION

Classify the following medications.

1. Aldactazide ______________________
2. coumadin ______________________
3. apresoline ______________________
4. Norvasc ______________________
5. Inderal ______________________
6. Zestril ______________________
7. Lasix ______________________
8. Procardia ______________________
9. Tenormin ______________________
10. Abbokinase ______________________

Dictionary Exercises

DICTIONARY EXERCISE 1

Use your dictionary to find the pronunciation and definition of the following words.

	Word	Pronunciation	Definition
1.	precordium	______	______
2.	atrophy	______	______
3.	auricle	______	______
4.	bigeminal	______	______
5.	bundle branch block	______	______
6.	Purkinje fibers	______	______
7.	cardiac massage	______	______
8.	cardiomotility	______	______
9.	cor pulmonale	______	______
10.	dilatation	______	______
11.	cusp	______	______
12.	lumen	______	______
13.	occlusion	______	______
14.	pneumopericardium	______	______
15.	sinus arrest	______	______
16.	ventricular septal defect	______	______
17.	atresia	______	______
18.	ductus arteriosus	______	______
19.	patent ductus arteriosus	______	______
20.	transposition	______	______
21.	hemodynamics	______	______
22.	bruit	______	______
23.	coarctation	______	______
24.	pallor	______	______
25.	percutaneous	______	______
26.	gradient	______	______
27.	hypokinesia	______	______
28.	circumflex	______	______
29.	intracoronary	______	______
30.	hypercholesterolemia	______	______

DICTIONARY EXERCISE 2

Pronunciation of the words below is provided. Using your dictionary, find the correct spelling and definition of the words.

	Word	Pronunciation	Definition
1.	______________	ăth"ĕr-ō-sklē-rŏt'ĭk	______________
2.	______________	păr"ŏk-sĭz'măl ā'trē-ăl	______________
	______________	tăk"ē-kăr'dē-ah	______________
3.	______________	kăr'dē-ak tăm"pŏn-ād'	______________
4.	______________	kăr'dē-ō-vĕr"zhŭn	______________
5.	______________	kŏm'ĭ-shūr	______________
6.	______________	dē-fĭb"rĭ-lā'tŏr	______________
7.	______________	dĭsp'nē-ah	______________
8.	______________	prē-kŏr'dē-ah	______________
9.	______________	pŭl-mŏn'ĭk stĕ-nō'sĭs	______________
10.	______________	păl-pĭ-tā'shŭn	______________
11.	______________	rē-sŭs"ĭ-tā'shŭn	______________
12.	______________	sī'nŭs ah-rĭth'mē-ah	______________
13.	______________	tĕ-trăl'ō-jē of făl-ō'	______________
14.	______________	sĭn'kō-pē	______________
15.	______________	ah-năs"tō-mō'sĭs	______________
16.	______________	klaw"dĭ-kā'shŭn	______________
17.	______________	eks-trăv"ah-sā'shŭn	______________
18.	______________	plăk	______________
19.	______________	văs"ō-kŏn-strĭk'shŭn	______________
20.	______________	pĕr-fū'zhŭn	______________
21.	______________	ăn"ah-săr'kah	______________
22.	______________	hī"pŏks'ē-ă	______________
23.	______________	văs"ō-kŏn-strĭk'shŭn	______________
24.	______________	sī-ă-nō'sĭs	______________
25.	______________	thrŏm-bŏt'ĭk ŏ-kloo'zhŭn	______________

DICTIONARY EXERCISE 3

Rewrite the following sentences in your own words. Provide the pronunciation of the italicized words where indicated.

1. The patient arrived in *cardiac arrest* and *resuscitation* (______________) measures were performed.

   ____

2. Diagnosis suggested *aortic regurgitation* (______________).

   ____

3. The doctor heard a *gallop rhythm*.

   ____

4. The patient experienced *paroxysmal ventricular tachycardia* (________________).

5. Her doctor suspected *subacute bacterial endocarditis* (________________).

6. *Sinus rhythm* was normal.

7. Problems may be attributed to a *heart block*.

8. The physician heard *atrial fibrillation* (________________).

9. Unfortunately the baby was born with an *atrial septal defect* (________________).

10. *Central venous pressure* was elevated.

11. *Coronary artery perfusion* will be performed on Monday.

12. The patient's problem arose from an *embolus* (________________).

13. Upon physical examination, the patient was noted to have *pitting edema* in her ankle.

14. The physician prescribed *digitalis* (________________).

15. *Ischemia* (________________) resulted in *necrosis* (________________) of part of the myocardium.

16. His doctor believed the next step was a *percutaneous transluminal coronary angioplasty* (________________).

17. The doctor noted there were no rubs, *bruits* (________________), or *thrills*.

18. Mrs. Krasnowski took her prescription for a *beta blocker* to the pharmacy.

19. Hal complained of *claudication* (________________).

20. Madelyn discovered her new medication was a *statin*.

*Study*WARE™ Connection

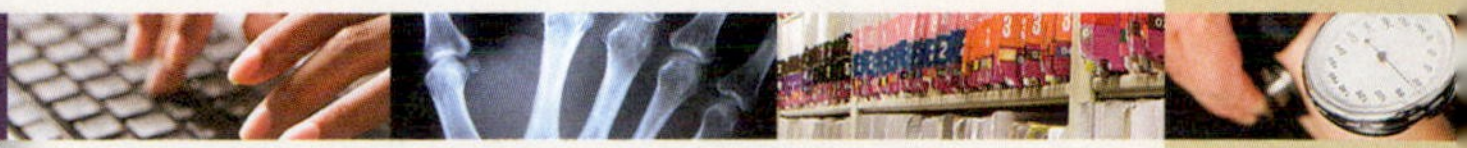

To play interactive games that reinforce the content in this chapter, go to your StudyWARE™ CD-ROM.

Listening Exercise

INSTRUCTIONS

1. Review the spelling, pronunciation, and meaning of the words provided in the preview.
2. Go to your StudyWARE™ CD-ROM and listen to **Listening Exercise 8-1**. Fill in the blank in the report as the word is dictated.
3. At the end of the activity, check your spelling against the preview words. They appear in the preview in the order in which they are encountered in the activity.
4. Review and practice the words you missed.
5. Look up words that are not familiar.

PREVIEW OF WORDS FOR LISTENING EXERCISE 8-1

Word	Pronunciation	Meaning
thrombolytic therapy	thrŏm"bō-lĭt'ĭk	treatment designed to break up a thrombus
ventriculogram	vĕn-trĭk'ū-lō-grăm	radiogram of the ventricles of the heart
percutaneous	pĕr"kū-tā'nē-ŭs	accomplished through the skin
gradient	grā'dē-ĕnt	an increase or decrease of varying degrees
hypokinesia	hī"pō-kī-nē'zē-ă	decreased motor activity
circumflex	sĕr'kŭm-flĕks	curved like a bow; spiraling around arteriosclerotic
heart disease	ăr-tē"rē-ō-sklĕ-rŏt'ĭk	heart disease produced by coronary artery disease

Listening Exercise 8-1

StudyWARE™ Connection

Listen to this report being read on your StudyWARE™ CD-ROM. Fill in each blank as the word is dictated.

Cardiac Catheterization and Angiography Report

PATIENT PROFILE: The patient is a 51-year-old woman with an acute anterior wall myocardial infarction treated with

_________________________.

PROCEDURE: Left heart catheterization with left _________________________ and coronary arteriography with _________________________ transluminal coronary angioplasty of the proximal left anterior descending and placement of an intracoronary stent and intracoronary nitroglycerin administration was performed without complication.

FINDINGS: Left ventricular pressure prior to left ventriculogram was 119/-1, 11 mm/Hg and following left ventriculogram was 121/0, 9 mm/Hg. Aortic pressure following left ventriculogram was 121/63 mm/Hg with a mean of 87 mm/Hg. There was no systolic _________________________. The left ventriculogram demonstrated mild _________________________ of the anterior wall of the left ventricle with an overall normal ejection fraction of 61%. There was no mitral insufficiency. The coronary arteriogram demonstrated no significant disease of the left main and left _________________________ coronary arteries. There was an 80% proximal stenosis of the left anterior descending coronary artery before the septal perforator branch and a 50% proximal stenosis of a small intermediate coronary artery. There was no significant disease of the right coronary artery. The left anterior descending coronary artery was dominant. The 80% proximal stenosis of the left anterior descending coronary artery was reduced to a residual 0% stenosis following placement of a 3.0 mm J&J stent that was deployed at 6 atmospheres and extended at 14 atmospheres with a 3.0 mm noncompliant Ranger balloon catheter.

IMPRESSION:

1. _________________________ _________________________ _________________________, acute anterior wall myocardial infarction treated with thrombolytic therapy, mild hypokinesia of the anterior wall of the left ventricle with a normal ejection fraction, normal left ventricular filling pressure with a significant proximal stenosis of the left anterior descending coronary artery.
2. Successful angioplasty of the proximal left anterior descending coronary artery using an intracoronary stent.

____

Chan Zhou, MD

CHAPTER 9

The Blood and Lymph Systems

"Blood is a very special juice."

—Goethe

OBJECTIVES

When you have completed this study of the blood and lymph systems, you should be able to

1. Spell and define major system components and explain how they operate.
2. Identify the meanings of related word elements.
3. Spell and define diagnostic procedures, diagnoses, treatment procedures, and abbreviations.
4. Spell the names of commonly used medications.
5. Use a dictionary as a tool in processing medical documents.
6. Hear how medical terminology is used in actual medical reports.

INTRODUCTION

Blood is essential to our existence. It travels literally miles in our veins and arteries, performing many functions grouped primarily into transportation and protection. Blood transports oxygen, carbon dioxide, nutrients, glucose, amino acids, fats, waste products, hormones, electrolytes, and heat from one part of the body to another. When disease or infection invades the body, chemical substances called antibodies move within the blood and take defensive action where needed.

Because blood flows through, around, and among body tissues, organs, and other blood vessels, certain diseases can be diagnosed with the aid of specific blood tests. The study of blood, **hematology** (hē"mah-tŏl'ō-jē), requires knowledge about the bone marrow, spleen, lymph nodes, and all the components of blood. Physicians who specialize in the study and treatment of the blood system are called **hematologists** (hē"mah-tŏl'ō-jĭsts).

COMPOSITION OF BLOOD

bas/o	base	hemat/o, hem/o	blood
blast/o	primitive cell	leuk/o	white
cyt/o	cell	mega-	large
-emia	blood condition	neutr/o	neutral
erythr/o	red	sangui/o	blood

The average adult has about six quarts of blood. Blood is composed of two prime elements, a liquid called plasma and a solid called formed elements, or cells.

PLASMA

Plasma is the fluid component of blood. About fifty-five percent of blood is plasma, and the plasma itself is composed of about ninety percent water. The remaining part of the plasma contains approximately 100 different substances dissolved or suspended in this watery medium. The largest component, about seven percent, is a group of proteins made up of **serum albumin** (ăl-bū'mĭn), **serum globulin** (glŏb'ū-lĭn), **fibrinogen** (fī-brĭn'ō-jĕn), and other coagulation proteins such as **prothrombin** (prō-thrŏm'bĭn). There are three types of globulin: alpha, beta, and gamma. They are identified by a process called **electrophoresis** (ē-lĕk"trō-fō-rē'sĭs). The gamma globulin fraction is especially important because it contains antibodies.

Sodium, calcium, potassium, magnesium, phosphorus, and other minerals comprise about one percent of the plasma; they are the **inorganic constituents**. Major **organic constituents** are amino acids, glucose, neutral fats (phospholipids [fŏs"-fō-lĭp'ĭds] and cholesterol [kō-lĕs'ter-ŏl]), and waste products (urea, uric acid, creatinine [krē-ăt'ĭ-nĭn], ammonia, and lactic acids). Plasma carries the nutrients to body cells for nourishment purposes and returns with waste products such as carbon dioxide, which it takes to the kidneys, bowels, intestines, lungs, or skin for excretion. Internal secretions, or hormones, antibodies, and enzymes, make up the remainder of the plasma.

CELLS

The basic unit of the body, the **cell**, varies in size and purpose. (For a review of cells, see Chapter 2.) Three types of blood cells flow freely suspended in the plasma shown in Figure 9-1: erythrocytes, leukocytes, and platelets (thrombocytes). They are formed in the red bone marrow found in the ends of long bones and in the pelvic and other flat bones.

Erythrocytes

Erythrocytes (ĕ-rĭth'rō-sīts) (1) are tiny disk-shaped red blood cells with a central area that is thinner than the edges. On average there are 4.5 million to 6 million erythrocytes per cubic millimeter of blood. Erythrocytes live for about 120 days in the bloodstream; then some of the elements are recycled as new ones are produced.

The main purpose of red blood cells is to carry oxygen from the lungs to the tissues. **Hemoglobin** (hē'mō-glō"bĭn), the primary ingredient of these cells, absorbs oxygen. Hemoglobin also carries about ten percent of the body's carbon dioxide back to the lungs. The normal hemoglobin measurement in the blood of males is from 14 to 18 grams per 100 milliliters; in the blood of females, it is from 12 to 16 grams per 100 milliliters. Iron is an essential constituent of hemoglobin. If iron is lacking, the size, color, and number of red blood cells are affected.

A **hematocrit** (hē-măt'ō-krĭt) is a measurement of red blood cells. It is done by comparing the volume of red blood cells with the total volume of blood. The normal range for men is forty to fifty-four percent; for women, it is thirty-seven to forty-seven percent.

Leukocytes

Leukocytes (lū'kō-sīts) (3) are white blood cells, pale in color with an irregular, ball-like shape, that contain nuclei of varying shapes and sizes. The normal number of leukocytes per cubic centimeter of blood ranges from 5,000 to 10,000.

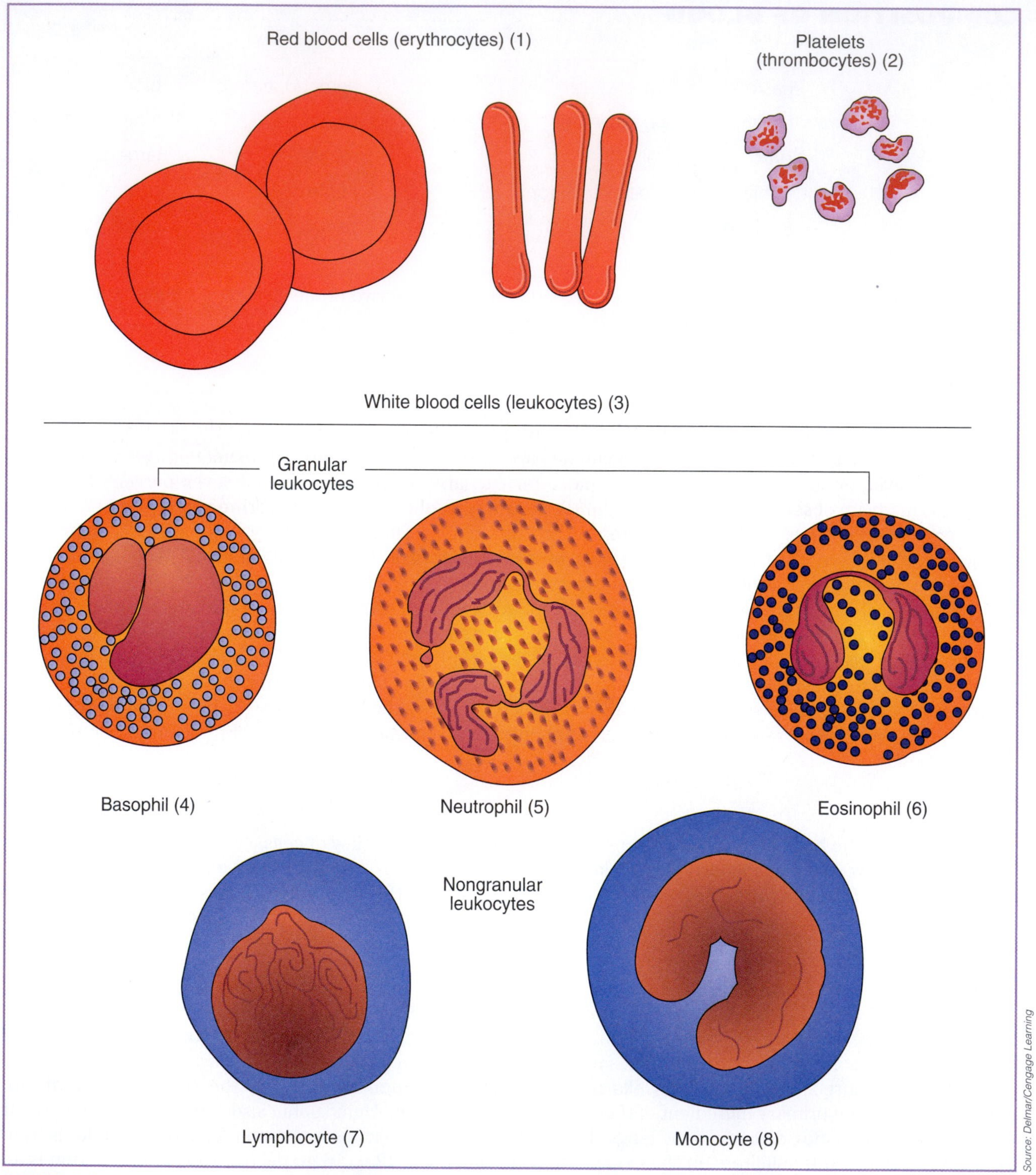

FIGURE 9-1 The Classification of Blood Cells

There are two major types of leukocytes: granular and nongranular (or agranular). Figure 9-1 shows both types. Granular leukocytes are the more numerous of the two types and are called **granulocytes** (grăn'ū-lō-sīts"), or a **polymorphonuclear** (pŏl"ē-mor"fō-noo'klē-ar) **leukocytes**. A granulocyte is classified as basophil (bā'sō-fĭl) (4), neutrophil (nū'trō-fĭl) (5), and eosinophil (ē"ō-sĭn'ō-fĭl) (6) based on their various staining qualities with specific dyes.

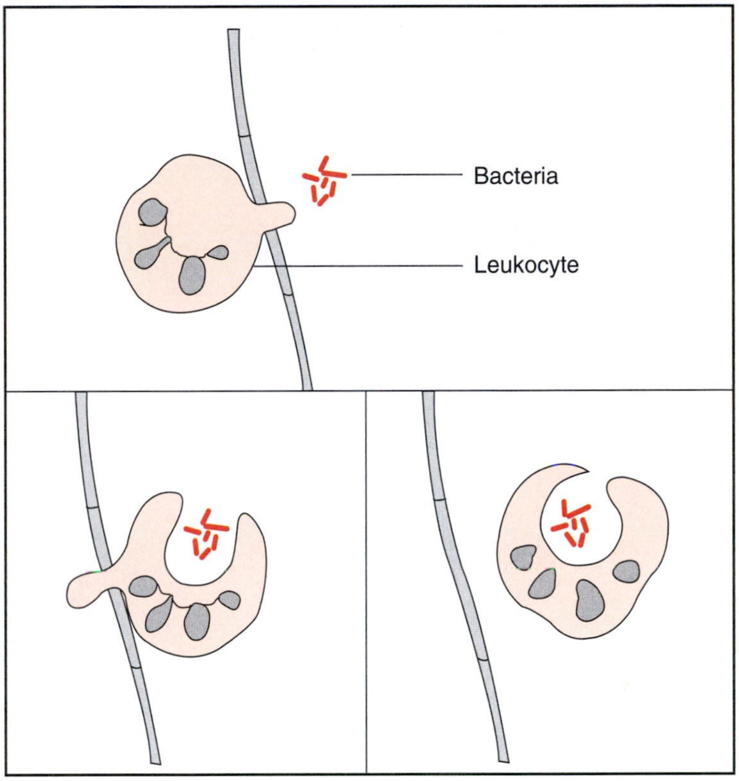

FIGURE 9-2 Body's Process of Fighting Infection: leukocytes pass through blood vessel walls and other cell membranes to engulf bacteria

Source: Delmar/Cengage Learning

Granulocytes are produced in the red bone marrow. When infection invades the body, production of granulocytes in the blood increases. As shown in Figure 9-2, these cells then pass through blood vessel walls and gather in the area of infection. The cells then form pus or a purulent discharge.

The other type of leukocyte is an **agranulocyte** (ă-grăn'ū-lō-sīt), or **mononuclear** (mŏn-ō-nū'klē-ăr) **cell**. It includes lymphocytes (7) and monocytes (8), as shown in Figure 9-1. Lymphocytes contain B cells and T cells and react to specific infecting agents. T cells are attack cells. B cells produce antibodies as their contribution to the body's defense. Some T cells instruct the B cells on which antibodies to make. Monocytes respond to many different types of infections and defend the body by engulfing foreign substances.

Platelets

Platelets, or **thrombocytes** (thrŏm'bō-sīts) (2) (see Figure 9-1), are essential for coagulation. If it were not for them, we would bleed to death from even the slightest cut. When a blood vessel is damaged, the platelets gather at that point and form a plug that closes the hole in the vessel (see Figure 9-3). At the same time, platelets release a chemical that helps activate the formation from fibrinogen (1) of a protein called **fibrin** (fī'brĭn). Fibrin (2) has the appearance of fine threads tangled together. As red cells are caught in the tangle of fibrin threads, they form the clot and give it its characteristic red color.

Platelets, or thrombocytes, are produced in the bone marrow from a white blood cell called a **megakaryocyte** (mĕg ah-kăr'ē-ō-sīt). This cell is many times larger than other white blood cells and forms small particles in the cytoplasm around its nucleus as it develops. Once particles break out of the cell and enter the bloodstream, they are called platelets.

StudyWARE™ Connection

View an animation on **Blood** on your StudyWARE™ CD-ROM.

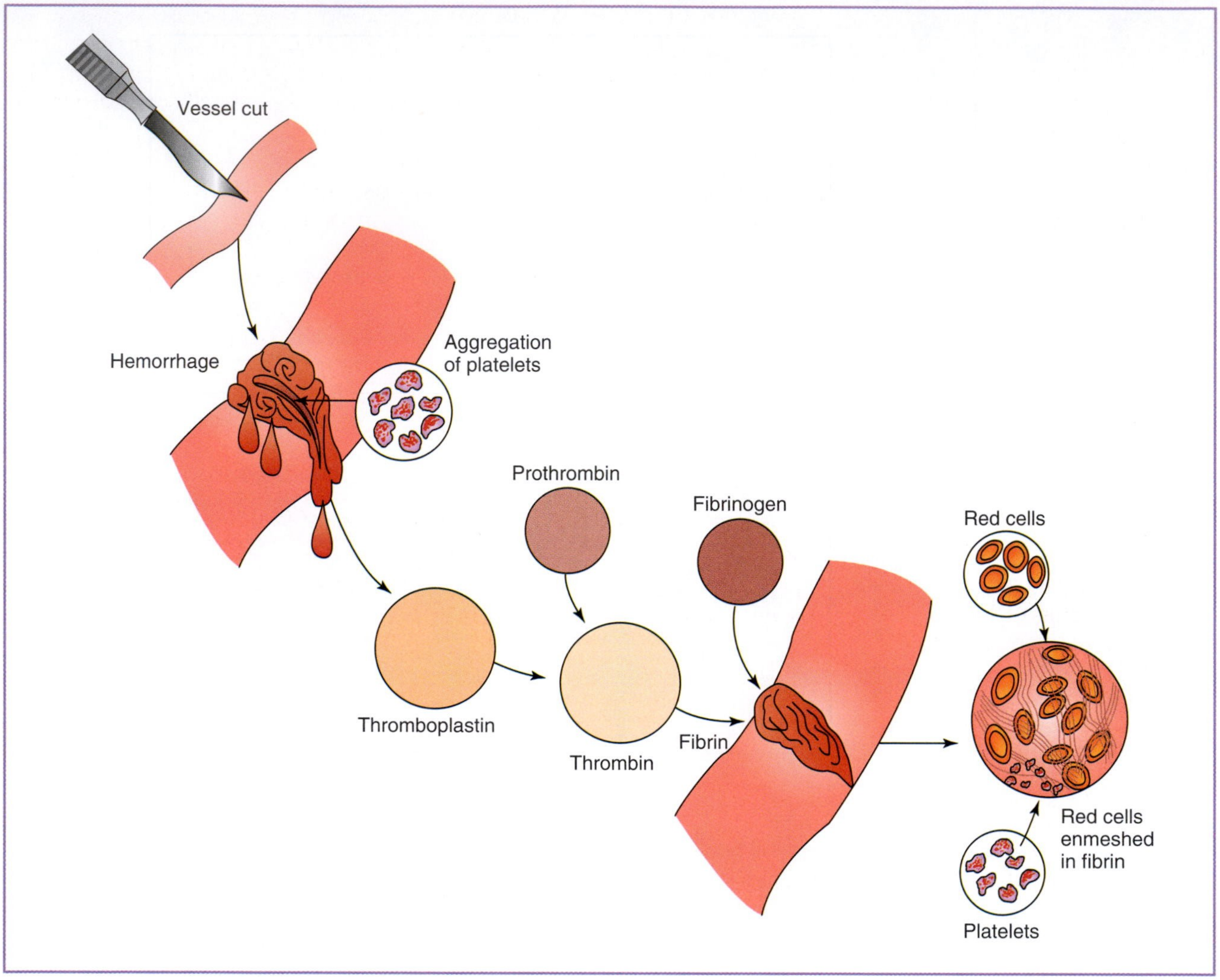

FIGURE 9-3 The Stages of Blood Clotting

BLOOD TYPING AND TRANSFUSIONS

agglutin/o	clumping, sticking together

There are many protein substances, or **antigens** (ăn'tĭ-jĕns), on the surface of the red blood cell that cause the blood of one person to be different from that of another. Antigens are substances that induce the formation of antibodies, which interact specifically with the antigens. The major antigens are referred to as A, B, and Rh. The presence or absence of the A and B antigens determines a person's blood type or group. Here is a summary of the characteristics of the four blood types.

Blood Type	Contains
A	A antigens and anti-B antibodies
B	B antigens and anti-A antibodies
AB	A and B antigens, but *neither* anti-A nor anti-B antibodies
O	neither A nor B antigens, but *both* anti-A and anti-B antibodies

The **transfusion** of blood may become necessary for injuries involving a severe loss of blood volume, during a surgical procedure, or for treatment of certain diseases. But with fourteen different blood groups (this varies by ethnic group) and more than 100 antigens, the composition of each person's blood is unique. This introduces an element of risk to the transfusion process because the blood of the donor may contain substances that will damage red blood cells of the recipient. In this case the donor is said to have **incompatible blood**. For example, if type A blood is transfused into a type B recipient, the A antigens from the type A blood (donor) will react adversely with the anti-A antibodies in the type B blood (recipient). Two kinds of reaction that may occur are **agglutination** (ă-gloo"tĭ-nā'shŭn) (clumping of cells) or **lysis** (lī'sĭs) (destruction of cells). (Lysis is also called hemolysis.)

People with AB blood type—who have neither anti-A nor anti-B antibodies—are considered *universal recipients*: They can receive blood from any blood type. Those with blood type O are considered *universal donors* because they have no antigens that antibodies may attack. But the notion of universal recipients or donors is theoretical because there are many other factors in blood that may result an adverse reaction during a transfusion.

The other major antigen group is designated the **Rh factor**. The Rh factor is designated as positive when it is present and negative when it is not. When an Rh negative woman with an Rh positive mate produces an Rh positive infant, some of the blood of the mother and infant may intermix at birth. The mother's blood will then form anti-Rh antibodies. In a future pregnancy, the antibodies may enter the fetus' bloodstream and can result in **hemolytic** (hē"mō-lĭt'ik) **disease of the newborn** (formerly erythroblastosis fetalis [ĕ-rĭth'rō-blăs-tō'sĭs fĕ-tă'lĭs]) or neonatal jaundice. In this case, the child may be stillborn or, if alive, may require a replacement transfusion at birth. Today these mothers can be given Rho(D) immune globulin (human), called RhoGAM, a drug to prevent this antibody formation from occurring.

BLOOD DERIVATIVES

Blood can be separated into its various components and used for a number of purposes. Plasma, serum, and gamma globulin are three that are used frequently. Plasma is the fluid portion of the blood that remains after all the cells have been removed; ninety-one percent is water. Since it has no red cells, it can be transfused without compatibility problems. **Serum** is the clear, thin, sticky fluid portion of blood that is left after blood has clotted. The difference between plasma and serum is that plasma contains fibrinogen and serum does not. Serum does contain many valuable protein substances, including **gamma globulin**, which is the protein fluid that contains most of the antibodies.

The various formed elements (cells) are also separated and transfused for specific needs.

LYMPH SYSTEM

aden/o	gland	splen/o	spleen
immun/o	immune, protection	thym/o	thymus
lymph/o	lymph		

The lymphatic system is part of the infection-fighting system of the body and is closely associated with the blood and cardiovascular systems, bone marrow, spleen, and thymus. The combination of vessels and glands form a vast network throughout the body.

Blood, although contained in vascular channels, is constantly interchanged with fluids outside the vessel walls. This fluid, which leaves the blood vessels and comes into direct contact with tissue cells, is called **lymph**. Lymph itself is an almost colorless fluid rich in white blood cells, called lymphocytes, and similar in appearance to blood plasma.

The lymph system serves as a drainage system that transports proteins and fluids into the bloodstream. It absorbs lipids (fats) from the small intestine and transports them to the bloodstream. It is related to the **immune system**, the body's defense system against foreign organisms, through the processes of defense, attack, and removal of pathogens. It also helps the body to remove aging or dead cells and other debris.

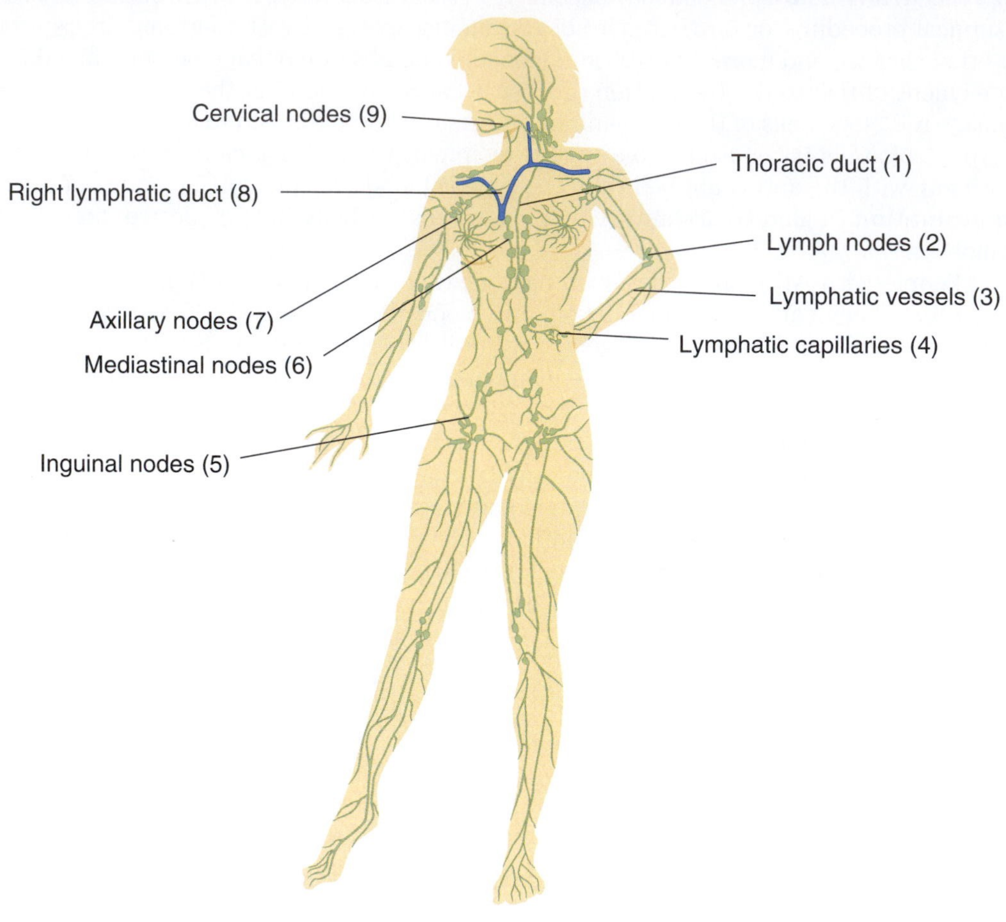

FIGURE 9-4
Lymphatic System

Source: Delmar/Cengage Learning

In Figure 9-4, note that lymphatic capillaries (4) and lymphatic vessels (3) are located in every part of the body except the brain, spinal cord, eyeball, internal ear, nails, and hair. They usually follow the path of the small blood vessels and run along with the nerves. Then they empty first into the chains of interconnected lymph nodes and finally into larger collecting lymphatic vessels, such as the thoracic duct.

The lymphatic vessels, thin-walled and delicate, are constructed with valves to prevent backflow. There are superficial (surface) and deep sets of vessels. The surface lymphatics are immediately below the skin, often continuing near the superficial veins. The deep vessels are larger and accompany the deeper veins. All lymphatic vessels form networks and at certain points carry lymph to and from small filtering stations called lymph nodes. Figure 9-5 shows this process.

LYMPH NODES

Lymph nodes (2) (see Figure 9-4) are made of a specialized tissue that removes impurities, manufactures lymphocytes, and produces antibodies. The nodes filter the lymph once it is drained from the tissues, as shown in Figure 9-6. Each node also has a fibrous connective tissue capsule from which partitions extend into the substance of an organ. Inside the nodes are masses of lymphatic tissue with space set aside for the production of lymphocytes and/or antibodies.

Lymph nodes are usually found in groups of 2 to more than 100. They are named according to their location, as illustrated in Figure 9-4. Some of the more common nodes and locations are as follows:

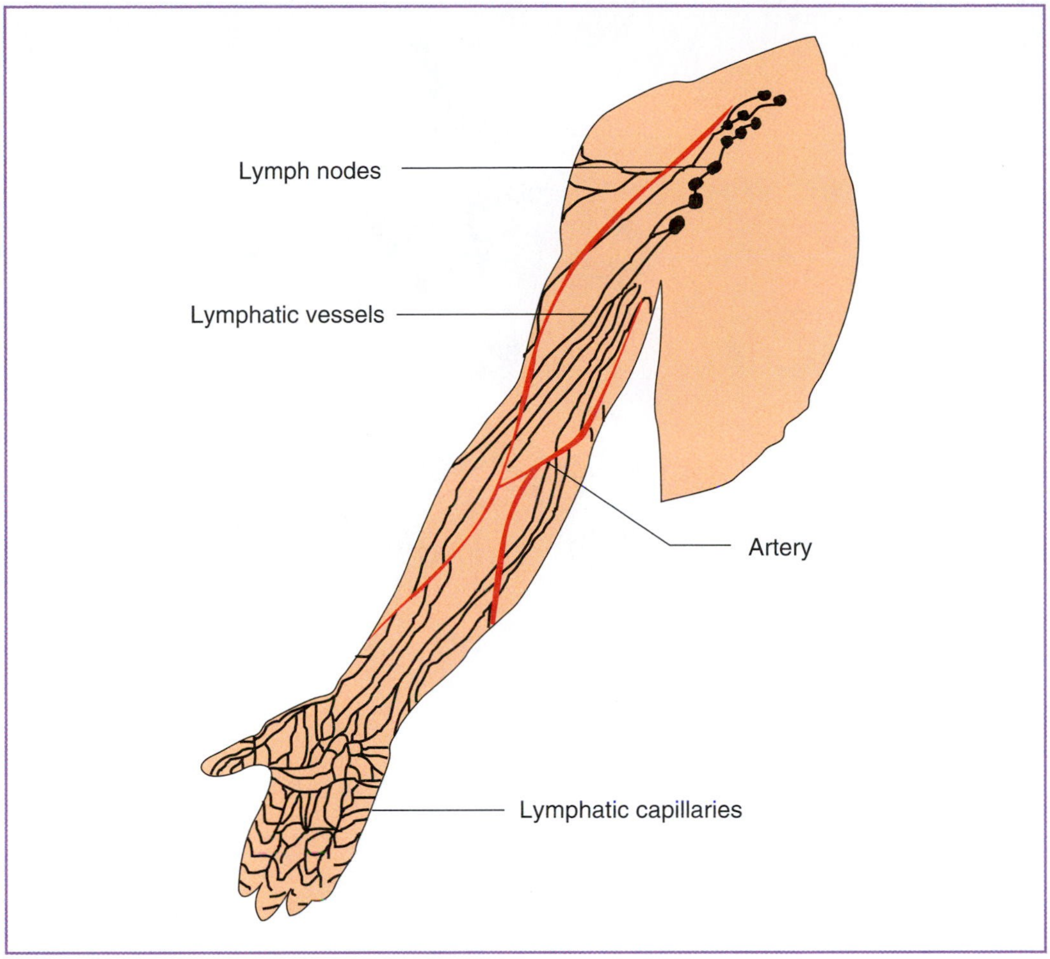

FIGURE 9-5
A Section of the Lymphatic System

Axillary nodes (7)
Nodes located in the armpits; they become enlarged from infections of the upper extremities and breasts; they often are invaded by cancer cells from the breasts.

Cervical nodes (9)
Nodes located in the neck that drain various parts of the head and neck; they often become enlarged during upper respiratory infections.

Tracheobronchial, mediastinal (6), and hilar nodes
Nodes located in the center of the chest between major organs such as the heart and lungs.

Inguinal nodes (5)
Nodes located in the groin.

Celiac, mesenteric, and retroperitoneal nodes
Nodes found behind the peritoneum within the abdomen.

LYMPH DUCTS

Ultimately the lymph vessels drain into two principal **lymph ducts**—the **thoracic** and **right lymphatic ducts**. The thoracic duct (1) (See Figure 9-7) drains most of the body. The beginning of this tube in the abdomen is enlarged to form a temporary storage pouch called the **cisterna chyli** (sĭs-ter'nah kī'lē). It empties into the left subclavian

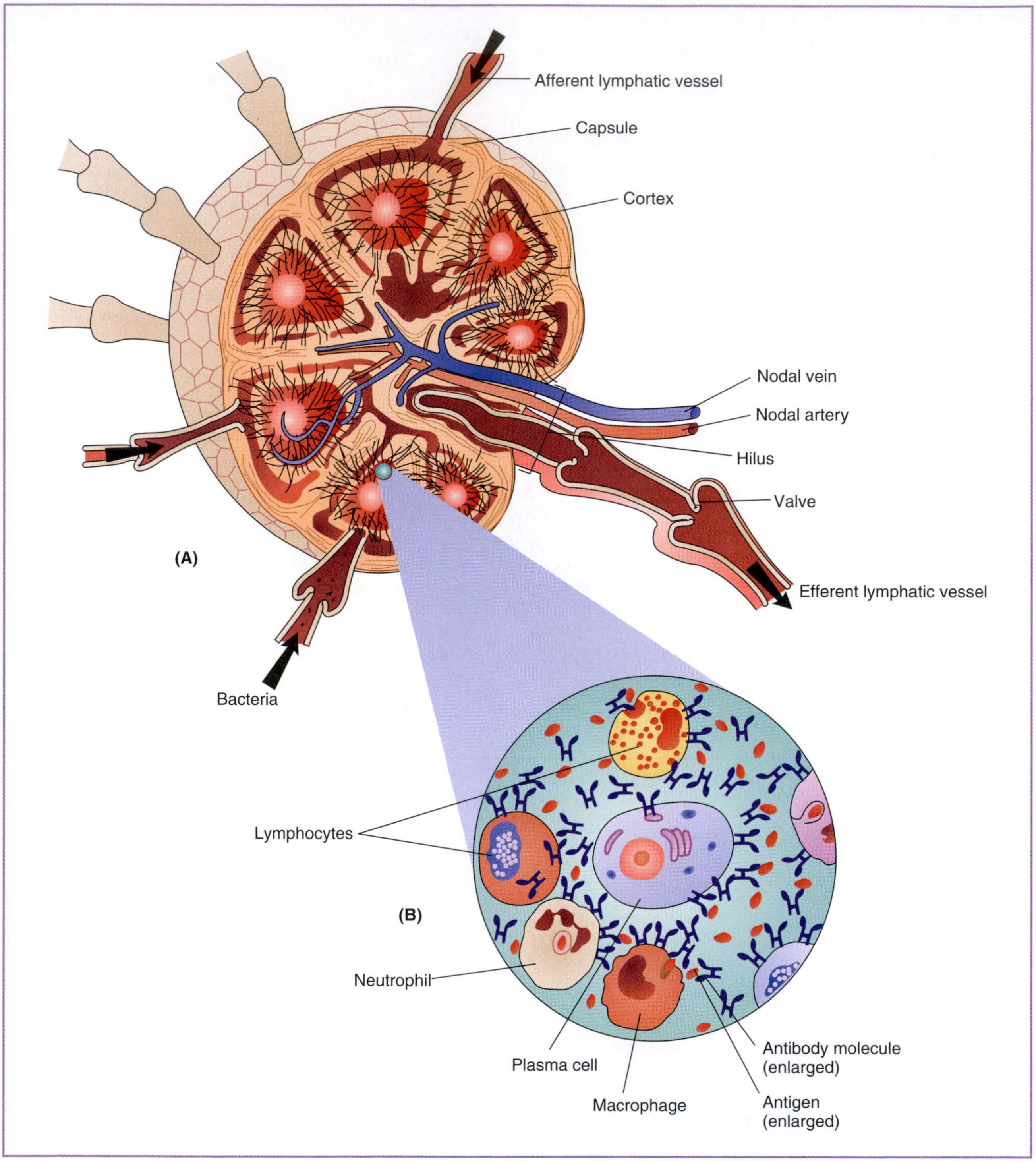

FIGURE 9-6 Lymph node (A) Section through a lymph node showing the flow of lymph. (B) Microscopic detail of bacteria being destroyed within the lymph node

vein. The right lymphatic duct (8) receives lymph from the right side of the head, neck, thorax, and right upper extremity. This empties into the right subclavian vein.

LYMPHOID ORGANS

The lymphoid organs include the thymus, spleen, and tonsils. These lymphoid organs, which are not strictly lymph nodes, perform many similar functions. From fetal life through adolescence, the **thymus** (thī'mŭs) is especially

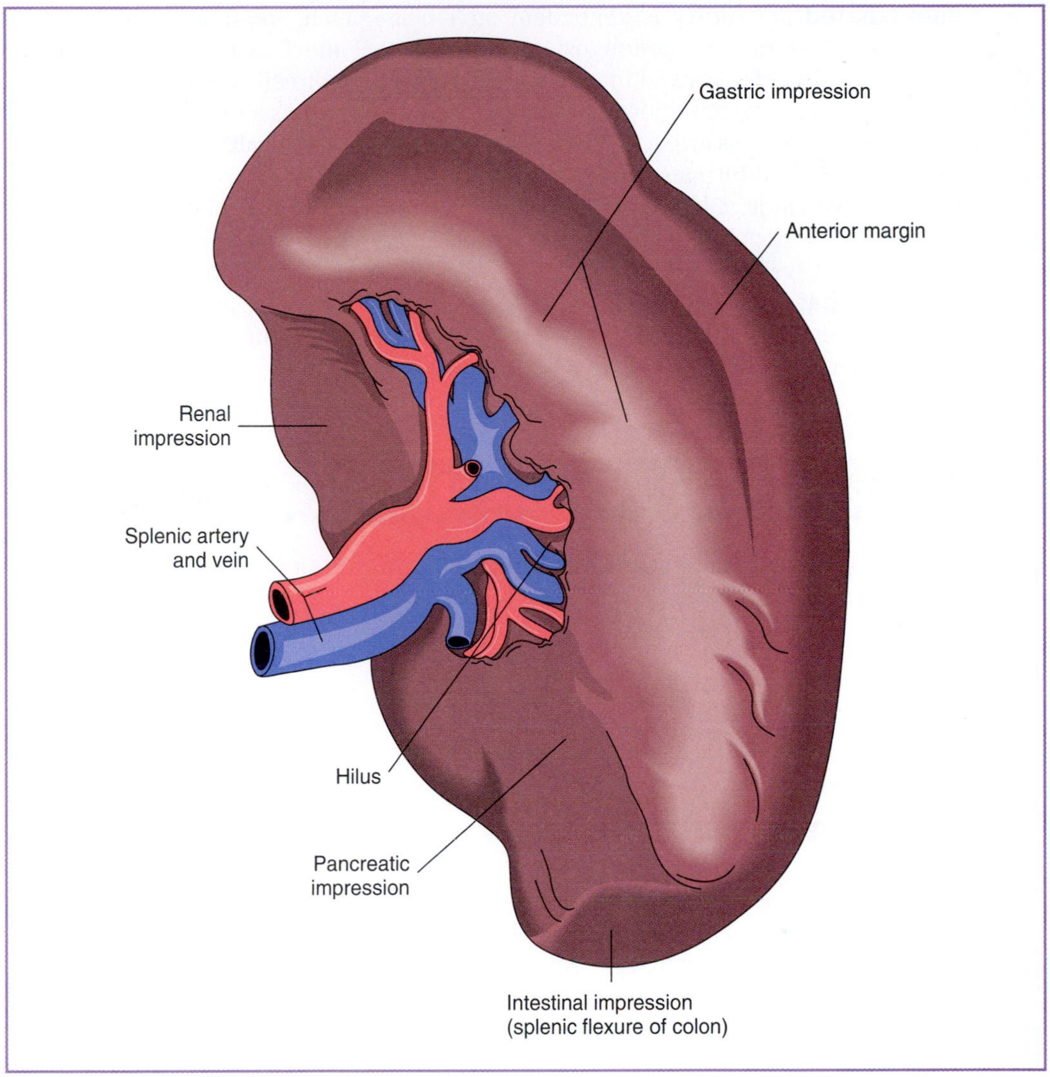

FIGURE 9-7
External View of the Spleen

important in directing the body's development of antibodies and other immune functions. It also tells lymph nodes how to work in early life. After adolescence, the thymus gradually reduces in size.

The **spleen**, as shown in Figure 9-7, is essentially a large lymph node with an extensive network of blood vessels added. The size of the spleen increases through childhood, but remains fairly stable in adults. Any increase in size is usually the result an underlying condition or disease. This enlargement displays no symptoms and is called **splenomegaly** (splē-"nō-mĕg'ăh-lē).

The spleen is not essential to maintain life, even though it serves several functions. Its chief function is the formation of lymphocytes and monocytes and the destruction of bacteria, white blood cells, and aging red blood cells. Splenomegaly may cause the destruction of blood cells passing through the spleen (hypersplenism), leading to low blood counts (pancytopenia). Splenic absence (asplenia) may cause increased susceptibility to bloodstream infection (septicemia).

Tonsils, located on either side of the pharyngeal wall of the throat, play a part in the manufacture of lymphocytes. They too can be removed without endangering one's existence.

Although blood and lymph are essentially two different substances and systems, they intertwine in a way that assists the body in defending itself. This is referred to as the immune system. When bacteria enter the body, the first attack comes from **phagocytes** (făg'ō-sīts), a neutrophil (or monocyte) that attacks bacteria. If that fails, B and T cells (two major types of lymphocytes) are the next line of defense.

Humoral (hū'mor-al) **immunity** is an immune response based on B cells that are transformed into plasma cells. They secrete antibodies called **immunoglobulins** (ĭm"ū-nō-glob'ū-lĭns) and activate a complex series of proteins (such as complement proteins) that aid antibodies in destroying antigens.

Cell-mediated immunity is dependent on T cells which, when activated, surround and digest the antigen (such as a cancer cell, virus, fungus, or bacterium). Some T cells produce chemicals called **lymphokines** (lĭm'fō-kīns) (e.g., interferons and interleukins) that help other cells respond to antigens. Essentially the T cells act as helper cells to promote antibody synthesis by B cells or act as suppressor cells to inhibit antibody synthesis. Also involved in this process are dendritic cells. These cells are specialized white blood cells that process antigens and then transport this information to the T cells.

There are two kinds of **immunity**: natural and acquired. A **natural immunity** is one that exists from birth. Acquired immunities develop from either an active or passive event occurring after birth. An **active acquired immunity** is generally long term in nature and is the result of having a particular disease or having a vaccination for the disease. A **passive acquired immunity** usually provides only short-term protection and is the result of an injection of antibodies or immunoglobulins produced by another human or an animal. Antibodies passed from the mother to the fetus is an example of passive acquired immunity.

StudyWARE™ Connection

To watch an animation on the **Lymphatic System,** go to your StudyWARE™ CD-ROM.

INTERNET ASSIGNMENT

Medem is a physician-patient communication network on the Internet that seeks to sell secure communications and Web-based services for a physician's practice. As a service to physicians and the general public, they have partnered with medical societies such as the American Academy of Ophthalmology, the American Medical Association, and the American Psychiatric Association. The health care information provided is peer reviewed for accuracy. Access to this information is through the Medical Library entry.

Four general topic areas are available: Life Stages, Diseases and Conditions, Therapies and Health Strategies, and Health and Society. All listed items under each general topic are coded from simple to complex to provide the visitor with an indication of the difficulty of the information included.

ACTIVITY

Visit Medem at **www.medem.com.** Select for Patients and Medical Library. Then follow Medical Library link through Diseases and Conditions to Blood Disorders which will present a list of topics. Click on Sickle Cell Anemia and select one of the links. Read the information you find and summarize that portion that is new to you in a report to your instructor.

Review The Blood and Lymph Systems

- Blood has two prime elements: liquids (or plasma) and solids (or cells).
- Three types of cells flow in the plasma: erythrocytes (red), leukocytes (white), and platelets (thrombocytes).
- Antigens and antibodies on the surface of the red cell create an element of risk in the transfusion of blood from one person to another.
- The lymph system, composed of lymph nodes, ducts, and organs, is closely associated with the blood and cardiovascular systems, bone marrow, spleen, and thymus.
- The lymph system is related to the immune system, the body's defense system against foreign organisms.

Key Terminology Review

Word	Definition
agglutination	clumping of cells
agranulocytes (mononuclear cells)	white blood cells classified as lymphocytes or monocytes; nongranular leukocytes
antigen	substance that induces the formation of antibodies, which interact with the antigens
cell	basic unit of the body; circulating blood cells are: erythrocytes, leukocytes, and platelets
cell-mediated immunity	immune response based on T cell activity
cisterna chyli	enlarged portion of the main lymph duct in the abdomen
electrophoresis	technique that distinguishes between beta, alpha, and gamma globulins and other proteins
erythrocytes	red blood cells
fibrin	protein that allows blood to clot; formed from fibrinogen
fibrinogen	a protein element of blood
gamma globulin	protein plasma that contains most of the antibodies
granulocytes (polymorphonuclear leukocytes)	white blood cells classified as neutrophils, eosinophils, or basophils according to the granules they contain

continues

Word	Definition
hematocrit	measurement of the volume of red blood cells compared to the total volume of blood
hematologist	physician specializing in the study and treatment of the blood system
hematology	study and treatment of blood
hemoglobin	primary carrier of oxygen in red blood cells; the red pigment of erythrocytes and blood
hemolytic disease of the newborn	condition where antibodies of the mother's blood may enter the bloodstream of the fetus and destroy the fetal erythrocytes; formerly erythroblastosis fetalis
humoral immunity	immune response based on B cell activity and antibody production
immune system	body's defense system against foreign organisms
immunity • *natural (native)* • *active acquired* • *passive acquired*	 immunity one is born with the result of having a particular disease or having a vaccination for the disease; generally long term in nature the result of an injection of antibodies or immunoglobulins produced by another human or an animal; protection usually short term (e.g., mother to fetus)
immunoglobulins	antibodies secreted by B cells
incompatible blood	transfused blood containing an antigen against which a person has an antibody
inorganic constituents of plasma	sodium, calcium, potassium, magnesium, phosphorus
leukocytes	white blood cells; two major types are polymorphonuclear and mononuclear
lymph	almost colorless fluid rich in lymphocytes
lymph ducts, left (or thoracic) and right lymphatic	channels that drain lymph from the body
lymph nodes	specialized tissue that filters lymph after it has drained from the tissues and removes impurities, manufacturers lymphocytes, and produces antibodies
lymphokines	chemicals that help other cells respond to antigens; interferons and interleukins
lysis	destruction of cells
megakaryocyte	giant cell of bone marrow that produces platelets
mononuclear cells	one of two kinds of leukocytes in plasma that may be classified as monocytes or lymphocytes
organic constituents of plasma	amino acids, ammonia, cholesterol, creatinine, glucose, lactic acids, phospholipids, urea, uric acid
phagocytes	cells that attack bacteria or eat another cell
plasma	fluid component of blood
platelets (thrombocytes)	cells that coagulate blood

continues

Word	Definition
prothrombin	a protein element of blood made in the liver that controls blood clotting
Rh factor	a major antigen group in the red blood cells; positive (+) or negative (–)
serum	clear, thin, sticky fluid portion of blood remaining after blood has clotted
serum albumin	main protein found in blood; related to nutritional state and liver function
serum globulin	protein element of the blood that contains antibodies
spleen	lymphoid organ with an extensive network of blood vessels that forms lymphocytes and monocytes and destroys bacteria, white blood cells, and aging red blood cells
splenomegaly	enlargement of the spleen
thymus	lymphoid organ that tells the lymph nodes how to work in early life and directs the body's development of antibodies and cellular immunity
tonsils	lymphoid organs that play a part in the manufacture of lymphocytes
transfusion	transfer of a blood component from one person's body to another
type A, B, AB, and O blood	blood groups

Key Terminology Practice Exercises

COMPLETION

Complete the following statements.

1. The physician who studies and treats blood is called a ____________________.
2. The average adult has ____________________ quarts of blood in his or her body.
3. The two prime elements in blood are ____________________ and ____________________.
4. ____________________ is the primary ingredient of red cells.
5. ____________________ is a nearly colorless fluid rich in white blood cells called lymphocytes.
6. The lymph nodes located in the armpits are the ____________________ nodes.
7. The lymph nodes located in the neck are the ____________________ nodes.
8. The lymph nodes located in the groin are the ____________________ nodes.
9. ____________________ are made of a specialized tissue that removes impurities, manufactures lymphocytes, and produces antibodies.
10. ____________________ is an immune response based on T cell activity.
11. Creatinine, glucose, and cholesterol are examples of the ____________________ constituents of plasma.
12. The protein element of blood that contains antibodies is ____________________.

13. ____________________ is a protein element of blood.
14. A/n ____________________ measures the volume of red blood cells compared to the total volume of blood.
15. Sodium, calcium, and potassium are ____________________ constituents of plasma.

SHORT ANSWER

Supply a short answer to the following.

1. Name the three types of cells found in the blood and briefly define each.

____

____

____

2. Name the two ducts into which the lymph vessels and nodes empty.

____

____

____

3. Name the four blood types; tell what the differences are among them.

____

____

____

DEFINITION

Define the following terms.

1. agglutination ______________________________
2. lysis ______________________________
3. Rh factor ______________________________
4. cisterna chyli ______________________________
5. immunoglobulins ______________________________
6. lymph ______________________________
7. prothrombin ______________________________
8. splenomegaly ______________________________

MATCHING

Match the terms to their meanings.

1. _________	the most numerous types of leukocytes	a. active acquired immunity
2. _________	another name for platelets	b. passive acquired immunity
3. _________	protein substances on the surface of red blood cells	c. antigens
4. _________	clear, thin, sticky fluid portion of blood that is left after blood has clotted	d. electrophoresis
5. _________	protein fluid that contains most of the antibodies in serum	e. fibrin
6. _________	body's defense system against foreign organisms	f. gamma globulin

7.	________	organ that directs the body's development of antibodies and other immune functions	g. granulocytes
8.	________	a large lymph node with an extensive network of blood vessels added	h. hematology
9.	________	source of first attack on bacteria entering the body	i. humoral immunity
10.	________	chemicals produced by T cells	j. immune system
11.	________	study of blood	k. lymphokines
12.	________	largest component of plasma	l. lymph nodes
13.	________	process to identify the three types of globulin	m. megakaryocyte
14.	________	a protein forming fine threads that form clots when needed	n. phagocytes
15.	________	produces platelets in bone marrow	o. RhoGAM
16.	________	a drug to prevent formation of antibodies in an Rh negative mother	p. serum
17.	________	found in groups of two to more than 100	q. spleen
18.	________	immune response based on B cells that are transformed into plasma cells	r. thrombocyte
19.	________	immunity achieved by receiving a vaccination	s. thymus
20.	________	immunity received from antibodies passed to the fetus from the mother	t. water

Word Element Review

Root	Meaning	Example	Definition
aden/o	gland	**adenoid** (ăd'ĕ-noyd)	lymphoid; having the appearance of a gland
agglutin/o	clumping, sticking	**agglutination** (ah-gloo"tĭ-nā'shŭn)	clumping together of particular elements in the blood
bas/o	base	**basophil** (bā'sō-fĭl)	granular leukocyte
blast/o	primitive cell	**blastoma** (blăs-tō'mah)	new, abnormal growth of tissue composed of immature cells derived from the blastema of an organ or a tissue
coagul/o	clotting	**coagulant** (kō-ag'ū-lănt)	agent accelerating the formation of a clot
cyt/o	cell	**cytogenic** (sī-tō-jĕn'ĭk)	forming cells
eosin/o	red	**eosinopenia** (ē"ō-sĭn"ō-pē'nē-ah)	abnormal deficiency of eosinophils in the blood
erythr/o	red	**erythematous** (ĕr-ĭ-thĕm'ah-tŭs)	characterized by redness of the skin

continues

Root	Meaning	Example	Definition
granul/o	granules	**granuloblast** (grăn'ū-lō-blăst")	immature granulocyte
hemat/o, hem/o	blood	**hematoma** (hēm"ah-tō'mah)	localized collection of blood in an organ, a space, or a tissue; a bruise
immun/o	immune, protection	**immunosuppression** (ĭm"ū-nō-sŭ-prĕsh'ŭn)	artificial prevention of the immune response
kary/o	nucleus	**karyomegaly** (kăr"ē-ō-mĕg'ah-lē)	abnormal enlargement of a cell nucleus
leuk/o	white	**leukocytogenesis** (loo"kō-sī"tō-jĕn'ĕ-sĭs)	formation of white cells (leukocytes)
lymph/o	lymph	**lymphogranulomatosis** (lĭm"fō-grăn"ū-lō" mah-tō'sĭs)	Hodgkin's disease
mon/o	single	**monocyte** (mŏn'ō-sīt)	mononuclear, phagocytic leukocyte
myel/o	bone marrow	**myeloma** (mī"ĕ-lō'mah)	tumor composed of cells of the type normally found in the bone marrow
neutr/o	neutral	**neutrophil** (nū'trō-fĭl)	leukocyte that stains easily with neutral dyes
phag/o	eat, swallow	**phagocyte** (făg'ō-sīt)	any cell that eats another
sangui/o	blood	**sanguineous** (săng-gwĭn'ē-ŭs)	bloody; having an abundance of blood
splen/o	spleen	**splenic** (splĕn'ĭk)	pertaining to the spleen
thym/o	thymus	**thymectomy** (thī-mĕk'tō-mē)	surgical removal of the thymus

Prefix	Meaning	Example	Definition
mega-	large	**megakaryocyte** (mĕg"ă-kăr'ē-ō-sīt")	large bone marrow cell with large nuclei

Suffix	Meaning	Example	Definition
-blast	immature	**myeloblast** (mī'ĕ-lō-blăst")	immature cell of bone marrow
-cytosis	abnormal condition of cells	**leukocytosis** (loo"kō-sī-tō'sĭs)	temporary abnormal increase in the number of circulating white cells
-emia	blood condition	**anemia** (ah-nē'mē-ah)	reduction in the number of erythrocytes, quantity of hemoglobin, or volume of packed red cells
-lytic	pertaining to destruction	**thrombolytic** (thrŏm"bō-lĭt'ĭck)	pertaining to destruction of a blood clot

continues

Word Element Review continued

Suffix	Meaning	Example	Definition
-penia	deficiency	**neutropenia** (nu"trō-pē'nē-ah)	diminished number of neutrophils in the blood
-philia	attraction for	**eosinophilia** (ē"ō-sĭn"ō-fĭl'ē-ah)	formation of an abnormally large number of eosinophils in the blood
-phoresis	carrying	**electrophoresis** (ē-lek"trō-fō-rē'sĭs)	technique involving movement of charged particles suspended in a liquid under the influence of an applied electric field
-poiesis	formation	**erythropoiesis** (ē-rĭth"rō-poi-ē-sĭs)	formation of erythrocytes (red cells)
-stasis	stop, control	**hemostasis** (hē"mō-stā'sĭs)	arrest of bleeding

Word Element Practice Exercises

COMPLETION

Complete the following statements.

1. Two of the word elements stand for blood; they are __________________ and __________________.
2. Two of the elements refer to cells; they are __________________ and __________________.
3. Two elements designate color. Red is indicated by __________________ and __________________, and white is indicated by __________________.
4. Four elements refer to parts of the lymph system; they are __________________, __________________, __________________, and __________________.
5. "Sticking together" is designated by the word element __________________.
6. A word element that may serve as a root and a suffix is __________________.

MATCHING

Match the terms to their meanings.

1. ________ agent accelerating the formation of a clot		a. coagulant
2. ________ a bruise		b. erythropoiesis
3. ________ abnormal enlargement of a cell nucleus		c. granuloblast
4. ________ pertaining to the spleen		d. hematoma
5. ________ tumor composed of cells of the type normally found in bone marrow		e. hemostasis
6. ________ pertaining to destruction of a blood clot		f. karyomegaly
7. ________ formation of red cells or erythrocytes		g. leukocytogenesis
8. ________ formation of white cells		h. myeloma
9. ________ arrest of bleeding		i. phagocyte
10. ________ an immature granulocyte		j. splenic
		k. thrombolytic

SPELLING

Rewrite the misspelled words.

1. neutraphil ______
2. annemia ______
3. megacaryocyte ______
4. sanguneous ______
5. electroforesis ______
6. myeloblast ______
7. leukocytosis ______
8. eosinophillia ______
9. monocyte ______
10. phagacyte ______
11. neutropennia ______
12. agglutinatation ______

WORD ELEMENT MEANINGS

Give the meaning of each word element. Then use your dictionary to find a new word that contains each of theword elements. Specify whether the new word is a noun or an adjective by placing N or A in the last column.

Word Element	Meaning	Word	N or A
1. aden/o	______	______	______
2. agglutin/o	______	______	______
3. bas/o	______	______	______
4. blast/o	______	______	______
5. -blast	______	______	______
6. coagul/o	______	______	______
7. cyt/o	______	______	______
8. -cytosis	______	______	______
9. -emia	______	______	______
10. eosin/o	______	______	______
11. erythr/o	______	______	______
12. granul/o	______	______	______
13. hemat/o	______	______	______
14. hem/o	______	______	______
15. immun/o	______	______	______
16. kary/o	______	______	______
17. leuk/o	______	______	______
18. lymph/o	______	______	______
19. -lytic	______	______	______
20. mega–	______	______	______

21. mon/o	______	______	______
22. myel/o	______	______	______
23. neutr/o	______	______	______
24. -penia	______	______	______
25. phag/o	______	______	______
26. -philia	______	______	______
27. -phoresis	______	______	______
28. -poiesis	______	______	______
29. sangui/o	______	______	______
30. splen/o	______	______	______
31. -stasis	______	______	______
32. thym/o	______	______	______

Working Practice

DIAGNOSTIC PROCEDURES		
Word	**Pronunciation**	**Definition**
General		
bone marrow aspiration and biopsy	bī'ŏp-sē	Physician-ordered examination of bone marrow (where blood cells are formed) to aid in diagnosis. It can be obtained by two methods: (1) *aspiration*, which means inserting a large needle into the sternum or iliac crest to aspirate marrow, as illustrated in Figure 9-8, or (2) *biopsy*, which means using a large cutting to remove a small core of cancellous bone (or, rarely, making an open incision to excise a piece of bone). Aspiration and needle biopsy are commonly done as a combined procedure.
Nuclear Medicine		
chromium$_{51}$ RBC survival	krō'mē-ŭm	test that determines the length of life of red blood cells survival
chromium$_{51}$ RBC volume		test that determines the total body blood volume
radioisotope scan	rā"dē-ō-ī'sō-tōp	production of a two-dimensional record or picture of emissions of a radioactive isotope concentrated in a specific site in the body
Schilling test	shĭl'ĭng	test to assess the gastrointestinal absorption of vitamin B_{12} in order to diagnose primary pernicious anemia

continues

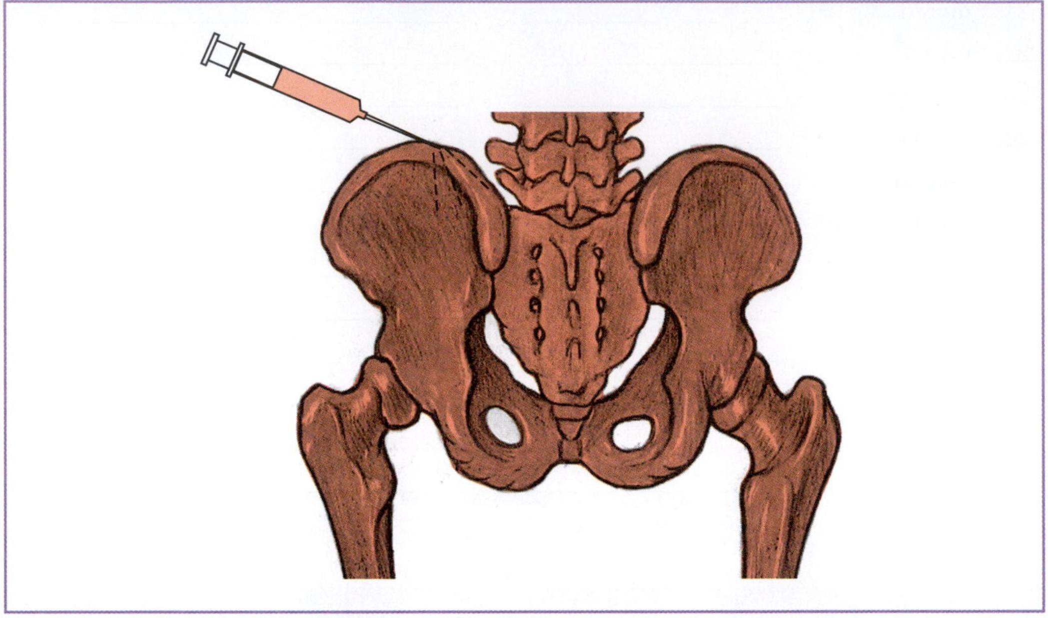
Source: Delmar/Cengage Learning

FIGURE 9-8
Bone Marrow Aspiration

DIAGNOSTIC PROCEDURES		
Word	Pronunciation	Definition
Radiology		
lymphangiogram	lĭm-făn'jē-ō-grăm	x-ray that is taken after dye is injected into lymph vessels in the foot; x-rays are taken to show the path of lymph flow as it moves into the chest region; other procedures are ordered depending on the suspected site
computed tomography (CT) or computed axial tomography (CAT) scan	tō-mŏg'ră-fē, ăk'sē-ăl	evaluating abnormalities of lymphoid (and other) organs by producing an image of the target organ using a computer to analyze the variance in absorption of a radio-graphic beam
magnetic resonance imaging (MRI)		making images of tissues and organs using the characteristic behavior of protons when placed in powerful magnetic fields
Blood Tests		
antiglobulin test	ăn"tĭ-glŏb'ū-lĭn	test for the presence of antibodies in human blood or on blood cells
bleeding time		time required for bleeding to stop after a small lancet cut
coagulation (clotting) time		time required for venous blood to clot in a test tube
complete blood count (CBC)		series of tests performed on peripheral blood; includes red and white blood cell counts (with differential), hemoglobin, hematocrit, and red cell indices—MCH, MCV, MCHC (See Table 9-1)
Coomb's test (direct and indirect antiglobulin tests)	ăn"tĭ-glŏb'ū-lĭn	blood test to discover the presence of antierythrocyte antibodies on red blood cells or in the serum

continues

TABLE 9-1 NORMAL VALUES FOR COMPLETE BLOOD COUNT		
Cells	Values	
Erythocytes	*Males*	4.6–6.3 million/mm^3
	Females	4.2–5.4 million/mm^3
Hematocrit	*Males*	40–54%
	Females	38–47%
Hemoglobin	*Males*	13.5–18 g/dl
	Females	12–16 g/dl
Red Blood Cell Indices		
• *MCV*	80–96 μm^3	
• *MCH*	21–31 pg	
• *MCHC*	32–36%	
Leukocytes 4500–11,000 mm^3		
Differential		
• *Myelocytes*	0 mm^3	
• *Band neutrophils*	1,500–3,000 mm^3	
• *Segmented neutrophils*	300–500 mm^3	
• *Lymphocytes*	50–250 mm^3	
• *Monocytes*	15–50 mm^3	
• *Eosinophils*	15–50 mm^3	
• *Basophils*	15–50 mm^3	
Platelets	150,000–350,000 mm^3	
Reticulocytes	25,000–75,000 mm^3	
Key:		
μm^3 = cubic micrometers	g/dl = grams per deciliter	
mm^3 = cubic millimeters	pg = picograms	

DIAGNOSTIC PROCEDURES		
Word	Pronunciation	Definition
Blood Tests (*Continued*)		
enzyme immunoassay (EIA)	ĭm"ū-nō-ăs'sā	enzyme immunochemical test for determining the presence of antigens or antibodies in the blood; one of the primary diagnostic tests for many infectious diseases, including the human immunodeficiency virus (HIV); after a second test that is also HIV positive, the Western blot test is perform to verify HIV

continues

DIAGNOSTIC PROCEDURES		
Word	Pronunciation	Definition
Blood Tests (*Continued*)		
erythrocyte sedimentation rate (sed rate, ESR)	ē-rĭth'rō-sīt sĕd"ĭ-mĕn-tā'shŭn	simple test that determines the rate at which red blood cells will settle to the bottom of a test tube when mixed with a small amount of an anticoagulant
ferritin	fĕr'ĭ-tĭn	test used to determine how much iron the body has stored
hematocrit and indices (Hct)	hē-măt'ō-krĭt, ĭn'dĭ-sēz	measurement of the percentage of erythrocytes in a volume of blood
hemoglobin concentration (Hgb)	hē"mō-glō'bĭn	measurement of the number of grams of hemoglobin in a given volume of blood
immunoelectrophoresis	ĭm"ū-nō-ē-lĕk"trō-fō-rē'sĭs	test that separates human immunoglobulins
lipid profile	lĭ'pĭd	measurement of lipids in the blood
partial thromboplastin time (PTT)	thrŏm"bō-plăs'tĭn	one simple test that determines all but two of the thirteen blood-clotting factors and screens for blood-clotting abnormalities
platelet count	plāt'lĕt	number of platelets per cubic millimeter of blood
prothrombin time, protime (PT)	prō-thrŏm'bĭn	coagulation test of the blood to help identify blood-clotting and liver diseases and to monitor blood-thinning medications
red blood cell count (RBC)		measurement of the circulating number of red blood cells in one cubic millimeter of peripheral blood; includes red cell indices—MCH, MCV, MCHC
red blood cell morphology	mŏr-fŏl'ō-jē	stained blood smear to determine shape or form of red cells
reticulocyte count	rē-tĭk'ū-lō-sīt	measurement of how rapidly the bone marrow is releasing reticulocytes (immature erythrocytes) into the blood
Schilling test	shĭl'ĭng	test to assess the gastrointestinal absorption of vitamin B_{12} in order to diagnose primary pernicious anemia
serum iron and iron-binding capacity (Fe and IBC)		determination of the amount of iron present and the percentage of saturation in the serum
transferrin	trăns-fĕr'ĭn	test for transferrin to evaluate a patient's nutritional status or liver function; done instead of a total iron binding capacity test
Western blot		test to confirm the presence of HIV or other antibodies
white blood count (WBC)		cell measurement of circulating number of white blood cells in one cubic millimeter of peripheral blood
white blood differential count		test that determines the number of different types of leukocytes, both immature and mature forms; may "shift" either to increase or decrease

DIAGNOSES		
Word	**Pronunciation**	**Definition**
Disorders of Red Blood Cells		
anemia	ah-nē'mē-ah	condition marked by decreased red blood cells, hemoglobin, and/or hematocrit values
• *hemolytic*	hē"mō-lĭt'ĭk	red blood cells are broken down faster than bone marrow can produce new ones
• *aplastic*	ā-plăs-tĭk	anemia caused by failure of bone marrow to produce blood components; often also affects WBCs and platelets
• folic acid deficiency		causes a decrease in the number of oversized red cells
• *hemorrhagic*	hĕm"ō-răj'ĭk	anemia caused by acute loss of large amount of blood
• *iron-deficiency*		insufficient iron in the blood to permit manufacture of hemoglobin
• *pernicious*	pĕr-nĭsh'ŭs	caused by the inability of the digestive tract to absorb vitamin B_{12}
• *sickle cell*		hereditary condition caused by an abnormal type of hemoglobin in the red cell found predominantly in dark-skinned individuals of African and Mediterranean descent
• *thalassemia*	thăl-ă-sē'mē-ah	inherited defect in the ability to produce hemoglobin; most common in persons of Mediterranean origin
erthyrocytosis	ĕ-rĭth"rō-sī-tō'sĭs	increase in red blood cells
hemochromatosis	hĕ"mō-krō"mă-tō'sĭs	genetic disease marked by excessive absorption and accumulation of iron in the body
hemosiderosis	hē"mō-sĭd-ĕr-ō'sĭs	iron overload due (usually) to multiple transfusions of red blood cells
polycythemia vera	pŏl"ē-sī-thē'mē-ah	disorder that occurs when bone marrow produces too many red blood cells; a myleoproliferative disorder
rouleau	roo-lō'	group of red blood cells that are stuck together
Disorders of White Blood Cells and Bone Marrow		
agnogenic myeloid metaplasia	ăg-nō-jĕn'ĭk mī'ĕ-loyd	condition in which the bone marrow gradually becomes scarred and less able to manufacture blood cells
agranulocytosis	ă-grăn"ū-lō-sī-tō'sĭs	abnormal decrease in the number of granulocytes in the blood
granulocytosis	grăn"ū-lō-sī-tō'sĭs	abnormal increase number of granulocytes in the blood
leukemia	loo-kē'mē-ah	malignant disease of the bone marrow characterized by an unrestrained growth of leukocytes; may be classified as acute or chronic (See Figure 9-9)
• *lymphocytic*	lĭm-fō-sĭ'tĭk	
acute (ALL)		leukemia predominated by immature lymphocytes; found frequently in children
chronic (CLL)		exceptional amounts of abnormal lymphocytes found in the spleen, bone marrow, lymph nodes, and (usually in older adults) blood
• *myelogenous*	mī-ĕ-lōj'ĕn-ŭs	
acute (AML)		leukemia predominated by immature granulocytes
chronic (CML)		sustained increase in the number of granulocytes existing in the bloodstream and bone marrow

continues

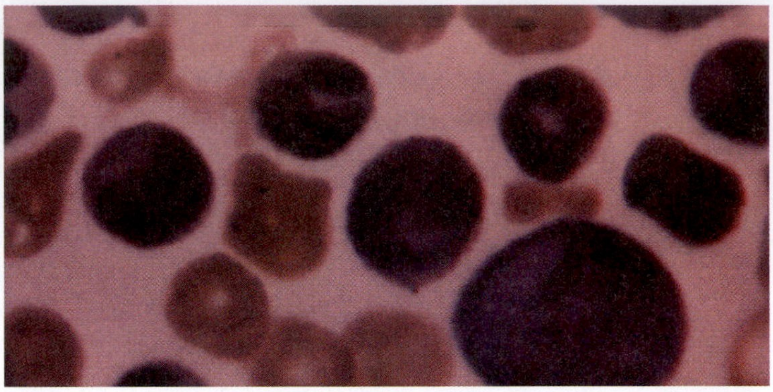

FIGURE 9-9
Leukemia: Unrestrained Growth of White Blood Cells (Leukocytes) in Bone Marrow

DIAGNOSES		
Word	**Pronunciation**	**Definition**
Disorders of White Blood Cells and Bone Marrow (*Continued*)		
leukocytosis	loo"kō-sī-tō'sĭs	increased white blood cell count
leukopenia	loo"kō-pē'nē-ă	abnormal decrease of white blood cells
mononucleosis	mŏn-ō-nū"klē-ō'sĭs	acute infectious disease caused by the Epstein-Barr virus manifested by an enlargement of the lymph nodes and spleen and an increased number of lymphocytes in the bloodstream
multiple myeloma	mī-ĕ-lō'mah	tumor characterized by uncontrolled multiplication of plasma cells in the bone marrow (see Figure 9-10)

continues

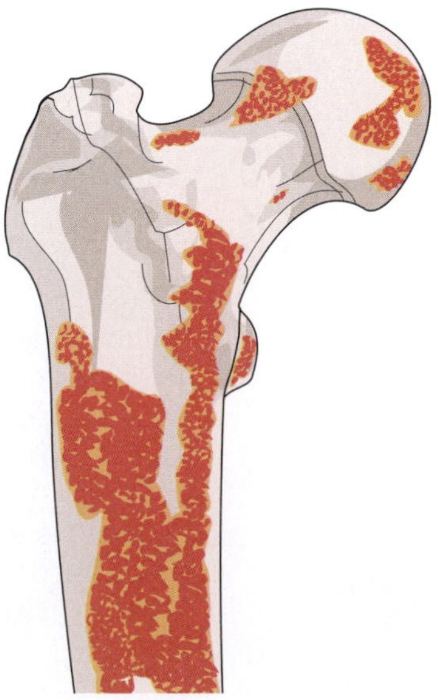

FIGURE 9-10
Multiple Myeloma

DIAGNOSES		
Word	Pronunciation	Definition
Disorders of White Blood Cells and Bone Marrow (*Continued*)		
myelodysplasia	mī"ĕl-ō-dĭs-plā'zē-a	subnormal production of blood cells by the bone marrow
myelodysplastic syndrome	mī"ĕl-ō-dĭs-plăs'tĭc	group of diseases of the bone marrow that can cause cytopenia and sometimes transform into acute leukemia
von Willebrand's disease (angiohemophilia)	ăn"jē-ō-he"mō-fĭl'ē-ah	chronic bleeding disorder (considered the most common hereditary bleeding disorder)
Disorders of Platelets/Blood Clotting		
disseminated intravascular coagulation (DIC)		nonhereditary bleeding disorder that results from excessive coagulation
hemophilia	he"mō-fĭl'ē-ah	hereditary condition characterized by impaired coagulability of the blood and a strong tendency to bleed
purpura	pŭr'pū-ră	multiple small hemorrhages and an accumulation of blood under the skin
thrombocytopenia	thrŏm"bō-sī"tō-pē'nē-ah	abnormal decrease in the number of blood platelets often resulting in increased bleeding or petechiae
thrombocytosis	thrŏm"bō-sī-tō'sĭs	increased platelets may lead to increased clotting or, less frequently, bleeding
Immune Deficiency Disorders		
acquired immunodeficiency syndrome (AIDS)		advanced stage of an HIV-positive infection where the immune response system has become nearly ineffective; the individual is now easy prey to most bacteria, parasites, and diseases that attempt to invade the body; these opportunistic infections (See Table 9-2) may affect multiple body systems at one time; this stage is nearly always fatal
human immunodeficiency virus (HIV)		infectious disease that kills cells of the immune system resulting in the suppression or deficiency of the immune response system; virus attacks the immune system (especially the T cells) and continues until the system has little ability to fight life-threatening infections and malignancies; transmission of the virus between individuals occurs through contact with infected body fluids; common means of transmission are shared needles and syringes for intravenous drug use, sexual contact with an infected partner, improperly screened blood transfusions, or by an infected mother to a child during pregnancy or birth; Table 9-2 presents some of the more common opportunistic infections related to AIDS

continues

TABLE 9-2 SOME OF THE MORE COMMON OPPORTUNISTIC INFECTIONS RELATED TO AIDS	
lymphadenopathy	a disease involving the enlargement of lymph nodes
persistent generalized lymphadenopathy (PGL)	continued presence of enlarged lymph nodes
Kaposi's sarcoma	cancer arising from the cell lining of the capillaries; may spread into the skin, mucous membranes, lymph nodes, and viscera
aspergillosis	fungal infection that may cause inflammation or lesions in or on any organ
candidiasis	infection caused by the *Candida* species of fungus
cryptococcus	yeastlike infection causing lung, brain, and blood infections
cytomegalovirus	infection caused by a large, herpes-type viruses
herpes simplex	viral infection marked by small blisters on the skin of the lips, nose, or genitals
Mycobacterium avium-intracellulare (MAI)	bacterial disease found in soil, water, and unpasteurized dairy products
norcardiosis	infection characterized by pneumonia and chronic abscesses of the brain
Pneumocystis carinii pneumonia (PCP)	one-celled organism causing a form of pneumonia
toxoplasmosis	infection from a parasite characterized by lesions of the central nervous system
tuberculosis	bacterial disease involving the lungs

DIAGNOSES

Word	Pronunciation	Definition
Immune Deficiency Disorders (*Continued*)		
HIV stages		
• acute infection		begins 1–3 weeks after initial infection; may be misdiagnosed as influenza
• asymptomatic HIV		no chronic signs or symptoms displayed, but lymphadenopathy and headache may occur intermittently; may last for 10–12 years depending on drug therapy and individual resistance
• symptomatic HIV		in the early phase a variety of symptoms affecting any or all body organs may be present; when T-cell count drops to less than 200 cells per microliter, the Centers for Disease Control diagnose this as AIDS, with a life expectancy of 3–5 years
• advanced		popularly known as AIDS and is nearly always fatal; every possible symptom or disease may be present because the individual's immune system has deteriorated (See Table 9-2)
Disorders of the Lymphatic System		
lymphadenitis	lĭm-făd"ēn-ī'tĭs	inflammation of the lymph nodes

continues

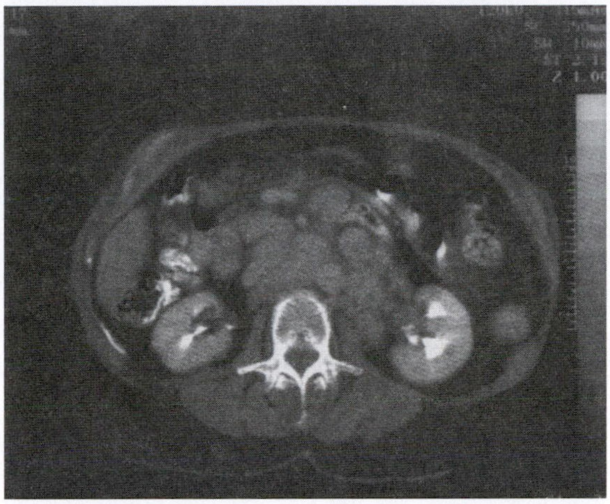

FIGURE 9-11 CT Showing Lymphoma

Source: Delmar/Cengage Learning

DIAGNOSES

Word	Pronunciation	Definition
Disorders of the Lymphatic System (*Continued*)		
lymphadenopathy	lĭm-făd"ĕ-nŏp"ă-thē	enlargement of the lymph nodes
lymphangitis	lĭm-făn-jī'tĭs	a condition of swelling of the lymphatic vessel due to inflammation
lymphedema	lĭmf-ĕ-dē'mah	abnormal collection of lymph fluid usually observed in the extremities
lymphoma	lĭmf-ō'mah	general term for a growth of malignant lymphoid tissue (See Figure 9-11)
• *Hodgkin's disease*		a type of malignant tumor arising in lymphatic tissue, such as the lymph nodes and spleen
• *non-Hodgkin's lymphoma (NHL) (lymphosarcoma)*	lĭmf-ō'săr-kō'mah	a diverse group of malignant tumors that arise from lymphatic tissues
lymphopenia	lĭm-fō-pē'nē-ah	decrease in the number of lymphocytes
Hypersensitivity Disorders		
allergies		a disorder resulting from an overreaction of the immune system to an antigen or allergen as in hay fever, asthma, urticaria, anaphylaxis, food allergies, or contact dermatitis
autoimmune disorders	aw"tō-ĭm-mūn	hypersensitivity in which the body reacts against its own antigens (rheumatic fever, rheumatoid arthritis, myasthenia gravis, Type 1 diabetes mellitus, lupus erythematosus, or scleroderma)
isoimmune disorders	īs"ō-ĭm-mūn	hypersensitivity of one individual to another individual's tissues (blood transfusion reaction or hemolytic disease of the newborn)
organ rejection		rejection of transplanted tissue as foreign tissue by an individual recipient's immune system

continues

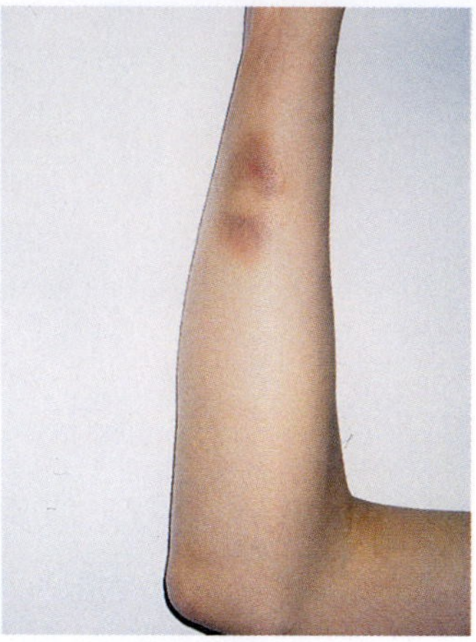

Source: Delmar/Cengage Learning

FIGURE 9-12
Ecchymosis

DIAGNOSES

Word	Pronunciation	Definition
Other Conditions		
ecchymoses	ĕk-ĭ-mō'sĭs	large areas of bruising (See Figure 9-12)
epistaxis	ĕp"ĭ-stăk'sĭs	nosebleed
hemarthrosis	hĕm-ăr-thrō'sĭs	bleeding into the joints
hematemesis	hĕm-ăt-ĕm'ĕ-sĭs	blood in the vomit
hematuria	hĕm-ă-tū-rē'ah	blood in the urine
hypersplenism	hī"pĕr-splĕn'ĭzm	increased activity of the spleen in which increased amounts of all types of blood cells are removed from the circulation
hypertension	hī-pĕr-tĕn'shŭn	blood pressure above the normal range
hypotension	hī"pō-tĕn'shŭn	blood pressure below the normal range
hypovolemia	hī"pō-vō-lē'mē-ah	low-blood volume
pancytopenia	păn"sī-tō-pē'nē-ah	decrease in all three major kinds of blood cells
petechiae	pē-tē'kē-ē	pinpoint purpura (red spots), usually caused by low platelet counts

TREATMENT PROCEDURES

Word	Pronunciation	Definition
apheresis	ă-fĕr'ē-sĭs	removal of blood from a patient or donor; separating and retaining certain components (such as plasma, platelets, or abnormal elements), some of which are retained; and then reinfusing elements into the donor
• *leukopheresis*	loo"kō-fĕr-ē'sĭs	removal of leukocytes only
• *plasmapheresis*	plăz"mă-fĕr-ē'sĭs	removal of noncellular materials
• *thrombopheresis*	thrŏm"bō-fĕr-ē'sĭs	reduction of platelet count

continues

TREATMENT PROCEDURES		
Word	**Pronunciation**	**Definition**
blood transfusion		after testing to ensure a close match of red cells or platelet type, whole blood or cells from an individual are infused into the recipient; may be *homologous* (from another) or *autologous* (from self)
bone marrow transplant		bone marrow cells from a donor whose tissue and blood cells closely match those of the patient are infused into the recipient; may be allogeneic from self or another person
erythrocytopheresis	ĕ-rĭth"rō-fĕr-ē'sĭs	procedure that removes abnormal red blood cells and replaces them with healthy red blood cells
hematopoietic	hē"mă-tō-po-ĕt'ĭk	placement of hematopoietic stem cells (from which all red and white blood cells evolve) from a compatible donor into a patient's vein
immunotherapy	ĭm"ū-nō-thĕr'ă-pē	treatment to suppress or enhance immunological functioning to identified allergens
phlebotomy	flĕ-bŏt-ō-mē	removal of blood from a vein
splenectomy	splē-nĕk'tō-mē	surgical removal of an enlarged spleen

MEDICATIONS PRESCRIBED	
Trade Name	**Generic Name**
Chemotherapeutic, Supportive, and Biologic Agents	
Adriamycin	doxorubicin HCl
Aloxi	palonosetron
Anzemet	dolasetron
Aranesp	darbepoetin alfa
Arimidex	anastrozole
Avastin	bevacizumab
BCNU, BiCNU	carmustine
Blenoxane	bleomycin sulfate
Camptosar	irinoteca
Casodex	bicalutamide
CeeNu, CCNU	lomustine
Cerubidine	daunorubicin
Cytoxan	cyclophosphamide
Decadron	dexamethasone
Deltasone, Orasone, Cordrol	prednisone
DTIC-Dome	dacarbazine
Eloxatin	oxaliplatin
Elspar	asparaginase
Emcyt	estramustine

continues

MEDICATIONS PRESCRIBED	
Trade Name	Generic Name
Chemotherapeutic, Supportive, and Biologic Agents (*Continued*)	
Emend	aprepitant
Epogen	epoetin alfa (synthetic)
Erbitux	cetuximab
Eulexin	flutamide
Fareston	toremifine
Femara	letrozole
Fludara	fludarabine
Gemzar	gemcitabine
Gleevec	imatinib mesylate
Herceptin	trastuzumab
Hycamtin	topotecan
Hydrea	hydroxyurea
IFEX	ifosfamide
Intron A, Roferon-A	interferon alfa
IVIG	intravenous immune globulin
Kytril	granisetron
Leucovorin	calcium folinic acid
Leukeran	chlorambucil
Leukine	sargramostim
Lupron	leuprolide acetate
Lysodren	mitotane
Matulane	procarbazine
Medrol	methylprednisolone
Megace	megestrol
MESNEX	mesna
Mithracin	plicamycin
Mustargen	mechlorethamine
Mutamycin	mitomycin
Myleran	busulfan
Navelbine	vinorelbine
Neulasta	pegfilgrastim
Neupogen	filgrastim (G-CSF)
Nexavar	sorafenib
Nolvadex	tamoxifen
Novantrone	mitoxantrone
Paraplatin	carboplatin

continues

MEDICATIONS PRESCRIBED	
Trade Name	Generic Name
Chemotherapeutic, Supportive, and Biologic Agents (*Continued*)	
Platinol	cisplatin
Procrit	epoetin alfa
Revlimid	lenalidomide
Rituxan	rituximab
Sandostatin	octreotide acetate
Solu-Cortef	hydrocortisone
Sprycel	dasatinib
Sutent	sunitinib malate
Tarceva	erlotinib
Taxol	paclitaxel
Taxotere	docetaxel
Temodal	temozolomide
Thalomid	thalidomide
Torisel	temsirolimus
Tykerb	lapatinib
Vectibix	panitumumab
Velban	vinblastine sulfate
Velcade	bortezomib
VePesid	etoposide
Xeloda	capecitabine
Zofran	ondansetron HCl
Zoladex	goserelin
5-FU	fluorouracil
AIDS Medications	
Crixivan	indinavir sulfate
Epivir	laminudine
Fortovase, Invase	saquinavir mesylate
Hivid	zalcitabine
Norvir	ruonavir
Rescriptor	delavirdine
Retrovir	zidovudine
Sustiva	efavirenz
Videx	didanosine
Viracept	nelfinavir mesylate
Viramune	nevirapine
Zerit	stavudine
Ziagen	abacavir

continues

MEDICATIONS PRESCRIBED	
Trade Name	Generic Name
Other Medications/Preparations	
Alupent	metaproterenol sulfate
Amicar, Immunex	aminocaproic acid
Aminophylline	aminophylline
Benadryl	diphenhydramine
Coumadin	warfarin sodium
Cyklokapron	tranexamic acid
DDAVP	desmopressin acetate
Fergon, Ferralet, Simron	ferrous gluconate
Feosol, Ferosul, Slow Fe	ferrous sulfate
Intropin	dopamine
Levophed	norepinephrine bitartrate
Mestinon	pyridostigmine bromide
Persantine	dipyridamole
Prostigmin	neostigine bromide
Proventil	albuterol
Streptase	streptokinase
Trental	pentoxifylline
Vitamin B_{12}	cyanocobalamin
Zyloprim	allopurinol

ABBREVIATIONS	
AIDS	acquired immune deficiency; acquired immunodeficiency syndrome
ALL	acute lymphocytic leukemia
AML	acute myelogenous leukemia
ARC	AIDS-related complex
baso	basophil(s)
CBC	complete blood count
CGL	chronic granulocytic leukemia
CLL	chronic lymphocytic leukemia
CML	chronic myelogenous leukemia
DIC	disseminated intravascular coagulation
diff	differential blood count
eos, eosins	eosinophil(s)
ESR, Sed rate	erythrocyte sedimentation rate
Hb, Hgb	hemoglobin
Hct	hematocrit

continues

ABBREVIATIONS	
HIV	human immunodeficiency virus
IgA, IgD, IgE, IgG, IgM	immunoglobulins
lymph	lymphocyte
MCH	mean corpuscular hemoglobin (amount of hemoglobin per cell)
MCHC	mean corpuscular hemoglobin concentration (average concentration of hemoglobin per red cell)
MCV	mean corpuscular volume (average volume of a red blood cell)
mono	monocyte
PMN, PMNL	polymorphonuclear neutrophil leukocytes
PT	prothrombin time
PTT	partial thromboplastin time
RBC	red blood cell, red blood count
WBC	white blood cell, white blood count

Working Practice Review Exercises

DEFINITIONS

Define the following diagnoses.

1. leukocytosis

____

2. lymphoma

____

3. multiple myeloma

____

4. lymphadenopathy

____

5. purpura

____

6. erthyrocytosis

____

7. mononucleosis

____

8. thrombocytosis

____

9. lymphadenitis

____

10. ecchymosis

____

COMPLETION

Provide the correct diagnostic or treatment procedure to complete these sentences.

1. A test that determines the length of life of red blood cells is ______________.
2. An x-ray taken after dye is injected into lymph vessels in the foot is a/n ______________.
3. A simple test for inflammation that determines the rate at which red blood cells will settle to the bottom of a test tube is ______________.
4. A test that separates human immunoglobulins is a/n ______________.
5. A stained blood smear to determine shape or form of red cells is ______________.
6. Removal of blood from a patient or donor is ______________.
7. Removal of abnormal red blood cells and replacement with healthy ones is ______________.
8. Removal of blood from a vein is ______________.
9. Surgical removal of an enlarged spleen is a/n ______________.
10. Transfer of bone marrow cells from a donor whose tissue and blood cells closely match the patient is a/n ______________.
11. A group of red blood cells that are stuck together is ______________.
12. Placement of peripheral stem cells from a compatible donor into a patient's vein is ______________.
13. A test to diagnose primary pernicious anemia is ______________.
14. Measurement of the number of circulating immature erythrocytes in the blood is ______________.
15. Test of the presence of antibodies in blood cells is ______________.

MATCHING

Match the terms to their meanings.

1. ________ x-rays follow dye injected into the foot as lymph moves into the chest	a. AIDS
2. ________ test to detect presence of HIV virus	b. allergies
3. ________ rate at which red cells settle to the bottom of a test tube when mixed with an anticoagulant	c. anemia
4. ________ decrease in red corpuscles or the iron in them	d. bone marrow aspiration and biopsy
5. ________ impaired coagulation of blood	e. $chromium_{51}$ RBC survival
6. ________ pinpoint hemorrhages under the skin	f. erythrocyte sedimentation rate
7. ________ determine the length of life of red blood cells	g. erythrocytopenia
8. ________ inserting a large needle to aspirate marrow or using a large cutting needle to remove a small core of bone	h. granulocytosis

9.	________ disorder resulting from overreaction of the immune system to an antigen or allergen	i.	hemophilia
10.	________ test for eleven of thirteen blood clotting factors	j.	hypovalemia
11.	________ abnormal increase in the number of granulocytes in blood	k.	lymphangiogram
12.	________ decrease in red blood cells	l.	partial thromboplastin
13.	________ advanced stage of HIV	m.	petechiae
14.	________ low blood volume	n.	polycythemia vera
15.	________ occurs when bone marrow produces too many red cells	o.	thrombocytopenia
16.	________ infection from a parasite characterized by lesions of the central nervous system	p.	toxoplasmosis
17.	________ bacterial disease involving the lungs	q.	transfusion
18.	________ abnormal decrease in the number of blood platelets	r.	tuberculosis
19.	________ chronic bleeding disorder	s.	van Willebrand's disease
20.	________ infusion of whole blood cells from one individual to another	t.	Western blot

Dictionary Exercises

DICTIONARY EXERCISE 1

Use your dictionary to find the pronunciation and definition of the following words.

Word	Pronunciation	Definition
1. agranulocytosis	____________	____________
2. antibody	____________	____________
3. elliptocytosis	____________	____________
4. erythropoiesis	____________	____________
5. granulopoiesis	____________	____________
6. erythroblast	____________	____________
7. viscosity	____________	____________
8. macrocytic anemia	____________	____________
9. metamyelocyte	____________	____________
10. Pel-Ebstein fever	____________	____________
11. poikilocytosis	____________	____________
12. hemolysis	____________	____________
13. thrombocytopenic purpura	____________	____________

14. anaphylaxis ______ ______
15. fibrin ______ ______
16. hemorrhage ______ ______
17. hemostasis ______ ______
18. septicemia ______ ______
19. stem cell ______ ______
20. sarcoidosis ______ ______

DICTIONARY EXERCISE 2

Select the correct meaning and provide the pronunciation where indicated.

1. elliptocyte (______)
   a. elliptical red blood cell
   b. cause of lupus erythematosus, a cutaneous or connective tissue disease
2. erythroblast (______)
   a. condition in which the capillary vascular channels are more fragile than normal
   b. immature red blood cell still having a nucleus
3. hematopoiesis (______)
   a. production and development of blood cells
   b. presence of red blood cells of a variety of shapes
4. hypochromic (______) anemia
   a. anemia in which red cells tend to be larger than normal
   b. anemia characterized by a hemoglobin deficiency in the red blood cells
5. phagocytosis (______)
   a. process of a cell engulfing and destroying bacteria
   b. any phagocyte cell involved in the defense against infection
6. polychromatophilia (______)
   a. disorder resulting from excess porphyrins in the blood
   b. quality of staining in which erythrocytes show various shades of blue or pink tinges
7. leukopoiesis (______)
   a. production of leukocytes
   b. passage of leukocytes through blood vessel walls
8. fibrinogen (______)
   a. coagulation factor
   b. resembling fibrin
9. reticulocyte (______)
   a. cells that mature in the thymus
   b. an immature erythrocyte
10. erythremia (______)
    a. abnormal increase in the number of red blood cells
    b. process of red blood cell production

DICTIONARY EXERCISE 3

Pronunciation of the words below is provided. Using your dictionary, find the correct spelling and definition of the words.

	Word	Pronunciation	Definition
1.	______	grăn"ū-lō-sī"tō-pē'nē-ah	______
2.	______	hĕt'ĕr-ō-fīl" antibody	______
3.	______	lĭp"ō-prō'tē-īn	______
4.	______	lĭm'foid tissue	______
5.	______	mī'ĕ-loid tissue	______
6.	______	pŏr-fē'rē-ah	______
7.	______	hī"pĕr-lĭp-ē'mē-ah	______

8. ______________________ hē"mō-glō"bĭ-nū'rē-ah ______________________
9. ______________________ ē"ō-sĭn"ō-fĭl'ē-ah ______________________
10. ______________________ ăn-ī"sō-sī-tō'sĭs ______________________
11. ______________________ ă-sī'tēz ______________________
12. ______________________ kō-ăg"ū-lā'shŭn ______________________
13. ______________________ kor'pŭs-ĕl ______________________
14. ______________________ dĭs-krā'zē-ă ______________________
15. ______________________ ī'ŏn ______________________

StudyWARE™ Connection

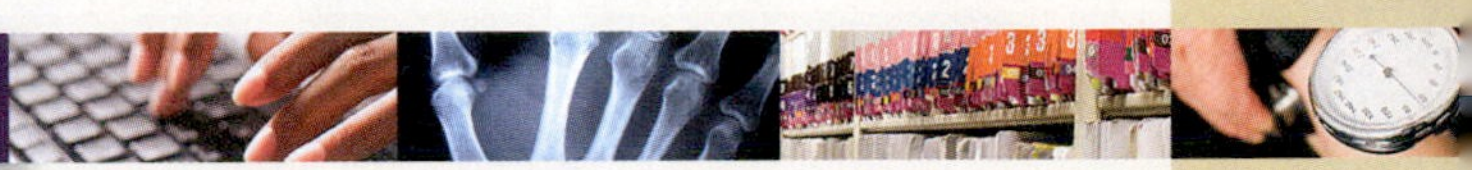

To take a practice quiz or play interactive games that reinforce the content in this chapter, go to your StudyWARE™ CD-ROM.

Listening Exercise

INSTRUCTIONS

1. Review the spelling, pronunciation, and meaning of the words provided in the preview.
2. Go to your StudyWARE™ CD-ROM and listen to **Listening Exercise 9-1**. Fill in the blank in the report as the word is dictated.
3. At the end of the activity, check your spelling against the preview words. They appear in the preview in the order in which they are encountered in the activity.
4. Review and practice the words you missed.
5. Look up words that are not familiar.

PREVIEW OF WORDS FOR LISTENING EXERCISE 9-1

Word	Pronunciation	Meaning
thrombocytopenia	thrŏm"bō-sī"tō-pē'nē-ă	decrease in the number of platelets in circulating blood
hematemesis	hĕm-ăt-ĕm'ĕ-sĭs	vomiting of blood
adenopathy	ăd-ĕ-nŏp'ă-thē	enlargement of glands, especially lymph nodes
cyanosis	sī-ă-nō'sĭs	bluish discoloration of skin due to excessive concentration of reduced hemoglobin in the blood
mentation	mēn-tā'shŭn	thinking, mental activity
lymphoproliferative	lĭm"fō-prō-lĭf'ĕr-ă-tĭv	a group of diseases characterized by generation of disorder lymphoid tissue

Listening Exercise 9-1

StudyWARE™ Connection

Listen to this report being read on your StudyWARE™ CD-ROM. Fill in each blank as the word is dictated.

History and Physical

CHIEF COMPLAINT: ____________

PRESENT ILLNESS: The patient indicates that she has had easy bruisability for many years. She has noticed some bleeding around the gums and some hemorrhoidal bleeding, but has not noted any submucosal hemorrhages in the mouth or eyes. She has had no melena or ____________. There has been no fever, night sweats, or weight loss. She has not noticed any. She saw Dr. Beyers for a routine physical on August 13, 20—, at which time laboratory studies showed a white blood count of 7,600, hemoglobin 15.4, hematocrit 45.4 with 50 segs, 37 lymphs, 10 monos, 2 eos, 1 baso, and platelet count of 40,000. The platelet count was repeated and was 31,000. Chemistry profile was normal except for an elevated cholesterol and triglycerides. The patient is seen at this time for evaluation of her thrombocytopenia.

PAST MEDICAL HISTORY: Surgeries include appendectomy in 1952, cholecystectomy in 1965, bladder suspension in 1980, coronary angioplasty in 1989, and cervical diskectomy in 1994.

Medical Illnesses: Hypothyroidism, hypertension for approximately 15 years, myocardial infarction 1989 with no recurrence of chest pain or episodes of congestive heart failure.

Medications: One aspirin daily, atenolol 25 mg daily, Dyazide 1 tablet daily, Synthroid 0.125 mg daily, Prempro 1 tablet daily. The aspirin, atenolol, and Dyazide were discontinued by Dr. Beyers when the low platelet count was found.

There are no known allergies. No transfusions. She does not use tobacco or alcohol. Reproductive: G-2, P-2, Ab-0.

Hospitalizations: Influenza. No injuries reported.

FAMILY HISTORY: Mother died at age 86 of unknown causes. Father died at age 46 from myocardial infarction. There are no known hematologic disorders within the family.

PHYSICAL EXAMINATION: In general the patient is a pleasant, Caucasian female who is not in any acute distress. BP: 140/90. PULSE: 84 & regular. Respiration, 14; temperature, 98.9; weight 249.

HEENT: There were telangiectasias on the face. EOMs were intact. Pupils were equal, round, and reactive to light. Funduscopic—no hemorrhages, exudates, papilledema. Pharynx was clear. External auditory canals and TMs clear.

NECK: There was no cervical adenopathy. Carotid impulse was normal. Thyroid was unremarkable. CHEST: Clear to percussion and auscultation. AXILLA: Free of adenopathy. BREASTS: No masses or tenderness were noted. HEART: There was regular rhythm. S1 and S2 were normal. No murmurs, gallops, or rubs were heard. No JVD or HJR. No edema.

ABDOMEN: Liver percussed and was not palpable. Spleen was not palpable. No masses or tenderness were noted within the abdomen.

RECTAL/PELVIC: No masses or tenderness.

continues

History and Physical

EXTREMITIES: Pulses were adequate and equal throughout. No clubbing or ______________. No joint deformity or muscle weakness.

NEUROLOGIC: Oriented to person, place, and time ______________ normal. Cranial nerves II–XII intact. Motor, sensory, and cerebellar exam negative. Deep tendon reflexes were 2+ and equal. Babinski sign is absent.

IMPRESSIONS:

1. Thrombocytopenia. The patient did not have any physical findings nor does she have any history that would suggest a cause for her thrombocytopenia. The atenolol and Dyazide have been associated with thrombocytopenia and they have been discontinued. She has not had any recent viral infections nor has she experienced any rheumatologic complaints that might suggest underlying diagnosis of lupus. She has had no lymphadenopathy or systemic symptoms that might suggest an underlying ____________________________. Based on these findings, I would think that the most likely diagnosis would be chronic ITP.

RECOMMENDATIONS:

1. Arrangements will be made for the other studies necessary.

Mark J. Black, MD

Comprehensive consult findings sent to: Vito Mansetti, MD

CHAPTER

10

Oncology

"The best of healers is good cheer."

—PINDAR

OBJECTIVES

When you have completed this chapter on oncology, you should be able to

1. Explain the development of cancer cells.
2. Identify and define three types of cancer.
3. Define tumor staging and grading.
4. Identify and define the tools for the diagnostic process: medical history and physical examination, laboratory tests, biopsy, and diagnostic imaging.
5. Identify and define methods of cancer treatment, including surgery, radiation therapy, chemotherapy, bone marrow/stem cell transplants, hormone therapy, and targeted therapies.
6. Spell common anticancer drug combinations.
7. Identify the meanings of related word elements.
8. Hear how medical terminology is used in actual medical reports.

INTRODUCTION

Oncology (ŏng-kŏl'ō-jē) is the sum of knowledge regarding tumors. **Tumors**, which may be benign or malignant, are abnormal masses of tissue that result from excessive cell division. Benign tumors are seldom a threat to life because they do not spread to other parts of the body. A malignant tumor, on the other hand, is referred to as *cancer*, and its growth is uncontrollable and marked by the spread of abnormal cells. When cancer cells break away from the primary site and start secondary growths in other parts of the body, the process is referred to as **metastasis** (mĕ-tăs'tah-sĭs). Physicians who specialize in the treatment of malignant tumors are called **oncologists** (ŏng-kŏl'ō-jĭsts).

BIOLOGY OF CANCER

The body is sustained over time by billions of cells that have special functions (referred to as cell differentiation). In a normal growth pattern, growth happens because of cell division. Only in recent years has research begun to provide answers as to what causes a normal cell to become cancerous. Building on this knowledge, expanded studies—particularly in the area of genome research—are expected to provide even more answers in the near future. To better understand this cell transformation process, it is necessary to look at basic cell biology.

ANATOMY OF A CELL

aden/o	gland	mutagen/o	causing genetic change
blast/o	embryonic, immature	onc/o	tumor
carcin/o	cancerous	plas/o	formation
meta-	beyond, change	sarc/o	flesh
mut/a	genetic change		

The **nucleus** (nū'klē-ŭs) (1) (Figure 10-1) is the structure within a cell that contains the chromosomes. Each cell contains 46 **chromosomes** (krō'mō-sōmz) (2)—23 from each parent—each composed of paired strands of deoxyribonucleic acid, or **DNA**, molecules (3) spiraled around one another in the form of a double helix.

DNA contains within its chemical structure a code that determines the sequence of amino acids in a protein. There only four chemical subunits—adenine (A), thymine (T), guanine (G), and cytosine (C)—that make up the code. They are strung out along a DNA strand in various combinations to identify the structure of a specific protein. This series of chemical codes is called a **gene** (4), the basic unit of heredity. It is the 50,000 to 100,000 genes scattered along a DNA strand that designs a protein that may function either as an enzyme or as a structural component of a cell. The total collection of genes is called the **human genome** (jē'nōm).

Although the full DNA is found in every cell, not all genes are active all of the time. It is the active genes, working in pairs, that dictate traits from eye color to the coding of the proteins that determine specific cell structure

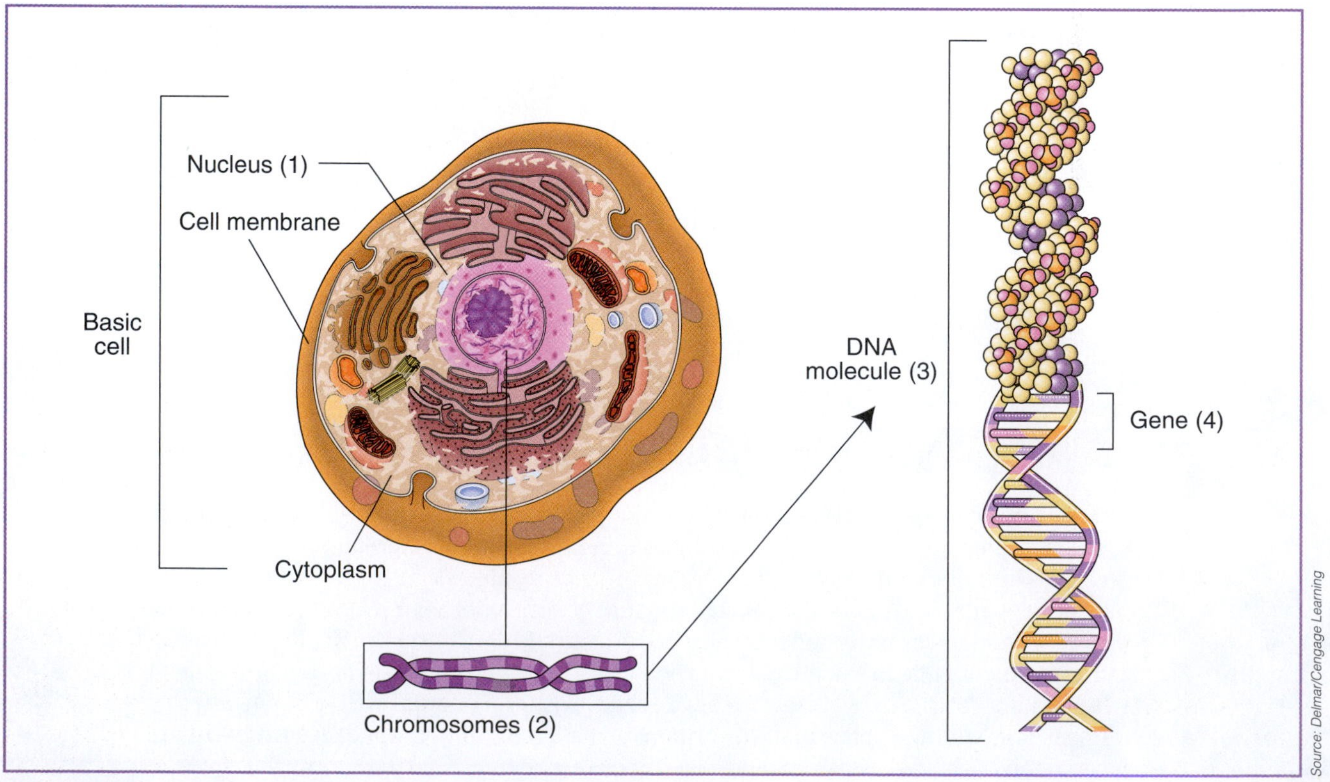

FIGURE 10-1 Basic Cell and DNA Molecule

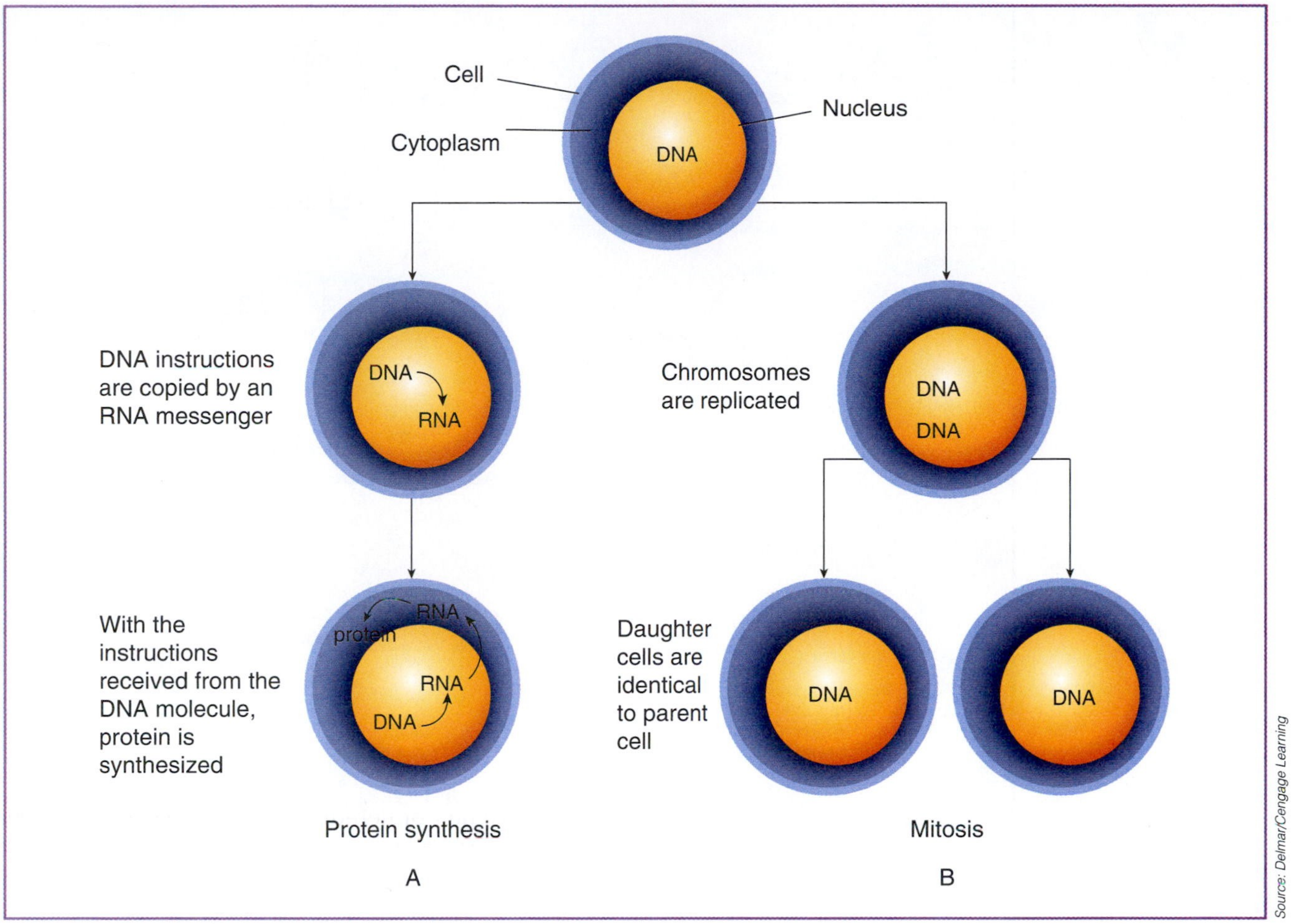

FIGURE 10-2 DNA in Action: (A) Protein Synthesis; (B) Mitosis

and function. For example, certain genes—referred to as "housekeeping" genes—perform similar basic functions in all cells. Other genes have more specific functions such as coding the proteins in muscle cells to decide whether they are to affect epithelial, connective, or nerve cells.

In a normal cell, the DNA has two functions: mitosis and protein synthesis. **Mitosis** (mī-tō'sĭs) is the process of cellular reproduction that occurs in the nucleus when it divides to form two identical nuclei called daughter cells. Between the cycles of mitosis, DNA manages the production of new proteins through a process called protein synthesis (Figure 10-2).

ROLE OF GENES IN MUTATION

Proto-oncogenes (prō'tō ŏng'kō-jēnz) are a family of normal genes that handle proteins during typical cell division. Under normal conditions, proteins called growth factors bind to receptors on the cell surface. In turn, a series of enzymes inside the cell activate special proteins called transcription factors located within the cell's nucleus.

Once activated, the transcription factors turn on the genes required for growth and proliferation. Proto-oncogenes are normally controlled by growth-factor proteins as they regulate cell division and differentiation, repair tissue, or even play a role in organ development.

When one of the components of a gene is changed or mutated, the result is an alteration in the control functions of proto-oncogenes. Genetic specialists call where that change occurs the **point mutation**. There are several possible sources for the mutation: oncogenes, tumor suppressor genes, and DNA repair genes. Each affects cell change in different ways.

Oncogenes (ŏng'kō-jēnz) arise when proto-oncogenes mutate. Although oncogenes physically resemble the proto-oncogenes, they differ in that they instruct cells to make proteins that stimulate excessive cell growth and cause cells to divide abnormally. Essentially, they code for an altered version of the growth-control proteins leading to hyperactivity within a cell. Sometimes more than one oncogene is present in a cell.

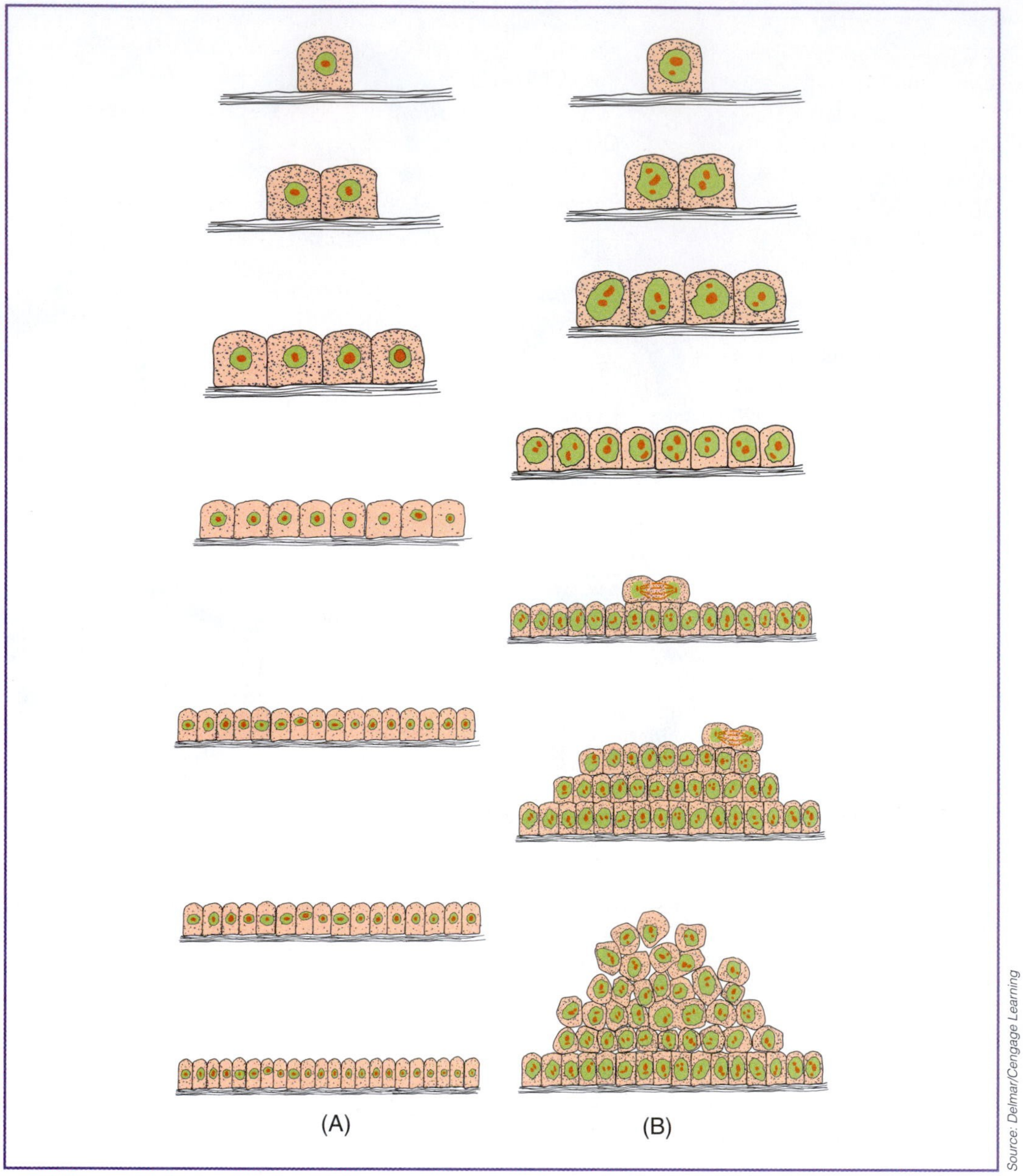

FIGURE 10-3
Cellular Growth Patterns: (A) Normal Cells; (B) Cancer Cells

Tumor suppressor genes (sometimes called antioncogenes) are normal genes whose function is to instruct cells to produce proteins that inhibit cell growth and division. If they are not present, the loss of the proteins they produce allows a cell to grow and divide uncontrollably and results in cancer. For example, the p53 protein coded by one of the suppressor genes can trigger cell suicide, thus preventing a genetically damaged cell from growing out of control.

DNA repair genes code proteins that will correct DNA cell duplication errors prior to cell division. If a mutation occurs in a DNA repair gene, the gene may fail to repair the DNA, thus allowing the mutations in the tumor suppressor genes and proto-oncogenes to accumulate.

An accumulation of mutations involving all three of these factors often leads to cancer. Figure 10-3 illustrates the difference between the growth of normal cells and cancerous cells.

MUTATIONS, HEREDITY, AND CARCINOGENS

Many disorders or diseases appear to stem from mutated genes received from the mother and/or father. These mutations are called **germline mutations** because the change exists in the reproductive cells of the parent. Estimates indicate about five percent of all cancers in the United States may be explained by inherited genetic mutations.

Another type of mutation is called an **acquired**, or **somatic**, **mutation**. This disruption of the normal genetic programming of a cell—with its potential of producing a malignancy—may occur any time in a person's life. This kind of mutation is passed only to direct descendants of an altered cell.

A random mutation may crop up during cell division or be the by-product of environmental stresses. The most common **carcinogen** (kăr"sĭn'ō-jĕn) results from the use of tobacco products. It causes as many as one of three deaths in any given year. In some cases, infectious, cancer-inducing viruses inject their own oncogenes into normal cells, which then seem to become unregulated by the normal cell process. Examples are cervical cancer, liver cancer, certain lymphomas, leukemia, and sarcomas. In other cases, bacterium such as *Helicobacter pylori* may be related to stomach cancer.

Prolonged or repeated exposure to certain types of radiation can cause cancer. Exposure to low-level sources such as sunlight—which delivers ultraviolet rays—most often results in skin cancer. Exposure to high-level radiation, such as those from x-rays or radioisotopes, is more likely to cause not-so-evident internal damage. (Note that dental x-rays and diagnostic body x-rays are considered low-level radiation and therefore not generally harmful when used with appropriate safety procedures.)

Chemicals also can be dangerous carcinogens. Examples include alkylating agents, arsenic, asbestos, benzene, hydrocarbons, and vinyl chloride. Many of these chemicals are "hidden" in common, everyday products. Others, like cigarette smoke, exhaust fumes from vehicles, insecticides, and asbestos insulation, are found in the environment.

GENETIC TESTING, MAPPING, AND SPLICING

Genetic testing can identify individuals or families with a possible predisposition to a disease or to confirm a suspected mutation. Testing is done by examining a person's DNA, which may be taken from cells in blood, tissue, or other body fluids. Several types of tests (with examples) are currently used: newborn screening (phenylketonuria), carrier testing (Tay-Sachs disease), prenatal diagnosis (Down syndrome), cancer/precancerous cells for early detection (familial adenomatous polyposis), diagnosis (leukemia), and prognosis (p53 tumor-suppressor gene).

Predictive gene testing is a newer development and focuses on identifying people who are at risk of getting a disease before any symptoms appear. To make this possible, a massive international collaboration called the Human Genome Project was undertaken in 1990. Its aim was to identify each of the tens of thousands of genes in the human DNA, as well as the sequence of the estimated 3 billion chemical bases. The project was completed in June 2003. Continuing exploration into the function of each human gene will affect the diagnosis, monitoring, and treatment of diseases. Molecular medicine has already aided researchers in dealing with dozens of genetic conditions. Genetic advances will ultimately help researchers to develop new ways to treat, cure, or even prevent thousands of diseases.

The potential for gene therapy to treat disease is an exciting arena. Since 1974, **gene-splicing technology** has allowed DNA from a different organism to be spliced or recombined to form a new organism. By 1983, a laboratory method for reproducing DNA quickly led to the identification of the first genetic marker for cystic fibrosis. And in 1986, tumor suppressor genes were discovered. Using these three key discoveries, coupled with genetic engineering, scientists can isolate and manipulate the action of individual cancer-causing genes to create models of human disease and pinpoint genes that are solely responsible for specific types of cancer.

Ongoing research is adding rapidly to our knowledge about the biology of cancer cells and the effect of various carcinogens in developing cancer.

TYPES OF CANCER

-blast	immature	-plasia	formation, growth
-oma	mass, tumor	-plasm	formation, growth

Currently recognized varieties of cancer can be grouped into three basic categories according to the type of tissue from which the tumor cells have arisen: carcinomas, sarcomas, and mixed-tissue tumors.

Carcinomas (kăr"sĭ-nō'mahz) are malignant new growths made up of epithelial (lining) cells that tend to infiltrate surrounding tissue (Figure 10-4). They are the largest group, accounting for approximately ninety percent of all malignancies. The two most frequently diagnosed types of carcinomas are **squamous** (skwā'mŭs)

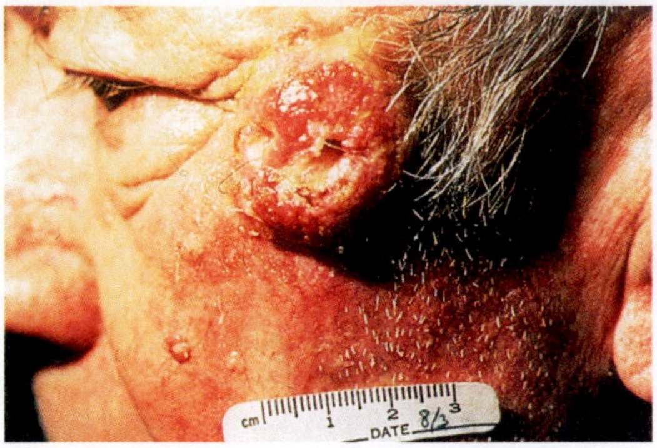

FIGURE 10-4 Squamous Cell Carcinoma

cell carcinoma (which develops primarily on the skin or in the mouth, lungs, bronchi, esophagus, or cervix) and **adenocarcinoma** (ăd"ĕ-nō-kăr"sĭnō'mah) (which arises from a glandular organ).

Sarcomas (săr-kō'mahz) are malignancies of the supporting tissues, such as bone, cartilage, muscle, or blood vessels. These account for approximately five percent of all malignant neoplasms (tumors).

Mixed-tissue tumors are the third type of cancer arising from tissue that is capable of differentiating into epithelial as well as connective tissue. Therefore, mixed tissue tumors are composed of several types of cells. They, too, represent about five percent of malignancies. The following table shows tissue types with some of their common malignancies.

Type of Tissue	Malignant Tumor
blood vessel tissue	hemangiosarcoma
bone	osteosarcoma (osteogenic sarcoma)
cartilage	chondrosarcoma
fat	liposarcoma
fibrous tissue	fibrosarcoma
gastrointestinal tract	
• *colon*	carcinoma of the colon
• *esophagus*	esophageal adenocarcinoma; squamous carcinoma
• *stomach*	gastric adenocarcinoma
glandular tissue	
• *adrenal glands*	carcinoma of the adrenal gland
• *breast*	carcinoma of the breast (see Figure 10-5)
• *pancreas*	carcinoma of the pancreas (pancreatic adenocarcinoma)
• *prostate*	carcinoma of the prostate
• *thyroid*	carcinoma of the thyroid
hematopoietic tissue	
• *leukocytes*	leukemia
• *lymphocytes*	Hodgkin's lymphoma; non-Hodgkin's lymphoma
• *plasma cells*	multiple myeloma

continues

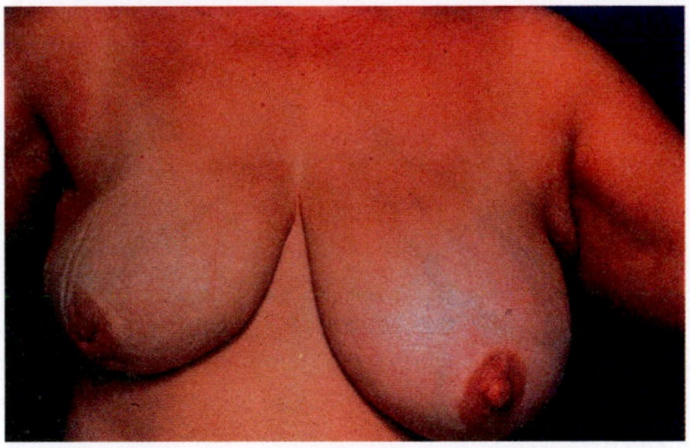

FIGURE 10-5 Asymmetry of Breasts Due to Cancer

Source: Courtesy of Dr. S. Eva Singletary, University of Texas, Anderson Cancer Center

Type of Tissue	Malignant Tumor
kidney	hypernephroma (renal cell carcinoma); Wilms' tumor (embryonal adenosarcoma)
lung	adenocarcinoma of the lung; epidermoid carcinoma; oat cell (small cell) carcinoma
muscle	
• *smooth (visceral) muscle*	leiomyosarcoma
• *striated (skeletal) muscle*	rhabdomyosarcoma
nerve tissue	
• *embryonic nerve tissue*	neuroblastoma; retinoblastoma
• *meningeal tissue*	meningeal sarcoma (meningioma)
• *neuroglial tissue*	astrocytoma (tumor of neuroglial cells called astrocytes)
reproductive organs	adenocarcinoma of the uterus; carcinoma of the penis; choriocarcinoma of the uterus or testes; cystadenocarcinoma of the ovaries; seminoma (carcinoma of the testes); squamous cell (epidermoid carcinoma of the vagina and cervix); teratoma (tumor composed of bone, muscle, gland cells, cartilage, etc.)

StudyWARE™ Connection

To watch an animation on **cancer metastasizing,** go to your StudyWARE™ CD-ROM.

DIAGNOSTIC PROCESS

The diagnostic process includes using various tools for evaluating a tumor and then staging and grading it as an aid to planning treatment.

TOOLS FOR DIAGNOSIS

Tools that can be used to diagnose cancer are the medical history and physical examination, laboratory tests, biopsy, and diagnostic imaging.

The process of diagnosing cancer begins with a *medical history and physical examination*. The physician will be looking for current physical complaints, prior health, the family history of illness (including cancer), and any environmental exposures that may have occurred to put the patient at risk.

Blood, urine, or other *laboratory tests* may be ordered to help rule out or diagnose a disease. Review Chapter 3 for the elements of a history and physical examination.

Biopsy is always necessary to make a cancer diagnosis. Three types of biopsy include needle biopsy (which may be either a **fine-needle biopsy** or **core biopsy**), endoscopic biopsy, or surgical biopsy.

In needle biopsy, the physician may use a thin needle to remove small particles of tissue or use a larger needle to remove a small, solid core of tissue.

Endoscopic biopsy is performed with an endoscope inserted into a natural body opening. Instruments can be inserted through the endoscope to remove tissue samples.

Surgical biopsy may be either excisional or incisional. Excisional biopsy removes an entire tumor, while an incisional biopsy removes only a portion of a tumor for examination.

The next step is *diagnostic imaging* to determine cancer location, size, and spread. These techniques include x-ray, computerized tomography (CT), magnetic resonance imaging (MRI), ultrasound, radionuclide scanning, positron emission tomography (PET), and single photon emission computerized tomography (SPECT). They are covered in Chapter 11 on radiology. However, depending on the size or location of a tumor, some cancers cannot be seen through imaging.

STAGING AND GRADING TUMORS

cyst/o	sac of fluid	papill/o	papillary
fibr/o	fibers	polyp/o	polyp
fung/o	fungus, mushroom	scirrh/o	hard
medull/o	soft, inner part		

Once a pathologist has diagnosed the type of cancer, the malignant tumor is categorized using a classification such as the American Joint Committee on Cancer (AJCC) or Union Internationale Contre le Cancer (UICC) classification. These classifications are based on the belief that cancers of similar **histology** (hĭs-tŏl'ō-jē) (the study of the microscopic structure of tissue) or site of origin share similar patterns of growth and extension. Determination of stage and grade will have an impact on treatment.

Stage

A **stage** is based on the extent of invasion or spread of an untreated primary cancer and is an important indicator of prognosis. The **TNM staging system** is commonly used. *T* (0–4) refers to the size of the primary tumor. It also indicates the degree to which it has invaded the local area. *N* (0–4) refers to the regional lymph nodes that have been involved by the tumor. *M* (0–3) refers to the presence or absence of distant metastasis of the tumor cells. This usually occurs when the cancer has existed undetected for an extended period of time and has spread to other parts of the body. Staging can be determined by clinical examination, but it might be classified differently after a surgical procedure and histologic examination. Staging of recurrent cancers may have different significance when considering therapy or determining prognosis.

Grade

Grade is an assessment of the extent to which a tumor resembles the normal tissue in a site and reflects an indication of prognosis. In general, the following classifications can be made.

GX	grade cannot be assessed
G1	well differentiated (least malignant)
G2	moderately differentiated
G3	poorly differentiated
G4	undifferentiated (malignant)

As indicated, the higher the grade the more serious the condition has become and the more difficult it is to treat. It should be noted that grading is not necessarily applied the same way to all types of cancer. One type—melanomas of the conjunctiva or adenocarcinomas—use only three grades. Also be aware that grading is not applied at all to some cancers, examples being carcinomas of the thyroid and some other locations.

Additional Descriptors

Cases needing separate analysis use the symbols *m*, *y*, *r*, and *a*. The *m* symbol in parentheses indicates the presence of multiple primary tumors in a single site. The *y* symbol is used during or following initial multiple methods of therapy. The *r* symbol is used when a patient has been staged *after* a disease-free interval. The *a* symbol indicates the classification was first determined during autopsy.

The following table lists the classification possibilities the TNM staging system offers.

TNM STAGING SYSTEM	
Tumor	**Meaning**
T_0	no evidence of primary tumor
T_{IS}	carcinoma in situ
T_1, T_2, T_3, T_4	progressive increase in tumor size and involvement
T_x	tumor cannot be assessed
Node	**Meaning**
N_0	regional lymph nodes not demonstrably abnormal
N_1, N_2, N_3, N_4	increasing numbers or increasing distant location of spread to regional lymph nodes
N_x	regional lymph nodes cannot be assessed clinically
Metastasis	**Meaning**
M_0	no evidence of distance metastasis
M_1, M_2, M_3	ascending degrees of distant metastasis

Other staging systems for tumors have the same general meaning. The most complete reference about tumor definitions is the *Atlas of Tumor Pathology*, published in many volumes by the Armed Forces Institute of Pathology, Washington, D.C.

METHODS OF TREATMENT

chem/o	chemical, drug	radi/o	rays, x-rays
immun/o	immune, immunity	-therapy	treatment

Early diagnosis is a key factor in successfully treating cancer. The American Cancer Society has developed seven cancer "early warning" signs. If any of these symptoms are a problem, one should seek a physician's advice.

1. Change in bowel or bladder habits
2. Sore that does not heal
3. Unusual bleeding or discharge
4. Thickening or lump in a breast or elsewhere in your body
5. Indigestion or swallowing difficulty
6. Obvious change in a wart or mole
7. Nagging cough or hoarseness

During examination, the physician can perform several tests to locate a malignancy. Common procedures are computed tomography (CT) scans, angiograms (to see if there are blockages or abnormal placement of blood vessels that may indicate a tumor is present), radioactive isotopes, ultrasound, special tests with tumor markers, laboratory tests, biopsies, or other diagnostic tests. These procedures are presented with each of the systems in this text.

Once a diagnosis has been made, there are several treatment options that may be used alone or in various combinations. Treatment is considered on an individual basis depending on the diagnosis and stage of the disease; the person's age, gender, and general health; and, in women, menopausal status.

Options are considered and a plan, or **protocol**, is developed for the treatment. Treatment options are surgery, radiation therapy, chemotherapy, bone marrow/stem cell transplants, hormone therapy, targeted therapies such as immunotherapy and biological therapies.

SURGERY

Surgery, often in the form of a biopsy, is done in more than ninety percent of all cases to extract a tissue sample from a suspected cancer. Diagnosis and staging of the suspect tissue is done by a specialist in a laboratory to determine whether the cancer has metastasized. Additional surgery is done in about sixty percent of all cases to remove cancerous growths or make the growth smaller (debulk the tumor) to improve the effectiveness of chemotherapy or radiation therapy.

Some of the more common procedures are outlined in the following table.

Procedure	Description
en bloc resection	removal of a tumor and a large area of surrounding tissue containing lymph nodes
exenteration	removing an organ of origin and surrounding tissue by a wide resection
fulguration	destruction of tissue with electric sparks
electrocauterization	destruction of tissue by burning
cryosurgery	destruction of tissue by freezing

When surgery is used for treatment, the tumor and some tissue adjacent to it are removed. Examination of this tissue can provide clues as to whether the cancer may return. If this is the case, other modalities of treatment need to be considered. This is also true when removal of the tumor is not possible or the patient cannot tolerate the surgery.

RADIATION THERAPY

Radiation therapy is a treatment that uses high energy carried by waves or streams of particles to treat cancer. Types of radiation include x-ray (either high-energy proton or low-energy electron), alpha and beta particles, and gamma rays. Radioactive substances include cobalt, iridium, iodine, and cesium. This procedure is sometimes referred to as radiotherapy, x-ray therapy, or irradiation. Such therapy affects only those cells within the radiation field and will not kill cancerous cells that have spread to other parts of the body.

Radiation therapy may be used during surgery at the completion of resection but before closure (intraoperative radiation), after surgery to shrink a tumor, after surgery to stop the growth of remaining cancer cells (postoperative radiation), or alone or in combination with anticancer drugs to destroy a malignant tumor. It may also be given to prevent cancer cells from growing in the area receiving radiation (prophylactic radiation therapy) or to help reduce symptoms that have spread to the bones or other parts of the body (palliative radiation therapy).

Simulation, performed by a radiation oncologist, is a process involving special x-ray pictures that are used to plan radiation treatment so the areas or fields to be treated are precisely located and marked for treatment and other tissues are protected by lead blocks. During simulation, the **treatment port** (the place on the body at which the radiation beam is aimed) is determined.

Radiation treatment is a team effort involving the radiation oncologist; a **radiation physicist** (fĭz'ĭ-sĭst), who makes sure the radiation machine delivers the right amount of radiation at the treatment site; and a **dosimetrist** (dō"sĭ-mĕt'rĭst), who plans and calculates the proper radiation dose for treatment. Dividing radiation into small, repeated doses—a process called **fractionation**—allows larger total doses to be given with less damage to normal tissue. These treatments are often administered five days a week on an outpatient basis by a **radiology technologist**.

Radiation therapy may come from an external or an internal source, or may be systemic radiation therapy. **External radiation** comes from outside the body from a machine called a linear accelerator. Sources of energy may be x-rays, gamma rays, or particle beams such as proton beam therapy. It can be used to treat most types of cancer or to relieve pain or other problems when cancers spread from the original primary site to other locations. It is also sometimes used during surgery to treat localized cancers. This procedure is referred to as **intraoperative radiation therapy**, which consists of a high dose of electronic beam therapy given directly to the tumor or tumor bed. This is done via a Lucite cone attached to the head of the treatment machine located in the operating room.

Internal radiation, sometimes called **brachytherapy** (brăk"ē-thĕr'ah-pē), may be delivered through the use of a radiation implant in the body. Doing so enables the doctor to give a greater dose of radiation than is possible with external radiation therapy and to save most of the healthy tissue around it. When the radioactive source is placed directly into tissue rather than a body cavity, the term **interstitial** (ĭn-tĕr-stĭsh'ăl) **implant** is used. It may also be inserted into the body with an applicator and is referred to as intracavity or intraluminal radiation therapy.

Unfortunately, radiation cannot distinguish between cancerous and noncancerous cells, so both are affected. Side effects are determined by location and amount of radiation used. Drugs called radiosensitizers and radioprotectors are currently being studied to alleviate this problem. **Radiosensitizers** make cancer cells more sensitive to radiation therapy. **Radioprotectors** protect noncancerous cells from radiation damage.

Currently new approaches to radiation therapy include using heat (hyperthermia) with radiation therapy. And researchers are studying the use of radiolabeled antibodies to deliver radiation directly to the cancer site (radioimmunotherapy). Clinical trials are currently underway to evaluate this technique.

CHEMOTHERAPY

Chemotherapy (kē"mō-thĕr'ă-pē) involves using anticancer drugs alone or in various combinations to treat cancer. These drugs may be administered by mouth, by injection, or intravenously. Some of the drugs may be given in cycles of treatment and rest. These drugs find their way into the bloodstream, which carries them through the entire body. Therefore, chemotherapy is called a **systemic treatment**. It, too, can affect normal tissue, especially in the bone marrow, gastrointestinal tract, reproductive system, and hair follicles.

When chemotherapy is used after potentially curative radiation or surgery in an attempt to kill remaining cancer cells, it is called **adjuvant** (ăd'jū-vănt) **chemotherapy**. Hair loss and other side effects may occur with some anticancer drugs, but these side effects are generally temporary.

Categories of chemotherapeutic agents are mitotic inhibitors, alkylating agents, antimetabolites, topoisomerase inhibitors, and anthracyclines.

Mitotic (mī'tō-tĭc) **inhibitors** may disrupt a kind of cell division called mitosis or inhibit cell growth by blocking protein-producing enzymes. These inhibitors include Velblan® (vinblastine sulfate) and Oncovin® (vincristine sulfate). They treat solid tumors, leukemia, and lymphoma.

Alkylating agents are combinations of synthetic compounds that interfere with the process of DNA synthesis by attacking the DNA molecules. Cisplatin®, Cytoxan® (cyclophosphamide), and Ifex® (ifosfamide) are examples of alkylating agents that damage the DNA of cancer cells which prevents the cells from dividing and multiplying.

Antimetabolites (ăn"tĭ-mĕ-tăb'ō-lītz) inhibit the synthesis of substances that are necessary components of DNA or they may block the replication of DNA. Common examples are Gemzar® (gemcitabine), 5-FU® (fluorouracil), Cytosar-U® (cytarabine), and Alimta® (pemetrexed). These agents are used to treat leukemia, ovarian and certain breast cancers, and cancer of the gastrointestinal tract.

Topoisomerase (tŏp"ō-ī-sŏm'ĕr-ās") **inhibitors** interfere with certain enzymes that play a role in the accurate replication on DNA. Examples are Camptosar® (irinoteca) and Hycaamtin® (topotecan).

Anthracyclines (ăn-thră-sī'klēnz), or anti-tumor antibiotics, bind to the DNA in a cell, promote DNA strand breaks, and prevent normal replication. These agents work in all phases of the cell cycle, unlike the antimetabolites which are only effective in a specific cycle of cell growth. Examples of the more commonly used anthracyclines are Adriamycin® (doxorubicin hydrochloride), Ellence® (epirubicin), and Daunomycine HCL® (daunorubicin hydrochloride).

Over the years **clinical trials**, an inherently slow process, have made important contributions in the treatment of cancer. With the introduction of a new drug, laboratory tests and animal studies are conducted. When the drug shows promise, a clinical trial is conducted with cancer patients to evaluate the safety and effectiveness of the treatment. Although progress in the treatment of cancer has improved in recent years, early diagnosis still remains the key to successful treatment. Survival rates are far better when intervention occurs early in the disease process.

The following table identifies medications used in cancer therapy. In addition to chemotherapy drugs, hormones, cell protectants, antidotes, and antiemetics are included. Note that some medications are used in the treatment of conditions or disease processes not related to cancer.

COMMON CHEMOTHERAPY AGENTS*

Generic name	Trade Name
carboplatin	Paraplatin
cisplatin	Platinol, Platinol-AQ
cyclophosphamide	Cytoxan, Neosar
docetaxel	Taxotere
doxorubicin	Adriamycin
erlotinib	Tarceva
etoposide	VePesid
fluorouracil	5-FU
gemcitabine	Gemzar
imatinib mesylate	Gleevec
irinotecan	Camptosar
methotrexate	Folex, Mexate, Amethopterin
paclitaxel	Taxol, Abraxane
sorafenib	Nexavar
sunitinib	Sutent
topotecan	Hycamtin
vincristine	Oncovin, Vincasar PFS
vinblastine	Velban

*For current information on cancer drugs, see **www.cancer.gov**, the National Cancer Institute's web site. Information is provided on drugs approved by the U.S. Food and Drug Administration (FDA).

The names of many of these drugs, because they are frequently used in combination, have been abbreviated to provide a quick way to refer to these long words. Some of the more common combinations are listed in the following table.

ABBREVIATIONS FOR FREQUENTLY USED COMBINATIONS	
Abbreviation	**Drug Combination**
CAE	cyclophosphamide, doxorubicin, etoposide
CAMP	cyclophosphamide, doxorubicin, methotrexate, procarbazine
CMF±P	cyclophosphamide, methotrexate, fluorouracil, prednisone
CVP	cyclophosphamide, vincristine, prednisone
FAC	fluorouracil, doxorubicin, cyclophosphamide
MOPP	mechlorethamine, vincristine, procarbazine, prednisone

BONE MARROW AND PERIPHERAL STEM CELL TRANSPLANTATION

Bone marrow transplantation (BMT) and **peripheral blood stem cell transplantation** (PBSCT) replaces bone marrow destroyed by very high doses of chemotherapy and/or radiation therapy used to destroy cancer cells.

Hematopoietic (hē"mă-tō-poy-ē'tĭk) or blood-forming **stem cells** are immature cells that can mature into blood cells. They are found in the bone marrow, the bloodstream, or the umbilical cord. Most are found in the bone marrow, but peripheral blood stem cells (PBSCs) are found in the blood stream.

Hematopoietic stem cells, unlike embryonic cells which can develop into every type of cell body, divide to form more blood-forming stem cells. They also can mature into white or red blood cells or platelets.

Both BMT and PBSCT can replace stem cells destroyed by treatment and are most commonly used in the treatment of leukemia and lymphoma. These transplants may be allogeneic, syngeneic, or autologous. An **allogeneic** (ăl"ō-jĕ-nē'ĭk) **transplant** uses a related or unrelated donor whose tissue type matches the patient's tissue. A **syngeneic** (sĭn-jĕ-nĕ'ĭk) **transplant** uses cells from an identical twin. An **autologous** (aw-tŏl'ō-gŭs) **transplant** uses the patient's own cells which were taken from the patient prior to treatment. One of the risks of allogenic transplants is **graft-versus-host disease**, or GVHD. In this case, the donor immune cells may attack certain of the patient's organs. Incidence of GVHD occurs in about one-third to one-half of all allogenic transplants.

Most hematopoietic stem cell transplants are now performed using stem cells collected from peripheral blood, rather than from bone marrow because it does not require the donor to be subjected to general anesthesia. Stem cell transplants have a lower mortality rate than bone marrow transplants because of the more rapid recovery of blood counts.

HORMONE THERAPY

Hormone therapy as a cancer treatment works in two ways: it reduces the hormones in your body and it changes the cancer's ability to use hormones. In hormone-sensitive cancers, this can make the tumors shrink. Cancers most likely to be hormone receptive are breast, prostate, ovarian, and endometrial cancers. Because hormones attach to receptor proteins in target tissue, they are key factors in stimulating cell growth of cancers found in these organs. Thus, drugs that prevent the formation of hormones or block their action can lead to tumor regression.

Hormone therapy may be given before beginning primary cancer treatment, in addition to primary treatment, or in cases of advanced cancers, as the main treatment.

There are several ways in which hormone therapy can be given. Surgery can reduce hormone levels by removing certain body parts. Radiation is used to stop or suppress the production of hormones. Drugs such as anti-hormones, aromatase inhibitors, and luteinizing hormone-releasing agents can alter the production of estrogen and testosterone.

Hormone therapy is similar to chemotherapy in that it is a systemic treatment and may affect cancer cells throughout the body. Men and women alike experience temporary side effects such as fluid retention, weight gain, nausea, vomiting, and changes in appetite. Permanent damage can be caused by surgery and radiation to the ovaries and testicles.

TARGETED THERAPIES

One of the problems with conventional cancer treatments such as chemotherapy or radiation therapy is the difficulty in distinguishing between normal cells and cancer cells, resulting in damage to otherwise healthy cells. A **targeted therapy** is designed to treat only the cancer cells, while minimizing danger to unaffected cells. They interfere with specific molecules that scientists call *molecular targets* and focus on molecular and cellular changes that are specific to cancer. Most are still in preclinical testing, some are in clinical trials, and some have been approved by the US Food and Drug Administration (FDA). The effect of targeted cancer therapies is that it provides doctors with a way to tailor cancer treatments to individual needs, which ultimately harms fewer normal cells, reduces side effects, and improves the quality of a patient's life.

Types of targeted therapy include monoclonal antibodies, angiogenesis inhibitors, tyrosine kinase inhibitors, proteasome inhibitors, and immunotherapy.

Monoclonal antibodies show promise as researchers have learned how to use fragments of antibodies instead of whole ones to better reach a tumor. These antibodies locate cancer cells, bind to them, and carry radioactive agents or poisons to them. Several of these antibodies have been approved for treatment, including Rituxan® (rituximab), Herceptin® (trastuzumab), Erbitux® (cetuximab), and Vectibix® (panitumumab). Currently, Zevalin® (ibritumomab tiuxetan), and Bexxar® (tositumomab) are the only radioactive antibody-based drugs approved by the FDA. They target a radioactive atom to the cancer cells.

Angiogenesis (ăn"jē-ō-jĕn'ĕ-sĭs) **inhibitors** starve tumors by preventing the formation of new blood vessels in the tumor, thus eliminating the tumor. Avastin® (bevacizumab) was the first successful angiogenesis inhibitor approved. Others include Revlimid® (lenalidomide), Thalomid® (thalidomide), Sutent® (sunitinib) and Nexavar® (sorafenib).

Tyrosine kinase (tī'rō-sĭn kĭn'ās) **inhibitors** are drugs that interfere with cell communication and growth. When used to treat cancer, it blocks growth. There are fewer side effects than with traditional chemotherapy.

Proteasome (prō-tē'sŏm) **inhibitors** are drugs that block the action of proteasomes, a large protein complex that helps destroy other cellular proteins when they are no longer needed. Velcade® (bortezomib) treats multiple myeloma inhibiting proteasomes and increases levels of proteins, thereby restoring some control over abnormal growth or metastasis of cells.

Immunotherapy is sometimes called **biotherapy** or **biological response modifier therapy**. These therapies use **biological response modifiers**, agents that boost, direct, or restore normal defenses of the body to fight cancer. They work through the **immune system** to stimulate production of T cells, which are specialized immune cells that recognize and kill cancer cells.

Naturally occurring substances in the body called cytokines use the body's immune system to fight cancer or to lessen the side effects that may be caused by some cancer treatments. **Interleukins** and **interferons**, two types of cytokines, can be produced in the laboratory for treating certain kinds of cancer. An interleukin is a protein substance that regulates cell growth. An interferon is a substance that stimulates the body's immune system to fight cancer cells.

INTERNET ASSIGNMENT

The American Cancer Society (ACS) is the nationwide, community-based voluntary health organization dedicated to eliminating cancer as a major health problem. It also has an international mission, which concentrates on developing cancer societies and on collaboration with cancer-related organizations throughout the world in conducting the strategic directions of the American Cancer Society.

The ACS consists of a National Society, with chartered divisions throughout the country and more than 3,400 local units with volunteers nationwide. The organization fights to conquer cancer through research, prevention, patient services, public policy, and advocacy programs. For example, the Society's advocacy initiative strives to influence public policies at all levels on issues such as

- the use, sale, distribution, marketing, and advertising of tobacco products, particularly to youth
- improved access for all Americans, particularly poor and underserved Americans, to a range of health care services for the prevention, early detection, diagnosis, and treatment of cancer and care of cancer patients
- increased federal funding and incentives for private sponsorship of cancer research to prevent and cure cancer, and
- advocacy for the rights of cancer survivors.

A visit to the ACS homepage at **www.cancer.org** finds information groups for Patients, Family, and Friends; Survivors; ACS Supporters; Health Information Seekers; and Professionals, in addition to current news items concerning cancer.

ACTIVITY

Access the American Cancer Society site at **www.cancer.org**. Select Site Index on the top bar of choices. Under For Patients, Survivors, Family, and Friends, click on Learn About Cancer. Then select All About Cancer. Finally, select Detailed Guide: Cancer (General Information). Look for the hyperlinks that provide answers for the following questions:

1. Who gets cancer?
2. How is cancer treated?
3. What are some of the questions you should ask your physician about cancer?
4. What did you learn about clinical trials?

Submit your answers in a report to your instructor.

Review *Oncology*

- DNA is composed of a sequence of four chemical subunits that instruct a cell to make a specific protein for a specific purpose.
- Chromosomes are composed of paired strands of DNA spiraled around one another in the shape of a double helix.
- Genes are the chemical subunits that identify a specific protein and are the basic unit of the heredity code.
- Changes in proto-oncogenes of cells cause the cells to grow abnormally and cause cancer.
- Three types of cancers are carcinomas (the largest group), sarcomas, and mixed tissue tumors.
- Tumor staging and grading refer to the extent of invasion of the cancer and degree to which a tumor resembles normal tissue.
- Cancer may be treated with surgery, radiation therapy, chemotherapy (including hormone therapy), and biological therapies (immunotherapy).
- Clinical trials provide opportunities to test experimental drugs on cancer patients to determine new safe and effective methods of treatment.

Key Terminology Review

Word	Definition
acquired mutations (somatic)	changes in DNA that develop throughout a person's life
adenocarcinoma	type of carcinoma that arises from a glandular organ
adjuvant chemotherapy	treatment used after radiation to kill remaining cancer cells
alkylating agents	combinations of synthetic compounds that attack DNA molecules
allogenic transplant	replacement using bone marrow or stem cells donated by a sibling or close relative
angiogenesis inhibitors	starve tumors by preventing the formation of new blood vessels in the tumor, thus eliminating the tumor
anthracyclines	agents that bind to DNA, promote strand breaks, and prevent normal replication of microorganisms
antimetabolite	agent that inhibits synthesis of substances that are necessary components of DNA or block replication of DNA
autologous transplant	replacement using the patient's own bone marrow gathered before treatment
biological response modifiers	agents that boost, direct, or restore the normal defenses of the body to fight cancer
bone marrow transplantation (BMT) or peripheral blood stem cell transplantation (PBSCT)	replacement of bone marrow destroyed by treatment using radiation or high-dose chemotherapy with healthy stem cells
carcinogens	factors that cause changes that lead to cancer
carcinoma	malignant new growth of epithelial cells
chemotherapy	treatment with anticancer drugs used alone or in combinations; may use alkylating agents, antibiotics, antimetabolics, antimitotics, or hormones
chromosomes	linear strands composed of DNA and proteins that carry genetic information
clinical trials	carefully designed and executed investigation to define the clinical efficacy and pharmacological effects of a drug
core biopsy	use of a larger needle to remove a small, solid core of tissue
DNA (deoxyribonucleic acid)	the chemical code that determines the sequence of amino acids in a protein
DNA repair genes	genes that code proteins that will correct DNA cell duplication errors prior to cell division
dosimetrist	health professional who calculates and plans the proper radiation dosage for treatment
endoscopic biopsy	use of an endoscope through which an instrument can be inserted to remove a sample tissue
external radiation	radiation treatment delivered by a linear accelerator
fine-needle biopsy	use of a fine needle to remove small particles of tissue
fractionation	division of radiation into safe, small doses thereby resulting in larger total doses with less damage to normal tissue
gene	basic unit of heredity found in DNA; carries coded instructions for producing a specific protein; each gene occupies a specific location on a chromosome

continues

Word	Definition
gene-splicing technology	splicing or recombining of DNA from different organisms to form a new organism
genetic testing	testing done by examining DNA taken from cells in blood, tissue, or body fluids
germline mutations	mutations in reproductive cells
grade	degree to which a tumor resembles normal tissue
graft-versus-host disease (GVHD)	attack on certain patient organs by donor immune cells during an allogenic transplant
hematopoietic stem cell	immature cells that can mature into blood cells
histology	study of the microscopic structure of tissue
hormone therapy	reduces the hormones in the body and changes a cancer's ability to use hormones
human genome	total collection of an individual's genes
immune system	complex groups of cells and organs that defend the body from foreign substances that might cause infection or disease
immunotherapy (biotherapy or biological response modifier therapy)	treatment that uses the body's own defense systems to fight cancer
interferon	substance that stimulates the body's immune system to fight cancer cells
interleukin	protein substance that regulates cell growth
internal radiation (brachytherapy)	treatment with an internally-placed source of radiation
interstitial implant	radioactive source placed directly into tissue rather than into a body cavity
intraoperative radiation therapy	treatment with a high dose of electron beams delivered directly to the tumor or tumor bed
metastasis	process whereby cancer cells break away from the primary site and begin secondary growths in other parts of the body
mitosis	process of cellular reproduction that occurs in the nucleus when it forms two identical daughter cells
mitotic inhibitors	disrupts cell division or cell growth by blocking protein-producing enzymes
mixed-tissue tumors	cancers arising from tissue that is capable of differentiating into epithelial and connective tissue
monoclonal antibodies	substances that locate cancer cells, bind to them, and carry radioactive agents or poisons to these cells
nucleus	core of a cell
oncogenes	special kind of genes that may cause cells to divide abnormally
oncologist	physician specializing in the treatment of malignant tumors
oncology	sum knowledge regarding tumors
palliative therapy	treatment to relieve cancer symptoms even though remission seems unlikely
point mutation	point where one of the components of a gene is changed
predictive gene testing	testing to identify individuals who are at risk of getting a disease *before* any symptoms appear

continues

Word	Definition
proteasome inhibitors	drugs that block the action of proteasomes, a large protein complex that helps destroy other cellular proteins when they are no longer needed
proto-oncogenes	normal form of an oncogene
protocol	plan for treatment
radiation physicist	technician who makes certain the machine delivers the right amount of radiation to a treatment site
radiation therapy	treatment that uses high energy radiation to treat cancer
radiology technologist	technician who administers radiation treatment to a patient
radioprotectors	drugs that protect noncancerous cells from radiation damage
radiosensitizers	drugs being studied that will boost the effect of radiation therapy
remission	temporary or permanent absence of cancer symptoms
sarcoma	malignancy of supporting tissues
simulation	process involving special x-ray pictures that are used to plan radiation treatment so the target area is precisely located
squamous cell carcinoma	type of carcinoma that develops primarily on the skin or in the mouth, lungs, bronchi, esophagus, or cervix
stage	extent of invasion of an untreated primary cancer
surgical biopsy	may be either excisional, which removes a whole tumor, or incisional, which removes a portion of a tumor
syngenic transplant	replacement using bone marrow or stem cells donated by an identical twin
systemic treatment	treatment of cancer by chemotherapy through the bloodstream
targeted therapy	therapy designed to treat only cancer cells, while minimizing danger to unaffected cells, by interfering with specific molecules (molecular targets) and focusing on molecular and cellular changes that are specific to cancer
TNM staging system	system used to refer to the size and degree of invasion of a tumor in the local area, nodes, or distant sites
topoisomerase inhibitors	substances that interfere with certain enzymes that play a role in the accurate replication of DNA
treatment port	place on the body at which radiation is aimed
tumor	abnormal mass of tissue resulting from excessive cell division
tumor suppressor genes	genes whose function is to instruct cells to produce proteins that restrain cell growth and division
tyrosine kinase inhibitors	substances that interfere with cell communication and growth used to block cancers

Key Terminology Practice Exercises

MATCHING

Match the terms to their meanings.

1. ________ point where one of the components of a gene is changed
2. ________ factors that cause changes that lead to cancer
3. ________ substance that stimulates the body's immune system to fight cancer cells
4. ________ agents that boost, direct, or restore the normal defenses of the body to fight cancer
5. ________ treatment of cancer by chemotherapy through the bloodstream
6. ________ treatment used after radiation treatment to kill remaining cancer cells
7. ________ body's defense system
8. ________ carefully designed and executed investigation to define the clinical efficacy and pharmacological effects of a drug
9. ________ substance that locates cancer cells and carries radioactive agents or poisons to them
10. ________ the study of the microscopic structure of tissue
11. ________ ways of referring to size and degree of invasion of a cancer
12. ________ normal form of an oncogene
13. ________ radiation treatment delivered by a linear accelerator
14. ________ temporary or permanent absence of cancer symptoms
15. ________ activity of immune system against foreign substances
16. ________ abnormal masses of tissue resulting from excessive cell division
17. ________ mutations in reproductive cells
18. ________ total collection of an individual's genes
19. ________ double strand spiraled into a helix composed of millions of chemical building blocks
20. ________ instructs cells to produce proteins that restrain malignant cell growth and division
21. ________ starve tumors by preventing the formation of new blood vessels in the tumor, thus eliminating the tumor
22. ________ agents that bind to DNA and prevent normal replication of microorganism
23. ________ protein substance that regulates cell growth
24. ________ transplant using the patient's own bone marrow gathered before treatment
25. ________ transplant using the bone marrow or stem cells donated by a sibling or close relative

a. adjuvant chemotherapy
b. allogeneic
c. angiogenesis
d. anthracyclines
e. autologous
f. biological response modifiers
g. carcinogens
h. clinical trial
i. DNA molecule
j. external radiation
k. germline mutations
l. histology
m. human genome
n. immune system
o. immune response
p. interferon
q. interleukin
r. monoclonal antibodies
s. point mutation
t. proto-oncogenes
u. remission
v. systemic treatment
w. TNM staging system
x. tumors
y. tumor suppressor gene

COMPLETION

Complete the following statements.

1. The process whereby cancer cells break away from the primary site and begin secondary growths at distant locations in the body is referred to as ____________________.
2. ____________________ is based on the extent of invasion of an untreated primary cancer; the degree to which a tumor resembles the normal tissue in a site is ____________________.
3. A cancer arising from tissue that is capable of differentiating into epithelial and connective tissue is said to be a ____________________ tumor.
4. Two types of carcinomas are ____________________ and ____________________.
5. Malignancies of epithelial cells are ____________________; malignancies of supporting tissues are ____________________
6. ____________________ mutations are changes in DNA that develop throughout a person's life; ____________________ mutations are in reproductive cells.
7. The sum of knowledge regarding tumors is ____________________.
8. The categories of chemotherapeutic agents are: ____________________, ____________________, ____________________, ____________________, and ____________________.
9. Linear strands composed of DNA and proteins that carry genetic information are called ____________________.
10. Subunits of DNA are called ____________________.
11. The core of a cell is the ____________________.
12. ____________________ is treatment with a source of radiation located within the body.
13. ____________________ is using the body's own defense systems to fight cancer.
14. A plan for treatment of cancer is called a ____________________.
15. Treatment to relieve cancer symptoms even though the possibility of remission seems unlikely is called ____________________.
16. ____________________ are drugs being studied that will boost the effect of radiation therapy.
17. A ____________________ is the place on the body at which the radiation beam is aimed.
18. ____________________ protect noncancerous cells from radiation damage.
19. ____________________ are substances that interfere with cell communication and growth, and when used to treat cancer, they block growth.
20. ____________________ reduces the hormones in the body and changes the cancer's ability to use hormones.
21. A transplant using bone marrow or stem cells donated by a sibling or close relative is a/n ____________________ transplant.
22. The process of cellular reproduction that occurs in the nucleus when it forms two identical daughter cells is known as ____________________.
23. Testing to identify individuals who are at risk of getting a disease before any symptoms appear is ____________________ testing.

SHORT ANSWER

Supply a short answer to the following:

1. Compare the three types of genes that are possible sources of proto-oncogene mutations.

____

____

____

2. Explain the difference between intraoperative radiation therapy and an interstitial implant.

____

____

____

3. What is the role of the immune system?

____

____

____

4. In brief, explain fractionation and its benefit to a patient.

____

____

____

5. Distinguish between fine-needle and core biopsies.

____

____

____

MATCHING

Match the terms to their meanings.

1. ________ transplant using the patient's own bone marrow gathered before treatment
2. ________ factors that cause changes that lead to cancer
3. ________ health professional whose calculations plan proper radiation dosage
4. ________ activity of immune system against foreign substances
5. ________ recombining DNA from different organisms to form a new organism
6. ________ replacement of stem cells derived from an umbilical cord
7. ________ chemical code that determines sequence of amino acids in a protein
8. ________ protein substance that regulates cell growth
9. ________ radioactive source placed directly into tissue instead of body cavity
10. ________ special kind of genes that may cause cells to divide abnormally
11. ________ physician specializing in the treatment of malignant tumors
12. ________ process using x-ray pictures to plan radiation treatment so target is precisely located
13. ________ technician who administers radiation treatment to a patient
14. ________ treatment with anticancer drugs
15. ________ testing done by examining DNA taken from cells in blood, tissue, or body fluids

a. autologous transplant
b. carcinogens
c. chemotherapy
d. cord stem cell transplant
e. DNA
f. dosimetrist
g. gene-splitting technology
h. genetic testing
i. immune response
j. interleukin
k. interstitial implant
l. oncogenes
m. oncologist
n. radiology technologist
o. simulation

Word Element Review

Root	Meaning	Example	Definition
aden/o	gland	**adenopathy** (ad"ĕ-nŏp'ah-thē)	enlargement of glands, especially lymph nodes
blast/o	immature, embryonic	**blastoma** (blăs-tō'mah)	neoplasm composed of immature cells derived from the blastema of an organ or a tissue
carcin/o	cancerous	**carcinogenic** (kăr"sĭ-nō-jĕn'ĭk)	causing cancer
		carcinomatous (kăr"sĭ-nŏm'ah-tŭs)	pertaining to cancer; malignant
chem/o	chemical, drug	**electrochemistry** (ē-lek"trō-kĕm'ĭs-trē)	study of chemical changes resulting from electric action
cyst/o	sac of fluid	**cystalgia** (sĭs-tăl'jē-ah)	pain in the bladder
fibr/o	fibers	**fibrinogen** (fī-brĭn'ō-jĕn)	kind of protein found in the blood
immun/o	immune, immunity	**immunogen** (ĭm'ū-nō-jĕn)	any substance capable of eliciting an immune response
medull/o	soft inner part	**medullization** (mĕd"ū-lī-zā'shŭn)	enlargement of marrow spaces
mut/a	genetic change	**transmutation** (trăns"mū-tā'shŭn)	evolutionary change of one species into another
mutagen/o	causing genetic change	**mutagenesis** (mū"tah-jĕn'ĕ-sĭs)	induction of genetic mutation
onc/o	tumor	**oncogenic** (ŏng"kō-jĕn'ĭk)	giving rise to tumors
papill/o	papillary	**papillated** (păp'ĭ-lāt-ĕd)	containing small, nipple-shaped projections or elevations
plas/o	formation	**plasma** (plăz'mah)	fluid portion of blood from which all solids have been removed
polyp/o	polyp	**polypoid** (pŏl'ē-poid)	resembling a polyp
radi/o	rays, x-rays	**radiotherapy** (rā"dē-ō-thĕr'ah-pē)	treatment of disease with x-rays, radium, and other radiations
sarc/o	flesh	**sarcomas** (săr-kō'măhs)	malignant tumors of supporting tissues
scirrh/o	hard	**scirrhous** (skĭr'ŭs)	hard or indurated
Prefix	**Meaning**	**Example**	**Definition**
meta-	beyond, change	**metastasis** (mĕ-tăs'tah-sĭs)	transfer of disease from one part of the body to another that is not directly connected to it

continues

Suffix	Meaning	Example	Definition
-blast	immature	**medulloblast** (mĕ-dŭl'ō-blăst)	undifferentiated cell of the neural tube that may develop into a neuroblast or spongioblast
-plasia	formation, growth	**neoplasia** (nē"ō-plā'zē-ah)	formation of a neoplasm (tumor)
-plasm	formation, growth	**neoplasm** (nē'ō-plăzm)	tumor; any new or abnormal growth
-therapy	treatment	**chemotherapy** (kē"mō-thĕr'ah-pē)	use of drugs to kill cancer cells

Word Element Practice Exercises

IDENTIFY WORD ELEMENTS

Write the word root of each of the following words and give its meaning.

	Word	Elements	Meaning
1.	adenopathy	____________	____________
2.	papillated	____________	____________
3.	scirrhous	____________	____________
4.	sarcomas	____________	____________
5.	blastoma	____________	____________
6.	immunogen	____________	____________
7.	medullization	____________	____________
8.	cystalgia	____________	____________
9.	fibrinogen	____________	____________
10.	polypoid	____________	____________
11.	oncogenic	____________	____________
12.	mutagenesis	____________	____________
13.	plasma	____________	____________
14.	radiotherapy	____________	____________
15.	carcinomatous	____________	____________
16.	metastasis	____________	____________
17.	chemotherapy	____________	____________
18.	neoplasm	____________	____________
19.	neoplasia	____________	____________
20.	medulloblast	____________	____________

IDENTIFY DEFINITIONS

Provide the terms for the following definitions.

1. causing cancer ____________
2. treatment of disease with x-rays, radium, and other radiations ____________
3. transfer of disease from one part of the body to another that is not directly connected to it ____________
4. resembling a polyp ____________
5. evolutionary change of one species into another ____________
6. induction of genetic mutation ____________
7. giving rise to tumors ____________
8. fluid portion of blood from which all solids have been removed ____________
9. study of chemical changes resulting from electric action ____________
10. pertaining to cancer ____________
11. formation of a neoplasm ____________
12. undifferentiated cells of the neural tube ____________
13. tumor; any new or abnormal growth ____________
14. use of drugs to kill cancer cells ____________
15. hard or indurated ____________

MATCHING

Match the word elements to their meanings.

1. ________ beyond, change
2. ________ treatment
3. ________ immature
4. ________ formation, growth

a. -blast
b. meta
c. -plasia
d. -plasm
e. -therapy

WORD ELEMENT MEANINGS

Give the meaning of each word element. Then use your dictionary to find a new word that contains each of the word elements. Specify whether the new word is a noun or an adjective by placing N or A in the last column.

Word Element	Meaning	Word	N or A
1. aden/o	________	________	____
2. blast/o	________	________	____
3. -blast	________	________	____
4. carcin/o	________	________	____
5. chem/o	________	________	____
6. cyst/o	________	________	____
7. fibr/o	________	________	____
8. immun/o	________	________	____

9. medull/o ____________ ____________ ____________
10. meta- ____________ ____________ ____________
11. mut/a ____________ ____________ ____________
12. mutagen/o ____________ ____________ ____________
13. onc/o ____________ ____________ ____________
14. papill/o ____________ ____________ ____________
15. plas/o ____________ ____________ ____________
16. -plasia ____________ ____________ ____________
17. -plasm ____________ ____________ ____________
18. polyp/o ____________ ____________ ____________
19. radi/o ____________ ____________ ____________
20. sarc/o ____________ ____________ ____________
21. scirrh/o ____________ ____________ ____________
22. -therapy ____________ ____________ ____________

Dictionary Exercises

Special vocabulary evolves with new procedures, and such terms may not appear in the dictionary. Study these words and then answer the exercise questions.

Word	Pronunciation	Definition
allogeneic transplantation	ăl"ō-jĕ-nē'ik	procedure in which bone marrow donor and recipient are not genetically identical
antithymocyte globulin	an"tĭ-thī'mō-sīt	protein preparation used to prevent and treat graft versus host disease
apoptosis	ă-pŏp-tō'sĭs	self-destruction
autologous	aw-tŏl'ō-gus	procedure in which marrow is removed from transplantation a patient and reinfused into that patient at a later time
B cells		white blood cells that develop in bone marrow and are the source of antibodies
marrow harvest		removal of a portion of the bone marrow for later transplantation
colony-stimulating factors		proteins that stimulate the development of cells in bone marrow
engraftment		process in which transplanted bone marrow begins to manufacture new white cells, red blood cells, and platelets in the patient's marrow cavities

continues

Word	Pronunciation	Definition
germ cell tumor		tumor arising from the reproductive cells
graft-versus-host disease		reaction of donated bone marrow or peripheral stem cells against the patient's own tissue
growth factor		agent that stimulates the growth of cells
human leukocyte antigen (HLA)	loo'kō-sīt	series of antigen tests used to assess the similarity of the tissue of different people
immunosuppression	ĭm"ū-nō-sū-prĕsh'ŭn	use of drugs or techniques that interfere with the body's immune response, thus making the body less able to fight infection; used in transplants to help protect against rejection of the tissue
morbidity	mŏr-bĭd'ĭ-tē	condition of being deceased
neoadjuvant therapy	nē-ō-ăd'jū-vănt	treatment given before the primary treatment
NK (natural killer) cells		large lymphocytes (lĭm'fō-sīts) that attack tumor cells and infected cells
purging		removal of tumor cells from marrow before autologous transplantation
severe combined immunodeficiency deficiency disease (SCID)	ĭm"ū-nō-dĕ-fĭsh'ĕn-sē	disorder characterized by complete absence or marked deficiency of B and T cells, types of white blood cells
stem cells		cells from which all blood cells develop
syngeneic transplantation	sĭn"jĕ-nē'ĭk	grafting between identical twins
T cells		white blood cells important in body's immune system

DICTIONARY EXERCISE 1

What relationships can you see between any of the words in the previous list?

Example: B and T cells are both white blood cells.

1. ______________________________
2. ______________________________
3. ______________________________
4. ______________________________
5. ______________________________
6. ______________________________
7. ______________________________
8. ______________________________
9. ______________________________
10. ______________________________
11. ______________________________
12. ______________________________

DICTIONARY EXERCISE 2

Pronunciation of the words below is provided. Using your dictionary, find the correct spelling and definition of these words.

	Word	Pronunciation	Definition
1.	____________	lĭm-fō'mah	____________
2.	____________	mĕl"ah-nō'mah	____________
3.	____________	pŏl'ĭp	____________
4.	____________	rē-frăk'tō-rē	____________
5.	____________	făg"ō-sī-tō'sĭs	____________
6.	____________	thrŏm"bō-sĭ"tō-pē'nē-ah	____________
7.	____________	kor"tĭ-kō-stĕr'oyd	____________
8.	____________	ăn'tĭ-jĕn	____________
9.	____________	ah-plăs'tĭk ah-nē'mē-ah	____________
10.	____________	ĭn-fū'zhun	____________
11.	____________	loo"kō-pē'nē-ah	____________
12.	____________	făg'ō-sīt	____________
13.	____________	ă-pŏp-tō'sĭs	____________
14.	____________	mŏr-bĭd'ĭ-tē	____________
15.	____________	ĕn-kăp'sŭ-lā"tĕd	____________
16.	____________	stĕr'oyd	____________
17.	____________	hēm	____________
18.	____________	făg"ō-sī-tō'sĭs	____________
19.	____________	sĭn-ĕr'ĕ-sĭs	____________
20.	____________	fī"brĭn-ŏl'ĭ-sĭs	____________

StudyWARE™ Connection

To take a practice quiz or play interactive games that reinforce the content in this chapter, go to your StudyWARE™ CD-ROM.

Listening Exercise

INSTRUCTIONS

1. Review the spelling, pronunciation, and meaning of the words provided in the preview.
2. Go to your StudyWARE™ CD-ROM and listen to **Listening Exercise 10-1**. Fill in the blank in the report as the word is dictated.
3. At the end of the activity, check your spelling against the preview words. They appear in the preview in the order in which they are encountered in the activity.
4. Review and practice the words you missed.
5. Look up words that are not familiar.

PREVIEW OF WORDS FOR LISTENING EXERCISE 10-1

Word	Pronunciation	Meaning
irradiation	ĭ-rā-dē-ā'shŭn	exposure to radiant energy for therapeutic purposes
adenocarcinoma	ăd"ĕ-nō-kăr"sĭn-ō'mă	cancer derived from glandular tissue
symptomatology	sĭmp"tō-mă-tŏl'ō-jē	the combined symptoms of a disease
fibrosis	fī-brō'sĭs	formation of fibrous tissue
organomegaly	or"gă-nō-mĕg'ă-lē	enlargement of organs
telangiectasias	tĕl-ăn"jē-ĕk-tă'zē-ă	vascular lesions formed by dilation of a group of small blood vessels

Listening Exercise 10-1

*Study*WARE™ Connection

Listen to this report being read on your StudyWARE™ CD-ROM. Fill in each blank as the word is dictated.

Letter of Consultation

Dr. Antonio Rameriz:

I had the opportunity to visit with our mutual patient, Katrina Switzgoebel, on 3/3/20—. She is now nine months after completion of her whole abdominal ____________, which followed her second-look laparotomy for a grade 2 ovarian ______________________.

I am glad you referred her to a dietitian who has been working with her to modify her diet and, therefore, has decreased her ______________. She has not had any vomiting since January and only intermittent cramping associated with certain foods. She denied the presence of blood in the stool, urine, or vagina. She does have a significant weight loss since we last saw her in December.

Her physical exam was remarkable for a weight of 61.7 kg, which is down from 70.8 kg on 9/6 of the previous year. She did not have any palpable lymphadenopathy. Breast exam was unremarkable. There was no back tenderness to percussion.

Her abdomen showed ___________ in the low abdominal area beneath the abdominal incision, but no masses or ________________________. Her pelvic exam was remarkable for an atrophic vagina, which presented dryness and ______________ consistent with her estrogen deficient state and postradiation status. Her laboratory evaluation was unremarkable except for an alkaline phosphatase of 260 (normal range 90–234), creatinine 1.2 (normal range 0.6–0.9). The creatinine level has not changed since her last visit and her alkaline phosphatase is actually down from 316 on 12/19. Her hemoglobin was 10.8. The rest of the hematology and chemistry panels were unremarkable.

Chest x-ray was normal, as were her mammograms. CA-125 level was 18.8.

Dr. Victor Montagno from GYN Oncology examined Katrina and agreed with my findings. It is our impression that she does not have evidence of recurrent ovarian cancer. She does present RTOG grade 2 gastrointestinal toxicity related to her postoperative irradiation.

I would advise that Katrina continue seeing her dietitian since diet modification has been the only thing that helped her gastrointestinal symptoms. We would like to see her again at the end of May.

Thank you for letting us participate in the care of your patient. If you have questions regarding her visit here, please do not hesitate to write.

Sincerely yours,

Lloyd Livermore, MD

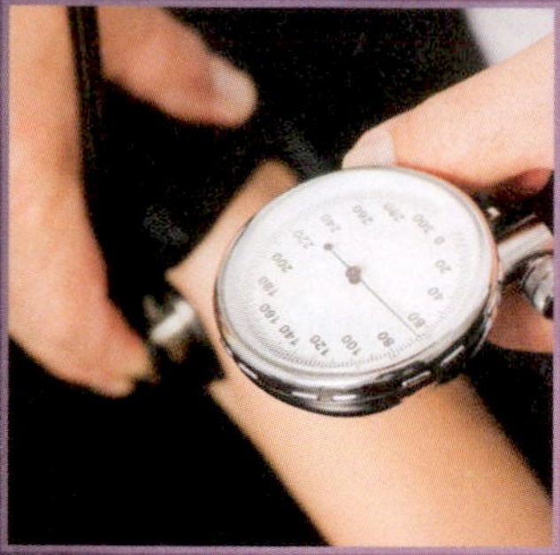

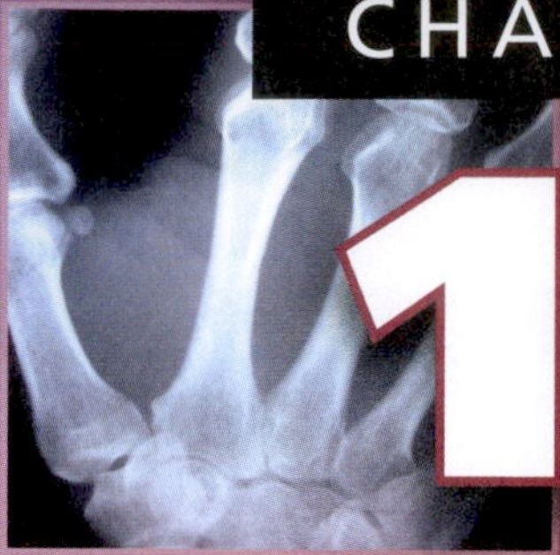

CHAPTER

11

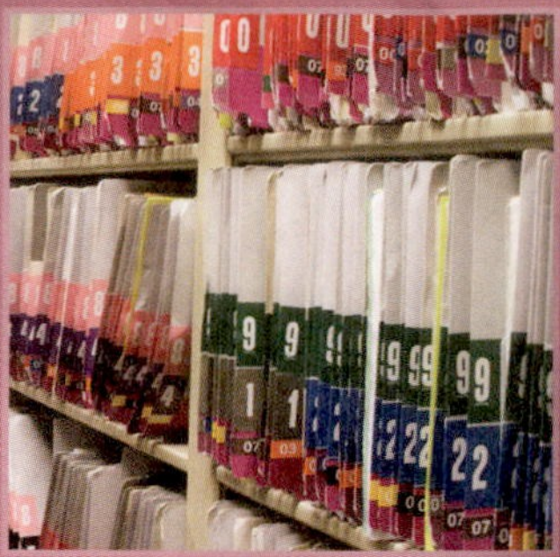

Radiology and Nuclear Medicine

"One look is worth a thousand listens."

—Merrill C. Sosman

OBJECTIVES

When you have completed this chapter on radiology and nuclear medicine, you should be able to

1. Identify and define the names of radiologic and nuclear medicine diagnostic techniques.
2. Identify and spell the positions for taking x-rays.
3. Identify and spell the names of radiographic contrast media.
4. Identify procedures that use barium, iodine, or other contrast media
5. Explain the role of radiopharmaceuticals.
6. Identify procedures that use labeled compounds
7. Identify interventional radiology and procedures that use interventional radiology techniques.
8. Identify abbreviations commonly used.
9. Identify the meanings of related word elements.
10. Hear how medical terminology is used in actual medical reports.

INTRODUCTION

Modern radiology is the outgrowth of two turn-of-the-twentieth-century discoveries. The first, in 1895, was the identification by Wilhelm Conrad Röntgen of types of radiation called **roentgen** (rĕnt'gĕn) **rays**. This discovery was of such importance that within 10 years radiology was being used all over the Western world. Then in 1903 Henri Becquerel and Marie Curie discovered radioactive properties in uranium. Curie recognized and diagrammed three different rays, called alpha and beta particles and gamma rays, which can be used to diagnose and treat disease. Such use of these radioactive substances is referred to as **nuclear medicine**.

There are several areas of specialization in the field of radiology, including the subfields of diagnostic, therapeutic, and interventional radiology. For example, a physician trained in the practice of diagnostic radiology is known as a **radiologist**. A physician or radiologist who focuses on the use of diagnostic nuclear medicine procedures is a **nuclear physician**. A physician who specializes in the practice of radiotherapy (treatment of disease using radiation) is a **radiotherapist** or technologist. Other subspecialties such as neuroradiology are divided by anatomic section.

The radiology report describes what the radiologist finds as a result of a radiologic examination. Other items included in the report are the name of the procedure performed, the name of the patient and date, and any other identification information the hospital or office may require.

When a contrast medium is used, it is noted in the report. The balance of the report details the findings and interpretations made by the radiologist who has reviewed the results of the study. More than one study may be included in one report.

An allied health professional must be aware of several types of information relating to radiology reports. This chapter discusses the use of radiology and nuclear medicine to diagnose and treat various medical problems, as well as x-ray positioning, contrast media, radioisotopes, and interventional radiology. Such information will help students to work with radiology reports in their specific medical environment.

DIAGNOSTIC TECHNIQUES USING RADIOLOGY

fluor/o	luminous	-opaque	obscure
-gram	a record	radi/o	ray
-graphy	process of recording	tele-	distant
is/o	same, equal	tom/o	to cut
-lucent	to shine		

A radiologist can use x-rays, sound waves, and magnetism to produce images that will assist in the diagnosis of medical problems.

IMAGES PRODUCED BY X-RAYS

The x-ray machine is one of the most basic and familiar tools in radiological diagnostics. It uses penetrating rays derived from high-energy electromagnetic sources rather than the chemical sources found in nuclear medicine. These machines are often used for evaluation of bony structures and soft tissues.

Body tissues and other substances vary in the way they accept x-rays. If x-rays pass through a substance, it is **radiolucent** (rā"dē-ō-lū'sĕnt). If a substance blocks the rays, it is **radiopaque** (rā"dē-ō-pāk'). The intensity of the rays used is determined by both the body part and the purpose (diagnostic or treatment) of the x-rays.

Radiographic examinations may consist of x-ray images or radiographs only. A technologist prepares the patient, takes the radiograph, and processes the image. Interpretation is then done by a radiologist. This is the familiar x-ray that is administered in a dentist's office, a laboratory, or a hospital. An example of a radiograph is shown in Figure 11-1. However, in the United States, the current trend is away from film and toward digital imaging displayed on a computer screen.

In a **fluoroscopic** (floo"rō-skŏp'ĭk) **examination** a continuous, moving picture gives the radiologist a means of observing how organs are functioning before and after a contrast medium has been introduced. The patient's position can be changed during the examination for a different or better view of the target area. A permanent record

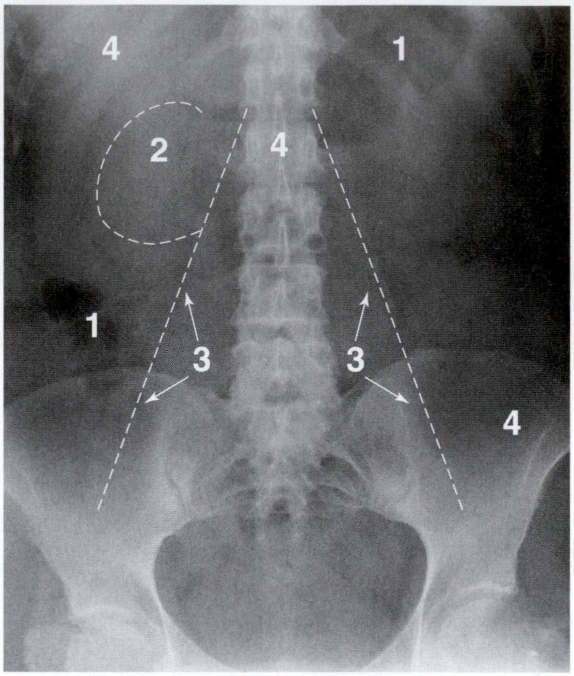

FIGURE 11-1 A Radiograph of the Abdomen Demonstrating (1) Air in the Stomach and Colon; (2) Fat Around the Kidneys; (3) Muscle to the Right and Left of the Spine; and (4) Ribs, Spine, and Pelvis

Source: Delmar/Cengage Learning

of a fluoroscopic (or x-ray) examination can be obtained by using a video recorder and/or a digital image capture device. Fluoroscopy is also used to assist in certain therapeutic procedures, such as installing catheters that deliver antibiotic or chemotherapy treatment or positioning tubes through the nasal passages to the stomach.

There is an inherent risk from the cumulative effect of continued exposure to radiation. The daily exposure which fluoroscopic and x-ray equipment operators face requires them to wear protective coverings such as lead-lined aprons, gloves, and thyroid shields. For individual patients who receive only the occasional x-ray, this poses no problem. *However, because radiation exposure to a pregnant woman in her first trimester may cause congenital problems for the fetus, x-rays are avoided. During the second and third trimesters, x-rays may be used cautiously for special reasons. A woman should tell her doctor or dentist if she suspects being pregnant.*

With **computerized axial tomography** (ăk'sē-al tō-mŏg'rah-fē) **(CAT)**, a layer or section of the body is exposed to thousands of small x-ray beams. The quantity of rays penetrating a given layer of tissue is recorded. A computer analyzes this series of cross-sectional, two-dimensional "slices" to generate a three-dimensional image. This procedure can also be used with a contrast medium. One of the advantages of this option is that it provides a three-dimensional view of a cross section of the body. The procedure is also known as **computed tomography (CT)** or **computer-assisted tomography (CAT)**. See Figure 11-2 for an example of a CT scan.

Another technique is **tomography**. This procedure permits visualization of a specific layer of the body while blocking out layers in front of and behind it. It is actually an x-ray slice taken at different depths of focus. Calcifications and solid lesions that are missed on conventional x-rays will often be identified on a **tomogram** (tō'mō-grăm), the picture produced by tomography (see Figure 11-3).

X-ray Positioning

X-ray positioning determines the view of an anatomical part being examined. X-rays of certain parts of the body can be taken only from specific body positions. The radiologist has special terms to refer to the direction of the x-ray beam in reference to the patient's position. The four most common terms are:

PA [posteroanterior (pŏs"ter-ō-ăn-tēr'ē-or) **projection]**
patient is positioned with back to the x-ray machine, front close to the film cassette; beam passes from back to front; an example is a chest x-ray (Figure 11-4)

AP [anteroposterior (an"tĕr-ō-pŏs-tēr'ē-or) **projection]**
patient is positioned with back to the film plate; beam passes from front to back; an example is a chest x-ray given to a very ill patient in bed (Figure 11-5)

lateral (lăt'er-ăl) **projection**
patient is held closely against the film plate; beam passes from one side of the body to the other; an example is an x-ray of the extremities, chest, or abdomen (Figure 11-6)

oblique (ŏ-blēk') **projection**
x-ray beam tube or patient is positioned at an angle that is *not* PA, AP, or lateral (Figure 11-7)

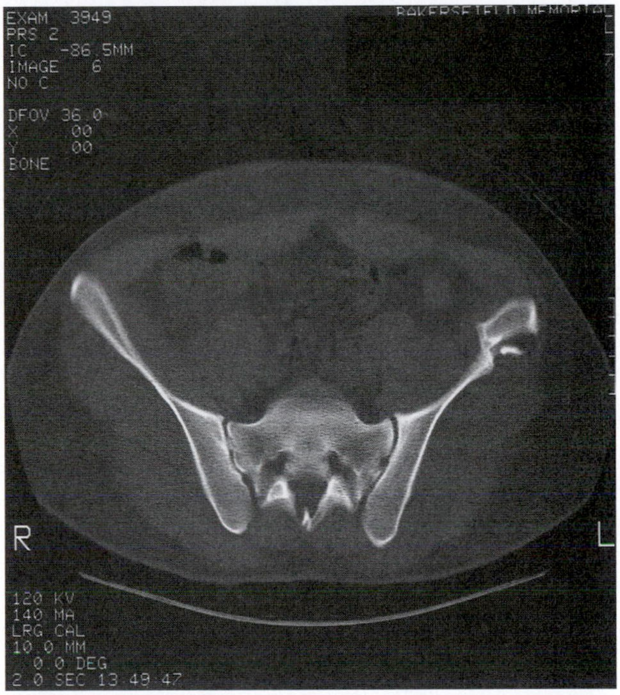

FIGURE 11-2
CT Image of Pelvis

Source: Delmar/Cengage Learning

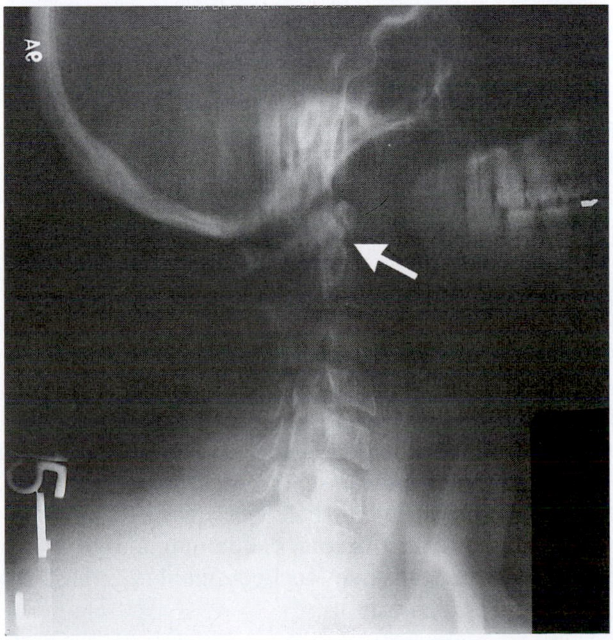

FIGURE 11-3
Conventional Lateral Tomogram of a Fracture of C1 as Indicated by the Arrow

Source: Delmar/Cengage Learning

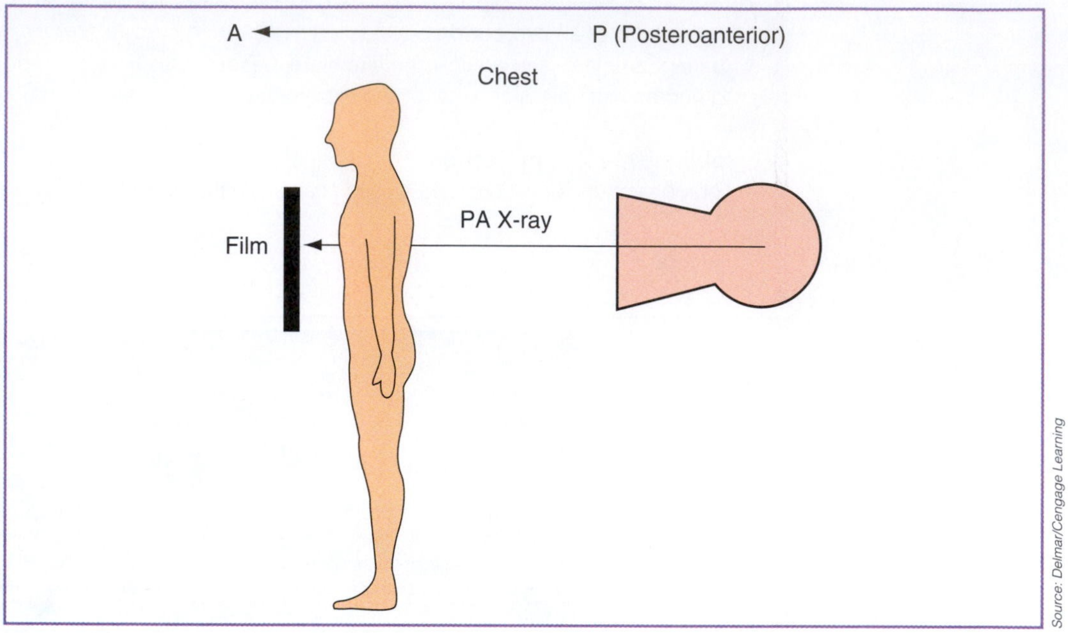

FIGURE 11-4
PA (Posteroanterior) Projection

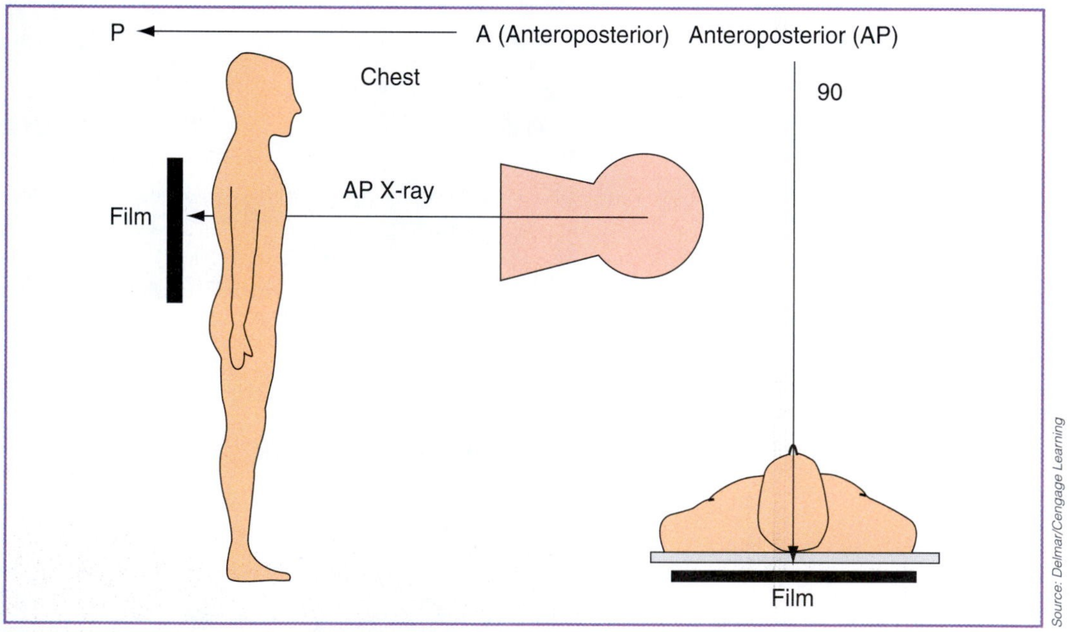

FIGURE 11-5
AP (Anteroposterior) Projection

Radiographic Contrast Media

To visualize organs or body parts that are not ordinarily seen, **radiographic contrast media** are used to help the radiologist. They differentiate the organ under study from the surrounding tissue. These media are injected, ingested, or administered by enema. Contrast media are radiopaque (not permitting passage of x-rays); most are barium- or iodine-based products. Other substances, such as oxygen, carbon dioxide, and air, are nonopaque and are classed as radiolucent (allowing passage of x-rays).

Barium sulfate, a contrast medium that does not permit x-rays to pass through it, causes the intestinal tract to stand out. Disorders of the esophagus, duodenum, and small and large intestines are primarily examined by swallowing barium or by barium enema. Most commonly performed tests are the upper GI series, small-bowel

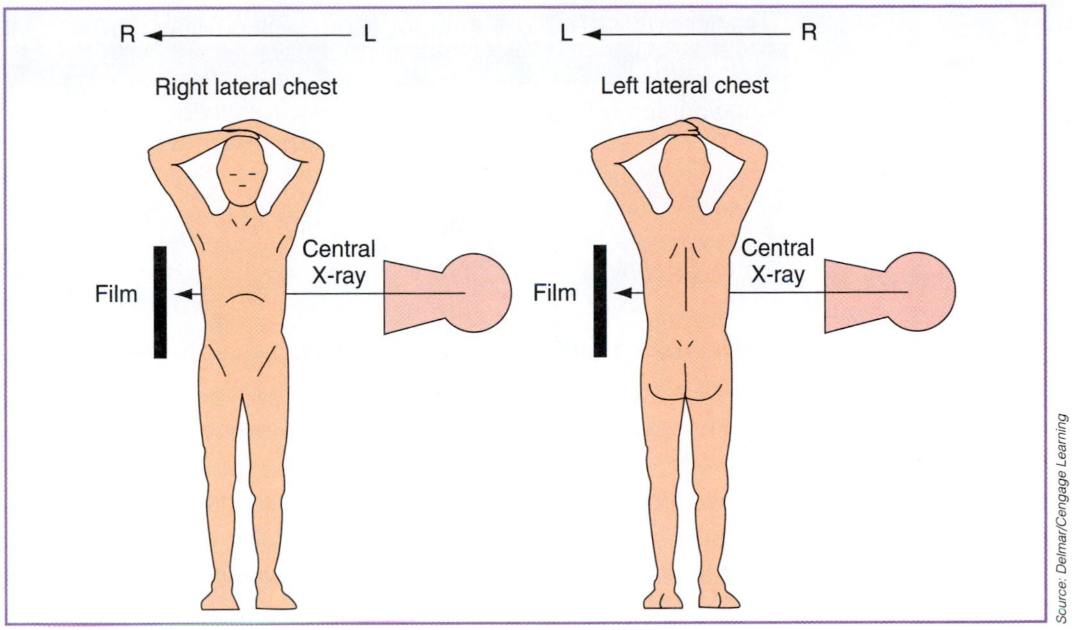

FIGURE 11-6
Lateral Projection

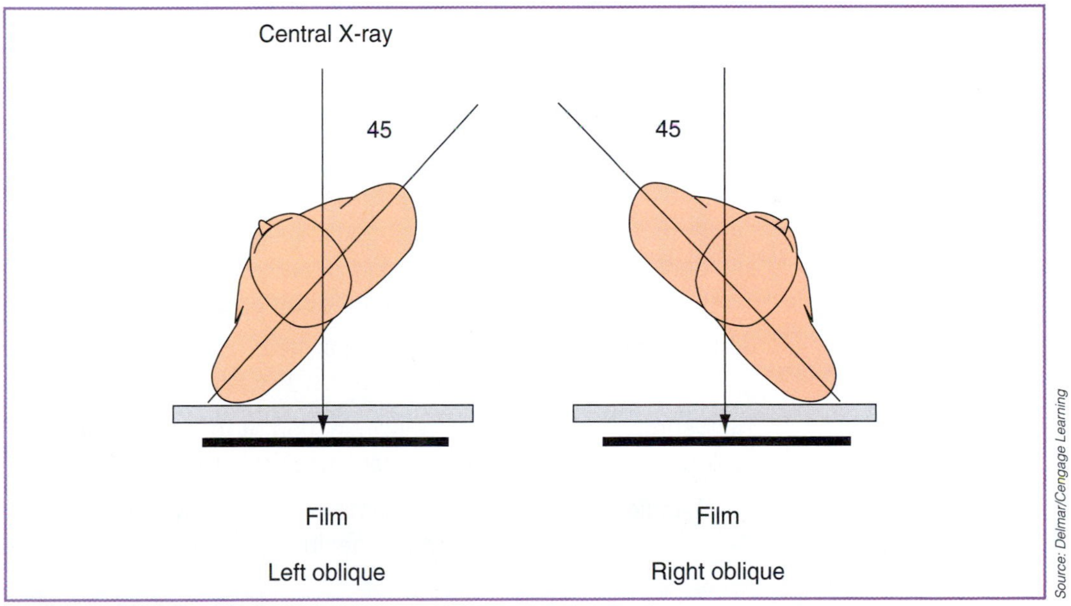

FIGURE 11-7
Oblique Projection

follow-through, and barium enema. Frequently, a double contrast study is prescribed. This procedure combines both a radiopaque and a radiolucent contrast medium.

For a variety of other diagnostic x-ray examinations, **iodinated substances** are combined with other compounds and used as the contrast medium. Some of the commonly used iodine-based contrast media are Diatrizoate (Hypaque 50), Metrizoate (Isopaque Coronar), Ioxaglate (Hexabrix), and Iopamidol (Isovue). Both Diatrizoate and Metrizoate have hyperosmolarity, while Ioxaglate and Iopamidol have hyposmolarity. All are water-soluble.

All iodinated contrast media may cause side effects that range from mild to severe. The reason for these adverse reactions is disputed.

PROCEDURES THAT USE BARIUM, IODINE, OR OTHER CONTRAST MEDIA	
Procedure	**Description**
angiography	a series of x-ray films follows the introduction of a contrast medium injected into an artery or vein
arteriography	a series of x-ray films after the introduction of contrast medium into an artery
arthrography	process of taking x-ray inside a joint space, after a contrast medium has been injected in the joint
barium enema (BE)	infusion of barium into the rectum while x-ray pictures are obtained
barium swallow	x-ray examination while the patient swallows a contrast medium
• *upper GI series*	examines the esophagus, stomach, and proximal small bowel
• *esophagram*	examines the esophagus only
cholangiography	radiography of the bile ducts (generally replaced by ultrasonography)
• *operative*	injection of a radiopaque dye directly into the ducts of the biliary tract during gallbladder surgery.
• *postoperative transhepatic (PTC)*	injection of a radiopaque dye through the skin directly into an intrahepatic bile duct
computed tomography, computed axial tomography (CT, CAT)	provides three-dimensional cross-sectional view of tissues; used for checking the pathology of tumors, stones, ducts, and other abnormalities in the chest, abdominal cavity, brain, or practically anywhere in the body
digital subtraction angiography (DSA)	procedure using before and after contrast medium pictures that allows blood vessels only to appear by a computerized digital video subtraction process (see Figure 11-8)
hysterosalpingography	x-ray after injecting contrast medium through the cervix and into the uterus and fallopian tubes
intravenous pyelography (IVP)	x-ray examination of the entire urinary tract after injection of contrast medium into a vein
lymphangiography	x-ray examination of the lymphatic vessels after injection of a contrast medium through the back of the hand or top of the foot
myelography	x-ray examination of the spinal space and vertebral canal following an injection of opaque contrast medium (See Figure 11-9)
small bowel follow through	x-ray examination of orally ingested contrast medium at timed intervals to observe progression of barium through the small intestine
voiding cystourethrography	radiopaque dye is placed in the bladder via urethral catheter and x-ray pictures are taken to observe the bladder and urethra as the bladder is filling and emptying.

To administer the contrast media or perform certain procedures, a variety of equipment is used. This equipment is divided into six groups. A few of the more common devices are listed on page 323.

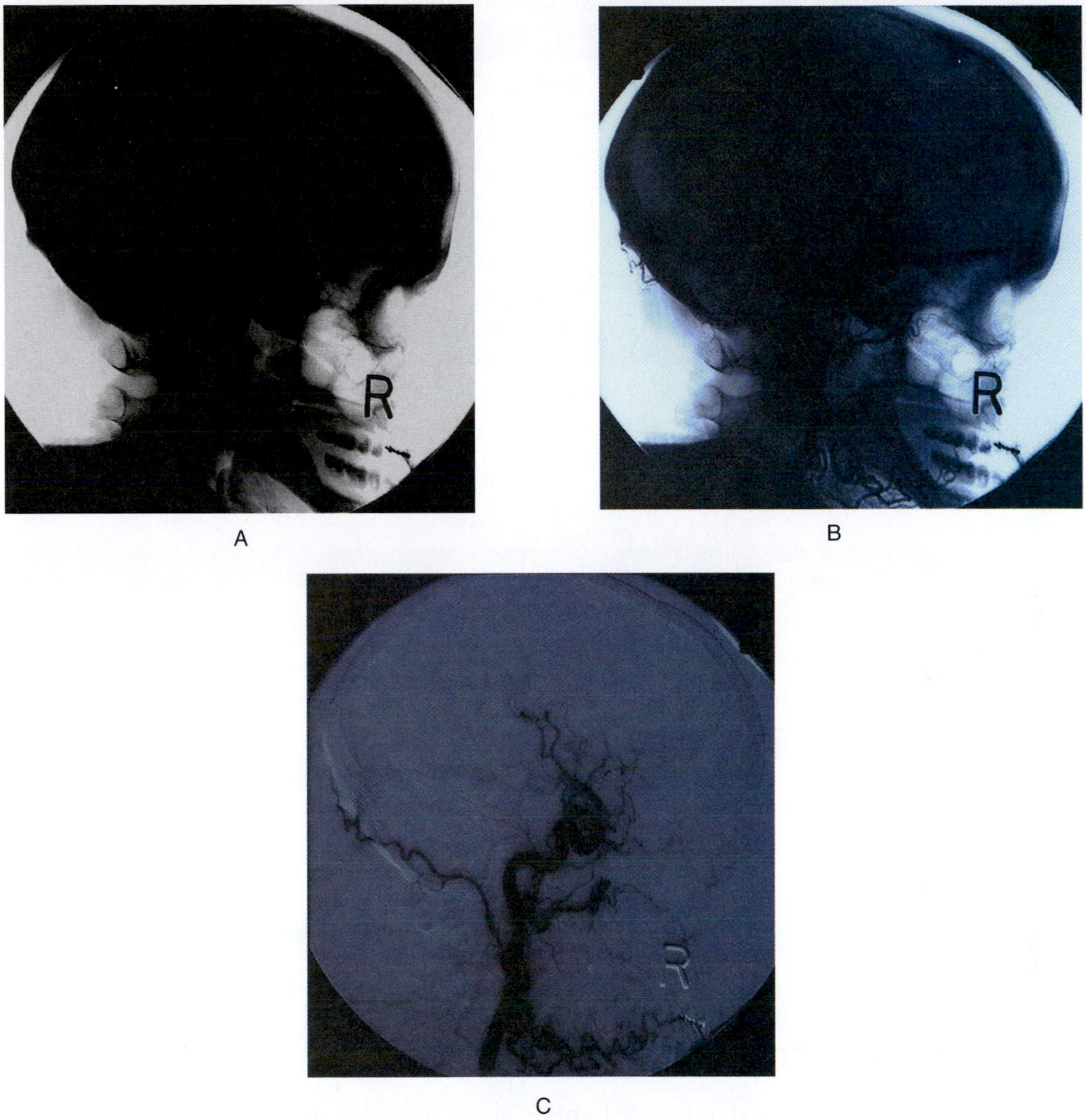

Source: Delmar/Cengage Learning

FIGURE 11-8 Digital Subtraction Angiography. This figure depicts the stages involved in digital subtraction angiography: (A) scout image; (B) injection image; and (C) resulting subtracted image

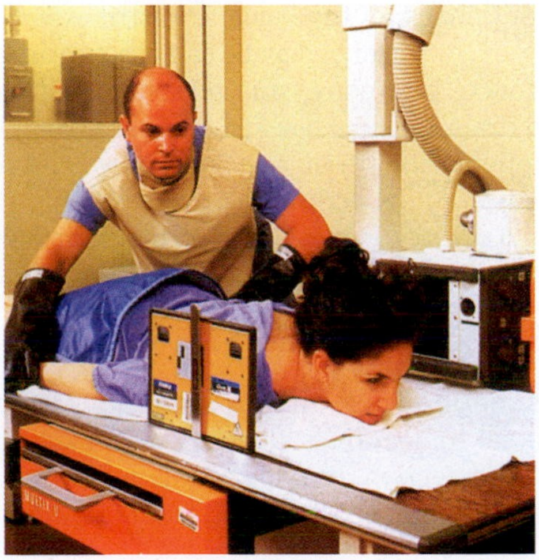

FIGURE 11-9 Cervical Myelography: can indicate the presence of cervical disk herniation, tumors (neurofibroma and astrocytoma), and inflammatory disease

Source: Delmar/Cengage Learning

DEVICES USED IN DIGITAL IMAGING		
Catheters		
Amplatz	Headhunter	Shepherd hook
Bentson	Hickman catheter	Simmons
Chuang	Judkins	Sones
Cobra	Kumpe	straight
Double J stent	Porta catheter	Swan Ganz
Grollman	Rosch	Van Aman
Needles	**Introducers**	**Embolization Materials**
Chiba	Greenfield	coils
Micropuncture	Bird	PVA (Ivalon)
Colapinto	S nest	glue
		gelfoam
Guidewires	**Stents**	
solid wire	Wall stent	
wrapped wire	Symphony	
fixed or movable core	Memotherm	
coated or noncoated	Palmaz	
J-tip	Z stent	
Tomcat		

As in other areas, this field also is affected by the advancement of technology and the resulting changes in procedures and equipment.

IMAGES PRODUCED BY SOUND WAVES

An **ultrasound** scan uses sound waves at ultrasonic levels to obtain images of specific parts of the body. Although it is limited by its inability to image through gases and solid (like air and bone), the process is generally safer—especially for obstetrical imaging—because it does not use ionizing radiation. Obstetricians and gynecologists employ it to evaluate fetal size and maturity, fetal and placental position, uterine tumors, and other pelvic masses. During the procedure, an ultrasonic beam is introduced into the body by an instrument called a **transducer** placed on the skin. Reflections, or echoes, of the beam as it strikes various substances can be detected, recorded, and photographed to produce a record, which may be called a **sonogram**, an ultrasound, or an **echogram**. Ultrasound scans can detect the differences between cystic and solid structures in the body and direct image-guided interventions such as biopsies and drainages. Such scans can also examine and evaluate abnormalities of the major blood vessels, organs in the abdominal and pelvic cavities, and small structures such as the eye.

An ultrasound procedure called **echocardiography** (ĕk"ō-kăr"dē-ŏg'rah-fē) is used to examine the heart to locate aortic aneurysms and diseased valves. An example of a sonogram is shown in Figure 11-10.

IMAGES PRODUCED BY MAGNETISM

Another diagnostic tool is **magnetic resonance imaging** (MRI). Some images created are similar to those produced by computerized axial tomography. However, the images, which better differentiate soft tissues, are far more detailed because one can section the body in multiple planes. In a CAT scan, the computer is linked to images produced by ionizing radiation; in the case of MRI, the computer is linked to images produced by magnetism.

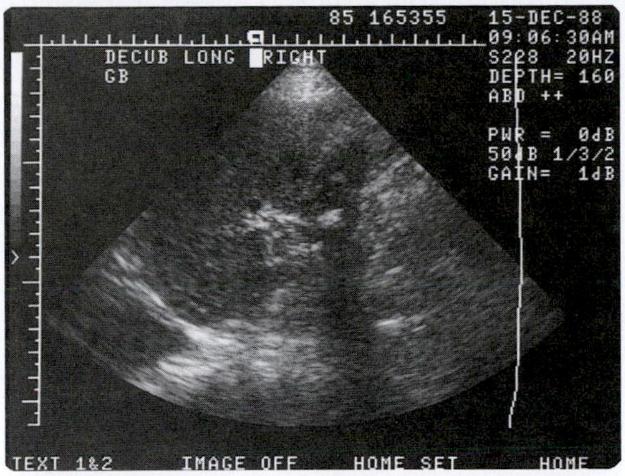

FIGURE 11-10 Sonogram of Gallbladder With Gallstones

Source: Delmar/Cengage Learning

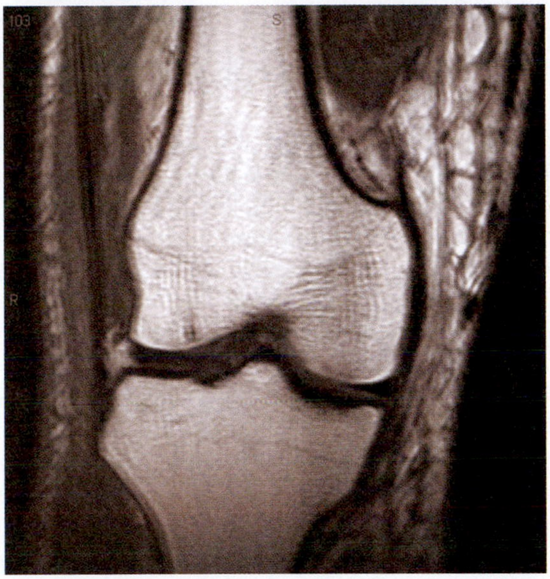

FIGURE 11-11 MRI of the Knee

Source: Delmar/Cengage Learning

Two types of contrast media may be used in clinical MRIs to improve the efficacy of the image. Intravenous gadolinium-DTPA and intravenous magnetic iron oxide particles both work by altering the magnetic properties of nearby atoms. The downside of using these contrast media is the prolonging of the examination.

A patient undergoing an MRI scan lies in a cylinder surrounded by a large magnet where the atoms are aligned according to the polarity of the magnet. Radiowaves are sent across the atoms. Each atom absorbs more or less energy from these radiowaves, thus altering the alignment and creating signals that are interpreted by the computer as images. The images are converted to visual displays on a computer screen.

The MRI makes it possible to distinguish between normal and abnormal tissue masses within the image. The process has decreased the need for some diagnostic procedures. It has also been especially useful in detecting edema in the brain, in finding tumors in the chest and abdomen, and in visualizing the cardiovascular system. An MRI of the knee can be seen in Figure 11-11.

DIAGNOSTIC TECHNIQUES USING NUCLEAR MEDICINE

vitr/o	glass	viv/o	life

Nuclear medicine is composed of diagnostic examinations that result in images of body anatomy and function. Its applications include bone scanning, staging cancers, myocardial perfusion imaging, and molecular imaging.

The process uses a **radiopharmaceutical** (rā"dē-ō-fărm"ă-sū'tĭ-kăl), or **labeled compound**, which is a specific radionuclide (or radioisotope) incorporated into a chemical substance. A **radionuclide** (rā"dē-ō-nū'klīd) gives off electromagnetic radiation as it disintegrates. The time it takes for this disintegration to occur is called its **half-life** or the time it takes for a substance to lose half of its radioactivity. To be effective, the half life must be long enough to allow for imaging, but short enough to prevent the patient from becoming overexposed to radiation.

These radioactive substances, called **tracers**, are given to the patient (orally or intravenously) and emit energy which produces images. The principal imaging device is the gamma camera which detects the radiation given off by the tracer in the body. In this way, tumors, infections, and other disorders can be detected by evaluating organ function.

Basically there are two types of tests: in vitro (ĭn vē'trō) and in vivo (ĭn vē'vō).

In vitro (a Latin phrase) refers to testing in a glass unit, such as a test tube, or other artificial environment. For example, laboratory procedures to analyze blood and urine specimens with radioactive chemicals would be in vitro procedures. A specific example is a radioimmunoassay (RAI), which combines radioactive chemicals and antibodies to detect hormones and drugs in a patient's blood. The development of the radioimmunoassay technique has facilitated research in endocrinology, pharmacology, and other branches of medicine.

In vivo refers to testing within a living body. In general, a radiopharmaceutical is introduced into the body where an organ or a tissue absorbs it at a rate referred to as the **uptake**. Then in a process called **scanning**, an image (or **scan**) of a target area is produced and subsequently analyzed by a radiologist.

Take the case of a radionuclide incorporated into a chemical substance and administered to the patient. This is what happens.

Gamma rays emitted from the administered radionuclide are detected by a gamma camera and translated into light flashes that indicate the frequency and intensity of the radiation. A photomultiplier reads these data and sends the information to a computer, which provides a statistical analysis of the test. The computer can also produce an image (a **scintiscan** (sĭn'tĭ-skăn) or **photoscan**) that depicts the distribution and intensity of the radionuclide in the organ or area under study. This latter process is referred to as **scintiphotography** (sĭn"tĭ-fō-tŏg'rah-fē).

One method of obtaining a scan involves an advancement in diagnostic nuclear medicine—**positron emission tomography** (PET). PET images register glucose metabolism in a cross section of the brain. The patient receives radioactive oxyglucose, which gives off radioactivity in the form of positrons. These positron emissions are picked up and transformed into a visual display by a computer. PET scans enable a physician to see how your tissues and organs are functioning and can detect changes often before a disease progresses. The level of chemical activity may indicate areas of disease not detected by other scanning methods. Currently, researchers are using PET scans to study strokes, epilepsy, migraine headaches, Alzheimer's disease, Parkinson's disease, and schizophrenia and to find metastasized cancers. An example of a PET scan is in Figure 11-12.

Another technique is **single-photon emission computed tomography** (SPECT). This procedure uses an intravenous injection of a radioactive tracer and a computer to construct a three-dimensional image of certain areas of the body. Liver tumors, cardiac ischemia, and bone disease of the spine are effectively evaluated with this technique.

Procedures such as PET and SPECT use labeled compounds, such as technetium-99m, iodine-131, xenon-133, and thallium-201, in a variety of ways for imaging various parts of the body. Some of the major procedures performed are described as follows.

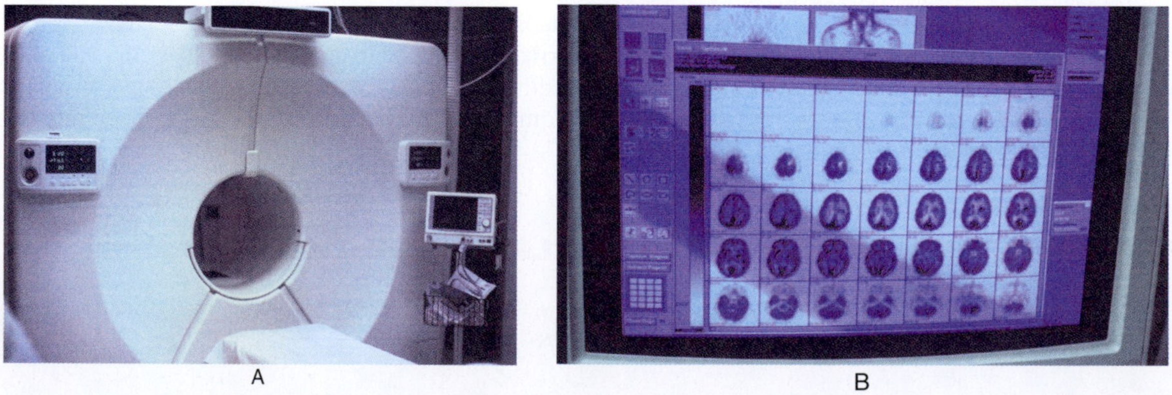

FIGURE 11-12 (A) Position Emission Tomography (PET) Scanner. (B) PET Scan Output Images

PROCEDURES USING LABELED COMPOUNDS	
Procedure	**Description**
bone scan	intravenously injected phosphate substance; helpful in locating skeletal abnormalities
brain scan	radionuclides enter the tumor or disease and allow it to be visualized
liver, spleen scan	radiopharmaceuticals injected intravenously; abnormalities such as cirrhosis, abscesses, tumors, hepatomegaly, hepatitis, and splenomegaly are spotted
lung scan	perfusion study: done by giving a labeled compound *intravenously*; ventilation study: done by the *inhalation* of radioactive gas
multiple gated acquisition scan (MUGA scan)	x-ray that uses radioactive isotopes injected into the blood vessels to evaluate the condition of the myocardium of the heart
positron emission tomography (PET)	computerized radiographic images of various body structures produced when radioactive substances are inhaled or injected
radioactive iodine up-take by thyroid gland	substance given orally by capsule; measures the rate of thyroid activity
sentinel node mapping	injection of radioactive material into breast tissue surrounding a cancer just prior to surgery; material migrates to the "sentinel lymph node," which is identified in the operating room by Geiger counter; node is removed and evaluated by the pathologist; results generally reflect the status of the remainder of the lymph nodes
thyroid scan	radionuclide administered intravenously; defines the size and shape of the thyroid gland
tumor imaging	radiopharmaceuticals administered to localize a tumor; includes peptides (small proteins), monoclonal antibodies (large proteins), and tumor-specific radioisotopes such as gallium-67 or thallium

INTERVENTIONAL RADIOLOGY

Interventional radiology is a clinical specialty that uses fluoroscopy, CT, ultrasound and MRI to guide procedures such as tissue biopsies, fluid draining, catheter insertion, and narrowed duct or vessel repair by dilation or stenting. The purpose is to gain access to the deep parts of most organs and organ systems in a minimally invasive manner. These new procedures are a major advance in medicine because they present a much lower risk to the patient than traditional surgery. They also reduce pain and recovery time, require no general anesthesia, and are cost effective.

Physicians who specialize in this area are called interventional radiologists. They are often joined by other types of doctors such as general surgeons, vascular surgeons, cardiologists, gastroenterologists, gynecologists, and urologists. Using tools such as balloons, catheters, microcatheters, stents and therapeutic embolization, these physicians have been responsible for the innovation and development of the minimally invasive procedures like interventional cardiology, vascular surgery, endoscopy, and laparoscopy that are commonplace today.

Some of the procedures that are performed are identified in the following chart.

PROCEDURES USING INTERVENTIONAL RADIOLOGY TECHNIQUES	
Procedure	**Description**
angiography	imaging the blood vessels to look for abnormalities with the use of various contrast media
balloon angioplasty; stent placement	opening of narrow or blocked blood vessels using a balloon; placement of metallic stents to keep a vessel open
biliary interventions	placement of catheters to bypass biliary obstructions and decompress the biliary system; placement of permanent, indwelling biliary stents
biopsy	taking of a tissue sample from the area of interest for pathological examination
chemoembolization	delivering cancer treatment directly to a tumor through its blood supply, followed by clot-inducing substances to block the artery to prevent wash out of the delivered chemotherapy
cryoablation	localized destruction of tissue by freezing
dialysis access/intervention	placement of tunneled hemodialysis catheters, peritoneal dialysis catheters, and revision of poorly functioning surgically placed AV fistulas and grafts
digital subtraction angiography (DSA)	technique used to clearly visualize blood vessels by subtracting a digital image taken before a contrast medium is administered (called a mark) from an image taken after introduction of a contrast medium; useful in diagnosing arterial and venous occlusions
drain insertions	placement of tubes into different parts of the body to drain fluids
embolization	blocking an abnormal blood vessel (to stop bleeding) or organ (to stop its function)
endovenous laser ablation of varicose veins	placement of thin laser fiber in varicose veins for non-surgical treatment of venous insufficiency
gastrostomy; gastrojejunostomy tube placement	placement of a feeding tube percutaneously into the stomach and/or jejunum
inferior vena cavae (IVC) filters	placement of metallic filters in the inferior vena cavae to prevent propagation of deep venous thrombus, both temporary and permanent
nephrostomy	placement of a catheter directly into the kidney to drain urine in situations where normal flow of urine is obstructed.
radiofrequency ablation (RFA)	localized destruction of tissue by heating
thrombolysis	dissolving blood clots by both pharmaceutical and mechanical means

continues

PROCEDURES USING INTERVENTIONAL RADIOLOGY TECHNIQUES	
Procedure	**Description**
transjugular intrahepatic portosystemic shunt (TIPS)	placement of a Transjugular Intrahepatic Porto-systemic Shunt for management of patients with critical end-stage liver disease and portal hypertension
venous access devices	insertion and management of specialized kinds of intravenous devices (e.g., PICC liintravenous nes, Hickman lines)
vertebroplasty	repair of a vertebrae by percutaneous injection of biocompatible bone cement inside fractured vertebrae

Current research is providing even newer techniques for imaging. One of the latest is molecular imaging. This is the noninvasive visualization of normal and abnormal cellular processes at a molecular level for specific disease processes in living animals and humans. The expansion in the field of interventional radiology will continue as computers offer new approaches to medical diagnosis and treatment.

ABBREVIATIONS

These abbreviations are commonly used in reference to radiology or nuclear medicine diagnostic or treatment procedures.

See Appendix C for additional abbreviations.

AP	anteroposterior
AV	atrioventricular node
Ba	barium
BBB	blood-brain barrier
BE	barium enema
CAT	computerized axial tomography, computer-assisted tomography
C-spine	cervical spine film
cGy	centigray
CT	computer tomography
DSA	digital subtraction angiography
DVI	digital vascular imaging
ERCP	endoscopic retrograde cholangiopancreatography
^{67}Ga	radioactive isotope of gallium*
^{123}I	radioactive isotope of iodine*
IVC	inferior vena cavae
IVP	intravenous pyelogram
KUB	kidney, ureter, bladder
MRI	magnetic resonance imaging
MUGA	multiple gated acquisition
NMR	nuclear magnetic resonance
NPO	nothing by mouth
PA	posteroanterior
PET	positron emission tomography
PICC	peripherally inserted central venous catheter
PTC	percutaneous transhepatic cholangiography
rad	radiation absorbed dose
RAI	radioimmunoassay
RFA	radiofrequency ablation
SBS	small bowel series
SPECT	single-photon emission computed tomography

^{99m}Tc	radioactive isotope of technetium*
^{201}Th	radioactive isotope of thallium*
TIPS	transjugular intrahepatic portosystemic shunt
UGI	upper gastrointestinal (series)
US, U/S	ultrasound

INTERNET ASSIGNMENT

Radiology Info (**www.radiologyinfo.org**) is the public information web site sponsored by the American College of Radiology (ACR) and Radiological Society of North America (RSNA). The site was established to inform and educate the public about radiologic procedures and the role of radiologists in health care. Each section of the site has been created with the guidance of a physician with expertise in the topic presented. All information contained in the web site is further reviewed by an ACR-RSNA committee comprised of physicians with expertise in several radiologic areas. Radiology Info is updated frequently and expanded to include new information as it occurs. The major sections of this web site are Diagnostic Radiology, Interventional Radiology, Radiation Therapy, and Radiation Safety. A glossary of terms and information about professions in radiation and about the RSNA and ACR are also included.

ACTIVITY

Access Radiology Info at **www.radiologyinfo.org**. Click on Diagnostic Radiology and a list of body systems and patient groups is displayed. Click on Abdomen and a new screen appears with specific procedures listed. Select CT–Abdomen. Scroll through the questions to What are some common uses of the procedure? Summarize the information you have found.

Go back to the top of the page and select Interventional Radiology from the list at the left. Heart and Vascular Procedures appears. Select Angioplasty & Vascular Stenting. Scroll through the questions until you get to What Are the Limitations of Angioplasty and Vascular Stenting? Summarize the information for this topic.

Next, go back to the top of the page again and select Glossary of Terms from the list at the left. Access to the glossary is through an A–Z index. Select a term from the words introduced in Chapter 11 of the text, click on the appropriate letter, and determine whether the web site provides additional information on the word. Summarize what you have found.

Submit all the information you have gathered to your instructor.

*Isotopes of chemical elements may be expressed in either of these formats: ^{201}Th or thallium-201.

Review *Radiology and Nuclear Medicine*

- The discoveries of Röntgen, Curie, and Becquerel at the turn of the twentieth century opened a new field of medicine that uses rays for diagnosis and treatment of a variety of medical conditions.
- Diagnostic techniques include x-ray images, fluoroscopic examination, computerized axial tomography, ultrasound, tomography, stereoscopy, and magnetic resonance imaging.
- Contrasts, usually barium or iodine, are used to enhance the images obtained in various radiological or nuclear medicine tests.
- Nuclear medicine utilizes radionuclides in two types of diagnostic tests: in vitro and in vivo.
- Interventional radiology allows physicians to diagnose and correct certain medical problems without high-risk invasive diagnostic procedures or surgery.

Key Terminology Review

Word	Definition
anteroposterior projection (AP)	x-ray position where the beam passes from front to back
barium sulfate	used as an opaque contrast medium in an x-ray of the digestive tract
computerized axial tomography (CAT), computed tomography (CT), computer-assisted tomography (CAT)	procedure that uses highly focused x-ray beams to generate a series of cross-sectional two-dimensional scans that are analyzed by a computer to generate a three-dimensional image
echocardiography	method of using ultrasound to examine the heart
echogram	record of an ultrasound scanning procedure
fluoroscopic examination	procedure that allows a radiologist to view body organs in motion
gamma rays	powerful photon rays given off by a radioactive substance
half-life	time required for a substance to lose half its radioactivity
in vitro	term referring to testing in a glass unit, such as a test tube, or other artificial environment
in vivo	term referring to testing within a living body
interventional radiology	use of minimally invasive fluoroscopy, CT, ultrasound and MRI to guide procedures such as tissue biopsies, fluid draining, catheter insertion, and narrowed duct or vessel repair by dilation or stenting

continues

Word	Definition
iodinated substances	water-soluble, iodinated contrast media
lateral projection	x-ray position where the beam passes from one side of the body to the other
magnetic resonance imaging (MRI)	use of magnetism to create images on a computer screen or tape to distinguish between normal and abnormal tissue changes within the area visualized
nuclear medicine	use of radioactive substances in the diagnosis and treatment of disease
nuclear physician	radiologist who uses diagnostic nuclear medicine procedures
oblique projection	x-ray position where the beam passes at an angle that is not PA, AP, or lateral
positron emission tomography (PET)	procedure that registers glucose metabolism in a cross section of the brain
posteroanterior projection (PA)	x-ray position where the beam passes from back to front
radiograph	film on which an image of a body part is produced through exposure to x-rays
radiographic contrast media	radiopaque or radiolucent substances used to differentiate organs under study from the surrounding tissue
radiologist	physician who specializes in the practice of diagnostic radiology
radiolucent	permitting the passage of x-rays
radionuclide	radiopharmaceutical substance that gives off high-energy particles as it disintegrates
radiopaque	not permitting the passage of x-rays
radiopharmaceutical (labeled compound)	combination of a radionuclide (radioisotope) with a chemical substance, which is used for diagnostic or therapeutic purposes
radiotherapist	specialist trained in radiotherapy
roentgen rays	x-rays; types of radiation
scan	image produced by a scanning procedure
scanning	process of making an image
scintiphotography	process of producing an image that depicts the distribution and intensity of the radionuclide in the organ or area under study
scintiscan, photoscan	image that depicts the distribution and intensity of a radionuclide
single-photon emission computed tomography (SPECT)	technique that uses an intravenous injection of a radioactive tracer and a computer to construct a three-dimensional image of a certain area of the body
sonogram	record of an ultrasound scanning procedure
tomogram	picture produced by tomography
tomography	procedure permitting visualization of x-ray slices at different depths of focus
transducer	device which converts energy from one form into another
ultrasound	use of reflected sound waves at ultrasonic levels to record images of specific body parts
uptake	rate at which a tissue or an organ absorbs a radiopharmaceutical

Key Terminology Practice Exercises

COMPLETION

Complete each of the following statements.

1. The first type of radiation identified was ________________________.
2. Curie discovered three kinds of rays; they are ________________________, ________________________, and ________________________.
3. Radioactive materials emit ________________________ rays.
4. Radiation produces images by three methods; they are ________________________, ________________________, and ________________________.
5. Nuclear medicine tests done within a living body are called ________________________.
6. A diagnostic procedure that permits visualization of a specific layer of the body while blocking out layers in front and behind is ________________________.
7. A contrast medium used in a GI series is ________________________.
8. A ________________________ is a specific radionuclide combined with a chemical substance that gives off radioactivity.
9. An instrument that introduces ultrasonic beams into the body is a ________________________.
10. A radioactive isotope introduced into the body to mark a specific molecule is a ________________________.

SHORT ANSWER

Supply a short answer to each of the following.

1. What is the difference between a radiograph and fluoroscopic examination?

____

____

____

2. What does the word *scan* mean?

____

____

____

3. Explain how interventional radiology assists with organ biopsies.

____

____

____

4. Explain the difference between radiolucent and radiopaque.

____

____

____

CIRCLE

Circle the correct answer in each statement.

1. (Lateral, oblique) is the projection obtained when a beam passes from one side of the body to another.
2. (Posteroanterior, lateral) is the projection obtained when the rays pass from back to front of the body part.

3. (Lateral, oblique) is the projection when the tube is not positioned at a perpendicular angle to the body.
4. (Anteroposterior, posteroanterior) is the projection obtained when rays pass from the front of the body to the back.

MATCHING

Match the terms to their meanings.

1. _________ rate at which a tissue or an organ absorbs a radiopharmaceutical
2. _________ time required for a substance to lose half of its radioactivity
3. _________ an imaging technique using the computer to provide a three-dimensional cross-sectional view of tissues
4. _________ permitting the passage of x-rays.
5. _________ term referring to testing in an artificial environment
6. _________ use of sound to obtain an image of a part of the body
7. _________ use of radioactive materials in the diagnosis and treatment of disease
8. _________ reduces deposits of fat, cholesterol, and lipids in arteries
9. _________ uses injection of radioactive tracer and computer to construct three-dimensional images
10. _________ procedure to repair a compression fracture

a. angioplasty
b. computerized axial tomography
c. half-life
d. in vitro
e. nuclear medicine
f. radiolucent
g. SPECT
h. ultrasound
i. uptake
j. vertebroplasty

ABBREVIATIONS

Give the abbreviation for each of the following.

1. barium ______________________
2. anteroposterior ______________________
3. computerized axial tomography ______________________
4. radioactive iodine ______________________
5. intravenous pyelogram ______________________
6. posteroanterior ______________________
7. magnetic resonance imaging ______________________
8. positron emission tomography ______________________
9. radiofrequency ablation ______________________
10. atrioventricular node ______________________

DEFINITIONS

Define the following procedures.

1. MUGA scan ______________________
2. echocardiography ______________________
3. chemoembolization ______________________
4. radioactive iodine uptake study ______________________
5. molecular imaging ______________________
6. angiography ______________________

Word Element Review

Root	Meaning	Example	Definition
fluor/o	luminous	**fluorescence** (floo"ō-rĕs'ĕnts)	property of emitting light while exposed to light; usually ultraviolet
is/o	same, equal	**isodose** (ī'sō-dōs')	radiation dose of equal intensity to more than one body area
radi/o	ray	**radiogram** (rā'dē-ō-grăm")	film produced of an x-ray picture
		radioisotopes (rā"dē-ō-ī'sō-tōps)	radioactive forms of elements
strict/o	drawing tight, narrowing	**stricture** (strĭk'chur)	abnormal narrowing of a duct or passage
tom/o	cut	**tomography** (tō-mŏg'ră-fē)	any x-ray method that produces images by focusing on a single tissue plane
vitr/o	glass	**vitreous** (vĭt'rē-ŭs)	glassy
viv/o	life	**vividialysis** (vĭv"ĭ-dī-ăl'ĭ-sĭs)	dialysis through a living membrane

Prefix	Meaning	Example	Definition
ab-	away from, not	**abnormality** (ăb"nor-măl'ĭ-tē)	deviation from normal
ante-	before	**anterior** (ăn-tēr'ē-or)	situated in the front
en-	in, within	**encapsulated** (ĕn-kăp'sū-lāt-ĕd)	enclosed in a capsule
post-	after, behind	**posterior** (pŏs-tēr'ē-or)	situated in the back
pre-	before, in front of	**precancerous** (prē-kăn'ser-ăs)	pathological condition that tends to become malignant
sym-, syn-	together, with	**symphysis** (sĭm'fĭ-sĭs)	line of union between two bones
		syndrome (sĭn'drōm)	group of symptoms and signs that collectively characterize a particular disease or abnormal condition
tele-	distant	**teleradiography** (tĕl"ĕ-rā"dē-ŏg'rah-fē)	treatment with the radiation source about two meters from the body

Suffix	Meaning	Example	Definition
-desis	binding, fixation	**syndesis** (sĭn'dē-sĭs)	condition of being bound together
-ectasis	expansion, dilation, stretching	**atelectasis** (ăt"ĕ-lĕk'tah-sĭs)	collapse or incomplete expansion of the lung

continues

Suffix	Meaning	Example	Definition
-gram	record, tracing, picture	**venogram** (vē'nō-grăm)	x-ray of a vein
-graphy	process of recording	**radiography** (rā"dē-ŏg'ră-fē)	making of film records of the internal structure of the body by exposure of x-ray-sensitive film
-lucent	shine	**translucent** (trăns-lū'sĕnt)	allows partial penetration by light rays
-opaque	obscure	**opacity** (ō-păs'ĭ-tē)	condition of being opaque; shadiness
-plasia	developmental	**dysplasia** (dĭs-plā'sē-ah)	abnormal growth of tissue development
		hyperplasia (hī"per-plā'zē-ah)	excessive increase in tissue growth

Word Element Practice Exercises

MATCHING

Match the terms to their meanings.

1. __________ at the back
2. __________ deviation from normal
3. __________ collective symptoms characterizing a disease or abnormal condition
4. __________ equal measure of radiation to more than one body part
5. __________ x-ray of a vein
6. __________ line of union between two bones
7. __________ making a record of the internal structure of the body by exposure of x-ray-sensitive film
8. __________ collapse of lungs
9. __________ enclosed in a capsule
10. __________ produces images by focusing on a single tissue plane
11. __________ excessive increase in tissue growth
12. __________ situated in front
13. __________ glassy
14. __________ radioactive forms of elements
15. __________ abnormal narrowing of a duct or passage

a. abnormality
b. anterior
c. atelectasis
d. dysplasia
e. encapsulated
f. fluorescence
g. hyperplasia
h. isodose
i. opacity
j. posterior
k. precancerous
l. radiogram
m. radiography
n. radioisotopes
o. stricture
p. symphysis

16. __________ allows partial penetration by light rays
17. __________ shadiness
18. __________ film produced for an x-ray picture
19. __________ dialysis through a living membrane
20. __________ property of emitting light while exposed to light
21. __________ bound together
22. __________ abnormal changes in the nature of tissue
23. __________ growth not yet malignant but known to become so if left unattended
24. __________ treatment in which the source of the therapeutic agent is at a distance from the body

q. syndesis
r. syndrome
s. teleradiography
t. tomography
u. translucent
v. venogram
w. vitreous
x. vividialysis

COMPLETION

Provide the correct root, prefix, or suffix.

1. glassy ____________________ eous
2. radioactive forms of elements ____________________ isotopes
3. property of emitting light while exposed to light ____________________ escence
4. abnormal narrowing of a duct or passage ____________________ ure
5. group of symptoms and signs that characterize a disease/condition ____________________ drome
6. condition of being bound together syn ____________________
7. allows partial penetration by light rays trans ____________________
8. abnormal growth in development of tissue dys ____________________
9. x-ray of a vein veno ____________________
10. situated in the back ____________________ erior

WORD ELEMENT MEANINGS

Give the meaning of each word element. Then use your dictionary to find a new word that contains each of the word elements. Specify whether the new word is a noun or an adjective by placing N or A in the last column.

Word Element	Meaning	Word	N or A
1. ab-			
2. ante-			
3. -desis			
4. -ectasis			
5. en-			
6. fluor/o			
7. -gram			
8. -graphy			
9. is/o			
10. -lucent			
11. -opaque			

12. -plasia			
13. post-			
14. pre-			
15. radi/o			
16. strict/o			
17. sym-, syn-			
18. tele-			
19. tom/o			
20. vitr/o			
21. viv/o			

Dictionary Exercises

DICTIONARY EXERCISE 1

Use your dictionary to find the pronunciation and definition of the following words.

Word	Pronunciation	Definition
1. acoustic impedance		
2. erg		
3. proton		
4. quantum number		
5. rad		
6. radon		
7. rectilinear		
8. tagging		
9. atomic weight		
10. isotope		
11. cassette		
12. tracer studies		
13. Doppler effect		
14. ionization		
15. irradiation		

DICTIONARY EXERCISE 2

Use your dictionary to find the meaning and pronunciation (where indicated) of each term. Then write a sentence that identifies the meaning in your own words.

1. blood-brain barrier (BBB)

   ____

2. radioactive contamination

   ____

3. Geiger counter (______________________)
____

4. lymphangiography (______________________)
____

5. mammography (______________________)
____

6. planigram (______________________)
____

7. radiation sickness
____

8. spot film
____

9. stopcock
____

10. urography (______________________)
____

11. venogram (______________________)
____

12. lethal
____

13. hyperosmolarity (______________________)
____

DICTIONARY EXERCISE 3

Pronunciation of the words below is provided. Using your dictionary, find the correct spelling and definition of each word.

	Word	Pronunciation	Definition
1.	______________	ah-tĕn"ū-ā'shŭn	______________
2.	______________	kal"ĭ-brā'shŭn	______________
3.	______________	ĭ-rā"dē-ā'shŭn	______________
4.	______________	fō'tŏn	______________
5.	______________	sĭn"tĭ-lā'shŭn	______________
6.	______________	dō-sĭm'ē-ter	______________
7.	______________	rĕnt-gĕn'ō-grăm"	______________
8.	______________	kō'bawlt therapy	______________
9.	______________	ăb-sŏrp'shŭn	______________
10.	______________	ăr-tē'rē-ō-grăm"	______________
11.	______________	nu'klē-on	______________
12.	______________	ŏr"thō-vŏl'tĭj mah-chēn'	______________
13.	______________	tăg'ing	______________
14.	______________	mī"ē-lō-sŭ-prĕsh'ŭn	______________
15.	______________	rā"dē-ō-thĕr'ă-pē	______________

DICTIONARY EXERCISE 4

Match the terms to their meanings.

1. ____________ a decrease in the number of radioactive atoms in a radioactive substance over time
2. ____________ smallest particle of an element capable of entering into a chemical reaction
3. ____________ encounter between two subatomic particles that changes the existing momentum and energy conditions
4. ____________ a device by which radiant energy can be evaluated
5. ____________ specific amount of roentgen rays or other radiation administered
6. ____________ determining the amount of ionizing radiation in an area or a substance
7. ____________ atom having either a positive or negative charge as a result of having lost or gained an electron
8. ____________ changes of direction that subatomic particles or photons undergo as a result of collision or interaction with matter
9. ____________ measurement of the ability of the thyroid gland to trap and retain the isotope following the oral ingestion of a tracer dose of radioactive iodine
10. ____________ method of introducing a catheter into a vein or an artery
11. ____________ a preliminary film taken to check technique, positioning, and patient preparation, as well as to determine what diseases are considered as diagnostic possibilities
12. ____________ any protective device used to prevent or reduce the passage of particles of radiation
13. ____________ production of an image or picture
14. ____________ name for the process of tagging radionuclides and following them through the body
15. ____________ number of protons in the nucleus of an atom
16. ____________ cyclic accelerator that produces high energy electrons for radiotherapy treatments
17. ____________ turning outward or inside out
18. ____________ radiotherapy in which needles and wires containing radioactive material are implanted directly into tumor area
19. ____________ turning inward
20. ____________ generation of voltage across a solid when a mechanical stress is applied

a. atom
b. atomic number
c. betatron
d. collision
e. dose
f. eversion
g. imaging
h. interstitial
i. inversion
j. ion
k. monitoring
l. piezoelectric
m. radioactive decay
n. radiation detector
o. radioactive iodine uptake determination
p. scattering
q. scout film
r. Seldinger technique
s. shield
t. tracer studies

StudyWARE™ Connection

To take a practice quiz or play interactive games that reinforce the content in this chapter, go to your StudyWARE™ CD-ROM.

Listening Exercises

INSTRUCTIONS

1. Review the spelling, pronunciation, and meaning of the words provided in the preview.
2. Go to your StudyWARE™ CD-ROM and listen to **Listening Exercises 11-1, 11-2, and 11-3**. Fill in the blank in the report as the word is dictated.
3. At the end of each activity, check your spelling against the preview words. They appear in the preview in the order in which they are encountered in the activity.
4. Review and practice the words you missed.
5. Look up words that are not familiar.

PREVIEW OF WORDS FOR LISTENING EXERCISES 11-1, 11-2, 11-3

Word	Pronunciation	Meaning
Exercise 11-1, Dx Chest, Two View		
pneumothorax	nū-mō-thō'raks	presence of air in the pleural space outside the lung, but inside the chest
infiltrate	ĭn-fĭl'trāt	an abnormal substance that accumulates gradually in cells or tissues
vasculature	văs'kū-lă-tūr"	the vascular system of the body or any part of it
Exercise 11-2, CT Pelvis, Without		
lobulated	lŏb'ū-lāt-ĕd	made up of lobules or small segments
ileostomy	ĭl"ē-ŏs'tō-mē	surgical creation of an opening into the ileum with a stoma on the abdominal wall
lymphadenopathy	lĭm-făd"ē-nŏp'ă-thē	disease of the lymph nodes
Exercise 11-3, Gallbladder Sonogram		
edema	ĕ-dē'mă	abnormal accumulation of fluid in the body
common bile duct		union of the hepatic and cystic duct, which leads to the duodenum

StudyWARE™ Connection

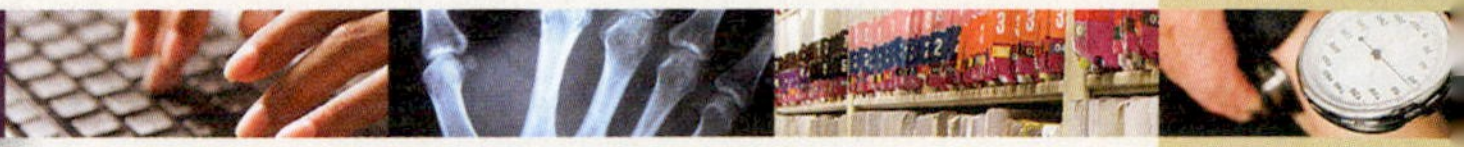

Listen to the reports on the next page being read on your StudyWARE™ CD-ROM. Fill in each blank as the word is dictated.

DX Chest, Two View

Clinical Data: PA/LAT CXR

Comparison is made to a study dated 8/3/20—. A central venous catheter is present with the tip in the distal superior vena cava. No ________________ is seen. The heart is normal in size. The lungs are free of ________________ with normal pulmonary ________________. Degenerative changes are seen in the thoracic spine.

IMPRESSION:

1. No change when compared to the study of 8/3/20—.
   No acute process is seen.

CT Pelvis, Without

Clinical Data: CT PELVIS WITHOUT CONTRAST

CT SCAN OF THE PELVIS WITHOUT INTRAVENOUS CONTRAST, 12/21/20—

INDICATIONS:

Rule out pelvic mass/fluid collection

DISCUSSION:

Comparison is with a study dated 12/11/20—. The patient was returned for additional imaging following infusion of contrast material into the bladder and into the rectum. Axial images were obtained prior to infusion of contrast material. Images were obtained following infusion of contrast material into the bladder. Finally, images were obtained following infusion of contrast material into the bladder and into the rectum.

The bladder is well opacified. The bladder is somewhat floppy and ______________. The areas previously questioned for the most part do opacify with rectal contrast. There is what appears to be unopacified loops of bowel just below the level of the ____________________. As they do not fill from below, they are probably jejunum and ileum. No definite fluid collections are identified. No _________________ is identified.

IMPRESSION:

1. While some unopacified loops of bowel are seen in the pelvis, specifically left side, no definite fluid collections or masses are identified to suggest an abscess.
2. Gallstones are noted incidentally.

Gallbladder Sonogram

ULTRASOUND OF THE GALLBLADDER:

There are no stones seen in the gallbladder. There is no ______________________or thickening of the wall. The ____________ is not dilated. Head and body of the pancreas appear normal.

IMPRESSION: 1. A normal study.

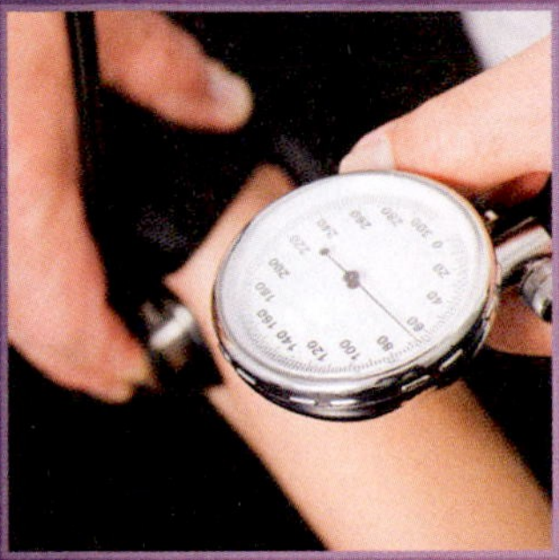
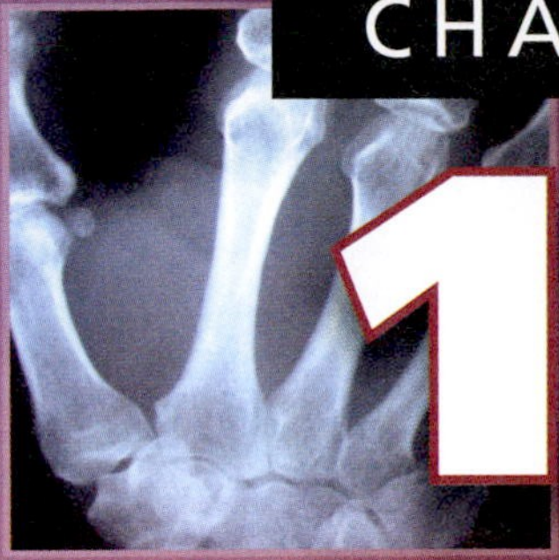

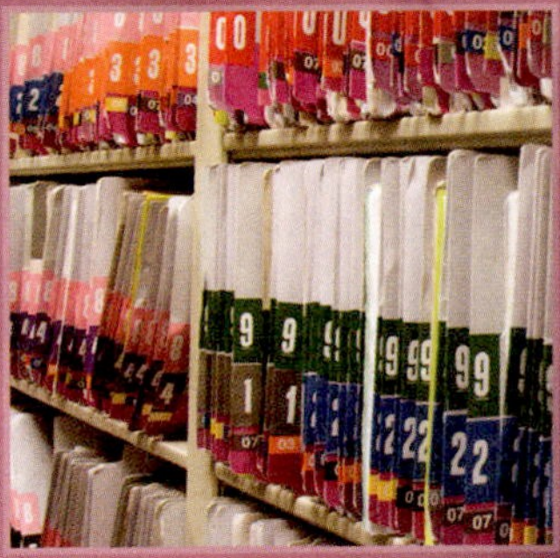

CHAPTER

12

The Respiratory System

"Some folk seem glad even to draw their breath."

—William Morris

OBJECTIVES

When you have completed this chapter on the respiratory system, you should be able to

1. Spell and define major system components and explain how they operate.
2. Identify the meanings of related word elements.
3. Spell and define diagnostic procedures, diagnoses, treatment procedures, and abbreviations.
4. Spell the names of commonly used medications.
5. Use a dictionary as a tool in processing medical documents.
6. Hear how medical terminology is used in actual medical reports.

INTRODUCTION

The respiratory system allows the blood to exchange oxygen and carbon dioxide. This gaseous exchange is known as respiration and is essential for life. Interruption of this cycle for more than a few minutes can cause brain damage or death. Physicians who specialize in the diagnosis and medical treatment of pulmonary or respiratory diseases are pulmonary disease or chest specialists. Surgeons who specialize in the surgical treatment of chest diseases are called chest or thoracic surgeons.

COMPOSITION OF THE RESPIRATORY SYSTEM

pector/o	chest	-thorax	chest
thorac/o	chest		

The principal organs of the respiratory system discussed in this chapter are the nose, pharynx, larynx, trachea, bronchi, alveoli, and lungs.

NOSE

nas/o nose	rhin/o nose

Figure 12-1 illustrates how air enters our nostrils and passes through two **nasal cavities** (2) that are separated by a partition called the **septum**. The septum and walls of the nasal cavity are constructed of cartilage covered with mucous membrane. There are numerous hairs in the nostrils that serve to filter out larger dirt particles as air passes through them. Smaller particles are caught by the mucus secreted by the mucous membranes.

Besides being filtered, inhaled air is conditioned as it moves through the nasal cavities. The airflow is warmed by capillaries in the mucous membrane lining to bring it closer to body temperature, and moisture is added from the membrane secretions.

The nasal cavity itself is separated from the mouth by a partition called the **palate** (păl'ăt) (3). Also within the facial bones are several mucous-membrane-lined, air-filled pockets called **sinuses** (1), which produce the mucus fluids.

PHARYNX

pharyng/o	pharynx, throat

The **pharynx** (far'inks) (13), which is called the throat, is used by both the digestive and respiratory systems. In the respiratory system, the pharynx allows air to pass from the nasal cavity and mouth into the larynx.

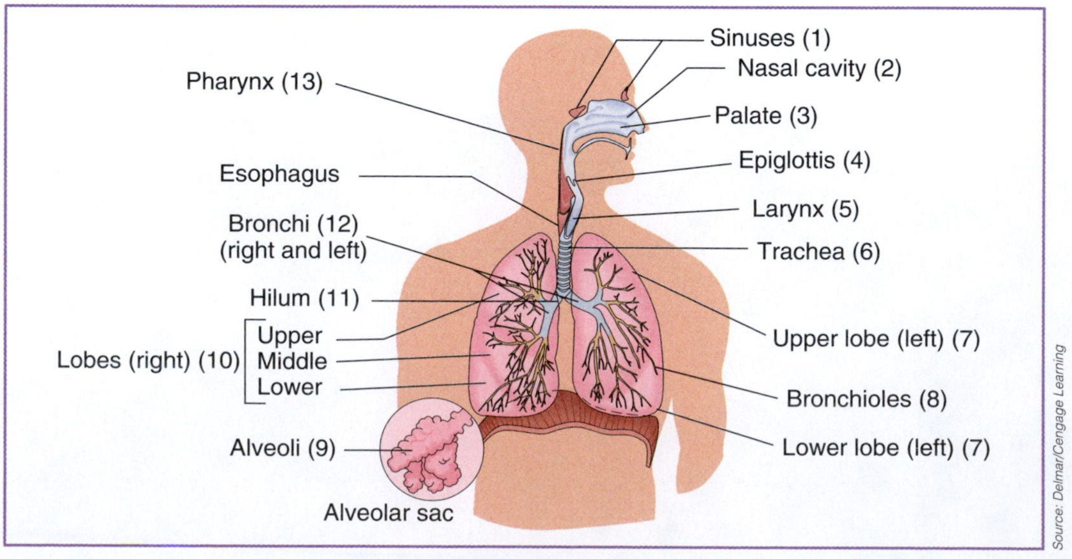

FIGURE 12-1
Respiratory System

LARYNX

epiglott/o	epiglottis	laryng/o	larynx

The **larynx** (lăr'ĭnks) (5), or voice box, is located between the pharynx and the windpipe. The two vocal cords and the opening between them is called the **glottis** (glŏt'ĭs), and the little leaflike structure that closes this opening during swallowing is called the **epiglottis** (ĕp"ĭ-glŏt'ĭs) (4). This way food is kept out of the respiratory tract.

TRACHEA

trache/o	neck

The **trachea** (trā'kē-ah) (6), or windpipe, is a tube that extends from the lower edge of the larynx to the level of the seventh thoracic vertebra. The trachea lies on the anterior (front) surface of the esophagus. The airway passage is kept open by a series of cartilage rings. Its purpose is to conduct air to and from the lungs by way of the bronchi.

BRONCHI AND ALVEOLI

alveol/o	alveolus, air sac	bronchiol/o	bronchiole
bronchi/o, bronch/o	bronchus		

At its lower end the trachea divides into the left and right **bronchi** (brŏng'kī) (12). These bronchi are separated by a tracheal ridge or structure called the **carina** (kah-rī'nah). One bronchus extends to each lung. The notch in the lung that allows the entry of the bronchus and pulmonary vessels is called the **hilum** (hī'lŭm) (11). Within the lung, the bronchus immediately subdivides into branches. These branches are referred to as the **bronchial** (brŏng'kē-ăl) **tree**. Each bronchial tree subdivides again and again into progressively smaller units. The smallest are called **bronchioles** (brŏng'kē-ōls) (8). At the end of the bronchial tree there is a whole cluster of air sacs known as **alveoli** (ăl-vē'ō -lī) (9). An alveolus (singular) is surrounded by networks of capillaries, through whose walls an exchange of carbon dioxide and oxygen takes place. There are an estimated 700,000 alveoli (see Figure 12-2).

LUNGS

lob/o	lobe	pneum/o, pneumon/o	lung, air
pleur/o	pleura, rib, side	pulmon/o	lung

The **lungs** are the organs in which respiration takes place. Blood and air meet at the point where the extremely thin and delicate alveoli and capillary walls adjoin. The lungs are encased in a double-folded membrane called the **pleura** (ploor'ah), which is divided into the **visceral** (vĭs'er-ăl) and **parietal** (pah-rī'ĕ-tăl) layers. The visceral pleura adheres to the lung, and the parietal pleura lines the wall of the chest cavity. Each lung occupies its own half of the thoracic cavity. The right lung (1) has three divisions called **lobes**—upper, middle, and lower—and is larger than the left lung (2) which has only two lobes. (See Figure 12-3 for a more detailed view of the interior of a lobule.)

StudyWARE™ Connection

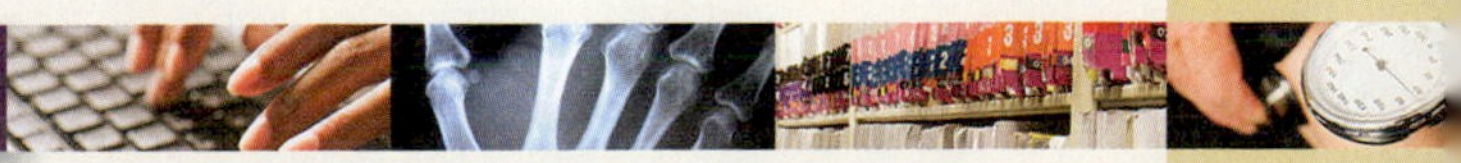

Play an interactive game labeling structures of the **Respiratory System** on your StudyWARE™ CD-ROM.

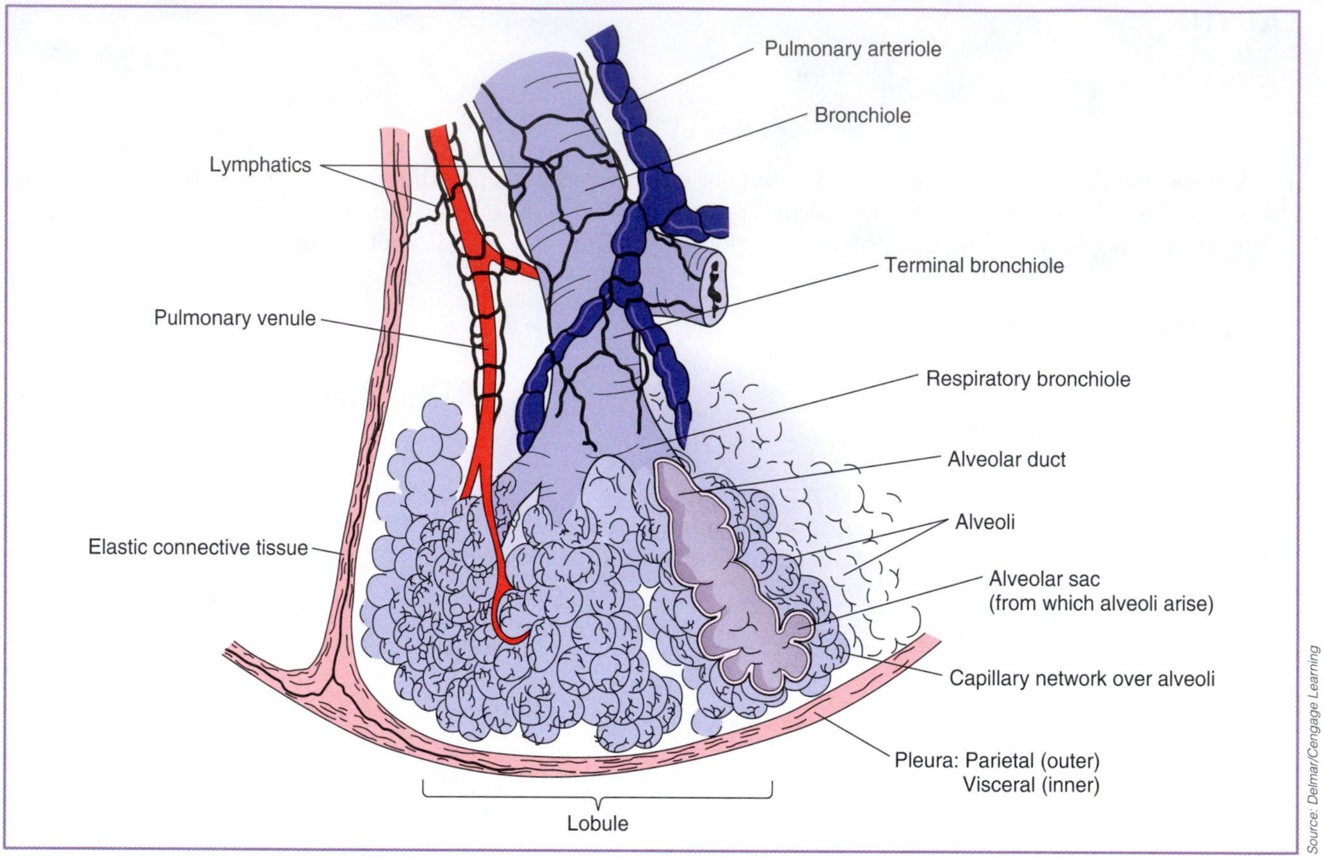

FIGURE 12-2 Anatomy of a Lobule of a Lung

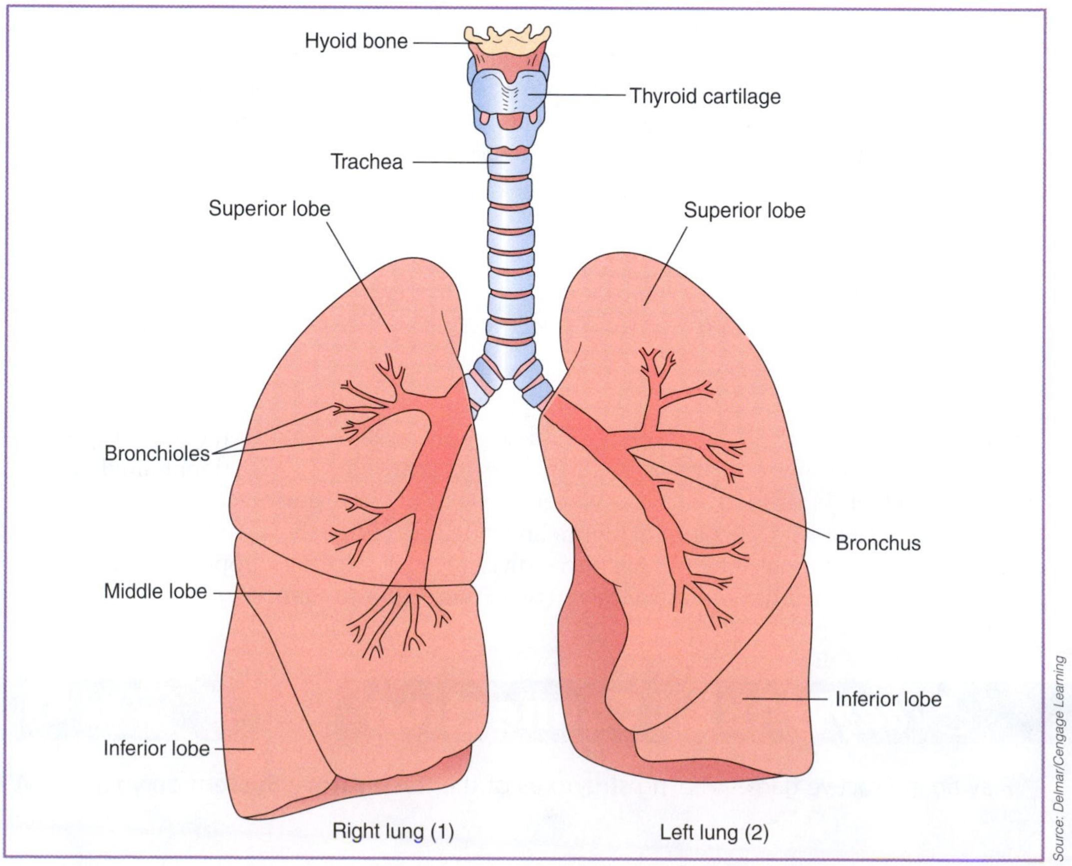

FIGURE 12-3 The Branching Bronchi and the Lobes of the Lungs

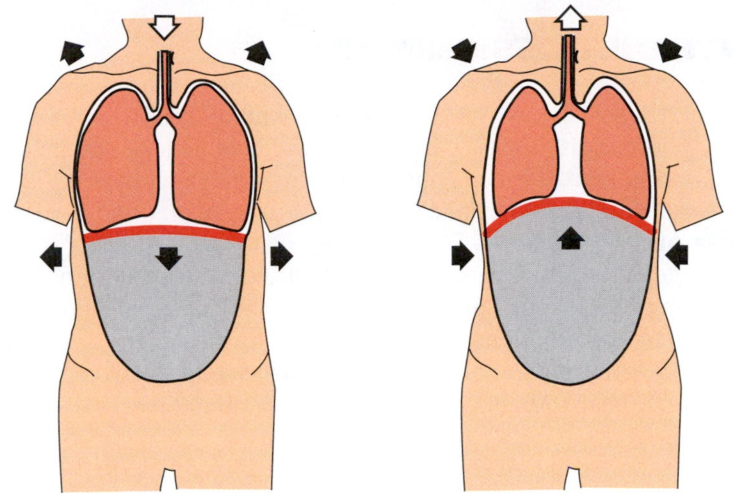

FIGURE 12-4
The Diaphragm in (A) Inspiration and (B) Expirartion

HOW RESPIRATION WORKS

aer/o	air	-pnea	to breathe, breathing
phren/o	diaphragm	spir/o	to breathe

The lungs are separated from the abdominal cavity by a muscular partition known as the **diaphragm** (dī'ah-frăm), which is the chief muscle of respiration. There are three cycles in respiration. **Inspiration** is the breathing of air into the lungs, as demonstrated in Figure 12-4A. Figure 12-4B shows **expiration**, or the exhalation of air from the lungs. **Rest** is the interval between expiration and inspiration.

As we breathe, the diaphragm moves down and then up to induce air movement. This is how it works. When the diaphragm contracts and descends, the ribs elevate. The result is a negative thoracic pressure causing air to be drawn into the lungs to equalize the pressure. The diaphragm then relaxes and is drawn upward. This increases the pressure in the thoracic cavity and forces air to be expelled from the lungs. The respiratory center in the brain controls the rhythmic movements produced by respiration.

Respiration involves the exchange of oxygen and carbon dioxide in the lungs. The amount of oxygen retained by the tissues and cells is dependent on several factors, including the needs of the tissues and cells, as well as the age, health, and activity level of the individual.

There are several terms used to indicate lung capacity and airflow rate. **Tidal volume** is the amount of air breathed in and out during quiet or unlabored respiration. **Total lung capacity** is the total volume of air in the lungs at the end of maximum inspiration. **Residual volume** is the amount of air remaining in the lung after a forced expiration. Other terms mentioned frequently in reference to volume studies are *expiratory reserve volume* and *inspiratory reserve volume.*

StudyWARE™ Connection

View an animation on **Respiration** on your StudyWARE™ CD-ROM.

INTERNET ASSIGNMENT

The American Lung Association (ALA), the oldest voluntary health organization in the United States, was founded in 1904 to fight tuberculosis. Today the ALA has widened its scope to include lung disease in all its forms, with special emphasis on asthma, tobacco control, and environmental health. ALA is funded by contributions from the public along with gifts and grants from corporations, foundations, and government agencies. Its web site is located at **www.lungusa.org**.

The homepage of the site shows its comprehensive nature. Click on the Lungs button at the top of the homepage. Align the cursor with Your Lungs at the top of the home page and several choices appear in a drop down menu. Select any one of the options to find out more about how the lungs work. The Human Respiratory System provides a helpful illustration and explanation of the system. Images of Lungs provides pictures of normal and abnormal lung tissue. Learn About Your Respiratory System takes you through an animated presentation about respiratory functions.

Return to the home page. At the top of the home page, click on the button labeled Diseases A to Z. Clicking here takes you to an index site that lists respiratory diseases. Specific information on a disease is obtained by clicking on the disease name.

ACTIVITY

Visit the American Lung Association web site at **www.lungusa.org**. Find and read the explanation of how the human respiratory system works. In a short report summarize any new information you found.

Access Images of Lungs and report on the illustrations included.

Access Diseases A to Z and select one of the diagnoses listed in Chapter 12. Click the first letter of that diagnosis and then select the diagnosis from the list. Summarize new information the description provides.

Submit all of your reports to your instructor.

Review *The Respiratory System*

- Respiration provides the oxygen that is essential to life.
- The components of the respiratory system assist in the exchange of oxygen and carbon dioxide through the walls of capillaries in the lungs.
- The nose, pharynx, larynx, and trachea carry inhaled (or inspired) air through the bronchi into the lungs.
- The chief muscle of respiration is the diaphragm, which descends during inspiration and ascends during expiration.

Key Terminology Review

Word	Definition
alveoli	clusters of air sacs at the end of the bronchial tree
bronchi	main branches leading from the trachea to the lungs for air movement
bronchial tree	branches of the bronchus after entering the respective lung
bronchioles	smallest divisions of the bronchial tree
carina	ridge at the lower end of the trachea, separating the two bronchi
diaphragm	chief muscle of respiration
epiglottis	leaflike structure that opens and closes over the glottis during swallowing
expiration	breathing of air out of the lungs
glottis	the two vocal cords and the opening between them
hilum	notch in the lung where the bronchi and pulmonary vessels enter
inspiration	breathing of air into the lungs
larynx	voice box
lobes	major divisions of the lungs; the right lung has three lobes and the left lung has two
lungs	organs in which respiration takes place
nasal cavities	two cavities—separated by the nasal septum—through which air passes
palate	partition separating the mouth from the nasal cavity
parietal pleura	membrane that lines the chest cavity on the inside of the ribcage
pharynx	airway between the nasal cavity and the mouth and larynx; throat
pleura	double-folded membrane that encases the lungs and lines the chest cavity
residual volume	amount of air remaining in the lung after a forced expiration
rest	interval between expiration and inspiration
septum	partition that separates the nasal cavities
sinuses	pockets in the facial bones
tidal volume	amount of air breathed in and out during quiet or unlabored respiration
total lung capacity	total volume of air in the lungs at the end of maximum inspiration
trachea	tube that extends from the lower edge of the voice box to the level of the seventh thoracic vertebra; windpipe
visceral pleura	membrane that adheres to the lungs

Key Terminology Practice Exercises

SELECTION

Select the correct word from the list below to complete each of the following statements.

alveoli	bronchi	bronchioles	carina	diaphragm	epiglottis	expiration
glottis	hilum	inspiration	larynx	lobes	lungs	nasal cavities
palate	pharynx	pleura	rest	septum	trachea	

1. The partition between the two nasal cavities is called the ____________________.
2. The ____________________ separates the nasal cavity from the mouth.
3. The passageway for food, liquid, and air is the ____________________.
4. The ____________________ extends from the lower edge of the voice box and conducts air to and from the lungs.
5. The ____________________ keeps food out of the respiratory tract.
6. The trachea divides into two ____________________ and forms the carina.
7. The membrane encasing the lungs is referred to as the ____________________.
8. The chief muscle of respiration is the ____________________.
9. The notch where the bronchi and vessels enter the lung is the ____________________.
10. Air sacs at the end of the bronchial tree are called ____________________.
11. Exhalation of air out of the lungs is known as ____________________.
12. Breathing air into the lungs is known as ____________________.
13. The smallest branches of a bronchial tree are the ____________________.
14. The bronchi are separated by a structure called the ____________________.
15. Each lung is divided into two or three ____________________.
16. The space between two vocal cords is the ____________________.
17. The voice box is the ____________________.
18. Organs in which respiration takes place are called ____________________.
19. Two cavities separated by the nasal septum through which air passes are the ____________________.
20. The interval between expiration and inspiration is known as ____________________.

DEFINITIONS

Define each of the following terms.

1. tidal volume

____

2. total lung capacity

____

3. residual volume

____

4. bronchial tree

____

Word Element Review

Root	Meaning	Example	Definition
aer/o	air	**aerial** (ār'ē-ăl)	pertaining to the air
alveol/o	alveolus, air sac	**alveolocapillary** (al-vē"ah-lō-kap'ĭ-lar-ē)	pertaining to pulmonary alveoli and capillaries
bronchi/o, bronch/o	bronchus	**bronchopneumonia** (brŏng"kō-nū-mō'nē-ah)	inflammation of the lungs, beginning at the end of the bronchi
bronchiol/o	bronchiole	**bronchiolitis** (brong"kē-ō-lī'tĭs)	inflammation of the bronchioles due to a viral infection
epiglott/o	epiglottis	**epiglottidectomy** (ĕp"ĭ-glŏt"ĭ-dĕk'tō-mē)	excision of the epiglottis
laryng/o	larynx	**laryngology** (lăr"ĭn-gŏl'ō-jē)	branch of medicine dealing with the throat
		otorhinolaryngology (ō"tō-rī"nō-lăr"ĭn-gŏl'ō-jē)	study of otology, rhinology, and laryngology
lob/o	lobe	**lobar pneumonia** (lō'ber nū-mō'nē-ah	inflammation of one or more lobes of the lung
nas/o	nose	**nasopharyngitis** (nā"zō-făr"ĭn-jī'tĭs)	inflammation of the nasopharynx
pector/o	chest	**pectoralis** (pĕk"tō-rā'lĭs)	one of four muscles of the anterior upper portion of the chest
pharyng/o	pharynx, throat	**pharyngocele** (fah-rĭng'gō-sēl)	hernial protrusion of a part of the pharynx
phren/o	diaphragm	**phrenitis** (frĕ-nī'tĭs)	inflammation of the diaphragm
pleur/o	pleura, rib, side	**pleurisy** (ploor'ĭ-sē)	inflammation of the pleura
pneum/o, pneumon/o	lung, air	**pneumonia** (nū-mō'nē-ah)	disease of the lungs
pulmon/o	lung	**pulmonary** (pŭl'mō-nĕr"ē)	pertaining to the lungs
rhin/o	nose	**rhinitis** (rī-nī'tĭs)	inflammation of the nose
spir/o	to breathe, breathing	**spirometer** (spī-rŏm'ĕ-ter)	instrument for measuring the volume of air inhaled and exhaled
thorac/o	chest	**thoracic surgeon** (thō-răs'ĭk)	surgeon who specializes in chest surgery
trache/o	windpipe	**tracheostomy** (trā"kē-ŏs'tō-mē)	creation of a new opening into the trachea

Suffix	Meaning	Example	Definition
-pnea	to breathe	**dyspnea** (dĭsp'nē-ah)	labored or difficult breathing
-thorax	chest	**hemothorax** (hē"mō-thō'răks)	collection of blood in the chest

Word Element Practice Exercises

CIRCLE AND DEFINE

Circle and define the word element in the following terms.

1. dyspnea ______________________
2. phrenitis ______________________
3. bronchopneumonia ______________________
4. epiglottidectomy ______________________
5. pharyngocele ______________________
6. nasopharyngitis ______________________
7. laryngology ______________________
8. tracheostomy ______________________
9. aerial ______________________
10. pulmonary ______________________
11. hemothorax ______________________
12. spirometer ______________________
13. otorhinolaryngology ______________________
14. alveolocapillary ______________________
15. bronchiolitis ______________________
16. lobar pneumonia ______________________
17. pectoralis ______________________
18. pleurisy ______________________
19. pneumonia ______________________
20. rhinitis ______________________

IDENTIFICATION

Give the term for the following definitions.

1. inflammation of the nose ______________________
2. hernial protrusion of a part of the pharynx ______________________
3. inflammation of the diaphragm ______________________
4. pertaining to pulmonary alveoli and capillaries ______________________
5. disease of the lungs ______________________
6. inflammation of the pleura ______________________
7. one of four muscles in the upper chest ______________________
8. inflammation of one or more lobes of the lung ______________________
9. inflammation of the bronchioles due to a viral infection ______________________
10. labored or difficult breathing ______________________
11. instrument for measuring volume of air inhaled/exhaled ______________________
12. surgeon who specializes in chest surgery ______________________
13. study of otology, rhinology, and laryngology ______________________
14. excision of the epiglottis ______________________

15. creation of a new opening into the trachea ____________________
16. pertaining to the air ____________________
17. study of the throat ____________________
18. pertaining to the lungs ____________________
19. collection of blood in the chest ____________________
20. inflammation of the nasopharynx ____________________

WORD ELEMENT MEANINGS

Give the meaning of each word element. Then use your dictionary to find a new word that contains each of the word elements. Specify whether the new word is a noun or an adjective by placing N or A in the last column.

Word Element	Meaning	Word	N or A
1. aer/o			
2. alveol/o			
3. bronchi/o			
4. bronch/o			
5. bronchiol/o			
6. epiglott/o			
7. laryng/o			
8. lob/o			
9. nas/o			
10. pector/o			
11. pharyng/o			
12. phren/o			
13. pleur/o			
14. -pnea			
15. pneum/o			
16. pneumon/o			
17. pulmon/o			
18. rhin/o			
19. spir/o			
20. thorac/o			
21. -thorax			
22. trache/o			

DIAGNOSTIC PROCEDURES		
Word	**Pronunciation**	**Definition**
General		
before and after (B/A) bronchodilator (by and after BCD)	brŏng"kō-dī-lā'tor	breathing test given before and after the use of a bronchodilator that causes dilation of the bronchi to check the effect on airflow
bronchoscopy	brŏng-kŏs'kō-pē	examination that allows direct bronchi through a bronchoscope
complete spirometry	spī-rŏm'ĕ-trē	measurement of the breathing capacity of the lungs
fiberoptic bronchoscopy	fī"ber-ŏp'tĭk	procedure using flexible, light-transmitting plastic fibers to visualize the bronchi (see Figure 12-5)
flow volume study		test lungs by breathing into a tube until expiration has been completed
laryngoscopy	lăr"ĭng-gŏs'kō-pē	visual examination of the larynx with a scope
lung biopsy	bī'ŏp-sē	biopsy of tissue taken from the lung by bronchoscopy for washing, cytology, and determination of malignancy
mediastinoscopy	mē"dē-ăs"tĭ-nŏs'kō-pē	visual examination of the mediastinum with an endoscope
pleural biopsy	ploor'-ăl	biopsy of tissue from the pleura
pulmonary function test (PFT)	pŭl'mō-nĕr"ē	one of several tests used to evaluate how the patient breathes and to determine lung volumes, pulmonary gas exchange, and flow rates
thoracentesis (thoracocentesis)	thō"rah-sĕn-tē'sĭs (thō"răk-ō-sĕn-tē'sĭs)	procedure in which the chest wall is punctured with a needle to obtain fluid for diagnostic studies
thoracoscopy	thō"ră-kŏs'kō-pē	visual examination of the pleural cavity by placing an endoscope through a small incision through the chest
tuberculin skin tests	too-bĕr'kū-lĭn	application of agents to the surface of the skin (Heaf and tine tests) or by intradermal injection (Mantoux test) to detect the presence of tuberculosis infection

continues

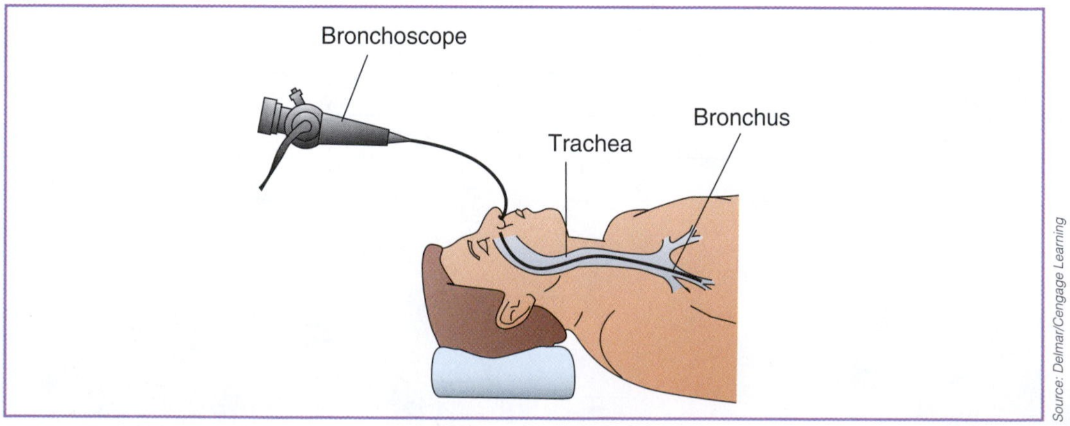

FIGURE 12-5 Fiberoptic Bronchoscopy

DIAGNOSTIC PROCEDURES		
Word	**Pronunciation**	**Definition**
Nuclear Medicine		
radioisotope perfusion and ventilation lung scan; ventilation-perfusion scan (V/Q scan)	rā"dē-ō'ī'sō-tōp pĕr-fū'zhŭn	techniques for diagnosing pulmonary embolism and demonstrating perfusion defects in normally ventilated areas of the lung
Radiology		
chest x-ray (PA/lat)		full view of the lungs and heart from the back and side
CT scan of the chest or lungs		computerized reconstruction of x-ray slices of the chest (see Figure 12-6)
MRI scan of the chest or lungs		procedure using magnetic fields to diagnose problems in the chest area (see Figure 12-7)

continues

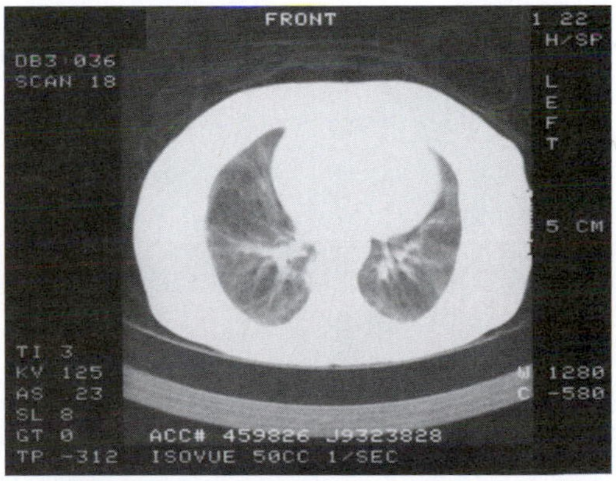

FIGURE 12-6
CT Scan of the Lungs

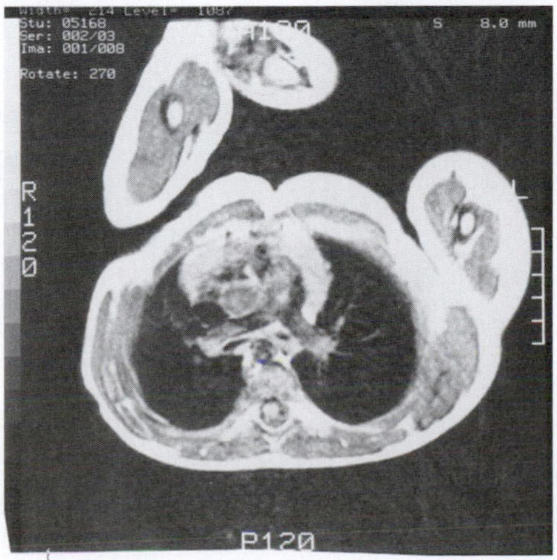

FIGURE 12-7
MRI Scan of the Lungs

DIAGNOSTIC PROCEDURES		
Word	**Pronunciation**	**Definition**
Radiology (*continued*)		
pulmonary angiography	ăn"jē-ŏg'rah-fē	x-ray technique for studying circulation in the lungs
sinus x-ray	sī'nŭs	face view of the sinus cavity
tomogram (laminogram)	tō'mō-grăm (lăm'ĭ-nō-grăm)	x-ray of a selected layer of the body made by body section roentgenography to examine lung fields
Laboratory Tests		
sputum culture and sensitivity	spū'tŭm	test requiring a patient to cough up sputum from the lungs for laboratory analysis; laboratory incubates the sputum sample to test for the presence and identification of microorganisms; if organisms are found, a determination is made about which antibiotics inhibit the growth of these organisms to aid the physician in prescribing drugs appropriately
sputum cytology	sī-tŏl'ō-jē	test for malignant cells in the sputum
Blood Tests		
arterial blood gases (ABGs)		measurements of hydrogen, carbon dioxide, pH, and oxygen pressures are obtained from a sample of arterial blood; aids in the determination of acid base balance, oxygen, and carbon dioxide level in arterial blood

DIAGNOSES		
Word	**Pronunciation**	**Definition**
Diseases of the Upper Respiratory System		
coryza	kŏ-rī'zah	common head cold; condition causing profuse discharge from nose
croup	kroop	condition seen in children and marked by obstruction, barking cough, hoarseness, and persistent stridor
diphtheria	dĭf-thē'rē-ă	infectious disease caused by bacterium *Corynebacterium diphtheriae* which affects nose, tonsils, uvula, soft palate, and posterior pharynx; rare
epistaxis	ĕp"ĭ-stăk'sĭs	nosebleed
laryngitis	lăr"ēn-jī"tĭs	inflammation of the larynx
pertussis	pĕr'tŭs'ĭs	whooping cough
pharyngitis	făr"ĭn-jī'tĭs	inflammation of the throat
rhinitis	rī-nī'tĭs	inflammation of the mucous membrane of the nose; may be acute (common cold) or allergic (hay fever), which is due to an allergy

continues

DIAGNOSES		
Word	**Pronunciation**	**Definition**
Diseases of the Upper Respiratory System (*continued*)		
sinusitis	sī"nŭ-sī'tĭs	inflammation of the sinuses, especially the nasal sinuses
tonsillitis	tŏn-sĭl-ī'tĭs	inflammation of a palatine (or faucial) tonsil
upper respiratory infection (URI)		broad term referring to several infectious diseases often caused by a group called *Rhinovirus*
Diseases of the Bronchi/Lungs		
acute respiratory distress syndrome (ARDS)		condition that may follow or accompany various serious diseases including pulmonary embolism or sepsis; shock lung
anthracosis	ăn-thră-kō'sĭs	black lung disease; accumulation of carbon deposits in the lungs due to breathing smoke or coal dust
asbestosis	ăs"bĕs-tō'sĭs	lung disease resulting from protracted breathing of asbestos particles
asthma	ăz'mah	condition marked by recurrent attacks of shortness of breath with wheezing due to spasms in the bronchi
atelectasis	ăt"ĕ-lĕk'tah-sĭs	collapse of the lung parenchyma due to obstruction from secretions, fluids, or other factors
bronchiectasis	brŏng"kē-ĕk'tah-sĭs	chronic distention of the bronchi or bronchioles
bronchiolitis	brŏng"kē-ō'lī'tĭs	respiratory infection that causes bronchioles to become inflamed and secrete an excessive amount of mucus
bronchitis	brŏng"kī'tĭs	inflammation of the bronchi; may be acute or chronic
bronchogenic	brŏng-kō-jĕn'ĭk	lung cancer
carcinoma	kăr"sĭ-nō'mă	
byssinosis	bĭs"ĭ-nō'sĭs	lung disease caused by inhalation of dust from cotton, flax, and hemp; brown lung disease
chronic obstructive pulmonary disease (COPD)		condition characterized by chronic obstruction to the airflow in the lungs
cor pulmonale (pulmonary heart disease)	kŏr pŭl-mŏn-āl'	hypertrophy of the right ventricle of the heart usually due to a chronic condition of airflow obstruction

continues

*Study*WARE™ Connection

View an animation on **Asthma** on your StudyWARE™ CD-ROM.

DIAGNOSES		
Word	Pronunciation	Definition
Diseases of the Bronchi/Lungs (*continued*)		
cystic fibrosis	sĭs'tĭk fī-brō'sĭs	hereditary disease affecting both the respiratory and digestive systems
emphysema	ĕm"fĭ-sē'mah	condition marked by presence of increased air in the intraalveolar tissue of the lungs due to distention of their walls and rupture of the alveoli (see Figure 12-8)
hyline membrane disease (respiratory distress syndrome [RDS])		severe impairment of respiratory function in a newborn
idiopathic	ĭd"ē-ō-păth'ĭk	formation of scar tissue in the connective
fibrosis	fī-brō'sĭs	inflammation of the alveoli
influenza (flu)	ĭn"flū-ĕn'zah	highly contagious viral upper respiratory infection
pneumonia	nū"mō'nē-ah	inflammation of the lungs; may be caused by bacteria, viruses, fungi, or mechanical, physical, or chemical irritants (Figure 12-9 shows comparison of alveoli in normal tissue to various abnormal alveoli.)
pulmonary abscess	pŭl'mō-nĕr"ē ăb'sĕs	collection of pus in the lungs (see Figure 12-10)
pulmonary edema	ĕ-dē'mah	filling of the air sacs and bronchioles with fluid

continues

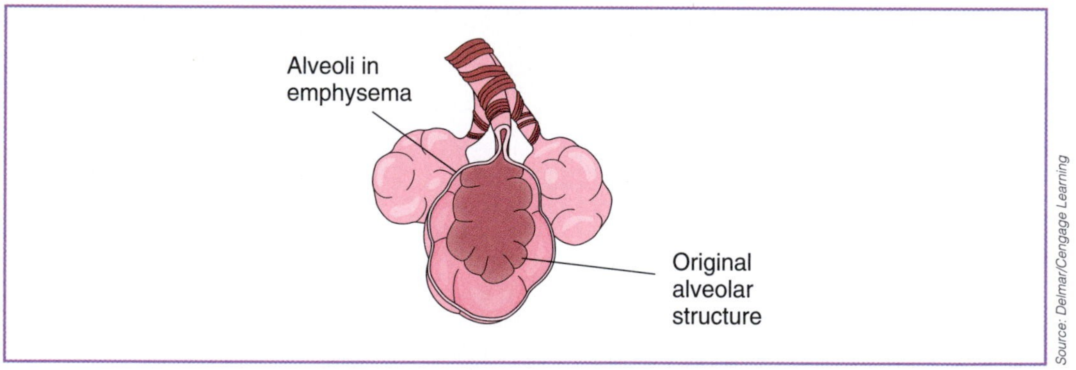

FIGURE 12-8
Emphysema

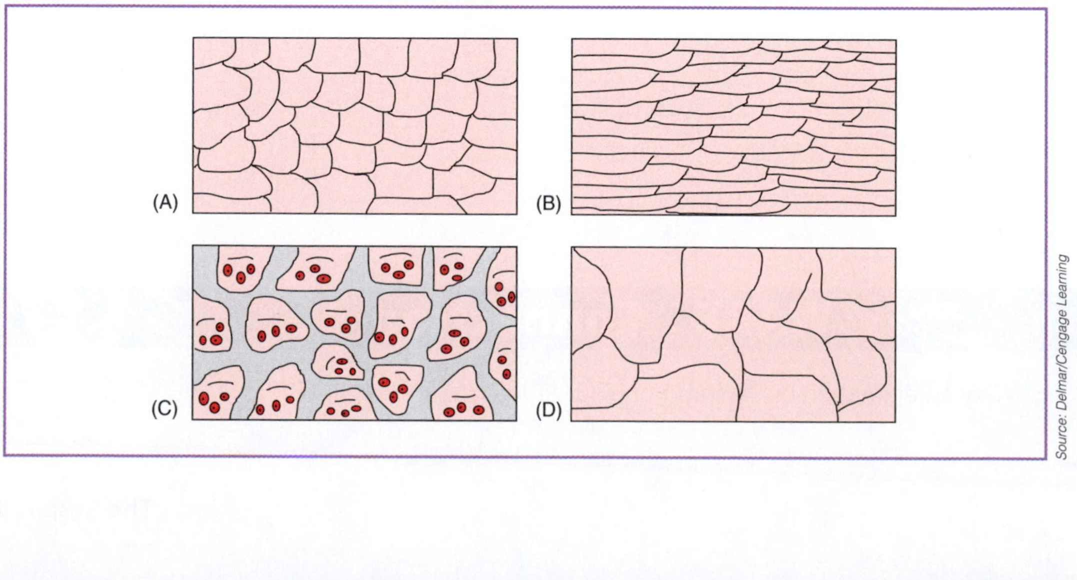

FIGURE 12-9
Alveoli: in (A) normal lung tissue; (B) atelectasis; (C) pneumonia; and (D) emphysema

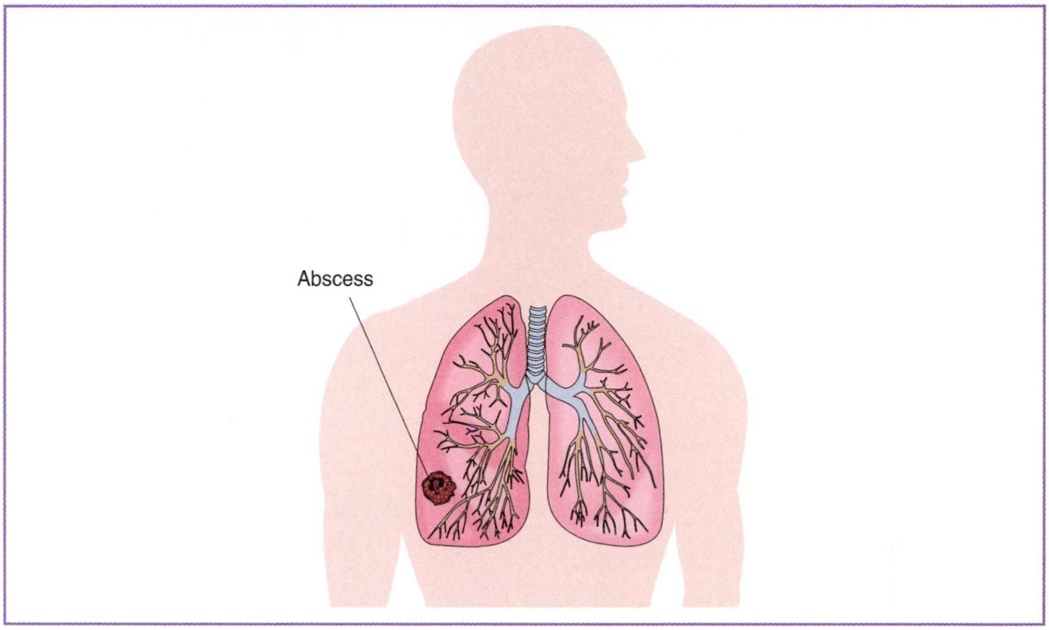

FIGURE 12-10
Pulmonary Abscess

Source: Delmar/Cengage Learning

DIAGNOSES

Word	Pronunciation	Definition
Diseases of the Bronchi/Lungs (*continued*)		
pulmonary embolism	ĕm'bō-lizm	obstruction of the pulmonary artery or one of its branches by a clot or foreign material
sarcoidosis	săr"koi-dō'sĭs	chronic, progressive, generalized granulomatous reticulosis involving the lungs
silicosis	sĭl-ĭ-kō'sĭs	lung disease caused by inhaling silica (quartz) dust
tuberculosis	too-bĕr"kū-lō'sĭs	chronic bacterial infection caused by inhaling droplets sprayed into the air by someone infected with Mycobacterium tuberculosis
Diseases of the Pleura and Chest		
empyema	ĕm"pī-ē'mah	condition marked by pus in the pleural space of the thoracic cavity
hemothorax	hē"mō-thō'răks	collection of blood in the chest cavity
mesothelioma	mēs"ō-thē-lē-ō'mă	malignant tumor derived from the mesothelial cells of the pleura, peritoneum, or pericardium; found in those exposed to asbestos
pleural effusion	ploo'răl ĕ-fū'zhŭn	presence of fluid in the pleural space of the thoracic cavity (See Figure 12-11)
pleurisy (pleuritis)	ploo'rĭs-ē (ploo-rī'tĭs)	inflammation of the pleura (covering of the lungs)
pneumothorax	nū"mō-thō'răks	presence of air in the pleural space outside the lung, but inside the chest due to a ruptured alveolus or bronchus (See Figure 12-12)

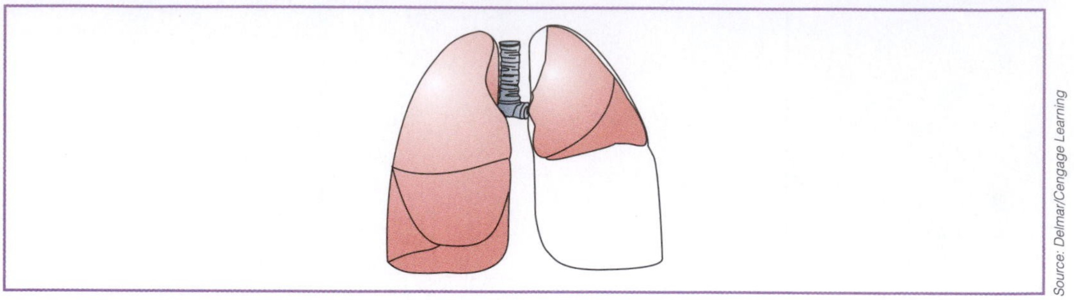

FIGURE 12-11
Pleural Effusion

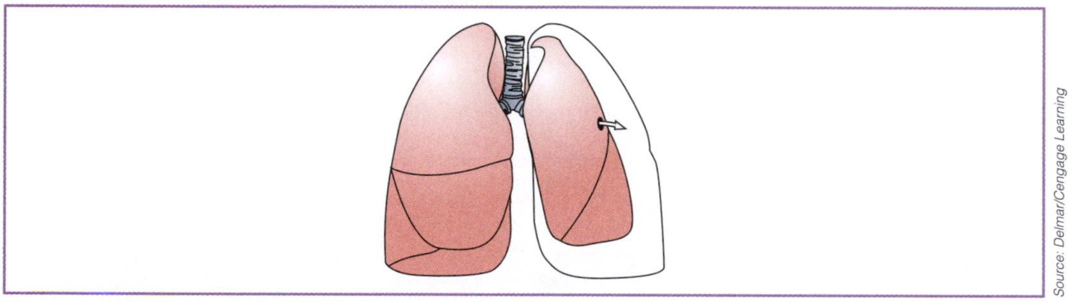

FIGURE 12-12
Pneumothorax

TREATMENT PROCEDURES		
Word	**Pronunciation**	**Definition**
endotracheal intubation	ĕn"dō-trā'kē-al ĭn"tŭ-bā'shŭn	procedure that establishes an airway with the insertion of a tube through the nose or mouth, pharynx, and larynx into the trachea
lobectomy	lō-bĕk'tō-mē	resection of a lobe of the lung
pleurectomy	ploor-ĕk'tō-mē	excision of a portion of pleura
pneumonectomy	nū"mō-nĕk'tō-mē	surgical removal of a lung—total or either right or left lung
thoracostomy	thō"rah-kŏs'tō-mē	surgical insertion of a tube or to aid diagnosis of a disease process
thoracotomy	thō"răk-ŏt'ō-mē	major surgical incision of the chest
tracheostomy	trā"kē-ŏs'tō-mē	emergency or elective surgical opening of the trachea to provide and secure an open airway
tracheotomy	trā"kē-ŏt'ō-mē	incision into the trachea airflow

MEDICATIONS PRESCRIBED	
Trade Name	**Generic Name**
Antiasthmatic, Antiallergic, Inhalant, or by Mouth	
Intal, Nasalcrom, Gastrocrom	cromolyn Na
Antibiotics	
Amoxil, Augmentin	amoxicillin
Ampicillin, Polycillin	ampicillin
Biaxin	clarithromycin
Ceclor	cefaclor
Ceftin	cefuroxime axetil
Cefzil	cefprozil monohydrate
Cipro	ciprofloxacin
Eryped	erythromycin ethylsuccinate
Keflex	cephalexin
Tequin	gatifloxacin
Antihistamines	
Benadryl	diphenhydramine
Claritin	loratadine
Claritin D	loratadine and pseudoephedrine sulfate
Phenergan	promethazine
Zyrtec	cetirizine hydrochloride
Bronchodilators	
Albuterol, Proventil, Ventolin	albuterol
Alupent, Metaprel	metaproterenol
Aminophylline	aminophylline
Atrovent	ipratropium
Brethine, Brycanyl	terbutaline
Isuprel	isoproterenol
Primatene, Bronkaid, Vaponephrine, Adrenalin	epinephrine

continues

MEDICATIONS PRESCRIBED	
Trade Name	Generic Name
Bronchodilators (*continued*)	
Serevant	salmeterol
Slo-Phyllin, Slo-bid, Theo-clear, Theo-Dur	theophylline
Spiriva	tiotropium
Combination Products	
Advair	fluticasone and salmeterol
Entex	phenylephrine and guaifenesin
Expectorants	
Humabid	guaifenesin
Organidin	iodinated glycerol
Inhalation Steroids	
Azmacort, Nasacort	triamcinolone
Beclovent, Vanceril	beclomethasone
Decadron	dexamethasone
Flovent	fluticasone propionate
Nasalide	flunisolide
Vancenase, Beconase	beclomethasone
Lung Surfactants	
Exosurf	colfosceril palmitate
Survanta	beractant
Nasal Decongestants	
Afrin, Sudafed	pseudoephedrine

ABBREVIATIONS

ABGs	arterial blood gases
A&P	auscultation and percussion
AP	anteroposterior; from front to back
ARD	acute respiratory disease
ARDS	acute respiratory distress syndrome
ARF	acute respiratory failure
Bronch	bronchoscopy
CO_2	carbon dioxide
COLD	chronic obstructive lung disease
COPD	chronic obstructive pulmonary disease
CPAP	continuous positive airway pressure
CPR	cardiopulmonary resuscitation
CTA	clear to auscultation
DOE	dyspnea on exertion
IPPB	intermittent positive pressure breathing
O_2	oxygen
PA	posteroanterior; from back to front
PE	pulmonary embolism
PFT	pulmonary function test
PND	paroxysmal nocturnal dyspnea
PPD	purified protein derivative (tuberculosis skin test)
SOB	shortness of breath
TB	tuberculosis
TPR	temperature, pulse, and respiration
URI	upper respiratory infection
V/Q	scan ventilation-perfusion scan

Working Practice Review Exercises

IDENTIFICATION/PROCEDURES

Identify the following procedures.

1. x-ray technique for studying circulation in the lungs ____________________
2. measurement of hydrogen, carbon dioxide, pH, and oxygen pressure from arterial blood ____________________
3. evaluates how a patient breathes ____________________
4. the chest wall is punctured with a needle to obtain fluid for diagnostic studies ____________________
5. examination of the bronchi with a scope ____________________
6. measurement of breathing capacity of lungs ____________________
7. determines obstruction in airflow to lungs ____________________
8. test for malignant cells in the sputum ____________________
9. use of flexible scope to visualize bronchi ____________________
10. visual exam of pleural cavity by placing the endoscope through small incision through the chest ____________________

MEANING

Give the meaning of the underlined words.

1. The patient suffered an <u>asthmatic</u> attack on Friday.

   ____

2. As a result of the automobile accident, she developed a <u>hemothorax</u>.

   ____

3. We have scheduled her for a <u>thoracostomy</u> tomorrow.

   ____

4. For the past six months the patient has suffered with <u>chronic obstructive pulmonary disease</u>.

   ____

5. (On an x-ray report) Impression: <u>Atelectasis</u>, left lung.

   ____

6. Her lungs were clear to <u>A&P</u>.

   ____

7. It was diagnosed as a <u>URI</u>.

   ____

8. I have ordered a <u>sputum culture and sensitivity</u>.

   ____

9. She will have a <u>V/Q</u> scan later today.

   ____

10. Unfortunately their son has <u>hyline membrane</u> disease.

    ____

11. There was evidence of <u>epistaxis</u>.

    ____

12. Have you seen the commercials on TV about mesothelioma?

____

13. A symptom of pleurisy is pain with coughing.

____

14. It was necessary to perform a tracheostomy.

____

15. The specialist identified silicosis as the diagnosis.

____

IDENTIFICATION/ABBREVIATIONS

Identify the following abbreviations.

1. ARDS _______________________________
2. COPD _______________________________
3. IPPB _______________________________
4. PFT _______________________________
5. ARF _______________________________
6. COLD _______________________________
7. CPR _______________________________
8. DOE _______________________________
9. SOB _______________________________
10. TB _______________________________
11. ARD _______________________________
12. CTA _______________________________
13. PE _______________________________
14. TPR _______________________________
15. O_2 _______________________________

MATCHING

Match to the correct diagnoses.

1. ____________ inflammation of mucous membrane of the nose
2. ____________ barking cough in children
3. ____________ a head cold
4. ____________ whooping cough
5. ____________ chronic distension of bronchi or bronchioles
6. ____________ condition characterized by chronic obstruction to the airflow in the lungs
7. ____________ hereditary disease affecting respiratory and digestive systems
8. ____________ inflammation of lungs
9. ____________ chronic, progressive, generalized granulomatous reticulosis involving the lungs

a. bronchiectasis
b. COPD
c. coryza
d. croup
e. cystic fibrosis
f. empyema
g. influenza
h. pertussis
i. pleurisy
j. pneumonia
k. pneumothorax
l. pulmonary abscess

10. ________________ pus in the pleural space
11. ________________ inflammation of the pleura
12. ________________ presence of air in the pleural space outside the lung but inside the chest
13. ________________ collection of pus in the lungs
14. ________________ filling of the air sacs and bronchioles with fluid
15. ________________ highly contagious viral upper respiratory infection

m. pulmonary edema
n. rhinitis
o. sarcoidosis

Dictionary Exercises

DICTIONARY EXERCISE 1

Use your dictionary to find the pronunciation and definition of the following words.

	Word	Pronunciation	Definition
1.	blastomycosis	________________	________________
2.	anthracosis	________________	________________
3.	coccidioidomycosis	________________	________________
4.	consolidation	________________	________________
5.	fibrosis	________________	________________
6.	hemopneumothorax	________________	________________
7.	rales	________________	________________
8.	bronchostaxis	________________	________________
9.	emphysematous bullae	________________	________________
10.	acid-fast bacillus	________________	________________
11.	hydropneumothorax	________________	________________
12.	rhonchi	________________	________________
13.	aspergillosis	________________	________________
14.	broncholith	________________	________________
15.	dysphonia	________________	________________

DICTIONARY EXERCISE 2

Select the correct meaning and provide the pronunciation where indicated.

1. bronchial brushing (__________)
   a. forming or containing pus
   b. scrapings from bronchial tubes used for cytologic and bacteriologic examinations
   c. crackling sound heard on auscultation in certain lung diseases
   d. accumulation of fluid in the chest
2. density
   a. quantity of a substance in a given space
   b. solidification, such as caused by the airlessness of the area of a lung affected with pneumonia
   c. growth of fibrous connective tissue
   d. failure of a lung to develop normally
3. diffusion
   a. blood and air in the pleural cavity
   b. accumulation of fluid in the chest
   c. crackling sound heard on auscultation
   d. process of becoming widely spread
4. effusion
   a. blood and air in the pleural cavity
   b. accumulation of fluid in the chest
   c. crackling sound heard on auscultation
   d. process of becoming widely spread
5. eupnea (________________________)
   a. temporarily without breath
   b. shortness of breath
   c. normal breathing
   d. difficulty in breathing unless sitting or standing
6. ventilation
   a. process of the exchange of air between the lungs and outside air
   b. process of becoming widely spread
   c. vibration felt in the chest wall during speaking when a hand is applied to the thorax
   d. normal breathing
7. interstitial tissue (________________)
   a. solidification
   b. thickness of a substance
   c. accumulation of fluid in the chest
   d. situated in the interspaces between and among epithelial structures
8. purulent (____________________)
   a. growth of fibrous connective tissue
   b. forming or containing pus
   c. accumulation of fluid in the chest
   d. material expelled from the chest by coughing or clearing the throat
9. cryptococcosis (________________)
   a. crackling sound heard on auscultation
   b. infection of the lungs from a yeastlike fungi
   c. growth of fibrous connective tissue
   d. accumulation of fluid in the chest
10. allergic alveolitis (________________)
    a. infection of the lungs from a yeastlike fungi
    b. expelling material from the chest by coughing or clearing the throat
    c. inflammation caused by exposure to organic dusts
    d. accumulation of fluid in the chest

DICTIONARY EXERCISE 3

Pronunciation of the words below is provided. Using your dictionary, find the correct spelling and definition for these words.

	Word	Pronunciation	Definition
1.	________________	ăp-nē'ah	____________________________
2.	________________	krĕp'ĭ-tănt rahlz	____________________________
3.	________________	hē-mŏp'tĭ-sĭs	____________________________

4. ________ nū"mō-kō"nē-ō'sĭs ________________________
5. ________ hī-pŏk'sē-ah ________________________
6. ________ pah-rĕng'kĭ-mah ________________________
7. ________ spū'tŭm ________________________
8. ________ nū"mō-thō'răks ________________________
9. ________ tăk'tĭl ________________________
10. ________ ĕk-spĕk'tō-rănt ________________________
11. ________ rī"nō-rē'ă ________________________
12. ________ kŭs'mawlz ________________________
    brēth'ĭng ________________________
13. ________ hī"pŏks'ēă ________________________
14. ________ ploo'răl ________________________
    frĭk'shŭn rŭb ________________________
15. ________ hwēz ________________________

DICTIONARY EXERCISE 4

Rewrite each sentence in your own words. Provide the pronunciation for the italicized words.

1. The child's lungs exhibited evidence of *aplasia* (________________).

   ____

2. The patient complained of *dyspnea* (________________).

   ____

3. The final diagnosis was *histoplasmosis* (________________).

   ____

4. One of her symptoms was *orthopnea* (________________).

   ____

5. Because of the *hypoxemia* (________________), he will undergo more extensive tests.

   ____

6. She is scheduled for *thoracoplasty* (________________) on Thursday.

   ____

7. One of her symptoms was *stridor* (________________), indicative of an obstruction.

   ____

*Study*WARE™ Connection

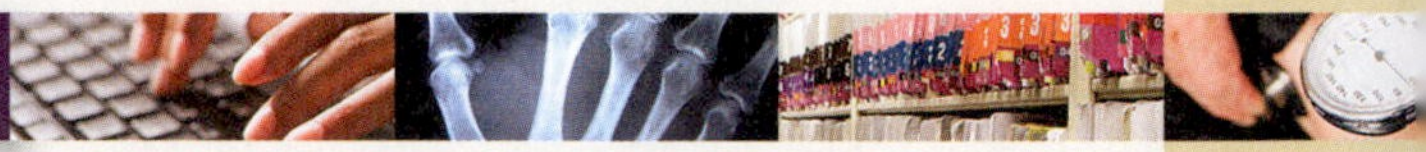

To take a practice quiz or play interactive games that reinforce the content in this chapter, go to your StudyWARE™ CD-ROM.

Listening Exercise

INSTRUCTIONS

1. Review the spelling, pronunciation, and meaning of the words provided in the preview.
2. Go to your StudyWARE™ CD-ROM and listen to **Listening Exercise 12-1**. Fill in the blank in the report as the word is dictated.
3. At the end of the activity, check your spelling against the preview words. They appear in the preview in the order in which they are encountered in the activity.
4. Review and practice the words you missed.
5. Look up words that are not familiar.

PREVIEW OF WORDS FOR LISTENING EXERCISE 12-1

Word	Pronunciation	Meaning
opacification	ō-păs"ĭ-fĭ-kā'shŭn	formation of areas that are not transparent
hemothorax	hē"mō-thō'răks	collection of blood in the pleural cavity
bronchus	brŏng'kŭs	one of the larger passages conveying air to and within the lungs
intubation	ĭn"tū-bā'shŭn	insertion of a tube into the respiratory tract
carina	kă-rī'nă	ridge at the lower end of the trachea, separating the two bronchi
patent	pā'tĕnt	open, unobstructed

Listening Exercise 12-1

StudyWARE™ Connection

Listen to this report being read on your StudyWARE™ CD-ROM. Fill in each blank as the word is dictated.

Operative Report

The patient is a 57-year-old white female who was referred by Dr. Steinger for evaluation of increasing shortness of breath as well as progressive ____________ of a left ____________. The patient was initially admitted and watched closely over the next hour-and-a-half after admission. The patient's respiratory rate increased remarkably and O_2 stats continued to drop. Initial films were obtained from Lakeview Hospital revealing a left lower lobe pneumonia. Repeat films tonight upon arrival here revealed increasing opacification with a left hemothorax. It was suspected there was marked mucous plugging of the left main stem ____________. After discussing options with the patient and her daughter, the patient was electively intubated with bronchoscopic evaluation following.

The patient was given Versed for ____________ and then Ativan. She underwent bronchoscopic evaluation for both diagnostic as well as therapeutic reasons.

On examination, the patient was in a fair amount of respiratory distress. The patient was given Ativan at 4 mg during the procedure. The P20 bronchoscope was gently inserted through the ET tube. This was held in place by the respiratory therapist and continuous O_2 monitoring as well as blood pressure and EKG monitoring were maintained. The patient was Ambued with 100% oxygen. The bronchoscope was gently inserted through the endotracheal tube. Initially, the endotracheal tube required pulling back approximately 2 cm because it was at the level of the ____________. Following this, the right upper, middle, and lower lobe segments were inspected. All segments were ____________. The carina was in the midline. The bronchoscope then was reentered into the left main stem bronchus. The entire left main stem bronchus was totally occluded with yellowish mucoid material. This was suctioned. All airways including the lingula, upper lobe, and lower lobe segments were totally occluded with mucus. Again multiple irrigations were instilled and these airways were suctioned. At the end of the procedure, all airways were patent. The bronchoscope was then withdrawn. The patient tolerated the procedure well. No endobronchial lesions were noted during the procedure. The specimens will be sent for Gram's stain and C&S as well as cytology when available.

IMPRESSION:

1. Total occlusion, left main stem bronchus, secondary to pneumonitis.
2. Heavy history of tobacco abuse.
3. Possible poliomyelitis syndrome.

The patient will be followed quite closely.

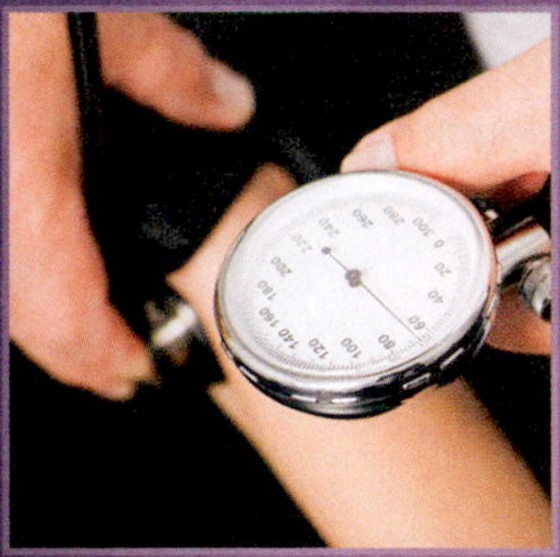

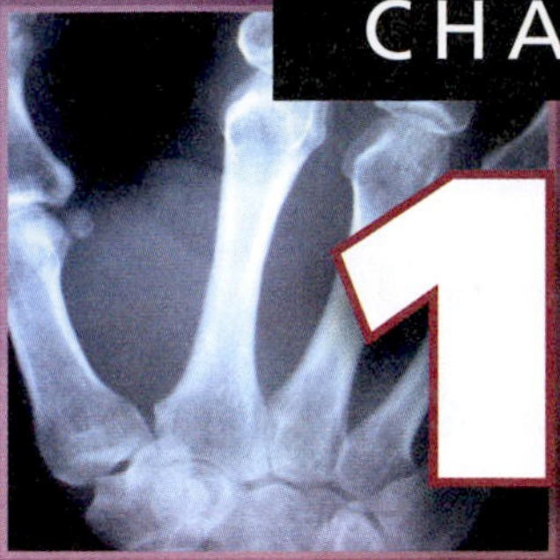

CHAPTER

13

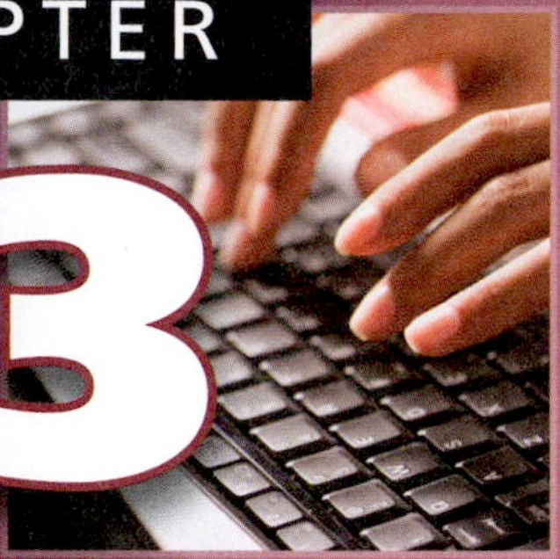

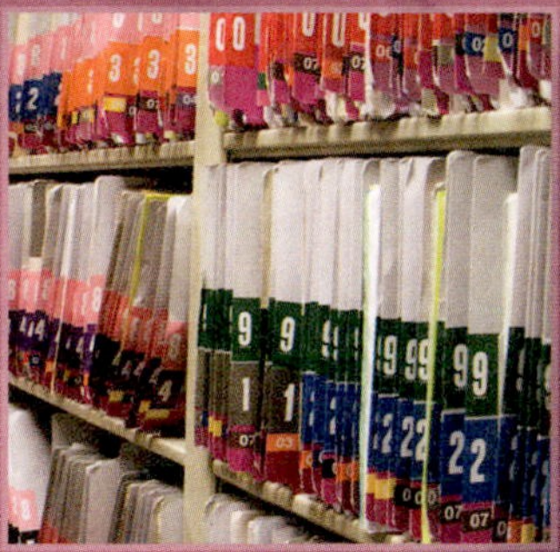

The Digestive System

"Now good digestion waits on appetite
And health on both!"

—William Shakespeare

OBJECTIVES

When you have completed this chapter on the digestive system, you should be able to

1. Spell and define major system components and explain how they operate.
2. Identify the meaning of related word elements.
3. Spell and define diagnostic procedures, diagnoses, treatment procedures, and abbreviations.
4. Spell the names of commonly used medications.
5. Use a dictionary as a tool in processing medical documents.
6. Hear how medical terminology is used in actual medical reports.

INTRODUCTION

The purpose of the digestive or gastrointestinal system is to receive and process food so that it nourishes the body and to eliminate solid waste. Physicians who specialize in the study of the digestive system are known as **gastroenterologists** (găs-trō-ĕn"tĕr-ŏl'ō-gĭst).

Terms that apply to this process include digestion, absorption, and elimination. **Digestion** is the process that converts food into nutrients; **absorption** is the process that transfers these nutrients into the bloodstream and body. **Elimination** is the process that concentrates and releases solid waste (feces). The process of digestion and absorption takes 36 hours or more.

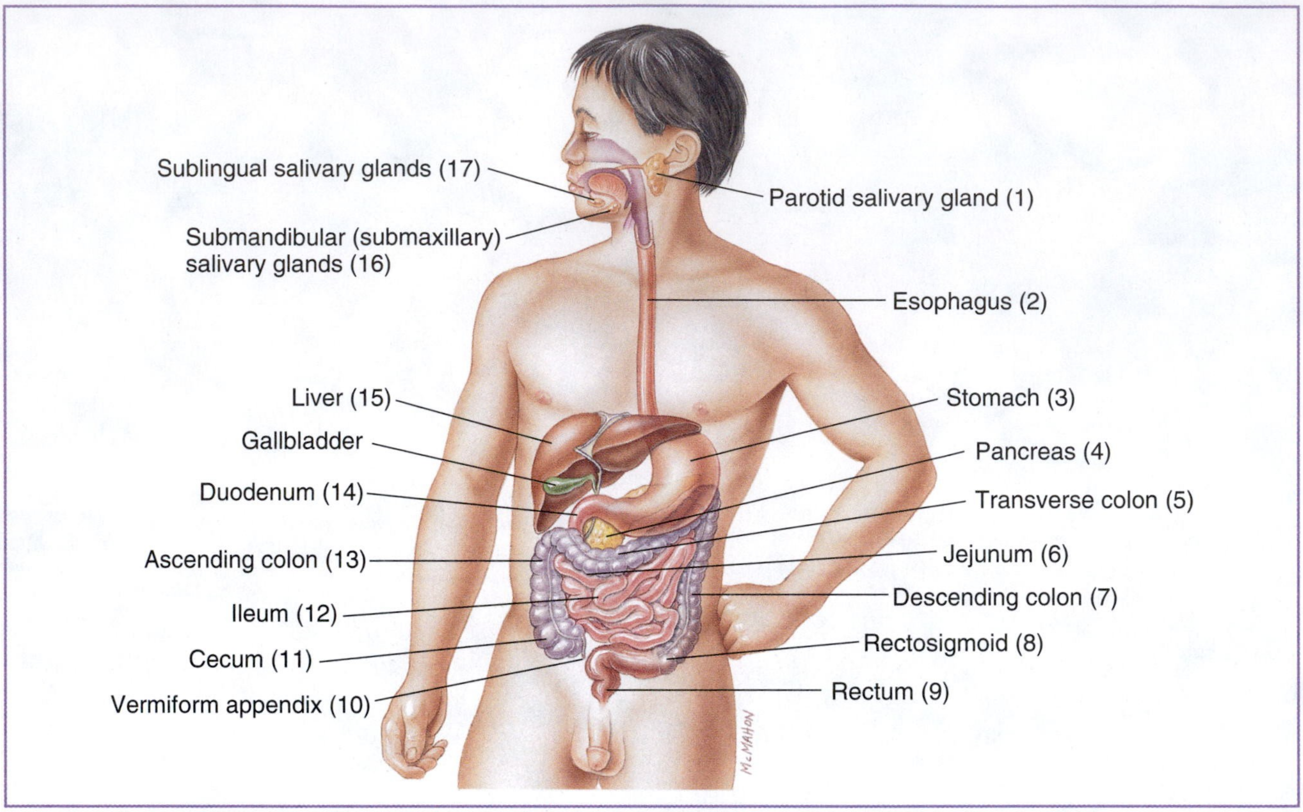

FIGURE 13-1 Alimentary Canal

COMPONENTS OF THE DIGESTIVE SYSTEM

The digestive system consists of the mouth or oral cavity, pharynx, esophagus, stomach, small intestine, and large intestine—all referred to as the **alimentary** (ăl"ĕ-mĕn'tăr-ē) **canal**, illustrated in Figure 13-1. This chapter discusses these organs.

ORAL CAVITY

cheil/o, chil/o	lip	peritone/o	peritoneum
gingiv/o	gum	phag/o	to eat
gloss/o	tongue	sial/o	salivary
odont/o	tooth	stomat/o, stom/o	mouth

The alimentary canal is a muscular digestive tube that starts in the oral cavity, or mouth, and extends through the entire body. Lodged in the mouth is a muscular organ called the tongue, which aids in chewing and swallowing, as well as in speech and breathing. **Saliva** is produced in the oral cavity and allows food to be swallowed more easily. This fluid is manufactured by three pairs of salivary glands, the first of several accessory organs that aid in the digestive process. The three pairs of major salivary glands are the **parotid** (pah-rŏt'ĭd) (1), **submandibular** (sŭb"măn-dĭb'ū-lăr) or **submaxillary** (sŭb-măk'sĭ-lĕr"ē) (16), and **sublingual** (sŭb-lĭng'gwăl) (17).

Like the rest of the alimentary canal, the oral cavity is lined with a moist mucous membrane.* Beneath this mucous membrane is a layer of connective tissue containing blood vessels and nerves. The parts of the alimentary canal that extend into the abdominal cavity have an additional covering or layer called the **peritoneum** (pĕr"ĭ-tō-nē'ŭm).

*mucous (adj.)—secreting mucus; mucus (n.)—free slime of the mucous membranes

PHARYNX

laryng/o	larynx	pharyng/o	pharynx

The **pharynx** (făr'ĭnks), which is situated directly behind the mouth, is the second part of the digestive system. The following seven cavities communicate with the pharynx: the two nasal cavities, the two tympanic cavities (middle ears via the eustachian tubes, commonly called the tympanopharyngeal canals), the mouth or oral cavity, the larynx, and the esophagus. The function of the pharynx in the digestive tract is to carry food to the esophagus.

ESOPHAGUS

esophag/o	esophagus

The **esophagus** (ē-sŏf'ah-gŭs) (2) is a passage that extends from the lower part of the pharynx through the diaphragm to the stomach (3). It is lined with stratified squamous epithelial cells. A loosely arranged coat of connective tissue and muscle lie beneath these cells. These layers of involuntary muscles produce a rhythmic, wavelike motion known as **peristalsis** (pĕr"ĭ-stăl'sĭs). This motion—which occurs along the entire length of the alimentary canal—begins in the esophagus where it directs food to the next organ, the stomach.

STOMACH

gastr/o	stomach	pyl/o, pylor/o	pylorus

The stomach is guarded by muscular valves called **sphincters** (sfĭngk'ters), which permit the passage of food in only one direction. The **cardiac valve**, more commonly called the lower esophageal sphincter (LES), encircles the lower end of the esophagus. The valve at the distal (or lower) end of the stomach, where it connects to the small intestine, is called the **pyloric** (pī-lor'ĭk) **sphincter**.

The stomach has folds called **rugae** (roo'gay) in the lining. As food is ingested, these folds expand to provide room for food to be mixed with the gastric juices (primarily hydrochloric acid and pepsin) that will begin the digestive process. When the gastric pressure exceeds that of the intestine, the pyloric sphincter relaxes and allows the passage of this slurrylike mixture of partially digested food and digestive secretions (called **chyme** [kīm]) into the small intestine. The sphincter then closes to prevent any backup.

SMALL INTESTINE

append/o, appendic/o	appendix	duoden/o	duodenum
		enter/o	intestine
bili/o	bile	hepat/o, hepatic/o	liver
celi/o, cel/o	abdomen	ile/o	ileum
cholangi/o	bile or hepatic duct	jejun/o	jejunum
choledoch/o	bile duct	lapar/o	abdominal wall
chol/e, chol/o	bile	pancreat/o	pancreas
cyst/o	bladder, sac	rect/o	rectum

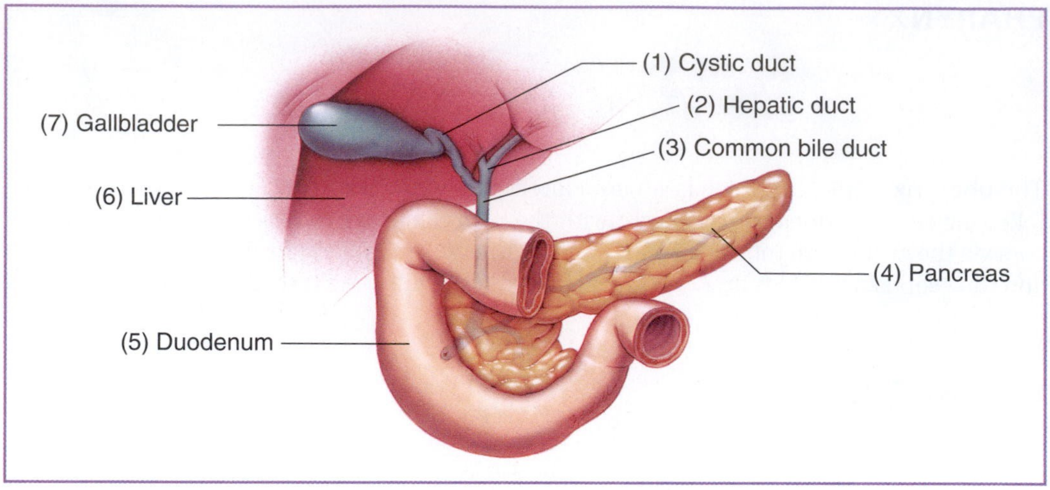

FIGURE 13-2
The Liver, Gallbladder, and Pancreas

The **small intestine** is the chief organ of digestion and absorption of food products. It is the longest part of the alimentary canal, averaging 20 feet. The lining of the small intestine, or the **mucosa** (mū-kō'sah), is covered with tiny fingerlike projections called **villi** (vĭl'lī).*

The first 10 to 12 inches of the small intestine is called the **duodenum** (dū"ō-dē'nŭm) (14). Secretions from the accessory organs—namely the pancreas (4) and the liver (15)—are received there.

One of the more important secretions is bile, which is produced by the liver and stored in a pouch called the **gallbladder** (7) (Figure 13-2). Bile assists the digestive processing of fats in two ways. Bile causes emulsification, or the break up, of large fat globules into millions of small fat droplets that provide large surface areas for the fat-digesting enzymes to work on. Subsequently, bile combines with the products of fat digestion to form spheres of bile salt molecules called micelles, which bring these end products into closer contact with the absorptive surface of the intestinal wall surface.

Aside from bile production, the **liver** (6)—the second largest glandular organ of the body—performs many other functions, including removal of poisons absorbed from the intestines, final treatment of fats, and storage of certain vitamins.

Bile moves through several ducts that are called the **biliary** (bĭl'ē-ā-rē) **tree**. The **hepatic** (hĕ-păt'ĭk) **duct** (2) (**right**, **left**, and **common**) leads from the liver to the duct draining the gallbladder, referred to as the **cystic duct** (1). These two ducts join to form the **common bile duct** (3), which leads to the duodenum. The opening of the common bile duct into the duodenum (5) is the **ampulla** (ăm-pŭl'lah) **of Vater**.

The **pancreas** (păn'krē-ăs) (4) is a gland situated under the stomach. It produces secretions that aid in the digestion of food and the neutralization of acid produced by the stomach. The main and accessory pancreatic ducts join with the common bile duct before they enter the duodenum through the ampulla of Vater.

Two more divisions of the small intestine (see Figure 13-1) are beyond the duodenum—the **jejunum** (jĕ-joo'nŭm) (6) and the **ileum** (ĭl'ē-ŭm) (12). The ileum joins the large intestine through another muscle valve called the **ileocecal** (ĭl"e-ō-sē'kăl) **valve**.

StudyWARE™ Connection

Play an interactive game labeling **Digestive System Structures** on your StudyWARE™ CD-ROM.

*villi (n.)—plural; villous (adj.); villus (n.)—singular

LARGE INTESTINE

an/o	anal	proct/o	anus, rectum
cec/o	cecum	sigmoid/o	sigmoid colon
col/o, colon/o	colon		

Once digestion and absorption have taken place in the small intestine, the residual liquid is passed to the **large intestine**, also referred to as the **colon**. Water is returned to the body through absorption of most of the fluids, and the residue becomes a solid called **fecal** (fē'kăl) **matter**.

The large intestine begins below the ileum and extends to the rectum (see Figure 13-3). It has five divisions in this order—**ascending** (3), **transverse** (4), **descending** (5), **rectosigmoid** (rĕk"tō-sĭg'moid) (which includes the **sigmoid** (sĭg'moid) **colon** (6) and the upper part of the rectum), and **rectum** (7). At the beginning of the large intestine is a pouch called the **cecum** (sē'kŭm) (2). Attached to the cecum is a small, blind tube called the **vermiform** (vĕr'mĭ-form) **appendix** (1). At the lower end the large intestine empties into the rectum. From the rectum, the **anal** (ā'năl) **canal** (8) leads out of the body, terminating in an opening called the **anus** (ā'nŭs) (9). The veins in this region are called **hemorrhoidal** (hĕm"ō-roi'dăl) **veins**.

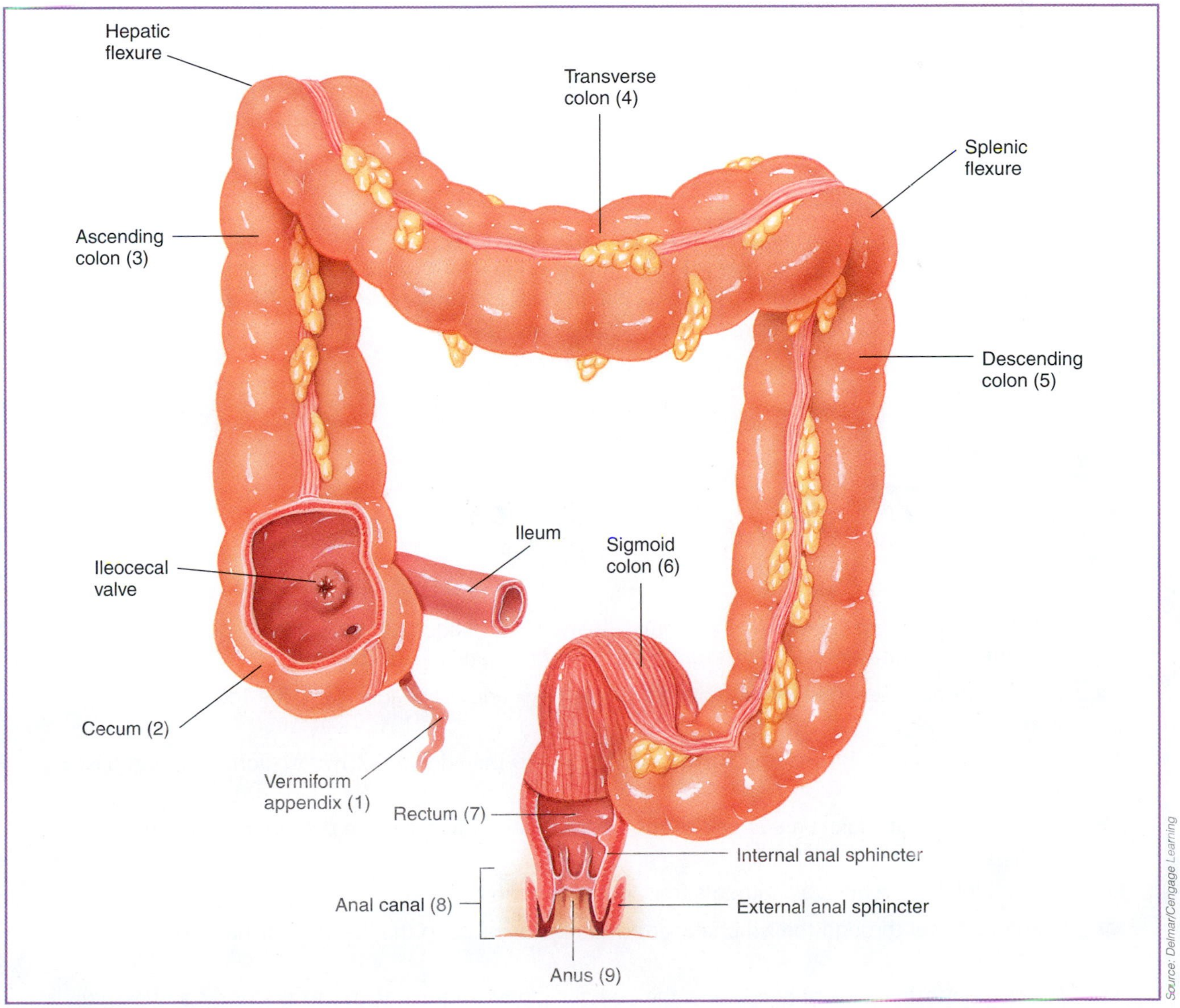

FIGURE 13-3 Anatomy of a Large Intestine

The **mesentery** (mĕs'ĕn-tĕr"ē) is a specialized, double-layered tissue that connects and suspends the intestines in the abdominal cavity. The portion of the mesentery connecting the lower border of the stomach to the transverse colon is called the **greater omentum** (ō-mĕn'tŭm). Sometimes it is referred to as the apron since it is elongated and extends freely into the pelvis. One of its functions is to control the spread of infection inside the abdominal cavity. The **lesser omentum** extends between the stomach and liver.

StudyWARE™ Connection

Play an interactive game labeling structures of the **Large Intestine** and watch an animation on **Digestion** on your StudyWARE™ CD-ROM.

INTERNET ASSIGNMENT

The American College of Gastroenterology is a professional organization of more than 10,000 gastroenterologists in 75 countries. Their mission is to advance the scientific study and medical treatment of disorders of the gastrointestinal tract. The College promotes the highest standards in medical education and is guided by its commitment to meeting the needs of clinical gastroenterology practitioners. One of their goals is to promote patient education on gastrointestinal conditions and digestive health. Their web site is at **www.acg.gi.org** where patient-related links for Patient Information, Site Map, and Site Search can be found at the bottom of the homepage. Other links are directed to clinical practitioners.

ACTIVITY

Visit the American College of Gastroenterology site at **www.acg.gi.org**. Click on Patient Information and note the link options available. Select an option that will take you to a digestive system problem or condition and read the information given. Summarize by providing bullets of important information and submit it to your instructor.

Review *The Digestive System*

- The digestive system consists of the mouth, pharynx, esophagus, stomach, gallbladder, small intestine, large intestine, and secretory glands (salivary glands, liver, pancreas).
- The mouth prepares food for swallowing; the pharynx and esophagus carry the food to the stomach.
- The stomach breaks up food by a churning action and the addition of hydrochloric acid and gastric juices.
- Bile and pancreatic juices are added to food after it passes through the pyloric sphincter into the duodenum.
- The small intestine absorbs nutrients from processed food.
- Nutrients travel through the lymphatic and vascular channels to the liver for further processing and distribution.
- The large intestine (colon) dehydrates the bowel contents, returns water to the body, and excretes the waste products as fecal material.

Key Terminology Review

Word	Definition
absorption	process that transfers nutrients into the bloodstream and body
alimentary canal	muscular digestive tube that starts in the oral cavity and extends through the entire body
ampulla of Vater	opening of the common bile duct into the duodenum
anal canal	passage leading to the body opening called the anus
anus	outlet of the anal canal
ascending colon	first section of the large intestine
biliary tree	system of ducts through which bile moves
cardiac valve	lower esophageal sphincter; muscular valve located at the lower end of the esophagus
cecum	pouch at the beginning of the colon or large intestine
chyme	slurry-like mixture of partially digested food and digestive secretions
colon	part of the digestive system that extends from the cecum to the rectum; large intestine
common bile duct	duct that leads to the duodenum; combination of the hepatic and cystic ducts
cystic duct	duct of the gallbladder
descending colon	third section of the large intestine
digestion	process that converts food into nutrients for the body
duodenum	first 10 to 12 inches of the small intestine
elimination	process that concentrates and releases solid waste (feces)
esophagus	passage from the pharynx through the diaphragm to the stomach
fecal matter	solid waste material left after food intake has been digested and absorbed
gallbladder	storage pouch for bile
gastroenterologist	physician who specializes in the study of the digestive system
greater omentum	portion of the mesentery connecting the lower border of the stomach to the transverse colon; sometimes called the apron
hemorrhoidal veins	veins in the region of the anus
hepatic duct	duct leading from the liver to the cystic duct for the gallbladder; has left, right, and common sections
ileocecal valve	muscular valve that joins the large intestine to the ileum
ileum	third division of the small intestine
jejunum	second division of the small intestine
large intestine	part of the digestive tract that turns residue into fecal matter; colon
lesser omentum	portion of the mesentary that extends between the stomach and liver
liver	second largest glandular organ of the body; produces bile and performs other functions
mesentery	specialized, double-layered tissue that connects and suspends the intestines in the abdominal cavity
mucosa	membrane that lines the alimentary canal

continues

Word	Definition
pancreas	gland that secretes juices that aid in the digestion of food and the neutralization of acid produced by the stomach
parotid glands	glands that produce saliva; located near the ear
peristalsis	rhythmic, wavelike motion produced by involuntary muscles of the alimentary canal to move food through its entire length
peritoneum	additional covering or layer on parts of the alimentary canal that extends into the abdominal cavity
pharynx	throat
pyloric sphincter	valve at the distal end of the stomach where the stomach connects to the small intestine
rectosigmoid colon	fourth section of the large intestine
rectum	lower part of the large intestine
rugae	folds found in the stomach lining
saliva	enzyme-containing secretion produced in the oral cavity to assist in chewing and swallowing
small intestine	chief organ of digestion and absorption
sphincters	ringlike muscular valves that encourage the passage of food in the stomach in only one direction
sublingual glands	glands that produce saliva; located under the tongue
submandibular (submaxillary) glands	glands that produce saliva; located in the lower jaw
transverse colon	second section of the large intestine
vermiform appendix	small, blind tube attached to the cecum
villi	tiny, fingerlike projections in the mucosa that line the small intestine

Key Terminology Practice Exercises

DEFINITIONS

Define the following terms.

1. digestion

   ____

2. absorption

   ____

3. peristalsis

   ____

4. rugae

5. alimentary canal

6. fecal matter

7. peritoneum

8. mesentery

9. greater omentum

10. pyloric sphincter

11. chyme

SHORT ANSWERS

Supply a short answer to the following.

1. Explain the difference between mucus and mucous.

2. Explain the difference between villi, villus, and villous.

3. Describe the biliary tree.

4. Explain the difference between the rectum and anus.

COMPLETION

Complete the following statements.

1. It usually takes food ____________________ hours to move from the mouth to the anus.
2. The longest part of the alimentary canal is the ____________________.
3. The chief organ of digestion, absorption, and elimination is the ____________________.
4. Food is carried to the stomach from the pharynx by the ____________________.
5. The gallbladder stores ____________________.
6. The second largest glandular organ of the body is the ____________________.
7. The portion of the mesentery that extends between the stomach and liver is the ____________________.
8. Two valves in the stomach ensure that food passes in only one direction; these are the ____________________ and the ____________________.
9. The three anatomic divisions of the small intestine are the ____________________, ____________________, and ____________________.
10. Bile is produced in the ____________________.
11. Saliva is produced in three glands; they are the ____________________, ____________________, and ____________________.
12. The large intestine is also known as the ____________________.
13. The five anatomic divisions of the colon are the ____________________, ____________________, ____________________, ____________________, and ____________________.
14. The fluid produced in the oral cavity that assists digestion is ____________________.
15. The stomach is guarded by muscular valves called ____________________.
16. The function of the ____________________ is to carry food to the esophagus.
17. The lining of the small intestine is the ____________________.
18. Tiny, fingerlike projections of the small intestine are ____________________.
19. A muscular valve that joins the large intestine to the ileum is the ____________________.
20. The ____________________ is the pouch at the beginning of the colon.

Word Element Review

Root	Meaning	Example	Definition
an/o	anal	**anus** (ā'nŭs)	opening of the anal canal
append/o, appendic/o	appendix	**appendectomy** (ăp"ĕn-dĕk'tō-mē)	surgical removal of the vermiform appendix
bil/i	bile	**biliary** (bĭl'ē-ā-rē)	pertaining to bile
		biliousness (bĭl'yŭs-nĕs)	discomfort characterized by constipation and indigestion

continues

Word Element Review

Root	Meaning	Example	Definition
cec/o	cecum	**cecocolostomy** (sē"kō-kō-lŏs'tō-mē)	colostomy consisting of joining the cecum and the colon
celi/o, cel/o	abdomen	**celiac** (sĕ'lē-ăk)	pertaining to the abdomen
cheil/o, chil/o	lip	**cheilitis** (kī-lī'tĭs)	inflammation of the lip
cholangi/o	bile or hepatic duct	**cholangitis** (kō"lăn-jī'tĭs)	inflammation of a bile duct
choledoch/o	bile duct	**choledochojejunostomy** (kō-lĕd"ō-kō-jĕ-jū-nŏs'tō-mē)	surgical anastomosis of the common bile duct to the jejunum
		choledocholithiasis (kō-lĕd"ō-kō-lĭ-thī'ah-sĭs)	calculi in the common bile duct
chol/e, chol/o	bile	**cholecystitis** (kō"lē-sĭs-tī'tĭs)	inflammation of the gallbladder
col/o, colon/o	colon	**colostomy** (kō-lŏs'tō-mē)	surgical creation of an opening to drain the intestines through the abdominal wall
cyst/o	bladder, sac	**cholecystectomy** (kō"lē-sĭs-tĕk'tō-mē)	excision of the gallbladder
duoden/o	duodenum	**duodenitis** (dū"ŏd-ĕ-nī'tĭs)	inflammation of the duodenum
enter/o	intestine	enteropathy (ĕn"ter-ŏp'ah-thē)	any disease of the intestines
esophag/o	esophagus	**esophageal** (ĕ-sŏf"ah-jē'ăl)	pertaining to the esophagus
gastr/o	stomach	**gastroenteric** (găs"trō-ĕn-tĕr'ĭk)	pertaining to the stomach and intestines
		gastrointestinal (găs"trō-ĭn-tĕs'tĭ-năl)	pertaining to the digestive system
gingiv/o	gum	**gingiva** (jĭn-jī'vah)	gum of the mouth
gloss/o	tongue	**hypoglossal** (hī"pō-glŏs'ăl)	underneath the tongue
hepat/o, hepatic/o	liver	**hepatology** (hĕp"ah-tŏl'ŏ-jē)	study of the liver
ile/o	ileum	**ileitis** (ĭl"ē-ī'tĭs)	inflammation of the ileum
		ileocecostomy (ĭl'ē-ō-sē-kŏs'tō-mē)	surgical opening between the ileum and cecum
jejun/o	jejunum	**jejunorrhaphy** (jē"joo-nor'ă-fē)	surgical repair of the jejunum

continues

Root	Meaning	Example	Definition
lapar/o	abdominal wall	**laparotomy** (lăp-ah-rŏt'ō-mē)	incision into the abdomen
laryng/o	larynx	**laryngitis** (lăr"ĭn-jī'tĭs)	inflammation of the larynx
		laryngoscope (lah-rĭng'gō-skōp)	instrument for viewing the larynx
odont/o	tooth	**odontic** (ō-dŏn'tĭk)	pertaining to the teeth
pancreat/o	pancreas	**pancreatalgia** (păn"krē-ā-tăl'jē-ă)	pain in the pancreas
peritone/o	peritoneum	**peritoneopathy** (pĕr"ĭ-tō-nē-ŏp'ăth-ē)	any disordered condition of the peritoneum
phag/o	to eat	**dysphagia** (dĭs-fā'jē-ah)	difficulty in swallowing
		phagocyte (făg'ō-sīt)	any cell that "eats" other cells
pharyng/o	pharynx	**pharyngeal** (făh-rĭn'jē-ăl)	pertaining to the pharynx
		pharyngitis (făr"ĭn-jī'tĭs)	inflammation of the pharynx
proct/o	anus and rectum	**proctology** (prŏk-tŏl'ō-jē)	branch of medicine dealing with the anus and rectum
pyl/o, pylor/o	pylorus	**gastropyloric** (găs"trō-pī-lor'ĭk)	pertaining to the stomach and pylorus
		pyloric (pī-lor'ik)	pertaining to the pylorus
rect/o	rectum	**rectoclysis** (rĕk-tŏk'lī-sĭs)	slow introduction of fluid into the rectum
sial/o	salivary	**sialogram** (sī-ăl'ō-grăm)	film produced by sialography
sigmoid/o	sigmoid colon	**sigmoidostomy** (sĭg-moyd-ŏs'tō-mē)	creation of an artificial anus in the sigmoid flexure
stomat/o, stom/o	mouth	**stomatic** (stō-măt'ĭk)	pertaining to the mouth

Word Element Practice Exercises

WORD ELEMENTS

Provide the correct word element to complete the following words.

1. branch of medicine dealing with the anus and rectum ______________ ology
2. underneath the tongue hypo ______________
3. any cell that "eats" other cells ______________ cyte
4. incision into the abdomen ______________ otomy
5. the gum of the mouth ______________ a
6. pertaining to the esophagus ______________ eal
7. any disease of the intestines ______________ pathy
8. pertaining to the abdomen ______________ iac
9. difficulty in swallowing dys ______________ ia
10. calculi in the common bile duct ______________ lithiasis

MATCHING

Match the word elements to their meanings.

1. ________ any disorder of the peritoneum
2. ________ colostomy that joins cecum and colon
3. ________ excision of gall bladder
4. ________ inflammation of the lip
5. ________ inflammation of the duodenum
6. ________ inflammation of ileum
7. ________ instrument for viewing the larynx
8. ________ pain in the pancreas
9. ________ pertaining to teeth
10. ________ pertaining to bile
11. ________ pertaining to the pharynx
12. ________ pertaining to the mouth
13. ________ slow introduction of fluid into the rectum
14. ________ study of the liver
15. ________ surgically created opening in the abdominal wall to drain intestines
16. ________ pertaining to the stomach and intestines
17. ________ pertaining to the digestive system
18. ________ pertaining to the pylorus
19. ________ film produced by sialography
20. ________ creation of a stoma in the sigmoid colon

a. biliary
b. cecocolostomy
c. cheilitis
d. cholecystectomy
e. colostomy
f. duodenitis
g. gastroenteric
h. gastrointestinal
i. hepatology
j. ileitis
k. laryngoscope
l. odontic
m. pancreatalgia
n. peritoneopathy
o. pharyngeal
p. pyloric
q. rectoclysis
r. sialogram
s. sigmoidostomy
t. stomatic

SPELLING

Rewrite the misspelled words.

1. biliousness ______
2. annus ______
3. laryngitis ______
4. apendectomy ______
5. cholesistitis ______
6. jejunorhaphy ______
7. gastropiloric ______
8. iliosecostomy ______
9. cholangitis ______
10. cholidochojejunostomy ______

WORD ELEMENT

Give the meaning of each word element. Then use your dictionary to find a new word that contains each of the word elements. Specify whether the new word is a noun or an adjective by placing N or A in the last column.

Word Element	Meaning	Word	N or A
1. an/o			
2. append/o			
3. appendic/o			
4. bil/i			
5. cec/o			
6. celi/o			
7. cel/o			
8. cheil/o			
9. chil/o			
10. choledoch/o			
11. chol/e			
12. chol/o			
13. cholangi/o			
14. col/o			
15. colon/o			
16. cyst/o			
17. duoden/o			
18. enter/o			
19. esophag/o			
20. gastr/o			
21. gingiv/o			
22. gloss/o			

Word Element	Meaning	Word	N or A
23. hepat/o	______	______	______
24. hepatic/o	______	______	______
25. ile/o	______	______	______
26. jejun/o	______	______	______
27. lapar/o	______	______	______
28. laryng/o	______	______	______
29. odont/o	______	______	______
30. pancreat/o	______	______	______
31. peritone/o	______	______	______
32. phag/o	______	______	______
33. pharyng/o	______	______	______
34. proct/o	______	______	______
35. pyl/o	______	______	______
36. pylor/o	______	______	______
37. rect/o	______	______	______
38. sial/o	______	______	______
39. sigmoid/o	______	______	______
40. stomat/o	______	______	______
41. stom/o	______	______	______

Working Practice

DIAGNOSTIC PROCEDURES

Word	Pronunciation	Definition
General		
cholangioscopy	kō"lăn-jē-ŏs'kō-pē	visual examination of the bile ducts with a fiberoptic endoscope
colonoscopy	kō"lŏn-ŏs'kō-pē	visual examination of the colon using a flexible colonoscope (see Figure 13-4)
endoscopic retrograde cholangiopancre-atophotography (ERCP)	ĕn-dō-skŏp'ĭk rĕt'rō-grād kō-lăn"jē-ō-păn"krē-ah-tŏg'rah-fē	visual examination of the bile and pancreatic ducts by injecting contrast medium through their opening into the intestinal tract by using an endoscope; if a blockage is found, the physician may be able to use one of the following procedures to remove or relieve the obstruction: sphincterotomy, duct dilation and stenting.

continues

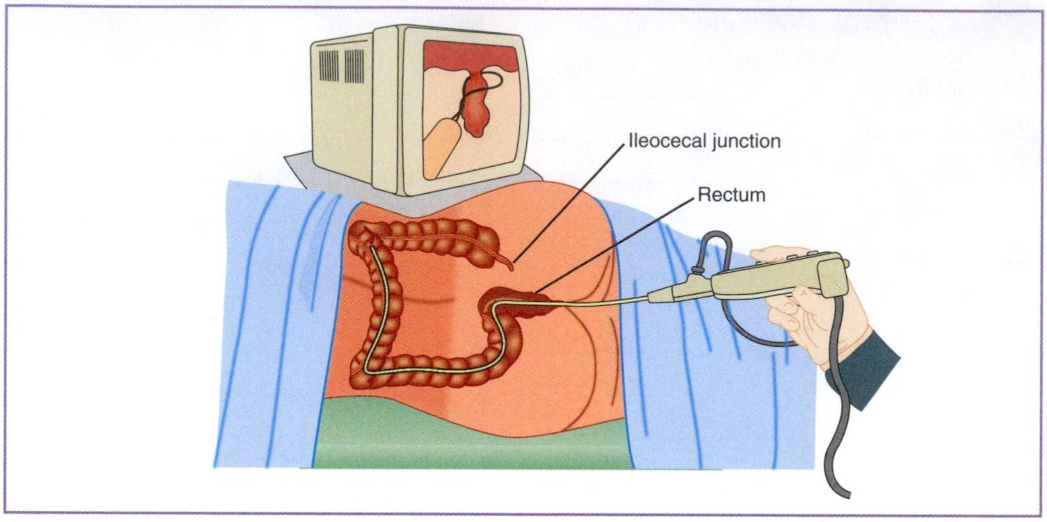

FIGURE 13-4
Colonoscopy

DIAGNOSTIC PROCEDURES		
Word	**Pronunciation**	**Definition**
enteroscopy	ĕn"tĕr-ŏs'kō-pē	visual examination of the small intestine using a long endoscope
esophageal motility	ĕ-sŏf"ah-jē'ăl mō-tĭl'ĭ-tē	diagnostic test that records movement and studies pressure in the esophagus; esophageal manometry evaluates swallowing problems
esophageal pH studies		records acid reflux events using a pH sensor attached to a catheter inserted through the nose or a pH sensor attached directly to the esophageal mucosa
esophagogastroduodenoscopy (EGD) (panendoscopy)	ĕ-sŏf"ah-gō-găs"trō-dū"ō-dĕ-nŏs'kō-pē (păn"ĕn-dŏs'kō-pē)	visual examination of the esophagus, stomach, and duodenum with a flexible gastroscope
esophagoscopy	ĕ-sŏf"ah-gŏs'kō-pē	visual examination of the esophagus using an esophagoscope
liver biopsy		removal of a tissue sample from the liver for microscopic examination
paracentesis (abdominocentesis)	păr"ah-sĕn-tē'sĭs (ăb-dŏm"ĭ-nō-sĕn-tē'sĭs)	needle puncture of the abdominal (peritoneal) cavity to remove fluid for laboratory examination
sigmoidoscopy (proctoscopy)	sĭg"moy-dŏs'kō-pē (prŏk-tŏs'kō-pē)	direct examination of the anus, rectum, and part of the sigmoid colon using a flexible sigmoidoscope
videocapsule endoscopy	ĕn-dŏs'kō-pē	visual examination of the esophagus, stomach, and small intestine by a miniature camera inside a capsule that is swallowed
Nuclear Medicine		
cholescintigraphy (HIDA scan)	kō"lē-sĭn-tig'ră-fē	nuclear medicine scanning procedure to evaluate gallbladder function

continues

DIAGNOSTIC PROCEDURES		
Word	Pronunciation	Definition
Nuclear Medicine *(continued)*		
gastric emptying study		a nuclear medicine imaging study done to evaluate the ability of the stomach to empty an ingested meal
liver scan		injection of a radioactive substance intravenously, which then circulates through the blood to the liver; a special camera takes a picture of the liver
Radiology		
abdominal magnetic resonance imaging (MRI)		visualization of the contents of the abdomen using magnetic resonance imaging
abdominal ultrasonogram	ŭl"tră-sŏn'ō-grăm	record made by imaging abdominal viscera from reflected sound waves
barium enema, air contrast		x-ray procedure that introduces first barium and then air into the colon to give added contrast
barium enema (BE)		infusion of barium, a radiopaque contrast medium, into the colon to better visualize the lower intestinal tract during x-ray examination (see Figure 13-5)
CT of the abdomen		detailed cross section of structures within the abdomen
fluoroscopy	floo"or-ŏs'kŏ-pē	real-time x-ray examination of organs to study their condition
intravenous cholangiography	ĭn-tră-vē'nŭs kō-lăn"iē-ŏg-ră-fē	x-ray procedure whereby a special dye is injected intravenously and then excreted into the bile ducts for study of the common bile duct primarily and the gallbladder secondarily

continues

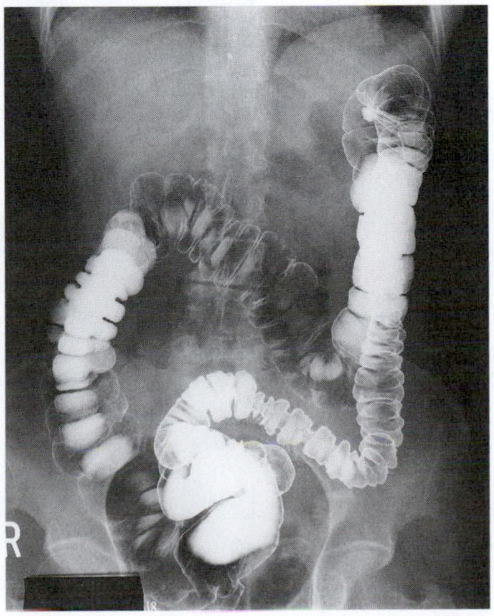

FIGURE 13-5
AP Colon with Barium Enema

DIAGNOSTIC PROCEDURES		
Word	**Pronunciation**	**Definition**
Radiology *(continued)*		
oral cholecystogram	kō"lē-sĭs'tō-grăm	x-ray of the gallbladder, which is made visible by orally administered dye; the dye is absorbed, excreted into the bile, and concentrated by the gallbladder
percutaneous transhepatic cholangiography (PTHC)	pĕr"kū-tā'nē-ŭs trăns-hĕ-păt'ĭk kō-lăn"jē-ŏg'rah-fē	x-ray procedure whereby a contrast medium is injected through the liver into the bile duct to detect an obstruction
small bowel follow-through (SBFT)		x-ray using barium to examine the small intestine at timed intervals
upper gastrointestinal series (UGI) (barium swallow)	găs"trō-ĭn-tĕs'tĭ-năl	x-ray study of the esophagus, stomach, and duodenum by orally administering a contrast medium (see Figure 13-6)
Laboratory Tests		
gastric analysis		study of acid secretion by the stomach
stool examination (ova and parasite [O&P])		analysis of stool to determine the presence or parasites
stool guaiac	gwī'ăk	chemical test for the presence of blood in stool
Blood Tests		
amylase	ăm'ĭ-lās	pancreatic enzyme that can be assayed in the blood to detect pancreatitis

continues

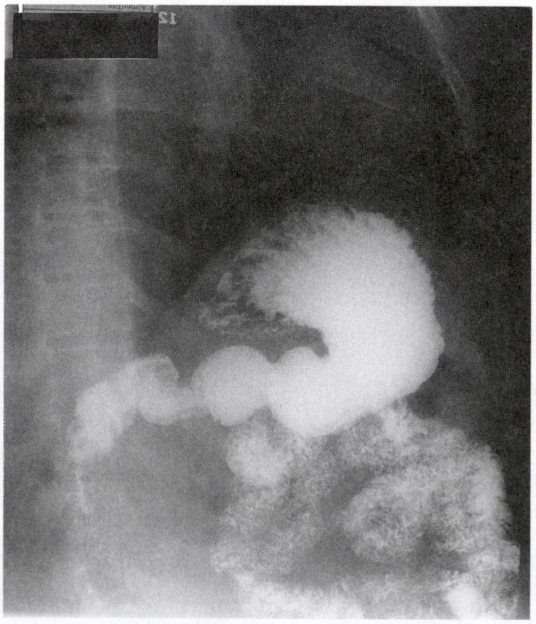

FIGURE 13-6
Single-Contrast Upper GI

Source: Delmar/Cengage Learning

DIAGNOSTIC PROCEDURES		
Word	Pronunciation	Definition
Blood Tests *(continued)*		
carcinoembryonic antigen (CEA)	kăr"sĭ-nō-ĕm"brē-ŏn'ĭk an'tĭ-gĕn	determination of whether an antigen is present in the patient's blood that is indicative of certain types of carcinoma when abnormally high, especially those arising in the colon; the antigen may also be elevated in other types of cancer and in some noncancerous conditions
total iron binding capacity (TIBC) and serum iron (SI)		tests used to diagnose hemochromatosis, a disorder of iron absorption that results in excess iron throughout the body; more often used to diagnose iron-deficiency anemia that may result from gastrointestinal blood loss
Liver Function Tests These tests are performed to diagnose liver-related problems.		
bilirubin and urobilinogen in urine	bĭl-ĭ-rŭ'bĭn ū"rō-bī-lĭn'ō-jĕn	
gamma-glutamyl transpeptidase (GGT)	trăns-pĕp'tĭ-dās	
5-nucleotidase	noo"klē-ŏt-ĭ'dās	
serum alkaline phosphatase (alkphos)	fŏs'fă-tās	
serum bilirubin (icterus index)		
aspartate aminotransferase (AST)	ă-spăr'tāt ă-mē"nō-trăns'fĕr-ās	
alanine aminotransfer-ase (ALT) (also SGPT)	ăl'ă-nēn ă-mē"nō-trăns'fĕr-ās	
serum lactate dehydrogenase (LDH)	dē-hī'drŏj-ĕn-ās	
Protein Metabolism Tests These tests measure the metabolism of proteins.		
albumin globulin ratio (A/G)		
prothrombin time (ProTime, PT)		
serum albumin (alb)		
serum globulin		
serum protein		
electrophoresis (SPEP)	ē-lĕk"trō-fō-rē'sĭs	
serum total proteins (TP)		

DIAGNOSES		
Word	Pronunciation	Definition
Esophagus		
achalasia	āk"ă-lā'zē-ă	disorder caused by lack of coordinated movement of esophageal muscles and by the failure of the sphincter muscle at the lower end of the esophagus to relax
esophageal varices	ē-sŏf"ah-jē'ăl văr'ĭ-sēz	unusually high pressure in esophageal veins that cause them to enlarge and occasionally hemorrhage
gastroesophageal reflux disease (GERD)	găs"trō-ē-sŏf"ah-jē'ăl	condition occurring when acid-containing stomach contents regurgitate from stomach to esophagus
hiatal hernia	hī-ā-tăl	a protrusion of part of the stomach through the diaphragm into the chest cavity (see Figure 13-7)
reflux esophagitis	ē-sŏf-ah-gī'tŭs	inflammation of the esophagus caused by backward flow of stomach acid into the esophagus
Stomach		
cancer of the stomach		malignant tumor of the stomach
dyspepsia (indigestion)	dis-pĕp'sē-ah	syndrome with upper abdominal pain, bloating, and nausea
gastritis	găs-trī'tĭs	inflammation of the stomach; may be acute or chronic; may be caused by Helicobacter

continues

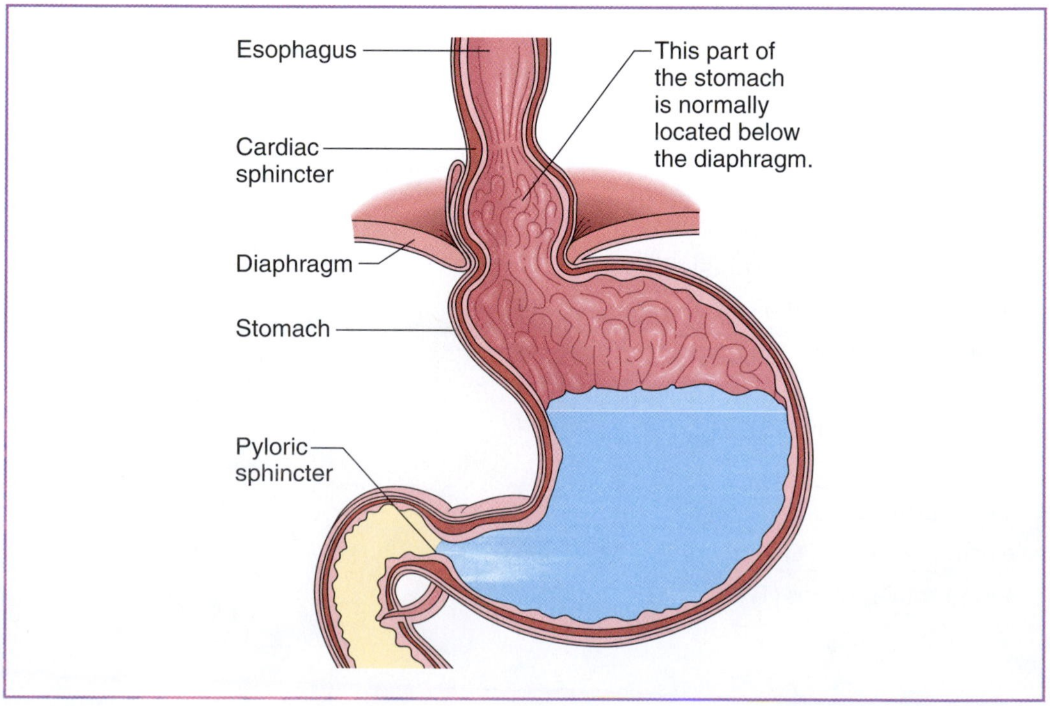

FIGURE 13-7
Hiatal Hernia

DIAGNOSES		
Word	**Pronunciation**	**Definition**
Stomach *(continued)*		
peptic ulcer		ulceration through the mucous membrane of the esophagus, stomach, or duodenum; called gastric ulcer in the stomach and duodenal ulcer in the duodenum (see Figure 13-8)
Zollinger-Ellison syndrome		condition caused by tuberous secretion of gastrin, a hormone that causes gastric hyperacidity with secondary ulcers and/or diarrhea
Small Intestine		
Viral Infections		
rotavirus	rō'tă-vī"rŭs	acute viral infection often found in child care centers and homes for the elderly
Norwalk virus		an acute viral infection, also called winter vomiting disease
cytomegalovirus	sī"tō-mĕg"ă-lō-vī'rŭs	an acute viral infection and common cause of diarrhea in individuals with AIDS; a species specific herpes virus
Bacterial Infections		
bacterial overgrowth		a condition characterized by diarrhea and malabsorption caused by accumulation of bacteria in the small intestine
Campylobacter infections	kăm"pĭ-lō-băk'tĕr	infections most commonly occurring in children younger than 1 year of age or in young adults; the source seems to be raw foods such as milk and poultry

continues

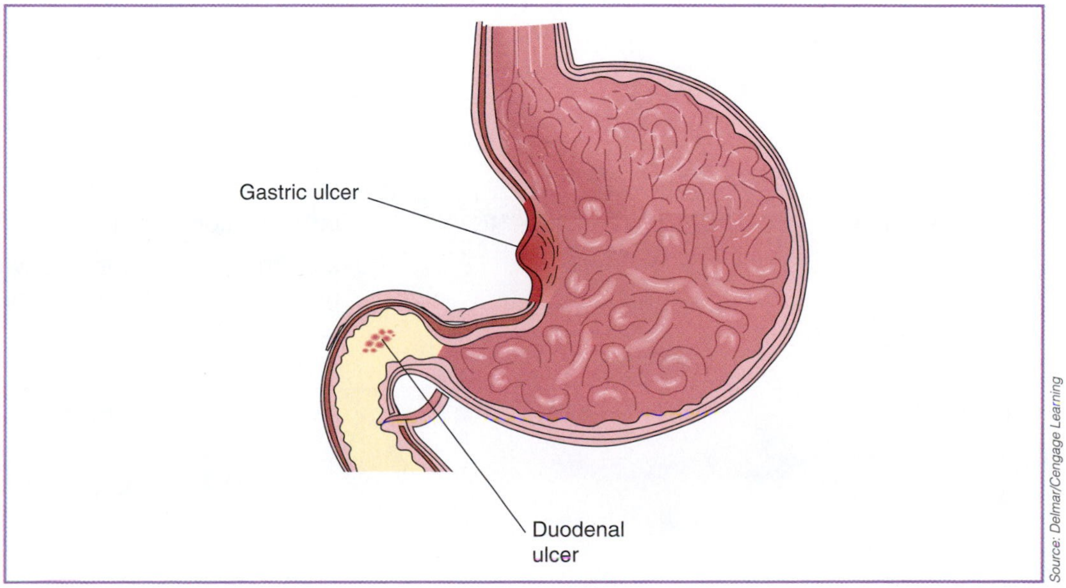

FIGURE 13-8
Peptic Ulcers

DIAGNOSES		
Word	**Pronunciation**	**Definition**
Small Intestine *(continued)*		
Helicobacter pylori (*H. pylori*)	hĕl"ĭ-kō-băk-tĕr pī-lor'ī	organisms responsible for most gastric and duodenal ulcers
Salmonella	săl"mō-nĕl'ah	a gram-negative bacteria that may cause intestinal infection; found in meats and dairy products; causes mild to fatal food poisoning
Shigella	shĭ-gĕl'lă	bacteria causing mild-to-fatal dysentery; found primarily in developing countries and in children ages 1 to 5 years
Parasitic Infections		
Cryptosporidium	krĭp"tō-spō-rĭd'ē-ŭm	an infection that is the common cause of diarrhea in AIDS patients; may occur in otherwise-healthy individuals
Entamoeba histolytica	ĕn"ta-mē'bă hĭs"tō-lĭt'ĭk-ah	a diarrheal infection that is common in the world but not in the United States; common in homosexual men
Giardia lamblia	jē-ăr'dē-ah lăm'blē-ah	infection that is one of the most common parasitic causes of diarrhea in the United States; the source is a contaminated water supply
Other GI-related Conditions		
antibiotic-associated diarrhea		antibiotics may alter the bowel environment resulting in certain bacterial growth and in inflammation
celiac sprue	sē'lē-ăk sproo	malabsorption and other difficulties from gluten (a wheat protein) intolerance
Crohn's disease (regional enteritis)	krōnz	chronic inflammatory bowel disease usually affecting the ileum, colon, or both structures; it is one type of inflammatory bowel disease (IBD)
duodenal ulcer	dŭ-ō-dē'năl	peptic ulcer in duodenum
food poisoning		a condition caused by eating contaminated foods, which results in the production of toxins such as those produced by *Staphylococcus aureus, Bacillus cereus*, and *Clostridium botulinum*
gastroenteritis	găs"trō-ĕn-tĕr-ī"tĭs	inflammation of both the stomach and intestines
inguinal hernia	ĭng'gwĭ-năl	a protrusion of a loop of bowel through the groin area; usually requires corrective surgery
malabsorption		inability of the small intestine to absorb nutrients and syndrome minerals
peritonitis	pĕr"ĭ-tō-nī'tĭs	an inflammation of the peritoneal lining

continues

DIAGNOSES		
Word	**Pronunciation**	**Definition**
Colon		
appendicitis	ă-pēn'dĭ-sī'tĭs	inflammation, swelling, and accumulation of pus in the appendix resulting in abdominal pain, nausea, and/or vomiting; usually requires surgery (see Figure 13-9)
colorectal cancer	kō"lō-rĕk'tăl	carcinoma of the colon or rectum
congenital megacolon (Hirschsprung's disease)		a congenital condition marked by enlarged colon (as a result of nerve damage) resulting in the inability of the colon to move feces
diverticulitis	dī"vĕr-tĭk"ū-lī'tĭs	inflammation of a diverticulum
diverticulosis	dī"vĕr-tĭk"ū-lō'sĭs	presence of diverticula (see Figure 13-10)
dysentery	dĭs'ĕn-tĕr"ē	acute inflammation caused by the invasion of microorganisms into the colon lining; results in often-times bloody diarrhea

continues

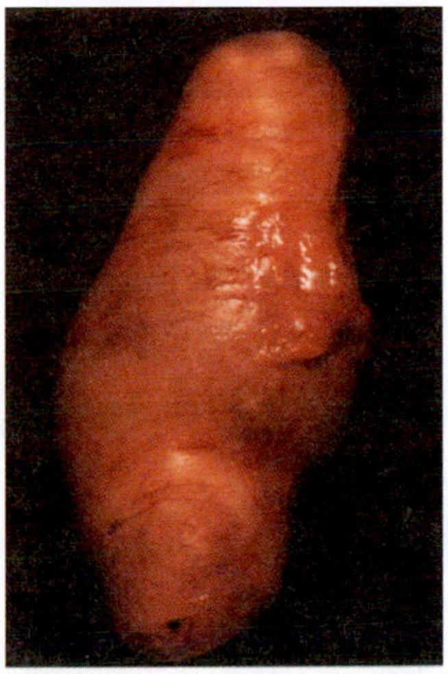

FIGURE 13-9
Inflamed Appendix After Surgical Removal

Source: Delmar/Cengage Learning

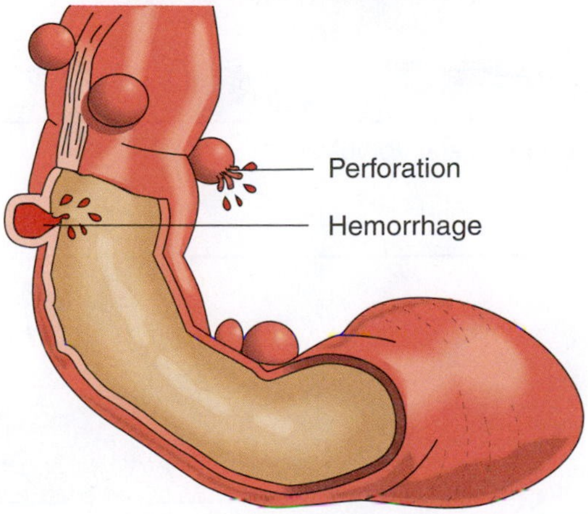

FIGURE 13-10
Diverticulosis

Source: Delmar/Cengage Learning

DIAGNOSES		
Word	Pronunciation	Definition
Colon *(continued)*		
granulomatous colitis	grăn"ŭ-lŏm'ă-tŭs kō-lī'tĭs	inflammation of the colon characterized by nodules of granular tissue; frequently involves all layers of the intestinal wall; also called Crohn's colitis
ileus	ĭl'ē-ŭs	disruption of intestinal activity because peristalsis slows or stops; commonly occurs after surgery (usually temporary)
inflammatory bowel disease (IBD)		descriptive term usually referring to ulcerative colitis or Crohn's disease
intestinal obstruction		partial or complete obstruction in small intestine or colon that prevents movement of the products of digestion
intussusception	ĭn"tŭ-sū-sĕp'shŭn	disorder occurring when a portion of the intestine telescopes into another segment of the intestine (See Figure 13-11A)
irritable bowel syndrome (IBS)		abnormally increased motility of the large and small (spastic colon) intestine that may be associated with emotional stress
polyps	pŏl'ĭps	small, tumorlike growths that project from the mucous membrane surface of the alimentary tract (see Figure 13-12)

continues

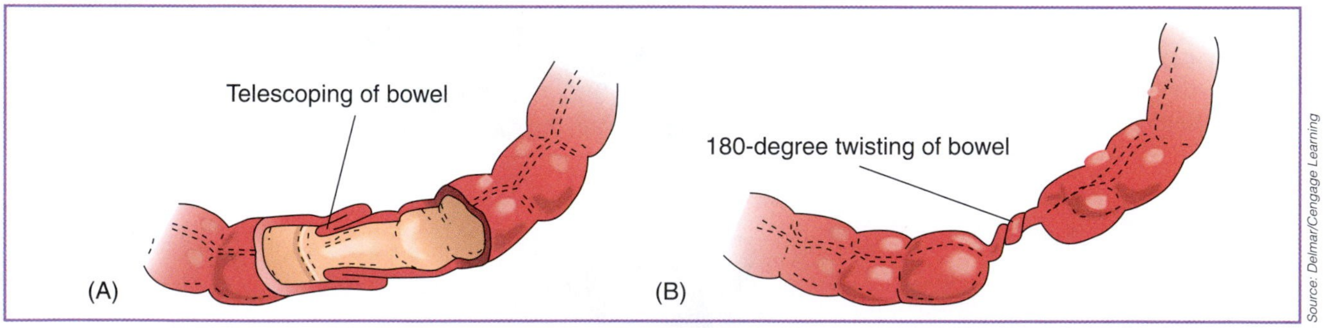

FIGURE 13-11 (A) Intussusception and (B) Volvulus

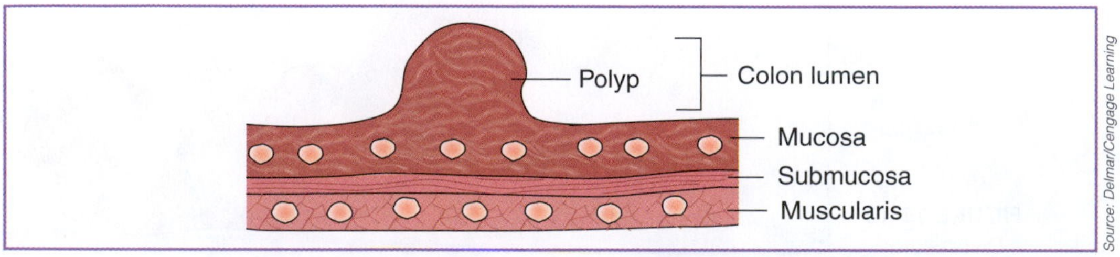

FIGURE 13-12 Colon Polyp

DIAGNOSES		
Word	**Pronunciation**	**Definition**
Colon *(continued)*		
scleroderma	sklē"rō'dĕr'mah	a condition marked by atrophy of the muscular walls of the intestines and esophagus resulting in impairment of movement of the intestine and the absorption of nutrients
short bowel syndrome		loss of a significant part of the intestines or disease involving a sufficient length of the small intestine with consequent impaired nutrient absorption
ulcerative colitis	ŭl'sĕr-ā-tĭv kō-lī'tĭs	ulceration of the colonic mucosa, cause unknown; it may cause diarrhea, loss of weight, or anemia, and increases the risk of developing colon cancer (see Figure 13-13)
volvulus	vŏl'vū-lŭs	twisting or looping of the intestine, often requiring emergency surgery (see Figure 13-11B)
Whipple's disease	(lĭp"-ō-dĭs'-trō-fē)	a disease characterized by fatty deposits caused by an (intestinal infectious organism, resulting in lipodystrophy) malabsorption of nutrients
Anus and Rectum		
abscess		collection of pus in tissue near the rectum, usually as a result of infected anal glands
fissure	fish'ūr	split in the epithelial surface of the anal canal
fistula	fĭs'tŭ-lah	abnormal passage between organs
hemorrhoids	hĕm'ō-roydz	varicose dilation of veins in the anal canal or rectum
pruritus ani	proo-rī'tŭs	itching around the anal area
rectal prolapse		a condition where the end of the rectum protrudes out of the anal canal

continues

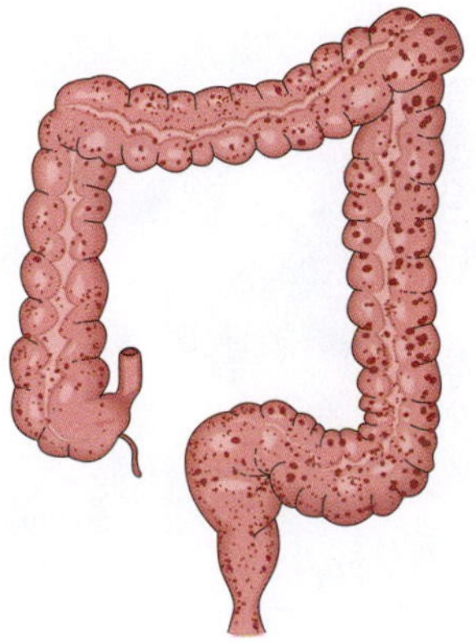

FIGURE 13-13
Ulcerative Colitis

Source: Delmar/Cengage Learning

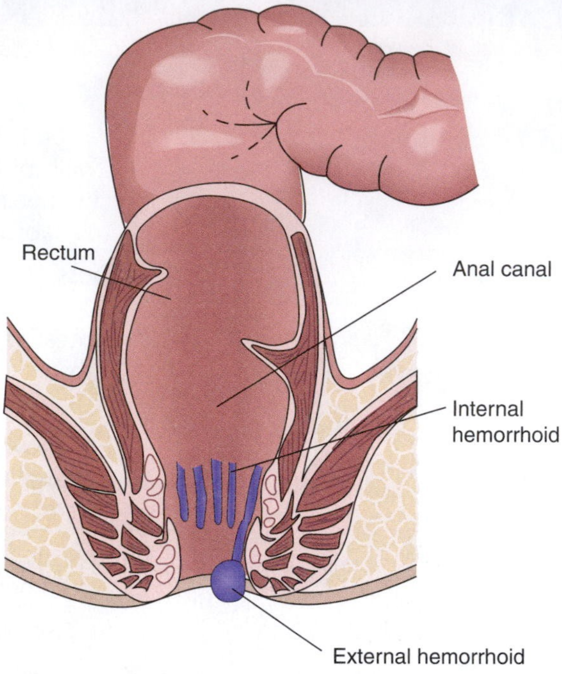

FIGURE 13-14 Hemorrhoids: Internal and External

DIAGNOSES		
Word	**Pronunciation**	**Definition**
Liver, Gallbladder, and Pancreas		
Liver		
cirrhosis	sĭ-rō'sĭs	scarring of the liver associated with a destruction of liver cells (see Figure 13-15); complications include varicosities, splenomegaly, GI hemorrhage, ascites, edema, jaundice, and hepatic encephalopathy
hepatitis	hĕp"ă-tī'tĭs	inflammation of the liver; may be acute or chronic hepatitis (A, B, and C are the most common)

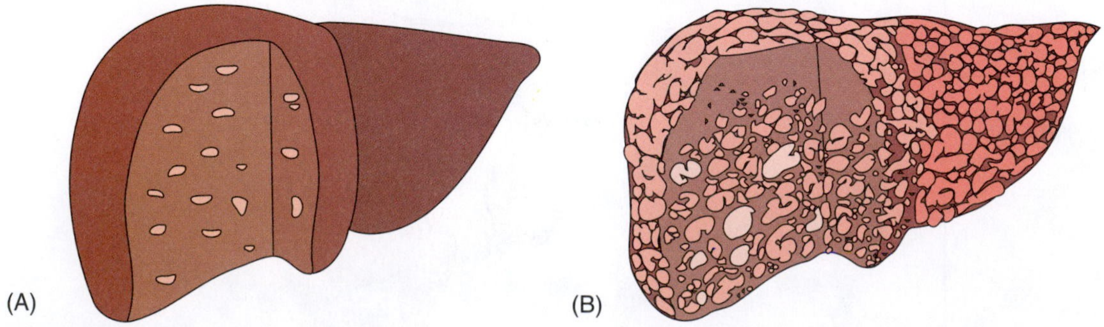

FIGURE 13-15 (A) Normal vs (B) Cirrhotic Liver

DIAGNOSES

Word	Pronunciation	Definition
Liver, Gallbladder, and Pancreas *(continued)*		
liver cancer		malignant tumor in the liver; usually occurs in the setting of cirrhosis
Gallbladder		
cholecystitis	kō"lē-sĭs-tī'tĭs	inflammation of gallbladder generally caused by obstruction of bile flow due to a gallstone
cholelithiasis	kō"lē-lĭ-thī'ă-sĭs	presence of gallstones in the gallbladder (see Figure 13-16)
choledocholithiasis	kō-lĕd"ō-kō-lĭ-thī'ă-sĭs	presence of gallstones in the common bile duct
Pancreas		
pancreatic cancer	păn'krē-ăt-ĭk	malignant tumor that occurs in the pancreas
pancreatitis	păn"krē-ă-tī'tĭs	inflammation of the pancreas; may be acute or chronic

TREATMENT PROCEDURES

Word	Pronunciation	Definition
anal fissurectomy	fĭsh-ūr-ĕk'tō-mē	removal of an anal fissure
appendectomy	ăp"ĕn-dĕk'tō-mē	removal of the appendix
argon plasma coagulation		procedure using an endoscope to deliver a burst of thermal energy or heat to a lesion in the stomach, esophagus, or intestine

continues

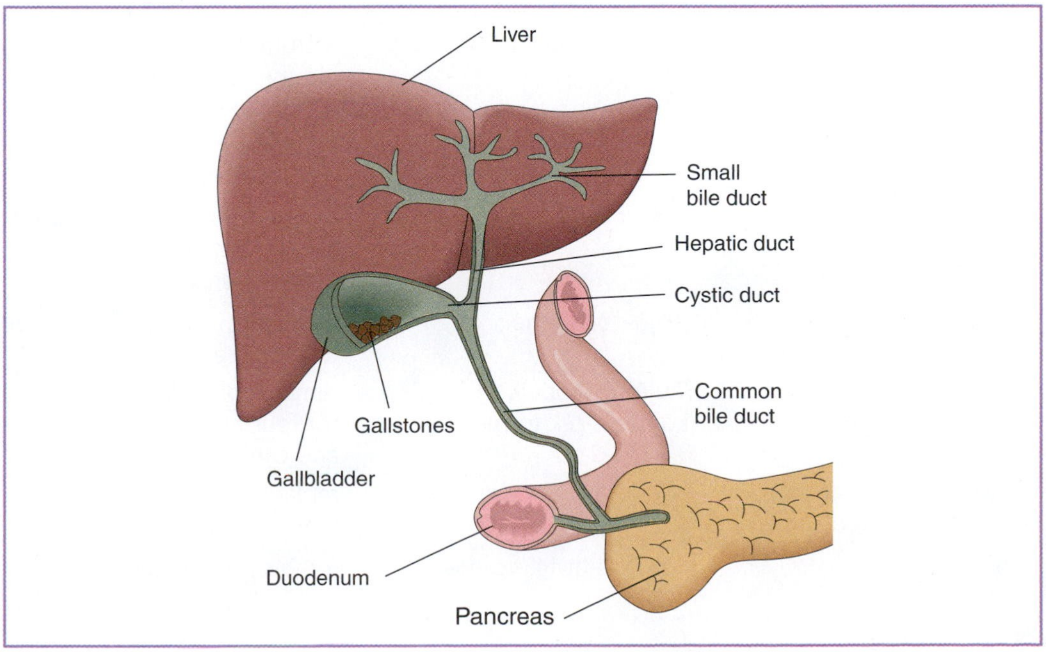

FIGURE 13-16
Cholelithiasis

TREATMENT PROCEDURES		
Word	**Pronunciation**	**Definition**
cholecystectomy	kō"lē-sĭs-tĕk'tō-mē	excision of the gallbladder
colectomy	kō-lĕk'tō-mē	excision of part or all of the colon
colostomy	kō-lŏs'tō-mē	surgical creation of an opening between the colon and body surface
duct dilation and stenting		procedure using a balloon catheter to stretch a narrowed opening
esophageal and colonic stent placement		procedure using an endoscope to place stents in the esophagus, duodenum and colon, as well as the bile duct system, or to open areas blocked by tumors or other obstructions
esophagogastrostomy	ē-sŏf"ă-gō-găs-trŏs'tō-mē	creation of an opening between the esophagus and stomach
esophagostomy	ē-sŏf"ă-gŏs'tō-mē	surgical creation of an opening in the esophagus
excision of Meckel's diverticulum	dī"vĕr-tĭk'ū-lūm	surgical removal of a congenital outpouching of the wall of the ileum
herniorrhaphy	hĕr-nē-or'ă-fē	surgical repair of a hernia
fistulectomy	fĭs"tū-lĕk'tō-mē	surgical removal of a fistula
gastrectomy	găs-trĕk'tō-mē	excision of all or part of the stomach
gastrostomy	găs-trōs'tō-mē	placement of a tube into the stomach; may be done endoscopically, radiologically, or surgically
hemorrhoid ligation	hĕm'ō-royd lī-gā'shŭn	removal of internal hemorrhoid groupings using a rubber band technique
hemorrhoidectomy	hĕm"ō-royd-ĕk'tō-mē	excision of a varicose dilation of a vein
extracorporeal shock wave lithotripsy (ESWL)	ĕks"tră-kor-pŏr'ē-ăl, lĭth'ō-trĭp"sē	ultrasound crushing of calculi in the gallbladder or kidney
ileo-anal anastomosis	ĭl"ē-ō-ā'năl ă-năs"tō-mō'sĭs	procedure to remove the entire colon and rectum through the abdominal wall, but preserving the sphincter muscles of the anus; a pouch is created in the ileum, which is then attached to the anus; a temporary ileostomy is used to collect fecal material until the juncture is healed
ileostomy	ĭl"ē-ŏs'tō-mē	a surgical passage through the abdominal wall into the small intestine (ileum) for drainage of fecal material
jejunostomy	jē"jū-nŏs'tō-mē	creation of an opening between the jejunum and the surface of the abdominal wall
laparoscopic cholecystectomy	lăp'ă-rō-skŏp"ĭk kō"lē-sĭs-tĕk'tō-mē	removal of gallbladder by making four punctures for four tiny tubes through which instruments and cameras are placed
liver transplantation		replacement of liver after other treatments have been exhausted
pancreatectomy	păn"krē-at-tĕk'tō-mē	removal of the pancreas

continues

TREATMENT PROCEDURES		
Word	**Pronunciation**	**Definition**
sphincterotomy	sfĭngk"tĕr-ŏt'ō-mē	a procedure to cut the muscle sphincter of the bile or pancreatic duct to remove stones
splenectomy	splē-nĕk'tō-mē	removal of the spleen
vagotomy	vā-gŏt'ō-mē	surgical transection of the fibers of the vagus nerve; frequently done to decrease acid secretion of the stomach in patients with ulcers

MEDICATIONS PRESCRIBED	
Trade Name	**Generic Name**
Anthelminthics	
Antepar	piperazine citrate
Antiminth	pyrantel pamoate
Vermox	mebendazole
Antibiotics	
Achromycin, Sumycin	tetracycline
Flagyl	metronidazole
Vancocin	vancomycin HCl
Anticholinergics/Antispasmodics	
Anaspaz, Levsin	l-hyoscyamine sulfate
Bentyl	dicyclomine HCl
Clindex, Clinoxide, Librax	clidinium, chlordiazepoxide
Donnatal	atropine, scopolamine, hyoscyamine, phenobarbital
Pro-Banthine	propantheline bromide
Robinul	glycopyrrolate
Antidiarrheals	
Bacid, Lactinex	lactobacillus
Imodium	loperamide
Lomotil	diphenoxylate with atropine
Pepto-Bismol	bismuth subsalicylate
Digestive Enzymes	
Ultrase, Pancrease	pancrelipase
Creon, Donnazyme	pancreatin
Gallstone Solubilizing Agents	
Actigall	ursodiol

continues

MEDICATIONS PRESCRIBED	
Trade Name	**Generic Name**
GI Stimulants	
Reglan	metoclopramide
$H_{(2)}$ Antagonists	
Axid	nizatidine
Pepcid	famotidine
Tagamet	cimetidine
Zantac	ranitidine
Proton Pump Inhibitors	
Aciphex	rabeprazole sodium
Nexium	esomeprazole magnesium
Prevacid	lansoprazole
Prilosec	omeprazole
Protonix	pantoprazole sodium
Other Medications that Lower Acid Secretion and/or Protect Mucosa	
Cytotec	misoprostol
Carafate	sucralfate
Over-the-Counter Antacids	
Alternagel	
Amphojel	
Gaviscon	
Maalox	
Milk of Magnesia (MOM)	
Mylanta	
Riopan	
Over-the-Counter Laxatives	
Cascara Sagrada	
Chronulac, Duphalac (lactulose)	
Citrucel	
Colace (docusate Na)	
Colyte, Golytely	
Dulcolax (bisacodyl)	
Ex-Lax	
Feen-a-mint	
Fleet Prep	

continues

MEDICATIONS PRESCRIBED	
Trade Name	**Generic Name**
Over-the-Counter Laxatives *(continued)*	
Metamucil	
Milk of Magnesia (MOM)	
Perdiem	
Senokot	
Surfak (docusate Ca)	
X-Prep	
Ulcer Protectant	
Carafate	sucralfate

ABBREVIATIONS	
Abdo, abd	abdomen; abdominal
A.C., a.c.	before eating
A/G	albumin globulin ration
alb	serum albumin
ALT	alanine aminotransferase
AST	aspartate aminotransferase
BE	barium enema
BW	body weight
CEA	carcinoembryonic antigen
DAT	diet as tolerated
EGD	esophagogastroduodenoscopy
ERCP	endoscopic retrograde cholangiopancreatography
GERD	gastroesophageal reflux disease
GGT	gamma-glutamyl transpeptidase
GI	gastrointestinal
IBD	inflammatory bowel disease
IBS	irritable bowel syndrome
IVC	intravenous cholangiogram
LDH	serum lactate dehydrogenase
MRI	magnetic resonance imaging
NG	nasogastric
NT	nastotracheal intubation
O&P	ova and parasite
PC	after eating

continues

ABBREVIATIONS	
ProTime, PT	prothrombin time
PTHC	percutaneous transhepatic cholangiography
RDA	recommended daily allowance
SBFT	small bowel follow-through
SPEP	serum protein electrophoresis
TP	serum total proteins
TPN	total parenteral nutrition
UGI	upper gastrointestinal series
VCE	videocapsule endoscopy

Working Practice Review Exercises

MATCHING

Match the terms to their meanings.

1. _______ studies the esophagus, stomach, and duodenum through the oral administration of barium
2. _______ x-ray using barium to examine the small intestine
3. _______ studies mainly the common bile duct
4. _______ needle puncture of a cavity to remove fluid for laboratory examination
5. _______ examination of the colon using barium
6. _______ x-ray visualizing the gallbladder by orally administering dye
7. _______ radiopaque substance flows to the liver, and an x-ray is taken
8. _______ x-ray procedure that uses contrast medium injected through the liver into the bile duct to detect an obstruction
9. _______ diagnostic test that records movement and pressure in the esophagus
10. _______ visual examination of the bile and pancreatic ducts by using an endoscope
11. _______ visual examination of the bile ducts with an endoscope
12. _______ nuclear medicine scanning procedure to evaluate gallbladder function

a. barium enema
b. cholangioscopy
c. cholescintigraphy
d. endoscopic retrograde cholangiopancreatography
e. esophageal motility study
f. gastric analysis
g. intravenous cholangiography
h. liver scan
i. oral cholecystogram
j. paracentesis
k. percutaneous transhepatic cholangiography
l. small bowel follow through
m. total iron binding capacity
n. upper GI series
o. videocapsule endoscopy

13. _______ visual examination of esophagus, stomach, and small intestine by a miniature camera that is swallowed
14. _______ study of acid secretion by the stomach
15. _______ test to diagnose hemochromatosis or iron-deficiency anemia

IDENTIFICATION

Identify the following diagnoses.

1. absence of peristalsis in the intestine ____________________
2. inflammation of the diverticulum ____________________
3. acute viral infection often found in child care centers and homes for the elderly ____________________
4. scarring of the liver and associated with destruction of liver cells ____________________
5. inflammation caused by a backward flow of stomach acid into the esophagus ____________________
6. indigestion ____________________
7. inflammation of the liver ____________________
8. varicose dilation of veins in the anal canal or rectum ____________________
9. acute viral infection and common cause of diarrhea in individuals with AIDS ____________________
10. infection that is one of the most common parasitic causes of diarrhea in the United States ____________________
11. protrusion of a bowel loop through the groin area ____________________
12. split in the epithelial surface of the anal canal ____________________
13. another name for Whipple's disease, which is characterized by fatty deposits caused by an infectious organism ____________________
14. removal of or disease in a significant part of the intestines, which impairs nutrient absorption ____________________
15. congenital condition marked by an enlarged colon ____________________
16. organisms responsible for most gastric and duodenal ulcers ____________________
17. itching around the anal area ____________________
18. condition where end of rectum protrudes out of anal canal ____________________
19. presence of gallstones in the common bile duct ____________________
20. abnormal passage between organs ____________________

COMPLETION

Provide the correct treatment procedure to complete these statements.

1. ____________________ is the endoscopic delivery of a burst of thermal energy or heat to a lesion in the stomach, esophagus, or intestines.
2. ____________________ is a procedure using a balloon catheter to stretch a narrowed opening.

3. ____________________ is a surgical removal of congenital outpouching of ileum wall.
4. ____________________ is the removal of internal hemorrhoid groupings using a rubber band technique.
5. ____________________ is a procedure that uses ultrasound to crush calculi in the gallbladder or kidney.
6. ____________________ is a procedure to remove entire colon and rectum through abdominal wall, but preserving sphincter muscles.
7. ____________________ is a procedure to cut the muscle sphincter of bile or pancreatic duct to remove stones.

WORD ELEMENTS

Provide the correct word element to complete the following treatment procedures.

1. excision of the gallbladder ____________________ ectomy
2. creation of a new opening between the colon and body surface ____________________ ostomy
3. excision of a varicose dilation of a vein in the anal canal ____________________ ectomy
4. creation of an opening between the jejunum and the surface of the abdominal wall ____________________ ostomy
5. surgical removal of a fistula ____________________ ectomy
6. removal of an anal fissure ____________________ ectomy
7. excision of the appendix ____________________ ectomy
8. excision of all or part of the stomach ____________________ ectomy
9. surgical passage through the abdominal wall into the small intestine for drainage of fecal material ____________________ ostomy
10. surgical transection of the fibers of the vagus nerve ____________________ otomy

ABBREVIATIONS

Provide the correct term for the following abbreviations.

1. NG ____________________
2. CEA ____________________
3. alb ____________________
4. TPN ____________________
5. PT ____________________
6. IBS ____________________
7. ERCP ____________________
8. PTHC ____________________
9. IVC ____________________
10. IBD ____________________
11. abd ____________________
12. a.c. ____________________
13. BW ____________________
14. DAT ____________________
15. VCE ____________________

Dictionary Exercises

DICTIONARY EXERCISE 1

Use your dictionary to find the pronunciation and definition of the following words.

	Word	Pronunciation	Definition
1.	achlorhydria	________	________
2.	anorexia	________	________
3.	ascites	________	________
4.	esophagoduodenostomy	________	________
5.	fundus of the stomach	________	________
6.	eructation	________	________
7.	islets of Langerhans	________	________
8.	Meckel's diverticulum	________	________
9.	viscera	________	________
10.	trichobezoar	________	________
11.	esophagitis	________	________
12.	hepatorenal	________	________
13.	cholesterosis	________	________
14.	lactose intolerance	________	________

DICTIONARY EXERCISE 2

Select the correct meaning and provide the pronunciation where indicated.

1. hematochezia (________)
   a. refers to blood in the stool
   b. bright red blood discharged from the rectum
   c. without teeth
   d. feeding by stomach tube
2. enterolysis (________)
   a. loosening adhesions of the intestine
   b. a condition in which cholesterol materials are deposited in tissues
   c. cramping and painful straining when passing a stool
   d. vomiting of blood
3. cholangitis (________)
   a. inflammation of stomach and duodenum
   b. inflammation of the intestine
   c. inflammation of the gallbladder
   d. inflammation of the bile ducts
4. varix (________)
   a. internal organs of any of the three great cavities of the body
   b. protrusion of part of an organ through the wall of its cavity
   c. enlarged vein
   d. jaundice
5. gavage (________)
   a. feeding by stomach tube
   b. telescoping of a tubular organ
   c. washing out of an organ or a cavity
   d. vomiting of blood
6. hematemesis (________)
   a. refers to blood in the stool
   b. vomiting of blood
   c. irrigation or washing out of an organ or a cavity
   d. passing of gaseous material from the stomach through the mouth

7. esophagitis (____________________)
   a. inflammation of the stomach
   b. inflammation of the intestine
   c. inflammation of the bile ducts
   d. inflammation of the esophagus
8. paralytic ileus (____________________)
   a. loss of peristalsis
   b. resection of the ileum
   c. islets of Langerhans
   d. inflammation of the ileum
9. melena (____________________)
   a. referring to the color black, especially with respect to blood in the feces
   b. without teeth
   c. benign tumor of the bile duct
   d. round mass of anything
10. hyperchlorhydria (____________________)
    a. failure of any part of the smooth muscle of the gastroenteric tract to relax where one section joins another
    b. absence of hydrochloric acid in the gastric juices
    c. difficulty in swallowing
    d. excessive amount of hydrochloric acid in the gastric juices
11. biliary colic
    a. pain from blocked cystic or common bile duct
    b. malabsorption caused by disease of the absorbing surfaces of the intestine
    c. disease caused by damage to the gallbladder
    d. congenital defect in diverticula of the ileum
12. Salmonella (____________________)
    a. excess fat in the feces
    b. various rod-shaped bacteria, many of which may cause food poisoning
    c. condition in which tumors form in the pancreas
    d. intestinal obstruction
13. jaundice (____________________)
    a. frequent thirst
    b. an enlarged vein
    c. yellowish coloration of the skin caused by bilirubin in the blood
    d. characteristic foul odor of breath due to disease of the liver
14. steatorrhea (____________________)
    a. cramping and straining feeling when passing stool
    b. redness of skin on palm of hand
    c. protrusion of part of an organ through the wall of its natural cavity
    d. excess fat in the feces

DICTIONARY EXERCISE 3

Pronunciation of the words below is provided. Using your dictionary, find the correct spelling and definition of each word.

Word	Pronunciation	Definition
1. __________	bē'zŏr	____________________
2. __________	bor"bō-rĭg'mŭs	____________________
3. __________	ē-dĕnt'ū-lŭs	____________________
4. __________	flăt'ū-lĕns	____________________
5. __________	dĕf-ĕ-kā'shŭn	____________________
6. __________	ŏb"stĭ-pā'shŭn	____________________
7. __________	fī"tō-bē'zŏr	____________________
8. __________	tĕ-nĕz'mŭs	____________________
9. __________	ĕp"ĭ-găs'trĭk	____________________

10. ______________ hĕp"ah-tō-mĕg'ah-lē ______________________________
11. ______________ dĕ"gloo-tĭsh'ŏn ______________________________
12. ______________ ĕ-sŏf"ah-jĕk'tō-mē ______________________________
13. ______________ hĕ-păt'ĭk-ĕn-sĕf"ă-lŏp'-ă-thē ______________________________
14. ______________ lăp-ah-rŏt'ō-mē ______________________________
15. ______________ la-vazh' ______________________________

DICTIONARY EXERCISE 4

Rewrite the sentences in your own words. Provide pronunciation marks for each italicized word.

1. The problem was related to *aphagia* (______________).

____

2. Failure of the alimentary canal to move the *bolus* (______________) caused a cramping feeling.

____

3. They discovered a *cholangioma* (______________).

____

4. It was necessary to perform a *choledocholithotomy* (______________).

____

5. She was experiencing *polydipsia* (______________), *eructation* (______________), and difficulties with *deglutition* (______________).

____

6. Besides dysphagia, the patient had *palmar erythema* (______________).

____

7. He was admitted with *icterus* (______________) and *asterixis* (______________).

____

8. The physician said she had trouble *defecating* (______________).

____

9. One of the symptoms was *fetor hepaticus* (______________).

____

10. The symptoms were indicative of *enteritis* (______________).

____

11. The digestive problem was directly tied to *emulsification* (______________) of fats.

____

12. The patient presented with *gastroduodenitis* (______________).

____

13. The patient reported *flatus* (______________) and *constipation* (______________).

____

14. The physician noted the pressure of *hyperbilirubinemia* (______________).

____

StudyWARE™ Connection

Remember, you can take a practice quiz or play interactive games on your StudyWARE™ CD-ROM that can help you learn the content in this chapter.

Listening Exercise

INSTRUCTIONS

1. Review the spelling, pronunciation, and meaning of the words provided in the preview.
2. Go to your StudyWARE™ CD-ROM and listen to **Listening Exercise 13-1**. Fill in the blank in the report as the word is dictated.
3. At the end of the exercise, check your spelling against the preview words. They appear in the preview in the order in which they are encountered in the exercise.
4. Review and practice the words you missed.
5. Look up words that are not familiar.

PREVIEW OF WORDS FOR LISTENING EXERCISE 13-1

Word	Pronunciation	Meaning
Hemoccult	hē'mō-kŭlt	trademark for guaiac reagent strip test for occult blood
colonoscopy	kō"lŏn-ŏs'kō-pē	visual examination of the colon using a special instrument
Helicobacter	hĕl"ī-kō-băk'tĕr	gram-negative, spiral bacterium that causes gastritis in humans
organomegular	or"gă-nō-mĕg'ŭ-lăr	visceral organs that have become enlarged
cholelithiasis	ko"lē-lī-thī'ă-sĭs	presence or formation of gallstones in the gallbladder
serology	sē-rŏl'ō-jē	the study of antibody reactions in infectious disease

Listening Exercise 13-1

*Study*WARE™ Connection

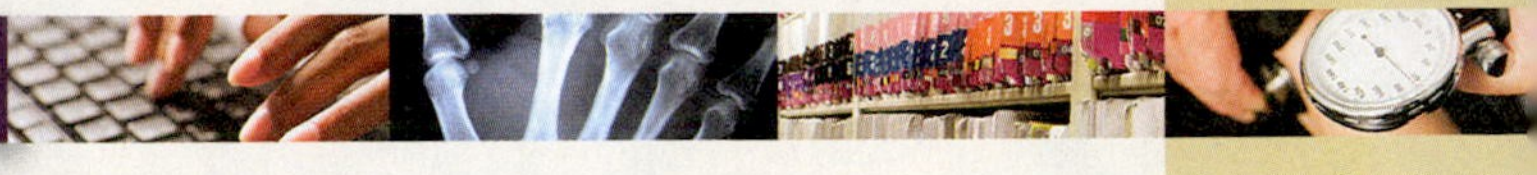

Listen to this report being read on your StudyWARE™ CD-ROM. Fill in each blank as the word is dictated.

Letter of Consultation

Dr. Rutherford Wiggins

1414 N. Cambria, Suite 245

Duluth, MN

Dear Dr. Wiggins:

Thanks for asking me to see your patient, Signe Nelstrom, because of her family history of early colon cancer. Her mother had that disease at age 24. As you know, we have seen Mrs. Nelstrom over the years for a variety of GI complaints. She had intermittent rectal bleeding, ____________________ positive stool. She last underwent ____________________ by Dr. Chan in 1992. The patient also was found to have gastritis due to ____________________ and was treated in 1994 with triple therapy.

Patient continues to have intermittent epigastric and right upper quadrant pain. It hasn't progressed, but it does bother her regularly. She has no food intolerance, no nausea or vomiting, no change in appetite or weight. Her bowels are still somewhat irregular and she occasionally notices some bright red blood. Her stools have not been tested for occult blood yet this year.

Review of the patient's family history shows no other family members with malignancies.

Physical exam; Weight 175, temperature 97.3, blood pressure is 120/82. Cardiorespiratory exam is negative. Her abdomen is soft. She has mild tenderness to deep palpation in the right upper quadrant. There is no ____________________ mass, guarding, or rebound. Bowel sounds are normal. Rectal exam is deferred.

IMPRESSIONS:

(1) Early colon cancer in first degree relative (mother—age 24) in a patient with chronically irregular bowel habits, abdominal pain, history of Hemoccult positive stool and intermittent bright red rectal bleeding.

(2) Right upper quadrant and epigastric pain. Rule out persisting or recurrent Helicobacter gastritis. Rule out ____________________.

PLAN: I am going to get ____________________ for Helicobacter and an ultrasound of the upper abdomen. If the serology is still significantly positive, I'll plan to do an upper GI endoscopy along with her colonoscopy. I agree with your recommendation for colonoscopy because of her family history, as well as her additional symptoms. I'll keep you informed of her progress.

Sincerely yours,

Hector Verandez, MD

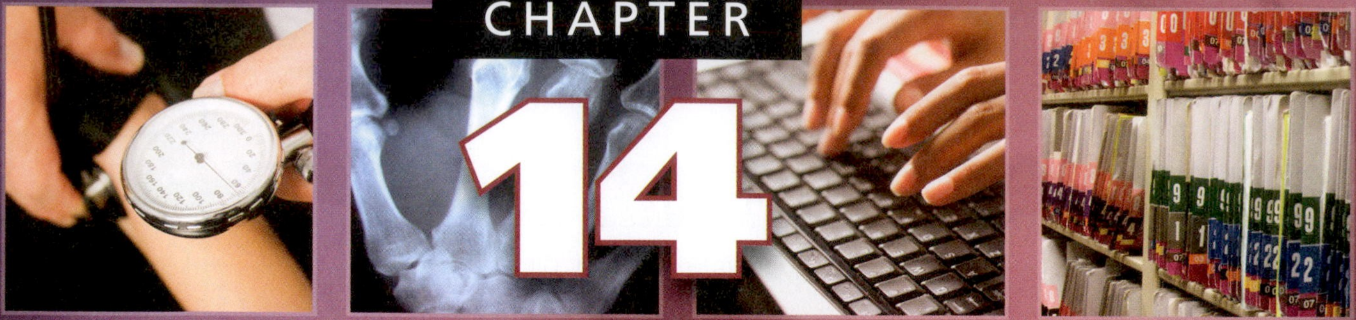

CHAPTER 14

Discharge Summaries

"Patients may not swear, curse, get drunk, behave rudely or indecently on pain of expulsion after the first admonition. There shall be no card playing or dicing and such patients as are able shall assist in nursing others, washing and ironing linen and cleaning the rooms and such other services as the matron may require"

—Regulation of the Philadelphia General Hospital, 1790

OBJECTIVES

When you have completed this chapter on discharge summaries, you should be able to

1. Define a Discharge Summary.
2. Identify and define the sections of a Discharge Summary.
3. Describe clinical uses of a Discharge Summary.
4. Identify administrative uses of a Discharge Summary.
5. Identify the meanings of related word elements.
6. Hear how medical terminology is used in actual medical reports.

INTRODUCTION

The Discharge Summary, or *Clinical Resumé*, is an important document in the patient's medical record. This document is usually associated with an episode of hospital care. In today's health care environment, many settings require a summarization of the care rendered to the patient. Nursing facilities, outpatient surgical clinics, community mental health centers, outpatient substance abuse centers, home health agencies, and large group practices or specialty centers are called upon to provide a summarization of patient care.

The Discharge Summary is one of the most frequently requested patient reports. It provides a clear description of the treatment the patient received, the patient's response to the treatment, and the condition of the patient at the conclusion of the episode of care. Review organizations, insurance companies, and other health care professionals are just a few of the groups that may need a copy of this document.

The Discharge Summary is usually dictated by the patient's physician. This summary may also be dictated by a nurse practitioner or physician assistant, but the report *must* be authenticated by the physician. Although specific headings in the report are determined by the health care agency, the health care industry has identified the types of information that should be included in a quality Discharge Summary. Regulatory and accrediting agencies have provided the impetus for improving the quality of this document.

Keep in mind that the headings used in the report and the organization of the report may vary from agency to agency. This chapter describes and defines the most frequently used and accepted components of a Discharge Summary.

COMPONENTS OF A DISCHARGE SUMMARY

The Discharge Summary includes several sections that provide Patient Identification, indicate the Diagnosis (Admitting and Discharge) and History, and give results of Laboratory Data and other Diagnostic Tests. A summary of the patient's Hospital Course, as well as the Discharge Disposition and Diagnosis, is included. These sections are discussed below. Italicized words used in the examples are defined in the Review of Terminology at the end of this section.

PATIENT IDENTIFICATION

The Patient Identification section must include the patient's name and case number. If the agency does not assign a case number, the date of birth or social security number is often used as secondary Patient Identification. The section usually includes the admission date and the discharge date. Ambulatory surgical centers may even include the time of admission and the time of discharge.

In addition to basic patient data and the admission and discharge dates, the section can include a brief notation about consultations, surgical procedures, and special procedures. If other active problems were addressed during the hospital stay, they should be included as well. Here is an example of a Patient Identification section.

EXAMPLE

PATIENT NAME: Juan Castilla
ADMITTED: March 19, 20—
CONSULTATIONS: Dermatologist
SURGICAL PROCEDURES: none

CASE NUMBER: 55-55-12
DISCHARGED: March 21, 20—
SPECIAL PROCEDURES: none

This first section tells the practitioner that this patient did not have any surgery or special procedures. There would be no need to page through the entire record to find this out. The notation about the consultation would be an indication that there should be a Dermatology Report.

DIAGNOSIS

The Diagnosis section can include the **Admitting Diagnosis** (the reason for the episode of care) and **Discharge Diagnosis** (the diagnosis that is made during the episode of care). When both diagnoses are given, this section is near the beginning of the report. Some agencies put the Admitting Diagnosis at the beginning of the report and the Discharge Diagnosis at the end.

Comparing these diagnoses is of particular interest to regulatory agencies and insurance companies. If there is a substantial difference between the Admitting and Discharge Diagnoses, the documentation in the patient record must clearly support that variation. In all cases, the diagnoses must always be supported by the information in the patient's record.

EXAMPLE

ADMITTING DIAGNOSIS:	Acute *erythematous* (er"ĭ-thĕm'ah-tŭs) rash, lower legs. *Ulcerations* (ŭl"sĕ-rā'shŭnz) with *exudate* (ĕks'ū-dāt)
DISCHARGE DIAGNOSIS:	*Cellulitis* (sĕl"ū-lī'tĭs) Staph infection

CONSULTANTS

Sometimes it is necessary to seek specialized knowledge from other individuals. If this is the case, the name and specialty of the physician should be included

EXAMPLE

CONSULTANTS: Dr. James Curian, Oncologist

PROCEDURES

Some hospitals require the names of procedures performed and a concise description of the results.

EXAMPLE

Echocardiography—ejection fraction 32%, global hypokinesia

COMPLICATIONS

The Complications section includes items not listed in the History and Hospital Course sections which need to be highlighted. If there were no complications, it is so noted.

EXAMPLE

COMPLICATIONS: None

HISTORY

The **History** section may or may not be a separate heading of the Discharge Summary. This section is most commonly used in hospitals and larger ambulatory care agencies. The History is a brief recap of the reason for the episode of care. A brief summary of the patient's current history and physical examination may also be included in the History section. Inclusion of the history and physical summary depends on agency policy and physician training and preference.

EXAMPLE

HISTORY: Mr. Castilla is a 40-year-old man who noticed a rash developing on his legs. He treated the rash with several ointments and creams. He noticed an increase in redness; and when the skin actually began to break down, he sought treatment.

LABORATORY DATA/DIAGNOSTIC TESTS

The **Laboratory Data and Diagnostic Tests** section is the most clinical and technical section of the Discharge Summary. The physician will describe and give the results of all tests performed initially. Pre-admission test results are reported under the History section and while subsequent tests may be recorded in the Hospital Course section. Careful attention must be given to the order of this information. Test results are usually presented in chronological order. Similar tests are grouped by date of service, with an explanation of the results. This information is taken from individual laboratory and Diagnostic Reports. The purpose of the summary is to consolidate all of this important information in one convenient location.

EXAMPLE

LABORATORY DATA: White count on 3/19 was 10,800 and 8,200 on 3/21. On 3/19 hemoglobin was 11 with a hematocrit of 33.3%. The hemoglobin was 12.8 on 3/21, with a hematocrit of 38.7. Culture taken on 3/19 revealed *Staphylococcus aureus* (stăf"ĭ-lō-kŏk'ŭs aw'rē-ŭs). Urinalysis was negative.

HOSPITAL COURSE

Discharge Summaries are usually associated with hospitalization. The patient's record will have many detailed reports that describe the treatment given and the patient's response. This section, called the **Hospital Course**, highlights the most significant aspects of the treatment process. Expect to find a chronological review of events justifying the hospital stay. This review would reflect on the severity of the illness and note any significant change in the patient's condition while in the hospital and when that change took place. It may also include a summary of important medications taken with the date and duration of their use. In the event that patient care is delivered in an outpatient or ambulatory setting, this section might be called *Treatment Course* or *Summary of Treatment.*

EXAMPLE

HOSPITAL COURSE: The patient was *febrile* (fēb'rĭl) on admission and started on antibiotic therapy. Culture revealed Staph aureus. An intramuscular injection of 1.2 million units of long-acting benzathine penicillin was given. The patient responded well to this treatment and was started on *cloxacillin* (klŏks"ah-sĭl'ĭn) 250 mg q.i.d. to be continued after discharge. On 3/21 lab work was within normal limits.

DISCHARGE DISPOSITION

The **Discharge Disposition** includes information about the condition of the patient and the plan for follow-up care. This section is mandated by regulatory and accrediting agencies. It may also be called the *Discharge Plan.* Specific information about dose and duration of medications, referrals, plans, and continued treatment is generally found in this section, as well as the name of the primary care or physician specialist who will have overall responsibility for the patient's follow-up care. Any additional appointments are also included. If applicable, identify physical limitations, capacity for self-care, and mental condition. There must also be a notation indicating that the discharge instructions were given to the patient. These instructions may be listed in the Discharge Disposition or documented on a separate form, signed by the patient, and placed in the patient's record.

EXAMPLE

DISCHARGE DISPOSITION: The patient was discharged on a regular diet. He is to stay off his feet as much as possible. He will continue with the cloxacillin 250 mg q.i.d. for 8 days. If he notices any changes in the condition of his legs, Mr. Castilla was advised to contact his attending physician immediately. He has been scheduled for a follow-up visit on March 30, 20—. Mr. Castilla was given discharge instructions, and a copy was placed in his record.

HILLCREST Medical Center

DISCHARGE SUMMARY

Patient Name: Dieter Stubinsky
Hospital No.: 65227

Admitted: December 14, 20—
Discharged: December 18, 20—

Consultations: Jose Medina, M.D.
Special Procedures: None

Surgical Procedure: Appendectomy
Complications: None

Discharge Diagnosis: Acute suppurative appendicitis

Admitting Diagnosis: Rule out acute appendicitis

HISTORY: This is a 45-year-old white man seen in my office on December 14 with the onset of acute abdominal pain at 10 a.m. that day. He was admitted directly to the hospital with a diagnosis of probable acute appendicitis.

LABORATORY DATA: Serum amylase was normal at 64. Cultures of peritoneal fluid at the time of discharge showed no growth. CBC performed as a follow-up on December 16 showed a white count of 12,400 (decreased from 21,000 on December 14). Hemoglobin today is 12 (decreased from 15.5 on the 14th). The remainder of the laboratory data was performed in the office prior to admission.

HOSPITAL COURSE: The patient was admitted and surgical consultation was obtained from Dr. Medina. The patient was taken to surgery the evening of admission where acute appendicitis with a small perforation was found. Pathology confirmed acute appendicitis. The patient convalesced without further difficulties, although he did have a low-grade fever with temperature of 100 F until the morning of December 17. He was discharged on the following medications: Darvocet N-100 one q.6h p.r.n. pain, Keflex 500 mg p.o. q.6h for three days. Diet at the time of discharge is as tolerated. Activities are as tolerated.

DISPOSITION: He will be seen by Dr. Medina in five days. He will be seen in my office in six weeks to be evaluated for possible hypercholesterolemia and possible hypothyroidism.

Ruth L. Samaan, M.D./XX

DD: 12-20-20—
DT: 12-22-20—

FIGURE 14-1
Discharge Summary

DISCHARGE DIAGNOSIS

Many agencies prefer to list the Discharge Diagnosis as a separate section at the end of the report. Location of the Discharge Diagnosis is dependent on agency policy and physician training and preference. This section is sometimes called *Final Diagnosis.*

EXAMPLE

DISCHARGE DIAGNOSES:
1. Cellulitis
2. Borderline hypertension
3. Psoriasis

The Discharge Summary *must* be authenticated by the physician. If the Discharge Summary is transcribed, the dates of dictation and transcription are required. This information is often checked by survey teams in order to verify compliance with accreditation standards.

Figure 14-1 shows an example of a completed Discharge Summary.

USES OF THE DISCHARGE SUMMARY

The Discharge Summary is a frequently requested report. Health care and administrative agencies can use this report to verify episodes of care, to communicate patient health information, and to monitor compliance with regulatory standards. Specific types of agencies and how they use the Discharge Summary are identified in this section.

HEALTH CARE AGENCIES

Patient care is provided in many different settings. Once a patient has been treated, there is a high probability that the results of that treatment will be sent to other health care professionals. Here are some examples of this process.

Physicians' Offices

Many patients receive services from specialists, regional medical centers, and ambulatory centers. Results of the treatment must be shared with the patient's family physician. The Discharge Summary can play an important role in communicating treatment results and aftercare plans.

Nursing Facilities

As the population ages, there is and will be greater demand for nursing facility care. In the past, nursing facilities were used as the end point of the health care process. Today these establishments may be used as a step between acute care and returning home. When a patient is transferred to a nursing or convalescent center, the Discharge Summary provides valuable information for the continuation of patient care. A thorough Discharge Summary will identify successful treatments, provide data about laboratory tests, and enumerate patient medications and followup plans.

Hospitals

Today's highly mobile population has resulted in the need to transfer and share patient information. Individuals may move from one community to another and take their health care concerns with them. Hospitals are able to transmit efficiently information about previous episodes of care with the Discharge Summary.

ADMINISTRATIVE AGENCIES

The Discharge Summary is used in many administrative settings. Various agencies that are involved in monitoring quality of care and cost-containment activities often need patient information. The Discharge Summary is a good way to provide that information. Here are some examples of the administrative uses of the Discharge Summary.

Insurance Companies

Reimbursement for patient care is a complex process. A common practice for health insurance companies is to request verification of patient services. Health care agencies may be able to charge the insurance companies for the cost of reproducing and sending information. If not, the agency must absorb the cost of sending this information; it may not charge the patient. By providing only the Discharge Summary instead of the entire patient record, the cost of reproduction may be controlled.

Peer-Review Organizations

Peer-review organizations are concerned with the quality and cost of health care services. These organizations review patient records to determine the adequacy of and charges for the care a patient receives. The Discharge Summary is a key document for this review process.

ACCREDITING, LICENSING, AND REGULATORY AGENCIES

Accrediting, licensing, and regulatory agencies use patient records as part of the survey process. These agencies look for accurate and timely documentation of patient care. The Discharge Summary is a required report and an important part of overall review activity. Incomplete or missing Discharge Summaries can have a negative impact on the licensing and accreditation process.

The Discharge Summary is an important part of the overall documentation of patient care. A quality report can contribute to continuity of patient care, reimbursement, and various administrative activities.

ABBREVIATIONS

Abbreviations are commonly used in medical reports. Although the use of abbreviations is acceptable, health care agencies, accrediting bodies, regulatory agencies, and various allied health professional organizations are actively discouraging their use, especially in the Discharge Summary. Abbreviations that relate to laboratory tests and medications are usually the only abbreviations found in a Discharge Summary. Generally accepted abbreviations for laboratory tests and medications are provided in each system chapter with more specific references in Chapters 3 and 4, respectively.

INTERNET ASSIGNMENT

The authoritative source about report guidelines is The American Health Information Management Association (AHIMA) at **www.ahima.org**. This organization was first identified in Chapter 3 of your text. The AHIMA represents more than 51,000 specially educated health information management professionals who work throughout the health care industry. They are specialists in administering information systems, managing medical records, and coding information for reimbursement and research. In addition to professional issues, the site has information for patients with regard to maintaining their personal medical record.

ACTIVITY

Access the American Health Information Management Association at **www.ahima.org**. Select Your Health Record from the options bar above the main text. Read the information about maintaining your own medical record. Summarize your findings for your instructor.

Review *Discharge Summaries*

- The Discharge Summary is a key document in the patient's record that recaps the treatment provided to the patient.
- Components of a Discharge Summary include Patient Identification, Admitting and Discharge Diagnoses, History, Laboratory and Diagnostic Test results, Hospital (or Treatment) Course, and Discharge Disposition.
- Nursing homes, physicians' offices, hospitals, and other health care agencies use the Discharge Summary to communicate clinical and medical information about the patient.
- The Discharge Summary is used as an administrative tool by insurance companies, professional review organizations, and accrediting and licensing agencies.
- The Discharge Summary must be accurate, complete, and produced in a timely manner. All information in the Discharge Summary must be supported by documentation elsewhere in the patient's record.

Key Terminology Review

Word	Definition
Admitting Diagnosis	reason for the current episode of care
cellulitis	inflammation of soft or connective tissue caused by infection
cloxacillin	penicillinase-resistant penicillin
Discharge Diagnosis	diagnosis that is made during the episode of care
Discharge Disposition	information about the condition of the patient and the plan for follow-up care
erythematous	characterized by the redness of skin due to congestion of the capillaries; rash
exudate	fluid filled with cellular debris and protein that has escaped from blood vessels as a result of inflammation
febrile	pertaining to fever; feverish
History	summary of the reasons for the episode of care
Hospital Course	summary of the most significant aspects of the treatment process in the hospital
Laboratory Data and Diagnostic Tests	results of all tests performed
Staphylococcus aureus	bacteria that causes infection
ulceration	circumscribed lesion of the skin resulting from necrosis caused by infection or inflammation

Key Terminology Practice Exercises

TERMS

Give the medical term for the following.

1. circumscribed lesion of the skin ______________________
2. inflammation of soft or connective tissue ______________________
3. pertaining to fever; feverish ______________________
4. redness of skin due to capillary congestion ______________________
5. fluid filled with cellular debris and protein ______________________

MATCHING

Match the terms to their meanings.

1. ________ diagnosis that is made during the episode of care
2. ________ bacteria that causes infection
3. ________ penicillinase-resistant penicillin
4. ________ reason for the episode of care
5. ________ summary of the reasons for the episode of care
6. ________ summary of the most significant aspects of the treatment process while in the hospital
7. ________ results of all tests performed
8. ________ information about patient and follow up plan
9. ________ another name for Discharge Disposition
10. ________ fluid filled with cellular debris and protein that has escaped from blood vessels as a result of inflammation

a. Admitting Diagnosis
b. cloxacillin
c. Discharge Diagnosis
d. Discharge Disposition
e. Discharge Plan
f. exudate
g. History
h. Hospital Course
i. Laboratory Data and Diagnostic Tests
j. Staphylococcus aureus

IDENTIFICATION

Check the headings that would be found in a discharge summary.

________ Chief Complaint
________ History
________ Patient Identification
________ Family History
________ Diagnosis
________ Plan
________ Discharge Disposition
________ Final Diagnosis
________ Review of Systems
________ Hospital Course
________ Laboratory Data
________ Social History

Word Element Review

Prefix	Meaning	Example	Definition
bi-	two	**bifurcation** (bi"fur-kā'shŭn)	separation into two branches
gemin-	two	**geminate** (jĕm'ĭ-nāt)	paired
hypo-	under, below	**hypotension** (hī"pō-tĕn'shŭn)	lowered blood pressure
macro-	large	**macrocyte** (măk'rō-sīt)	abnormally large erythrocyte
mal-	bad	**malformation** (măl"for-mā'shŭn)	deformity
malign-	bad	**malignant** (mah-lĭg'nănt)	tending to become progressively worse
meso-	middle	**mesiad** (mē'zē-ăd)	toward the median or center
micro-	small	**microcephaly** (mī"krō-sĕf'ah-lē)	abnormal smallness of the head
multi-	many	**multicystic** (mŭl"tĭ-sĭs'tĭk)	having many cysts
pan-	all	**panacea** (păn'ah-sē'ah)	remedy for all diseases
poly-	many	**polycythemia** (pŏl"ē-sī-thē'mē-ah)	excessive number of red corpuscles in the blood
semi-	half	**semilunar** (sĕm'ē-lū'năr)	shaped like a crescent or half-moon
tri-	three	**trigeminy** (trī-jĕm'ĭ-ne)	three pulse beats in rapid succession
uni-	one	**unicellular** (ū"nĭ-sel'ū-lar)	made up of a single cell

Suffix	Meaning	Example	Definition
-asthenia	weakness	**myasthenia** (mī"ăs-thē'nē-ah)	weakness of muscles
-coccus	berry-shaped organism	**Enterococcus** (ĕn"ter-ō-kŏk'ŭs)	any streptococcus of the human intestine
-penia	decrease, deficiency	**cytopenia** (sī"tō-pē'nē-ah)	deficiency of cellular elements of blood
-(r)rhea	discharge, flow	**rhinorrhea** (rī"nō-rē'ah)	free discharge of thin nasal mucus
-tropin	nourish, develop, stimulate	**somatotropin** (sō"mah-tō-trō'pĭn)	growth hormone

Word Element Practice Exercises

CIRCLE AND DEFINE

Circle and define the word element in the following terms.

1. myasthenia ______________________________
2. malformation ______________________________
3. malignant ______________________________
4. cytopenia ______________________________
5. panacea ______________________________
6. hypotension ______________________________
7. polycythemia ______________________________
8. macrocyte ______________________________

MATCHING

Match the word elements to their meanings.

1. ______ three		a. bi-, gemin
2. ______ large		b. tri
3. ______ bad		c. -penia
4. ______ half		d. mal-, malign
5. ______ under		e. macro
6. ______ two		f. poly-, multi
7. ______ all		g. pan
8. ______ weakness		h. hypo
9. ______ decrease, deficiency		i. -asthenia
10. ______ many		j. semi

MEANINGS

In the underlined words below, circle the word element presented in this chapter. Provide the meaning of the word.

1. Myasthenia gravis is an autoimmune disease that affects the legs and arms, as well as other body parts.

   ____

2. Blood tests revealed cytopenia, and the physician prescribed an appropriate treatment.

   ____

3. He required a myelosuppressive therapy to control his polycythemia.

   ____

4. The research team was looking for the ultimate panacea.

   ____

5. A biopsy performed indicated the tumor was malignant.

   ____

6. On examining the infant, the pediatrician noted a malformation of the right ear.

   ____

7. Examination of the blood sample determined the presence of a macrocyte.

____

8. Hypotension is often associated with long life.

____

MATCHING

Match the term to its definition.

1. separation into two branches	a. Enterococcus
2. any streptococcus of the human intestine	b. bifurcation
3. free discharge of thin nasal mucus	c. geminate
4. growth hormone	d. mesiad
5. paired	e. microcephaly
6. toward median or center	f. multicystic
7. abnormal smallness of the head	g. rhinorrhea
8. having many cysts	h. semilunar
9. shaped like a crescent or half-moon	i. somatotropin
10. made up of a single cell	j. trigeminy
11. three pulse beats in rapid succession	k. unicellular

WORD ELEMENTS

Give the meaning of each word element. Then use your dictionary to find a new word that contains each of the word elements. Specify whether the new word is a noun or an adjective by placing N or A in the last column.

Word Element	Meaning	Word	N or A
1. -asthenia			
2. bi-			
3. -coccus			
4. gemin-			
5. hypo-			
6. macro-			
7. mal-			
8. malign-			
9. meso-			
10. micro-			
11. multi-			
12. pan-			
13. -penia			
14. poly-			
15. -(r)rhea			
16. semi-			

17. tri- ______ ______ ______
18. -tropin ______ ______ ______
19. uni- ______ ______ ______

Dictionary Exercises

DICTIONARY EXERCISE 1

Use your dictionary to find the correct sign or symptom for each condition.

1. slow heart rate	a. anorexia
2. abnormally slow breathing	b. bradycardia
3. difficulty in speaking	c. bradypnea
4. labored, difficult breathing	d. dyspnea
5. excessive tissue fluid	e. dyspepsia
6. epigastric discomfort after eating	f. dysphagia
7. difficulty in swallowing	g. dysphonia
8. state of being extremely lean	h. edema
9. belching	i. emaciation
10. jaundice	j. enuresis
11. vague feeling of bodily weakness	k. eructation
12. drowsiness, mental sluggishness	l. icterus
13. urinary incontinence	m. lethargy
14. excessive thirst	n. malaise
15. loss of appetite	o. polydipsia

DICTIONARY EXERCISE 2

Define these children's communicable diseases and pathological conditions.

1. varicella ______
2. diphtheria ______
3. erythema infectiosum ______
4. impetigo ______
5. pertussis ______
6. rubella ______
7. rubeola ______
8. scarletina (scarlet fever) ______
9. asthma ______
10. cleft lip and palate ______

11. croup ______________________________
12. cryptorchidism ______________________________
13. Down syndrome ______________________________
14. hyaline membrane disease ______________________________
15. sudden infant death syndrome (SIDS) ______________________________

DICTIONARY EXERCISE 3

Rewrite each sentence in your own words. Provide the pronunciation for the italicized words.

1. Some diseases can be caused by specific *bacteria* (__________________).

   ____

2. A *cannula* (__________________) can be used by nurses and physicians when they provide care to the patient.

   ____

3. Once the infection had *disseminated* (__________________), several medications were needed to bring it under control.

   ____

4. Everyone involved in health care must take every precaution against *sepsis* (__________________).

   ____

5. Sometimes the *sequela* (__________________) is worse than the disease.

   ____

6. The *culture* (__________________) was positive for strep infection.

   ____

7. Her *disease* (__________________) process will sideline her for six months.

   ____

8. The patient's problem was really *functional* (__________________).

   ____

9. The patient's problem was definitely *organic* (__________________) in nature.

   ____

10. The skin *turgor* (__________________) of the hiker was showing strong signs of dehydration.

    ____

11. After the abdomen was opened, the surgeon requested a *trocar* (__________________).

    ____

12. The wound was oozing *pus* (__________________).

    ____

13. The lab report indicated that *Candida* (__________________) was present.

    ____

14. It was found that the young man's problem was protein decomposition caused by a *Proteus* (__________________) bacteria.

    ____

15. The patient had a *Pseudomonas aeruginosa* (__________________) infection.

    ____

StudyWARE™ Connection

Take a practice quiz or play interactive games that reinforce the content in this chapter, on your StudyWARE™ CD-ROM.

Listening Exercise

INSTRUCTIONS

1. Review the spelling, pronunciation, and meaning of the words provided in the preview.
2. Go to your StudyWARE™ CD-ROM and listen to **Listening Exercise 14-1.** Fill in the blank in the report as the word is dictated.
3. At the end of the activity, check your spelling against the preview words. They appear in the preview in the order in which they are encountered in the activity.
4. Review and practice the words you missed.
5. Look up words that are not familiar.

PREVIEW OF WORDS FOR LISTENING EXERCISE 14-1

Word	Pronunciation	Meaning
aspiration	ăs-pĭ-rā'shŭn	withdrawal of fluid by suction
suspension	sŭs-pĕn'-shŭn	solution where solid particles are *mixed* with the fluid, but *not dissolved* in it
aerosols	ĕr'ō-sŏlz	colloidal solutions suspended in a gas and dispensed in the form of a mist
lethargic	lĕ-thăr'jĭk	abnormally drowsy, sluggish, or indifferent
pulmonary toilet	pŭl'-mŏ-nĕ-rē	draining of fluids from the lungs

StudyWARE™ Connection

Listen to the reports on the next page being read on your StudyWARE™ CD-ROM. Fill in each blank as the word is dictated.

Listening Exercise 14-1

Discharge Summary

Date of Admission: 5/12/20—

Date of Discharge: 5/18/20—

DISCHARGE DIAGNOSIS:

1. Bronchitis.
2. Chronic respiratory insufficiency secondary to recurrent ________________________ and scarring of the lungs.
3. Cerebral palsy, severe.
4. Severe mental retardation.
5. History of seizure disorder.

RECOMMENDATIONS: The patient will be released on the following medications:

1. Bactrim ________________________ equivalent of a DS b.i.d. or 20 cc b.i.d.
2. Depakene 250 mg 5 cc at 2 p.m. and 10 cc b.i.d.
3. Organidin 4 cc q. 8 hours.
4. Valium 2 mg. h.s.
5. Beclovent 5 mg. q. 8 hours.
6. Reglan 5 cc q. 6 hours.
7. Theophylline syrup 80 mg in 15 cc, 25 cc q. 12 hours.
8. Albuterol ________________________ every 4 hours.
9. Nutren 3 cans 1.5 with one can of water.
10. 3 packs of ProMod over 14 hours daily.
11. Beclofen 5 mg t.i.d.
12. Theophylline 25 cc every 12 hours.
13. Natural Tears as needed.

The patient was also receiving 1,500 cc of free water. She is intolerant of Theragran.

Regina is a 15-year-old female who was admitted through the Emergency Room. The patient developed increasing shortness of breath and chest congestion. She had been on Cipro for the last 7–10 days without improvement. The patient has severe mental retardation. Her family was caring for her extremely well, but she continued to deteriorate. When seen in the Emergency Room, the patient was ________________________. She was in moderate respiratory distress. The patient was admitted for aggressive ________________________ ________________________ as well as IV antibiotics. We have attempted on a number of occasions to try to treat her as an outpatient on IV antibiotics, but access has been a major difficulty.

The patient was aggressively started on Fortaz as well as gentamicin. Gentamicin levels were followed closely. The patient continued to gradually improve. The patient over the next 48 to 72 hours improved enough that she was able to smile and her breathing was much improved. The patient is now released to be followed up as an outpatient.

Signature:______________________________

Katrina Zemstov, MD

CHAPTER 15

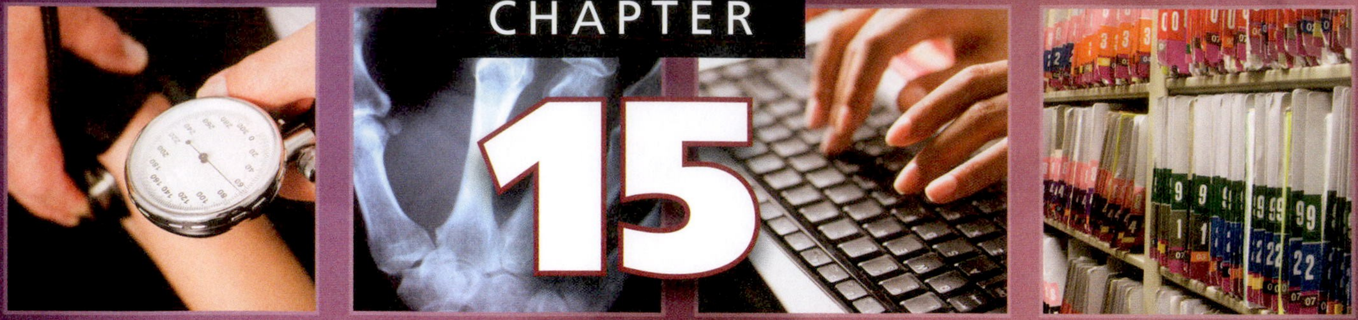

The Urinary System

"Bones can break, muscles can atrophy, glands can loaf, even the brain can go to sleep, without immediately endangering our survival; but should the kidneys fail... neither bone, muscle, gland, nor brain could carry on"

—Homer W. Smith

OBJECTIVES

When you have completed this chapter on the urinary system, you should be able to

1. Spell and define the major anatomical parts and explain how they operate.
2. Identify the meanings of related word elements.
3. Spell and define diagnostic procedures, diagnoses, treatment procedures, and abbreviations.
4. Spell the names of commonly used medications.
5. Use a dictionary as a tool in processing medical documents.
6. Hear how medical terminology is used in actual medical reports.

INTRODUCTION

The functions of the urinary system include filtration of the blood, recovery of useful products (such as sugar and salt), and elimination of fluid waste products. Every day about 1,700 quarts of blood flow through the kidneys to be cleansed. Without this critical process, waste products would accumulate and poison the bloodstream, which would lead to death.

Physicians who treat disorders and diseases of the urinary system are called urologists; those physicians trained in the medical treatment of the kidney and the urinary system are called **nephrologists** (nĕ-frŏl'ō-jĭsts). Nephrologists also provide treatment of systemic diseases involving the kidneys, such as hypertension, diabetes, and vasculitis.

COMPONENTS OF THE URINARY SYSTEM

The main parts of the urinary system are two kidneys, two ureters, a single urinary bladder, and a single urethra. This chapter discusses each of these organs.

KIDNEYS

cali/o, calic/o	calyx	nephr/o	kidney
glomerul/o	ball, cluster	pyel/o	trough, basin, pelvis
medull/o	medulla	ren/o	kidney

The **kidneys** have several functions, primary of which are filtration of blood, excretion of fluid waste products, maintenance of salt and water balance in body tissues, and regulation of an acid-base balance. The design of the kidneys is such that these functions occur without our conscious effort.

Figure 15-1 illustrates the position of the kidneys (4) in the upper abdomen between the muscles of the back (3) and the peritoneal cavity (1). The kidney area is separated from the peritoneal cavity by the peritoneum (7), the membrane lining the abdominal cavity.

In addition to the rib cage, the kidneys are surrounded and protected by three layers of tissue. The innermost layer covers the kidney surface. It is a fibrous connective tissue called the **renal capsule** (6). The next layer is the **adipose** (ăd'ĭ-pōs) **capsule** (5), which is filled with perirenal fat to cushion the kidney from external damage and to hold the kidney in place. Outermost is the **renal fascia** (făsh'ē-ah) (2), a double layer of thin, fibrous connective tissue that encloses the kidney and the renal and adipose capsules, anchoring them to the posterior abdominal wall and surrounding structures.

Each bean-shaped kidney (Figure 15-2) is about 4 1⁄2 inches long, 2 to 3 inches wide, and 1 inch thick with an indentation in the concave side called the **renal hilus** (hī'lŭs). The renal artery enters and the renal vein and ureter (5) emerge through the hilus.

Within each kidney are two general regions: the cortex and the medulla. The **cortex** (kŏr'tēx) (4) is the outer layer of the kidney and surrounds the medulla. The **medulla** (mē-dŭl'ah) (3) consists of eight to eighteen wedge-shaped areas called renal pyramids (1), which are composed of collecting tubules and blood vessels. The **renal papilla** (pă-pĭl'ah) (2), or tip, of each pyramid projects into the funnel-shaped opening of a **minor calyx** (kā'lĭks) (6), several of which join to form a **major calyx** (8). The major calyces, in turn, join to form the **renal pelvis** (7) (the expanded upper end of the ureter).

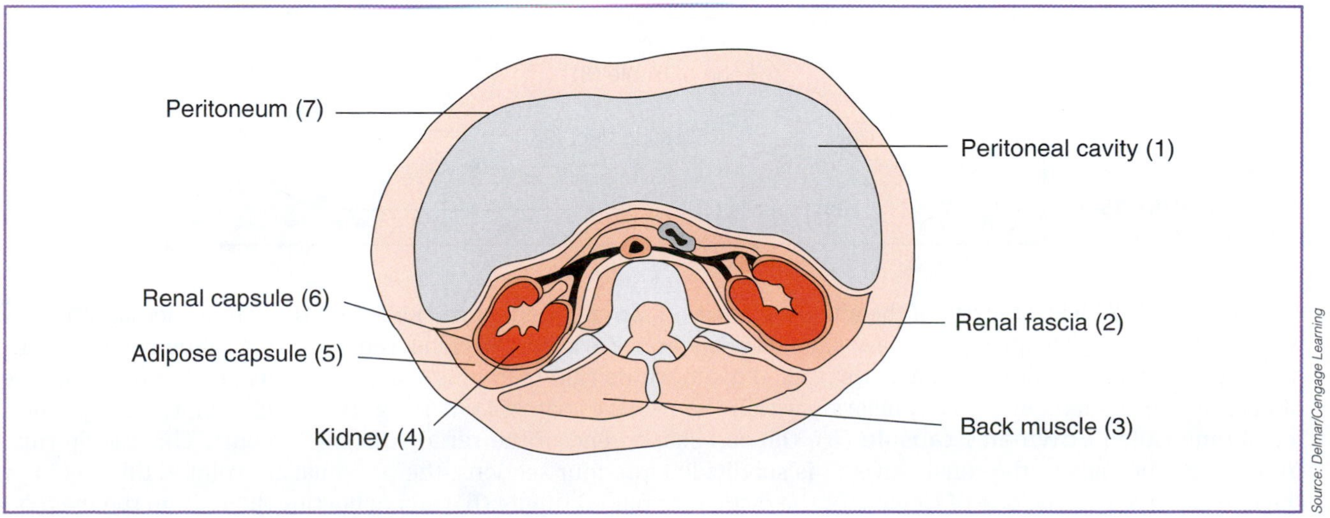

FIGURE 15-1 Transverse Section of the Body Trunk

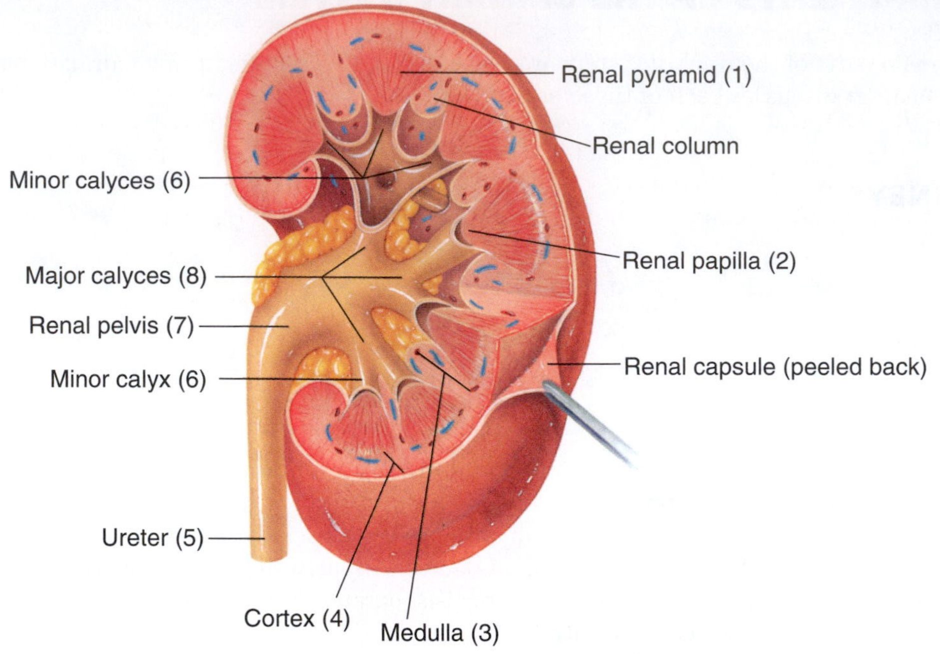

FIGURE 15-2
Internal Structure of the Kidney

Source: Delmar/Cengage Learning

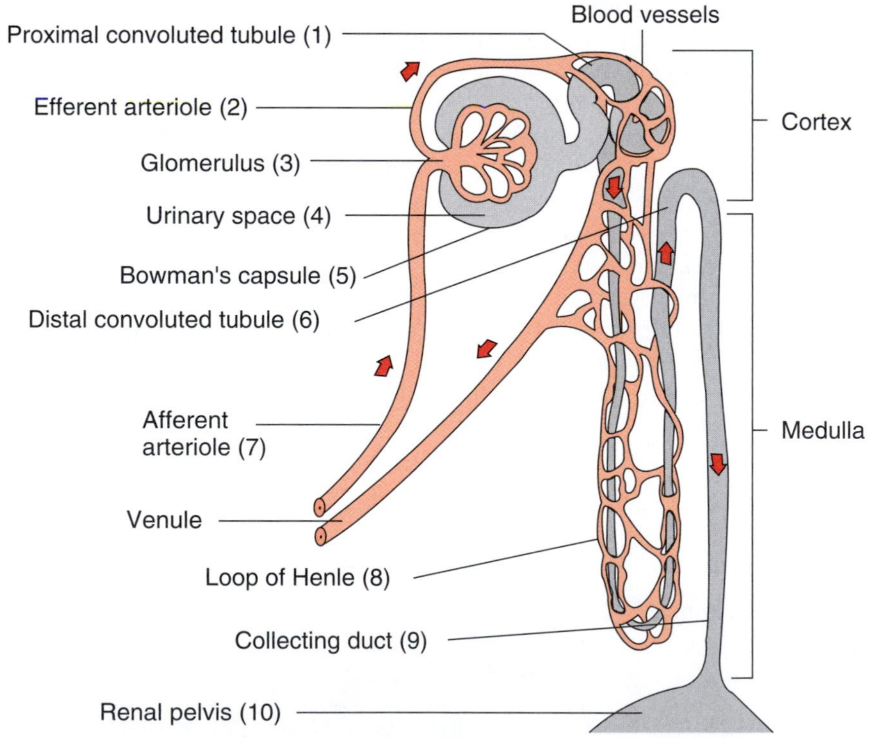

FIGURE 15-3
A Simplified Nephron

Source: Delmar/Cengage Learning

Figure 15-3 illustrates one of the million-plus urine-forming **nephrons** (nē'frŏns) that do the actual filtration work of the kidney. The process begins as blood flows from the aorta through a renal artery into the kidney where it is channeled into clusters of capillaries called **glomerulus** (glō-mĕr'ū-lŭs) (3). A glomerulus, the filtering unit of each nephron, is a cluster of capillaries within the urinary space (4). It is tightly encased in a double-walled membrane called **Bowman's capsule** (5), the cup-shaped end of the **renal tubule** (too'būl). This tubule runs from the glomerulus to the renal pelvis. It is subdivided into four sections: the proximal convoluted tubule (1) in the cortex area and the loop of Henle (8), the distal convoluted tubule (6), and collecting duct (9) in the medulla area. The glomerulus of each nephron has one blood vessel, the afferent arteriole (7), which branches from the interlobular artery to supply the cluster with blood, and another tiny vessel, the efferent arteriole (2), to drain the cluster. As blood passes through the capillary cluster, water, useful materials (such as sugar and salt), and waste materials pass directly from the blood through the capillary walls into the urinary space. These materials enter the tubule and make their way to the renal pelvis. During the passage most of the water and other useful materials are reabsorbed through the walls of the nephron tube into surrounding capillaries and sent back to the bloodstream.

The excess water and waste material (such as urea) remain in the filtrate. They are joined by other products (such as creatinine and medication by-products) secreted into the filtrate to become part of the urine. Through papillary ducts formed by uniting collecting ducts, the urine is emptied into the calyces of the renal pelvis (10). From the renal pelvis, urine is transported to the urinary bladder by the ureter.

URETERS

ureter/o	ureter

There are two **ureters** (ū-rē'tĕrs) (2), one originating from each kidney (1) as shown in Figure 15-4. (Occasionally a genetic malformation leads to a duplication.) The ureters are slender tubes about 10 to 12 inches long extending down to the urinary bladder (3) where they connect at the back. The ureter wall includes a lining of epithelial cells, a relatively thick layer of involuntary muscle, and an outer coat of fibrous connective tissue. The muscles of the ureter move the urine to the bladder by **peristalsis** (pĕr-ĭ-stăl'sĭs).

URINARY BLADDER

cyst/o	sac	vesic/o	bladder
ur/o	urinary tract, urine		

The **urinary bladder**, as shown in see Figure 15-5, is a reservoir for urine. It is located below the parietal peritoneum and behind the pubic joint when empty. When filled, it may extend well up into the abdominal cavity proper.

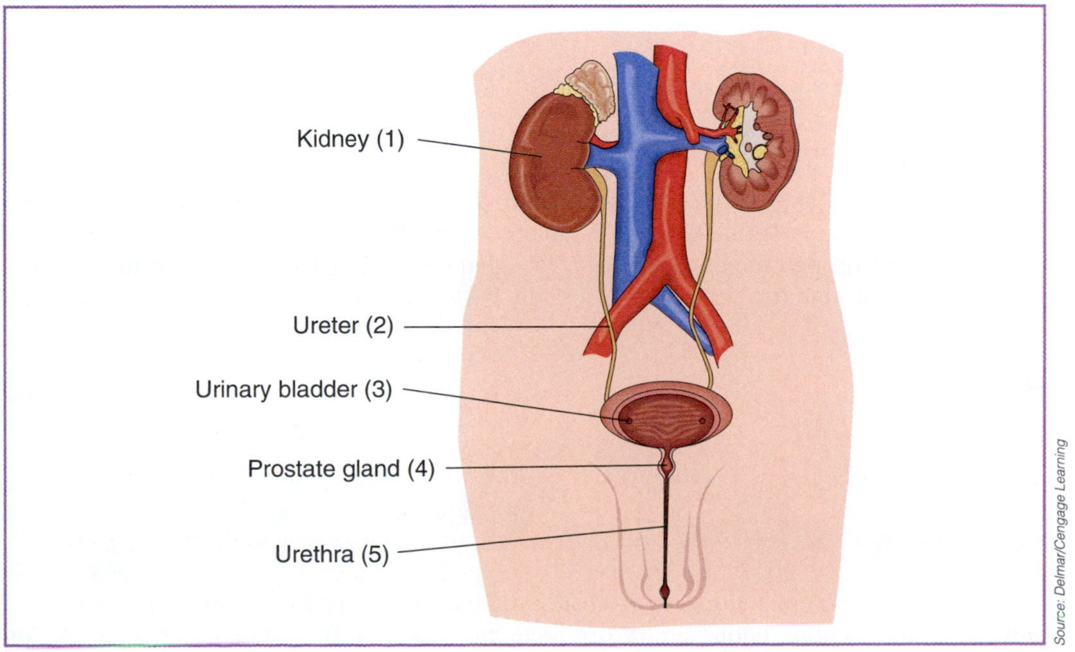

FIGURE 15-4
Urinary System

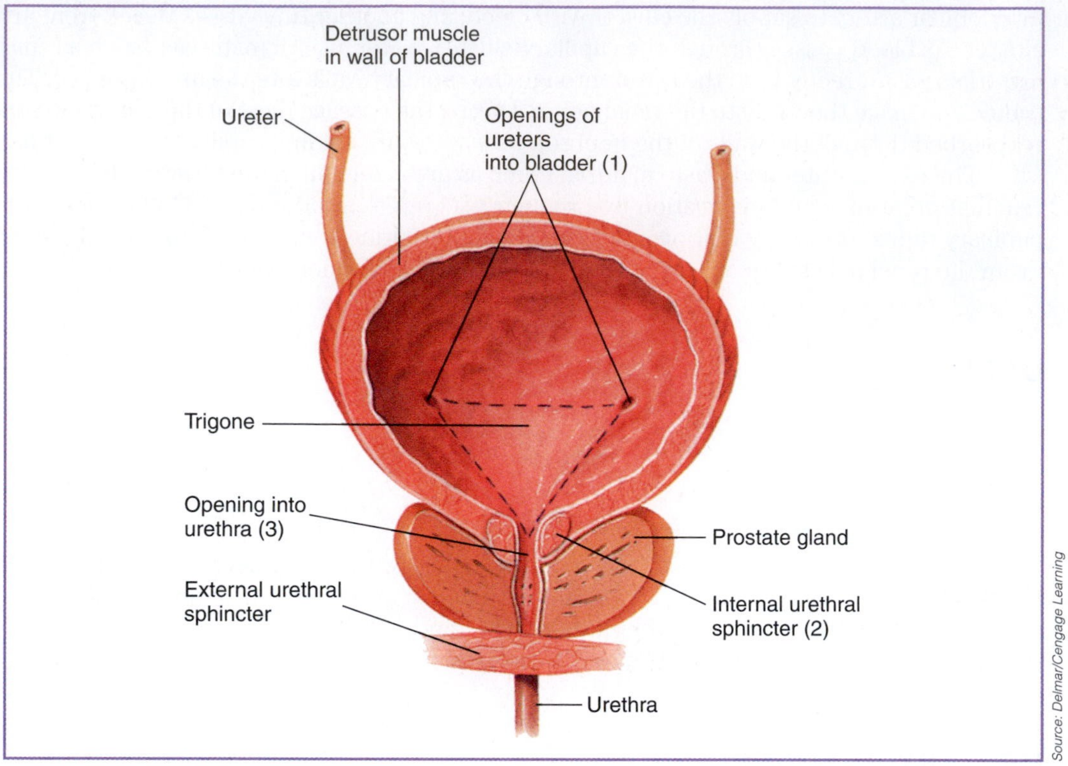

FIGURE 15-5
Anatomy of the Urinary Bladder

A bladder generally holds 700–800 ml of urine. However, at 200 to 400 ml, the stretch receptors of the bladder signal a conscious desire to urinate. The act of expelling urine from the bladder is known as **micturition** (mĭk-tū-rĭ'shŭn).

The bladder wall has many layers—mucous membrane, which is arranged into folds called **rugae** (roo'gay) when it is empty; connective tissue; a three-layered coat of involuntary muscle tissue; and an incomplete coat of peritoneum that covers only the upper portion of the bladder. Near the outlet of the bladder, the internal sphincter muscles (2) contract to prevent emptying at the wrong time.

There are three openings in the bladder—one for each ureter (1) and one opening to drain the bladder into the urethra (3). The smooth triangular region in the bladder outlined by these openings is the **trigone** (trī'gōn).

URETHRA

meat/o	meatus	urethr/o	urethra

The **urethra** (ū-rē'thrah) (5) is the tube leading from the bladder to the outside of the body. In a female it is embedded in the muscle of the front wall of the vagina between the clitoris and vaginal opening. It measures about 1.5 inches long. The external opening is called the **urethral** (or urinary) **meatus** (ū-rē'thral mē-ā'tŭs). The male urethra passes through the prostate (prŏs'tāt) gland (4) where two ducts carrying the male sex cells join it. From there it leads through the penis to the outside. In the male the urethra is about 8 inches long.

URINE

urin/o	urine	-uresis	urination
-uria	urination		

Urine is a yellowish concentration of waste product fluids. Gases dissolved in urine include carbon dioxide (CO_2) and ammonia. Nephrogenous waste products include urea, uric acid, creatinine, and other substances. Other waste products are excess sodium, potassium, chloride, bicarbonate, phosphates, sulfates, calcium, magnesium, and hydrogen ions (acid).

StudyWARE™ Connection

Watch an animation on the formation of **Urine** on your StudyWARE™ CD-ROM.

INTERNET ASSIGNMENT

The National Institute of Diabetes and Digestive and Kidney Diseases (NIDDK) conducts and supports research on many of the most serious diseases affecting public health. It is part of the National Institutes of Health.

NIDDK's Division of Intramural Research encompasses the broad spectrum of metabolic diseases including urology and renal disease. NIDDK extramural research is organized into five divisions. One is the Division of Kidney, Urologic, and Hematologic Diseases (KUH), which provides research funding and support for basic and clinical research about kidney diseases, urinary tract diseases, and disorders of the blood and blood-forming organs. Information comes from the National Kidney and Urologic Diseases Information Clearinghouse (NKUDIC), an information dissemination service of the National Institute of Diabetes and Digestive and Kidney Diseases.

ACTIVITY

Access the National Institute of Diabetes and Digestive and Kidney Diseases at **www.niddk.nih.gov**. Under Health Education, click on Learn About Diseases and Conditions. Then select Kidney and Urologic Diseases. Click on A-Z List of Topics. From this list, select one of the topics, write a short summary highlighting key points, and submit it to your instructor.

Review *The Urinary System*

- The primary functions of the urinary system are filtration of the blood, recovery of useful products (such as sugar and salt), and elimination of fluid waste products.
- The renal artery carries blood to the kidneys where it is channeled into a cluster of capillaries (the glomerulus) in the nephron.
- After the glomerulus filters out both reusable and waste products, it passes them into the urinary space.
- Reusable products are recovered or reabsorbed in the tubule portion of the nephron.
- Waste products in the form of urine are passed to the bladder through the ureters and are eliminated from the body through the urethra.

Key Terminology Review

Word	Definition
adipose capsule	fatty tissue that protects the kidneys
Bowman's capsule	double-walled membrane encasing the glomerulus
cortex	outer layer of the kidneys
glomerulus, *pl.* glomeruli	cluster of capillaries forming the filtering unit of a nephron
kidneys	two organs situated at the back of the abdominal cavity; their function is, among other things, to filter blood, to control excretion of waste products, to maintain salt and water balance in body tissues, and to regulate an acid-base balance
major calyx, *pl.* calyces	calyx formed from the joining of several minor calyces; major calyces join to form the renal pelvis
medulla	part of the kidney consisting of eight to eighteen triangular renal pyramids
micturition	act of expelling urine from the bladder
minor calyx	funnel-shaped part of the kidney that collects urine from the renal papilla
nephrologist	specialist in the treatment of kidneys and the urinary system
nephron	functional unit of the kidney consisting of the glomerulus and the renal tube
peristalsis	involuntary wavelike movement of muscles encircling a tube causing the contents of the tube to be forced onward
renal capsule	fibrous tissue that protects the kidneys
renal fascia	membrane sheet that protects the kidneys and anchors them to the posterior wall
renal hilus	indentation on the concave side of the kidney where the renal artery enters and the renal vein and ureter emerge
renal papilla, *pl.* papillae	tip of the renal pyramid that projects into the funnel-shaped opening of a minor calyx
renal pelvis	expanded upper end of the ureter
renal tubule	part of a nephron through which renal filtrate flows; divided into the proximal convoluted tubule, the loop of Henle, the distal convoluted tubule, and collecting duct
ruga, *pl.* rugae	fold that forms in the urinary bladder when it is empty
trigone	smooth, triangular region on the bladder outlined by the openings for the two ureters and the urethra
ureters	two long, slender muscular tubes extending from the kidney basin down to and through the lower part of the urinary bladder
urethra	tube leading from the bladder to the outside of the body
urethral meatus	external opening from the urethra to the outside of the body
urinary bladder	reservoir for urine
urine	yellowish fluid that contains dissolved waste product

Key Terminology Practice Exercises

SELECTION

Select the correct word from the list below to complete each of the following statements.

adipose	fascia	glomerulus	hilus	nephrologist	nephron
renal	rugae	ureters	urethral meatus	urinary bladder	urine

1. The basic unit in which the kidney's filtration work is actually done is the ________________.
2. The bladder, when it is empty, falls into folds called ________________.
3. The name of the external opening of the tube leading from the bladder to the outside of a female body is the ________________.
4. A physician who specializes in treating kidney diseases is a ________________.
5. The tubes that extend from the kidney to the urinary bladder are the ________________.
6. The protective substances around the kidneys are the ________________ capsule, ________________ capsule, and renal ________________.
7. Renal arteries, veins, and the ureter enter and leave the kidney in an area referred to as the renal ________________.
8. A cluster of capillaries in the kidney is called a ________________.
9. Urine is stored in a reservoir called the ________________.
10. The yellowish liquid containing dissolved waste products is called ________________.

MATCHING

Select the correct term for each of the following definitions.

1.	_____________	folds that form in the urinary bladder when it is empty	a. adipose capsule
2.	_____________	tube leading from the bladder to outside the body	b. Bowman's capsule
3.	_____________	reservoir for urine	c. cortex
4.	_____________	tip of renal pyramid projecting into a minor calyx	d. glomerulus
5.	_____________	membrane sheet that protects kidneys and anchors them to posterior wall	e. kidneys f. major calyx
6.	_____________	involuntary movement causing urine to be forced onward	g. medulla h. minor calyx
7.	_____________	specialist in the treatment of kidneys	i. nephrologist
8.	_____________	fatty tissue that protects kidneys	j. nephron
9.	_____________	outer layer of the kidneys	k. peristalsis
10.	_____________	two bean-shaped organs at back of abdominal cavity	l. renal capsule
11.	_____________	part of the kidney containing 8 to 18 renal pyramids	m. renal fascia
12.	_____________	yellowish liquid containing dissolved waste products	n. renal hilus
13.	_____________	external opening from urethra to outside the body	o. renal papilla
14.	_____________	two long tubes from the kidney basin to the bladder	p. renal tubule
15.	_____________	part of a nephron through which renal filtrate flows	q. rugae
16.	_____________	indentation on kidney for renal artery to enter	r. ureters
17.	_____________	fibrous tissue that protects the kidneys	s. urethra
18.	_____________	functional unit of kidney including glomerulus and renal tubule	t. urethral meatus

(continues)

19. ____________ funnel-shaped part of kidney that collects urine from renal papilla
20. ____________ calyx formed when joining several minor calyces
21. ____________ cluster of capillaries forming filtering unit of nephron
22. ____________ double-walled membrane encasing the glomerulus

u. urinary bladder
v. urine

COMPLETION

Complete the following statements.

1. The primary functions of the kidneys are ______________________________.
2. The tip of the renal pyramid that projects into the funnel-shaped opening of a minor calyx is the ______________________________.
3. ______________________________ encases the glomerulus in a double-walled membrane.
4. The involuntary movement of the muscles of the ureter to move urine to the bladder is ______________________________.
5. The tube leading from the bladder to the exterior of the body is the ______________________________.
6. The kidney is separated from the peritoneal cavity by the ______________________________.
7. The three layers of tissue protecting the kidneys are the ______________________________, ______________________________, and ______________________________.
8. The two general regions within each kidney are ______________________________ and ______________________________.
9. The kidney part that contains 8 to 18 renal pyramids is the ______________________________.
10. A glomerulus is encased in a double-walled membrane called ______________________________.
11. The act of expelling urine from the bladder is known as ______________________________.
12. The smooth triangular region in the bladder outline by the openings for the two ureters and the urethra is called the ______________________________.
13. In the male the urethra is about ______________________________ inches long.
14. The female urethra is about ______________________________ inches long.
15. The ______________________________ has three openings.

SPELLING

Rewrite the misspelled words.

1. cortex ______________________________
2. calyix ______________________________
3. glommeruli ______________________________
4. tubuole ______________________________
5. urethra ______________________________
6. ureteral meatus ______________________________

Word Element Review

Root	Meaning	Example	Definition
cali/o, calic/o	calyx (calix)	**calicectasis** (kăl"ĭ-sĕk'tă-sĭs)	dilation of a calyx of the kidney
cyst/o	sac; urinary bladder	**cystectomy** (sĭs-tĕk'tō-mē)	excision of a cyst
		endocystitis (ĕn"dō-sĭs-tī'tĭs)	inflammation of the membrane lining of the urinary bladder
glomerul/o	ball, cluster	**glomerulus** (glō-mer'ū-lŭs)	cluster of capillaries within the kidney
		glomeruli (glō-mer'ū-lī)	plural of glomerulus
meat/o	meatus	**meatotomy** (mĕ"ā-tŏt'ō-mē)	incision of the urinary meatus to enlarge the opening
medull/o	medulla	**medullary** (mĕd'ū-lār"ē)	pertaining to the medulla; one of the inner parts of the kidney
nephr/o	kidney	**nephrectomy** (nĕ-frĕk'tō-mē)	excision of the kidney
		nephrosis (nĕ-frō'sĭs)	any condition of the kidney in which there are degenerative changes without the occurrence of inflammation
pyel/o	trough, basin, pelvis	**pyelogram** (pī'ĕ-lō-grăm")	radiography of the renal pelvis and ureter after the injection of contrast material
		pyelonephritis (pī"ĕ-lō-nĕ-frī'tĭs)	inflammation of the kidney and its pelvis due to bacterial infection
ren/o	kidney	**renal insufficiency** (rē'năl ĭn"sŭ-fĭsh'ĕn-sē)	reduced capacity of the kidney to perform its function
ur/o	urinary tract, urine	**urogenital** (ū"rō-jĕn'ĭ-tăl)	pertaining to the urinary and reproductive organs
ureter/o	ureter	**ureteral** (ū-rē'ter-ăl)	pertaining to the ureter
		ureterectasis (ū-rē"ter-ĕk'tah-sĭs)	dilation of the ureter
urethr/o	urethra	**urethritis** (ū"rĕ-thrī'tĭs)	inflammation of the urethra
		urology (ū-rŏl'ō-jē)	study of the urinary tract of both sexes and the genital tract of the male
urin/o	urine	**urinoma** (ū"rĭ-nō'mă)	cyst containing urine
vesic/o	bladder	**vesicouterine** (vĕs"ĭ-kō-ū'ter-ĭn)	pertaining to the urinary bladder and uterus

continues

Suffix	Meaning	Example	Definition
-uresis	urination	**enuresis** (ĕn"ū-rē'sĭs)	involuntary discharge of urine
-uria	urination	**dysuria** (dĭs-ū'rē-ah)	painful urination
		hematuria (hĕm"ah-tū'rē-ah)	blood in the urine

Word Element Practice Exercises

MEANINGS

Give the meaning of the italicized words.

1. We'll be doing a *nephrectomy* tomorrow on Mr. Glover.

 ____

2. The patient complained of *dysuria*.

 ____

3. There is evidence of *ureterectasis*.

 ____

4. I have ordered a *pyelogram* for tomorrow.

 ____

5. The urologist performed a *meatotomy*.

 ____

IDENTIFICATION

Identify the following by providing the correct terms for each definition. Underline the word element in each term.

1. inflammation of the membrane lining of the urinary bladder ______________
2. pertaining to the ureter ______________
3. bacteria-caused infection of the kidney and its pelvis ______________
4. blood in the urine ______________
5. pertaining to the urinary bladder and uretus ______________
6. inflammation of the urethra ______________
7. dilation of the calyx of the kidney ______________
8. any change in the condition of the kidney without the occurrence of inflammation ______________
9. involuntary discharge of urine ______________

10. excision of a cyst ______________
11. pertaining to urinary and reproductive organs ______________
12. cyst containing urine ______________
13. plural of glomerulus ______________
14. cluster of capillaries within the kidney ______________
15. reduced capacity of kidney to perform its function ______________

MATCHING

Match the word elements to their meanings.

1. ________ ball, cluster	a. cyst/o
2. ________ urination	b. pyel/o
3. ________ urinary tract, urine	c. glomerul/o
4. ________ kidney	d. ur/o
5. ________ ureter	e. -uria
6. ________ sac	f. medull/o
7. ________ medulla	g. nephr/o, ren/o
8. ________ trough, basin, pelvis	h. ureter/o
9. ________ urethra	i. urethr/o
10. ________ bladder	j. vesic/o

WORD ELEMENTS

Give the meaning of each word element. Then use your dictionary to find a new word that contains each of the word elements. Specify whether the new word is a noun or an adjective by placing N or A in the last column.

Word Element	Meaning	Word	N or A
1. cali/o			
2. calic/o			
3. cyst/o			
4. glomerul/o			
5. meat/o			
6. medull/o			
7. nephr/o			
8. pyel/o			
9. ren/o			
10. ur/o			
11. -uresis			
12. ureter/o			
13. urethr/o			
14. -uria			
15. urin/o			
16. vesic/o			

DIAGNOSTIC PROCEDURES		
Word	**Pronunciation**	**Definition**
General		
catheterization	kăth"ĕ-tĕr-ĭ-zā'shŭn	introduction of a drainage tube through the urethra into the bladder to withdraw a urine sample which may be
• *sterile*		using aseptic techniques to remove urine via a catheter through the urethra
• *clean-catch*		patient uses antiseptic wipes
• *first-voided*		collection of first urine in the morning which is refrigerated until taken to laboratory
• *random*		collected at any time
• *residual*		removed by catheterization after patient has voided.
cystometrography	sĭs"tō-mĕ-trŏg'ră-fē	process for measuring the pressure in the bladder at varying stages of filling
cystoscopy	sĭs-tŏs'kō-pē	visual examination of the bladder with a cystoscope fitted with a light and small mirrors (see Figure 15-6)
cystoscopy with retrograde pyelogram	rĕt'rō-grād pī'ĕ-lō-grăm"	visual examination of the bladder followed by an x-ray of the kidney after the introduction of a contrast medium through the ureter
cystourethroscopy	sĭs"tō-ū-rē'thrō-skŏp"ē	insertion of lighted instrument through the urethra and bladder to view the interior surface
renal biopsy	rē'nal bī'ŏp-sē	removal of a piece of kidney for microscopic examination; usually done with a biopsy needle
transurethral biopsy	trăns"ū-rē'thrăl	removal of a sample of kidney tissue for microscopic examination; taken through the urethra

continues

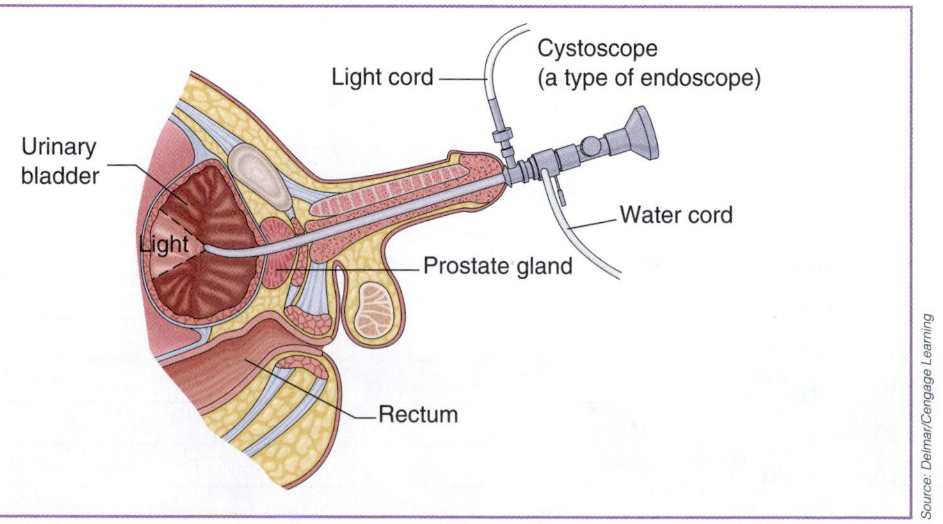

FIGURE 15-6
Cystoscopy

DIAGNOSTIC PROCEDURES		
Word	**Pronunciation**	**Definition**
Nuclear Medicine		
technetium cystogram	tĕk-nē'shē-ŭm sĭs'tō-grăm	x-ray of the urinary bladder after introducing a radioisotope so the outline of the organ can be seen
renal scan		scan taken after the injection of a radioactive isotope to evaluate renal blood flow, tubular function, diagnose obstructions, and determine the separate function of each kidney
Radiology		
cystography	sĭs-tŏg'rah-fē	contrast media study of the bladder
fistulogram	fĭs'tū-lō-grăm	x-ray taken after injection of contrast into an arteriovenous fistula
intravenous pyelography (IVP)	ĭn"trah-vē'nŭs pī"ĕ-lŏg'rah-fē	x-ray study of the kidney, ureter, and bladder using an intravenous contrast medium (see Figure 15-7)
nephrotomography	nĕf"rō-tō-mŏg'răh-fē	body section x-ray for visualization of the kidney
renal angiography	ăn"jē-ŏg'ră-fē	x-ray with contrast material to detect blood clots, tumors, or narrowing of arteries or veins of the kidney
renal artery Doppler		ultrasound study of the renal arteries to aid in the evaluation of renal blood flow
retrograde pyelography	rĕt'rō-grād pī"ĕ-lŏg'rah-fē	contrast media study of the urinary system via catheters introduced into the ureters through a cystoscope

continues

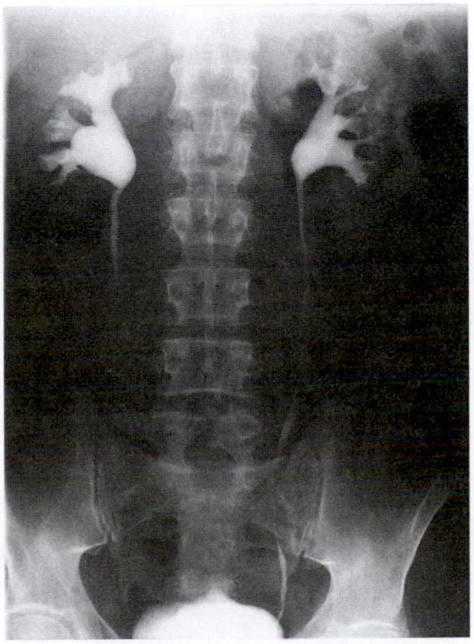

FIGURE 15-7 Intravenous Pyelography

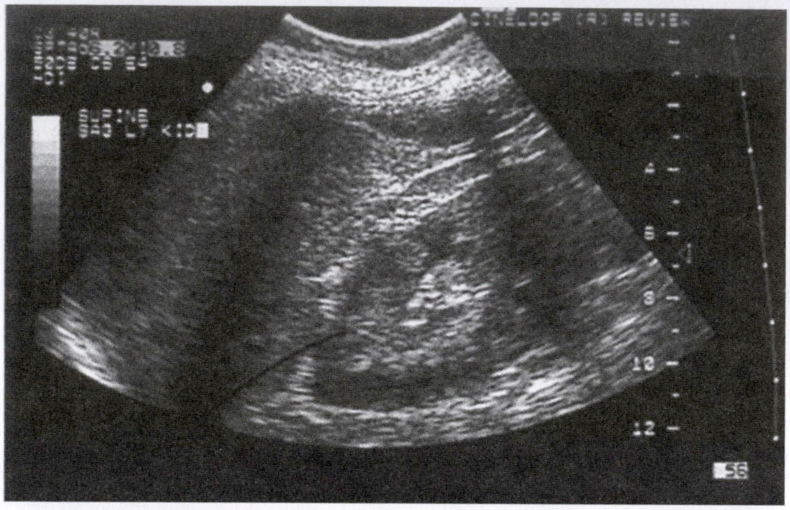

FIGURE 15-8
Renal Ultrasound: preferred imaging modality for suspected pyelonephritis

DIAGNOSTIC PROCEDURES

Word	Pronunciation	Definition
Radiology *(continued)*		
renal ultrasound	ŭl'trah-sownd	radiologic technique in which the structure of the kidneys is visualized by recording the reflection of ultrasound waves directed into the tissues (see Figure 15-8)
shuntogram	shŭnt'ō-grăm	x-ray taken after the injection of contrast into a GOR-TEX graft dialysis access
ureterography	ū-rē"ter-ŏg'rah-fē	contrast media study of the ureters
voiding cystourethrography	sĭs"tō-ū-rē-thrŏg'rah-fē	x-ray of the urinary bladder while the patient is voiding
x-ray of kidney, ureter, bladder (KUB)		radiogram done without injection of air or contrast media to demonstrate the size and location of the kidneys
Laboratory Tests		
24-hour specimen		collection of all of an individual's urine into a large container to evaluate kidney function, protein excretion, or the excretion of other substances by the kidney
urinalysis (UA)	ŭ"rĭ-năl'ĭ-sĭs	analysis of the urine to determine its physical, chemical, and microscopic properties; *physical* properties may include color, appearance, quantity, pH, and specific gravity; *chemical* properties are protein, sugar, ketone bodies, and bilirubin; a *microscopic* exam shows red and white blood cells, crystals, casts, and pus
urine culture and sensitivity (C&S)		test to determine the type of bacteria present and which antibiotic is the most effective for treatment

continues

DIAGNOSTIC PROCEDURES		
Word	Pronunciation	Definition
Blood Tests		
acid phosphatase	fŏs'fah-tās"	test that measures an enzyme in the blood when checking for prostate cancer
blood urea nitrogen (BUN)	ū-rē'ah nī'trō-jĕn	test that measures the concentration of urea in the blood
creatinine clearance	krē-ăt'ĭ-nĭn	test that measures the ability of the kidney to remove creatinine from the blood; used as an estimate of glomerular filtration rate
dysmorphic red blood	dĭs-mŏr'fĭk	test for misshapen blood cells in the urine, indicating an origin in the glomerulus as opposed to the renal collecting system
immunoelectrophoresis	ĭ-mū"nō-ē-lĕk"trō-fō-rē'sĭs	method of distinguishing proteins and antibodies in body fluid on the basis of their electrophoretic mobility and antigenic specificities

DIAGNOSES		
Word	Pronunciation	Definition
Urinary Tract Infections/Disorders		
cystitis	sĭs-tī'tĭs	inflammation of the urinary bladder (see Figure 15-9C)
nocturia	nŏk-tū'rē-ah	excessive urination at night
pyelonephritis	pī"ĕ-lō-nĕ-frī'tĭs	inflammation of the renal pelvis, usually due to infection (see Figure 15-9E)
stricture	strĭk'chŭr	narrowing of a urinary structure that interferes with flow of urine to the bladder
uremia	ū-rē'mē-ah	systemic result of the accumulation of toxins normally excreted by the kidneys
ureteritis	ū-rē"tĕr-ī'tĭs	inflammation of the ureter
urethritis	ū"rē-thrī'tĭs	inflammation of the urethra (see Figure 15-9B)
urinary calculi	kăl'kū-lī	stones occurring anywhere in the urinary tract
urinary tract infection (UTI)		infection of the urinary tract, especially the bladder and urethra; structural and systemic disorders affecting urine flow contribute to the problem (see Figure 15-9A)
vesicoureteral reflux	vĕs"ĭ-ko-ū-rē'tĕr-ăl	recurrent urinary tract infections, especially in children, where urine passes through the ureter from the bladder back to the kidney because the valve in the ureter is malfunctioning
Disorders/Disease of the Kidney		
cystinuria	sĭs'tī-nū'rē-ah	persistent excessive urinary excretion of certain amino acids due to impairment of their renal tubular reabsorption

continues

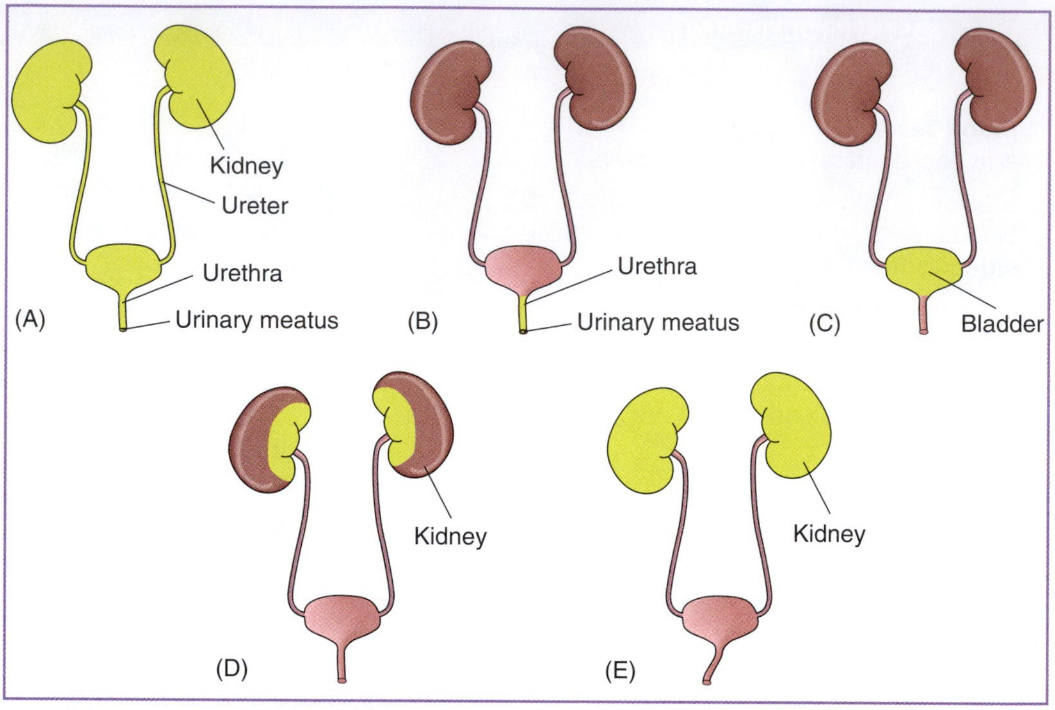

FIGURE 15-9 Sites of Urinary Tract Infections: (A) entire urinary tract infection; (B) urethritis; (C) cystitis; (D) pyelitis; (E) pyelonephritis

DIAGNOSES

Word	Pronunciation	Definition
Disorders/Disease of the Kidney *(continued)*		
end-stage renal disease (ESRD)		terminal kidney failure requiring dialysis or transplantation
glomerulonephritis	glō-mĕr"ū-lō-nĕ-frī'tĭs	inflammation of the glomeruli; may be acute or chronic
hydronephrosis	hī"drō-nĕ-frō'sĭs	dilation of the renal pelvis caused by obstruction of the ureter or lower urinary tract (see Figure 15-10)
interstitial nephritis	ĭn"tĕr-stĭsh'ăl nĕ-frī'tĭs	inflammation of the spaces between the glomeruli and tubules in the kidney
kidney cysts		fluid-filled masses in the kidney
medullary sponge kidney	mĕd'ū-lār-ē	multiple small cysts in the central kidney portion of the renal pyramids
nephrocalcinosis	nĕf-rō"kăl"sĭn-ō'sĭs	diffuse calcification of the kidney
nephrolithiasis (renal calculi)	nĕf"rō-lĭth-ī'ah-sĭs (rē'năl kăl'kū-lī)	presence of calculi in the kidney; kidney stones (see Figure 15-11)
nephropathy	nĕ-frŏp'ah-thē	any disease of the kidney, including inflammatory (nephritis), degenerative (nephrosis), and sclerotic kidney lesions
nephrotic syndrome (nephrosis)	nĕ-frŏt'ĭk (nĕf"rō'sĭs)	disorder characterized by protein loss from the kidneys, resulting in edema
polycystic kidney disease (PKD)	pŏl"ē-sĭs'tĭk	multiple cysts in the kidney (see Figure 15-12)

continues

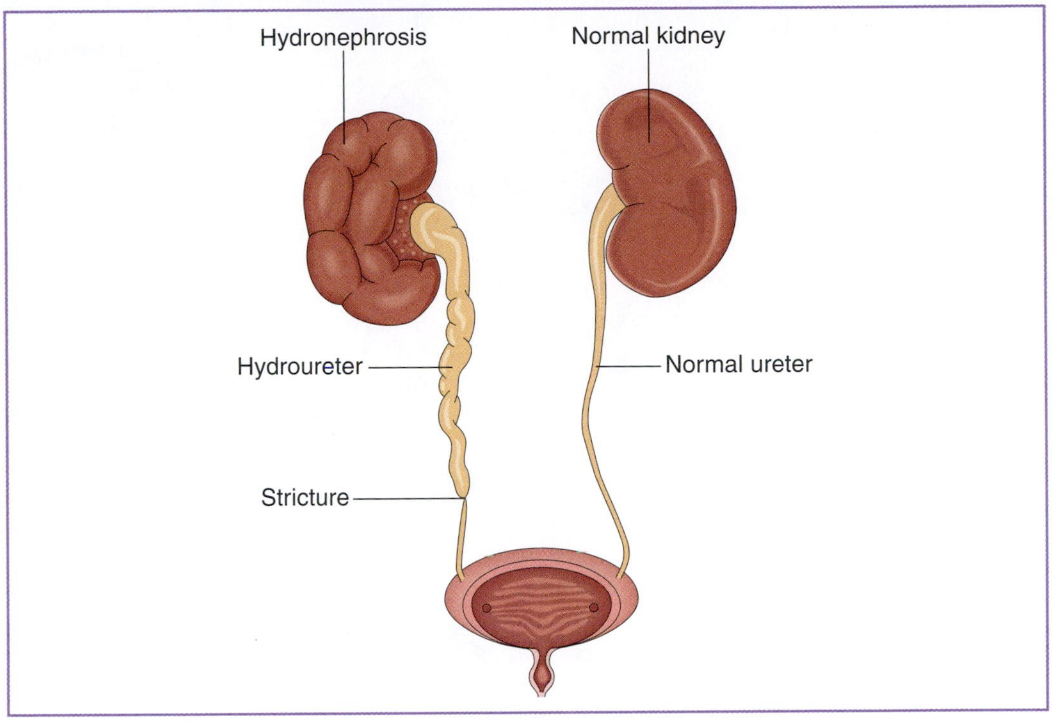

FIGURE 15-10
Hydronephrosis

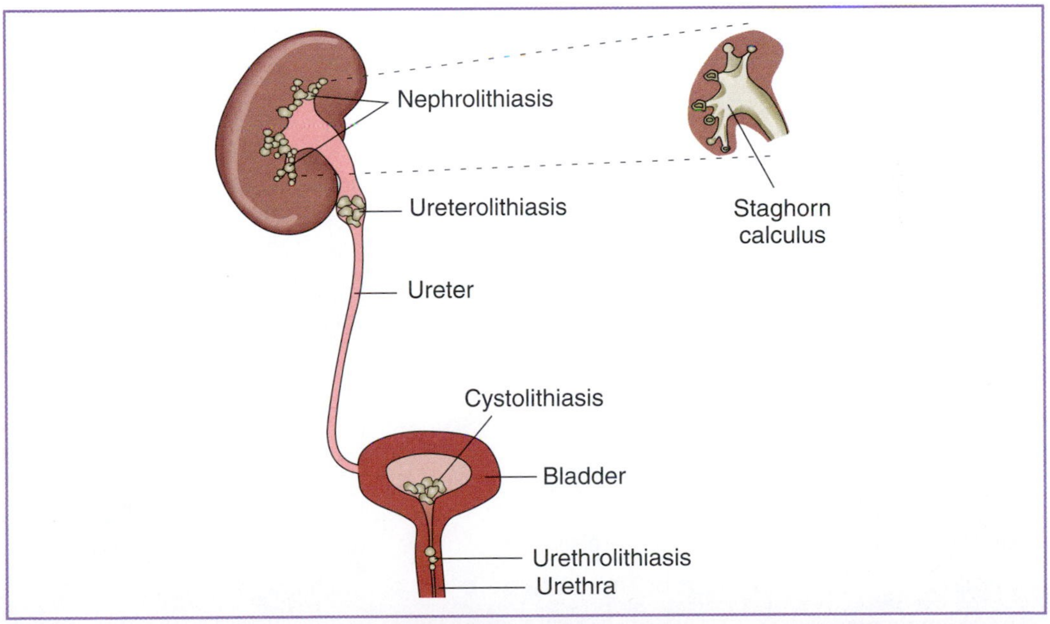

FIGURE 15-11
Types and Locations of Renal Calculi

DIAGNOSES

Word	Pronunciation	Definition
Disorders/Disease of the Kidney *(continued)*		
proteinuria	prō'tē-ĭn-ŭ'rē-ah	presence of abnormal amounts of protein in the urine
pyelitis	pī"ĕ-lī'tĭs	inflammation of the pelvis of the kidney (see Figure 15-9D)
pyelonephritis	pī"ē-lō-nĕ-frī'tĭs	inflammation of the kidney and renal pelvis

continues

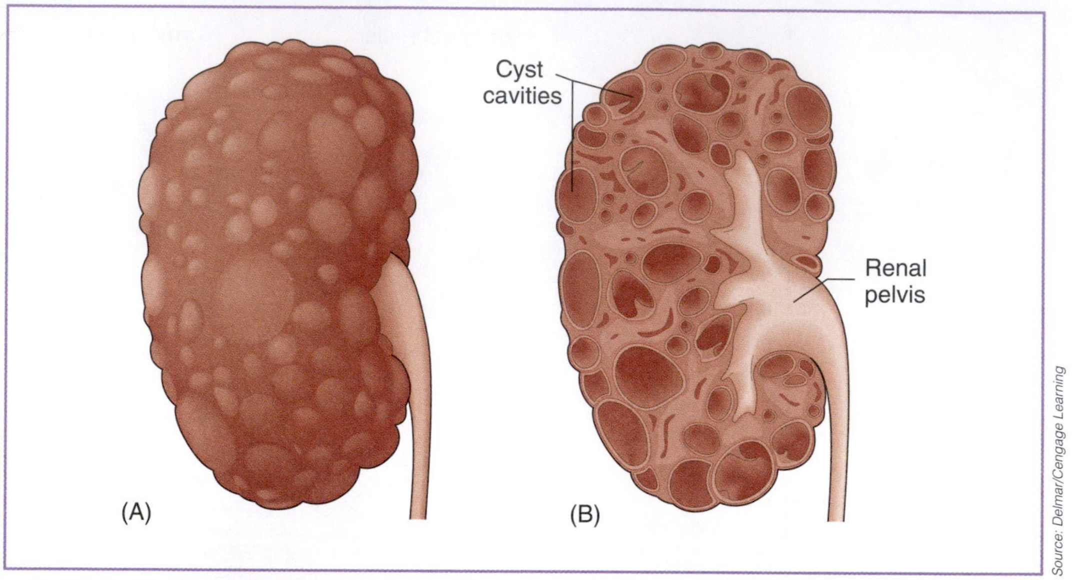

FIGURE 15-12
Polycystic Kidneys: (A) polycystic; (B) section through kidney

DIAGNOSES

Word	Pronunciation	Definition
Disorders/Disease of the Kidney *(continued)*		
renal cell carcinoma	kăr"sĭ-nō'mah	malignant growth of the renal parenchyma, composed of tubular cells in varying arrangements
renal failure		decreased function of the kidney
renal hypertension	hī"pĕr-tĕn'shŭn	high blood pressure resulting from kidney disease
renal tubular acidosis (RTA)	ăs"ĭ-dō'sĭs	accumulation of acid in the body due to a failure of the kidneys to appropriately acidify the urine; main types are: Type 1 distal RTA, Type 2 Proximal RTA, and Type 4 hyperkinetic RTA
Wilms' tumor	vĭlmz	tumor of the kidneys found in children
Disease/Disorders of the Bladder		
bladder cancer		malignant growth of the bladder
bladder stones		calculi usually formed of crystalline urinary salts that collect in the bladder and other organs
diuresis	dī"ū-rē'sĭs	urine excretion in excess of the usual amount
hematuria	hē"mă-tū'rē-ah	discharge of blood into the urine
neurogenic bladder	nū"rō-jĕn'ĭk	dysfunction due to injury of the nervous system supplying the urinary tract or bladder
urinary incontinence	ĭn-kŏnt'ĭn-ĕns	loss of control of the passage of urine from the bladder
• *nocturnal enuresis*	nŏk-tŭr'năl ĕn"ū-rē'sĭs	incontinence that occurs during sleep
• *overflow*		bladder does not empty properly; leaks when overfull
• *stress*		reaction to laughing, sneezing, coughing, etc.
• *total*		no urine can be retained in the bladder
• *urge*		uncontrollable urge to empty the bladder

continues

DIAGNOSES		
Word	**Pronunciation**	**Definition**
Blood Vessel Problems		
acute arterial occlusion	ăr-tē'rē-ăl ō-kloo'zhŭn	sudden, severe blockage of the renal artery
renal artery stenosis	stĕ-nō'sĭs	blockage of the renal artery before it enters the kidney
renal vein thrombosis	thrŏm-bō'sĭs	blood clot attached to the wall of the veins draining the kidneys
Trauma/Rare Diseases		
interstitial cystitis	ĭn"tĕr-stĭsh'ăl sĭs-tī'tĭs	inflammation of the spaces between the glomeruli and tubules in the kidney
straddle injuries		injury as a result of riding a bike, walking a beam, etc.
toxic injury		injuring results from factors such as drugs, lead-based paints, solvents and fuels, as well as the body's own overproduction of uric acid

TREATMENT PROCEDURES		
Word	**Pronunciation**	**Definition**
bilateral cutaneous ureterostomy	kūtā'nē-ŭs ū-rē"tĕr-ŏtō-mē	surgical procedures to implant ureters into the abdominal wall
bladder diverticulectomy	dī"ver-tĭk"ū-lĕk'tō-mē	removal of a diverticulum (sac) from the bladder
cystectomy	sĭs-tĕk'tō-mē	partial or complete resection of the urinary bladder
cystostomy	sĭs-tŏs'tō-mē	incision into the urinary bladder, usually for drainage
dialysis	dī-ăl'ĭ-sĭs	artificial means of removing waste products from the blood when kidneys have failed
• *hemodialysis*		waste removed directly from the blood
• *peritoneal*		uses peritoneal cavity in the abdomen to filter the blood
• *continuous ambulatory peritoneal dialysis* (CAPD)		abdominal cavity is infused four or five times per day
• *continuous cycling peritoneal dialysis*		automatic infusion of dialysis solution in and out of the peritoneal cavity, drains several times during the night or
• *intermittent peritoneal dialysis* (IPD)		performed several times a week, usually done at home
fulguration	fŭl-gū-rā'shŭn	procedure that uses high-frequency electric sparks to burn lesions off the bladder wall
GOR-TEX graft		artificial blood vessel made of GORE-TEX® used as an artery to a vein connection to create a vascular access for hemodialysis, or to connect an artery to another artery for the treatment of peripheral vascular disease

continues

TREATMENT PROCEDURES		
Word	**Pronunciation**	**Definition**
hemofiltration	hē"mō-fĭl-trā'shŭn	form of dialysis to remove excess metabolic products from the blood; usually done on a continuous basis using a hemofilter instead of a dialyzer; form of Continuous Renal Replacement Therapy (CRRT)
ileal conduit	ĭl'ē-ăl kŏn'doo-ĭt	surgical procedure to transplant the ureters into an isolated segment of the ileum, which is sutured closed on one end, and attaching the other end to the abdominal wall thus diverting urine through a stoma to a collection bag
kidney transplantation		replacement of a failed kidney with a kidney from an identical twin (isograft) or another compatible donor (allograft)
litholapaxy	lĭth-ŏl'ă-păks"ē	crushing of a calculus (stone) in the bladder, followed by immediate washing out of fragments through a catheter
lithotripsy	lĭth'ō-trĭp"sē	procedure to break up or crush stones in the urinary tract
• *extracorporeal shock wave lithotripsy*		the body is immersed in water and hundreds of shock waves are administered using the water as the carrier (the body is not harmed)
• *percutaneous ultrasonic lithotripsy*		uses a small ultrasound-producing unit inserted into the kidney through the abdomen
• *endoscopic lithotripsy*		uses an ultrasound-producing unit passed through the bladder and into the ureter
meatotomy	mē"ah-tŏt'ō-mē	procedure that increases the caliber of urinary meatus
nephrectomy	nĕ-frĕk'tō-mē	removal of a kidney
nephrolithotomy	nĕf"rō-lĭth-ŏt'ō-mē	removal of a calculus from a kidney
nephrostomy	nĕ-frŏs'tō-mē	surgical creation of an opening from the renal pelvis to the outside of the body
percutaneous nephrolithotomy	pĕr"kū-tā'nē-ŭs nĕf"rō-lĭth-ŏt'ō-mē	endoscopic procedure to remove kidney stones
pyelolithotomy	pī"ĕ-lō-lĭ-thŏt'ō-mē	incision into the renal pelvis for removal of calculi
pyeloplasty	pī'ĕ-lō-plăs"tē	repair of the renal pelvis
renal angioplasty	ăn'jē-ō-plăs"tē	dilation of narrowed areas in renal arteries and placement of a stent to keep the vessel open
suprapubic catheter	soo"pră-pū'bĭk	tube that permits direct urinary drainage from the bladder through the lower abdominal wall, from a surgically fashioned opening located just above the pubic symphysis
ureterolithotomy	ū-rē"ter-ō-lĭ-thŏt'ō-mē	incision of the ureter for removal of a calculus

continues

TREATMENT PROCEDURES		
Word	**Pronunciation**	**Definition**
ureterosigmoidostomy	ū-rē"tĕr-ō-sĭg-moyd-ŏs'tō-mē	procedure to implant ureter into the sigmoid colon and creation of a continent stoma with a pouch of bowel; may be Kock, Mainz, or Gilchrist ileocecal reservoir
urethropexy	ū-rē'thrō-pĕk"sē	fixation of the urethra to the posterior aspect of the pubic bone
urethroplasty	ū-rē'thrō-plăs"tē	reconstruction or operative repair of the urethra
urinary catheterization	kăth"ĕ-tĕr-ĭ-zā'shŭn	passing of a flexible tube through the urethra into the urinary bladder

MEDICATIONS PRESCRIBED	
Trade Name	**Generic Name**
Antibiotics, Antimicrobials	
Bactrim, Cotrim, Septra	sulfamethoxazole and trimethoprim
Ceftin	cefuroxime axetil
Cipro	ciprofloxacin
Diflucan	fluconazole
Duricef	cefadroxil
Fortaz	ceftazidime
Furadantin, Macrodantin	nitrofurantoin
Gantrisin	sulfisoxazole
Garamycin, Genoptic, Gentacidin, Gentak, Pediatric Gentamicin	gentamicin sulfate
Keflex	cephalexin
Monocid	cefonicid
Noroxin	norfloxacin
Omnipen, Principen, Totacillin	ampicillin
Rocephin	ceftriaxone
Tobramycin	aminoglycosides
Vancocin, Vancoled	vancomycin HCl
Anticholinergics/Anesthetics	
Detrol	tolterodine tarte
Prosed	methenamine, phenyl salicylate, atropine, hyoscyamine, benzoic acid, and methylene blue
Pyridium, Pyridiate, Baridium	phenazopyridine HCl
Urispas	flavoxate

continues

MEDICATIONS PRESCRIBED	
Trade Name	Generic Name
Antispasmodics	
Anaspaz, Cystospas, Levbid, Levsin, Levsinex	hyoscyamine sulfate
Ditropan	oxybutynin chloride
Pro-Banthine	propantheline bromide
Dialysis and Chronic Kidney Disease	
Aranesp	darbepoeten
Cathflo Activase	alteplase
DDAVP	desmopressin
Epogen	epoetin alfa
Ferrlecit	ferric gluconate
Fosrenol	lanthanum carbonate
Hectorol	doxercalciferol
Infed	iron dextran
PhosLo	calcium acetate
Renagel	sevelamer
Venofer	iron sucrose
Zemplar	paracalcitol
Renal Failure	
Accupril	quinapril
Aldomet	methyldopa
Apresoline	hydralazine HCl
Bumex	bumetanide
Calderol	calcifedial
Catapres	clonidine HCl
HydroDIURIL	hydrochlorothiazide HCl
Inocor	amrinone lactate
Kayexalate	sodium polystyrene sulfonate
Lanoxin	digoxin
Lasix	furosemide
Loniten	minoxidil
Procardia	nifedipine
Rocaltrol	calcitrol (synthetic vitamin D)
Vasotec	enalapril maleate

continues

MEDICATIONS PRESCRIBED	
Trade Name	**Generic Name**
Renal Transplantation	
CellCept	mycophenolate mofetil
Imuran	azathioprine
Myfortic	mycophenolic acid
Neoral	cyclosporine microemulsion
Prograf	tacrolimus
Rapamune	sirolimus
Rituxan	rituximab
Sandimmune	cyclosporine
Other Medications	
Azo Gantrisin	sulfisoxazole and phenazopyridine
Bicitra, Shohl's solution	sodium citrate, citric acid
Neosporin G.U. irritant	neomycin, polymyxin B
Prostigmin	neostigmine bromide
Renacidin Irrigation	citric acid, magnesium carbonate, gluconodelta-lactone
Urecholine, Duvoid	bethanechol

ABBREVIATIONS	
ACE	angiotensin-converting enzyme
ACEI	angiotensin-converting enzyme inhibitor
ADH	antidiuretic hormone
AKI	acute kidney injury
ANCA	antineutrophil cytoplasmic antibody
ARB	angiotensin receptor blocker
ARF	acute renal failure
A-V	arteriovenous
BUN	blood urea nitrogen
CAPD	continuous ambulatory peritoneal dialysis
cath	catheter, catheterization
CAVH	continuous arteriovenous hemofiltration
CCPD	continuous cycling peritoneal dialysis
CKD	chronic kidney disease
CRF	chronic renal failure
CRRT	continuous renal replacement therapy
C&S	culture and sensitivity
CVVH	continuous venovenous hemofiltration

continues

ABBREVIATIONS	
cysto	cystoscopic examination
ESRD	end-stage renal disease
ESWL	extracorporeal shock wave lithotripsy
GBM	glomerular basement membrane
GFR	glomerular filtration rate
GU	genitourinary
HD	hemodialysis
IPD	intermittent peritoneal dialysis
IVP	intravenous pyelogram
K^+	potassium ion (potassium electrolyte)
KUB	kidney, ureter, and bladder
MPGN	membranoproliferative glomerulonephritis
Na^+	sodium ion (sodium electrolyte)
PD	peritoneal dialysis
PKD	polycystic kidney disease
PTH	parathyroid hormone
RPGN	rapidly progressive glomerulonephritis
RTA	renal tubular acidosis
SIADH	syndrome of inappropriate antidiuretic hormone
SLE	systemic lupus erythematosus
SLEDD	sustained low-efficiency daily dialysis
UA	urinalysis
UC	urine culture
URR	urea reduction ratio
UTI	urinary tract infection
VCUG	voiding cystourethrogram

Working Practice Review Exercises

IDENTIFICATION

Identify the following diagnostic procedures and laboratory tests.

1. deep structures of the kidney are visualized by recording reflections of sound waves ______________________
2. x-ray of the urinary bladder while the patient is voiding ______________________

3. body section roentgenography of the kidney ______________
4. x-ray study of the kidney, ureter, and bladder using an intravenous contrast medium ______________
5. contrast medium study of the bladder ______________
6. visual examination of the bladder with a scope ______________
7. removal of a tissue sample from the kidney, usually done with a biopsy needle ______________
8. graphic recording of bladder volumes and changing pressure reactions ______________
9. analysis of urine ______________
10. measures urea in the blood ______________
11. measures the ability of the kidney to remove creatinine from the blood ______________
12. measures an enzyme in the blood to check for cancer of the prostate ______________
13. introduction of a catheter into bladder to remove sterile specimen of urine for testing ______________
14. ultrasound of renal arteries to evaluate renal blood flow ______________
15. x-ray of kidney, ureter, bladder ______________
16. x-ray of urinary bladder after introduction of a radioisotope ______________
17. collection of all of an individual's urine to evaluate kidney function, protein secretion, or excretion of other substances ______________
18. test to determine type of bacteria present and which antibiotic to use on it ______________
19. test to see if red blood cells in urine have an irregular shape ______________
20. method of distinguishing proteins and antibodies in body fluid on basis of electrophoretic mobility and antigenic specificities ______________

DEFINITIONS

Define and provide the pronunciation for the following surgical procedures.

1. cystostomy ______________

____

2. pyelolithotomy ______________

____

3. urethroplasty ______________

____

4. meatotomy ______________

____

5. nephrectomy ______________

____

MATCHING

Match the meanings to the correct diagnoses.

1. _______ more urine than usual	a. acute arterial occlusion
2. _______ any disease of the kidney	b. cystitis
3. _______ stones occurring anywhere in the urinary tract	c. diuresis
4. _______ decreased function of the kidneys	d. end-stage renal disease
5. _______ multiple cysts in the kidney	e. glomerulonephritis
6. _______ inflammation of the glomeruli	f. kidney cysts
7. _______ inflammation of the urinary bladder	g. medullary sponge kidney
8. _______ protein loss from the kidneys, resulting in edema	h. nephrotic syndrome
9. _______ multiple small cysts in the central portion of the renal pyramids	i. nephrolithiasis
10. _______ severe blockage of the renal artery	j. nephropathy
11. _______ terminal kidney failure requiring dialysis or transplantation	k. polycystic kidney disease
12. _______ fluid-filled masses in the kidney	l. pyelitis
13. _______ presence of calculi in the kidney	m. renal failure
14. _______ inflammation of pelvis of kidney	n. uremia
15. _______ systemic result of accumulation of toxins normally secreted by kidneys	o. urinary calculi

IDENTIFICATION/ABBREVIATIONS

Identify the following abbreviations.

1. IVP ______________________________
2. BUN ______________________________
3. UA ______________________________
4. GU ______________________________
5. GFR ______________________________
6. cath ______________________________
7. ESRD ______________________________
8. KUB ______________________________
9. UTI ______________________________
10. C&S ______________________________

Dictionary Exercises

DICTIONARY EXERCISE 1

Use your dictionary to find the pronunciation and definition of each of the following words.

	Word	Pronunciation	Definition
1.	diuretic	______	______
2.	aldosterone	______	______
3.	oliguria	______	______
4.	urinary retention	______	______
5.	glycosuria	______	______
6.	ketosis	______	______
7.	anuria	______	______
8.	urinary casts	______	______
9.	angiotensin	______	______
10.	azotemia	______	______

DICTIONARY EXERCISE 2

Select the correct meaning and provide the pronunciation where indicated.

1. albuminuria (______)
   a. painful urination
   b. frequent urination
   c. albumin in the urine
   d. pus in the urine
2. calculus (______)
   a. stone found in a body part
   b. tube for insertion into a duct or a cavity that allows the escape of fluid
   c. warty, dry, cauliflower-like lesions
   d. one of the layers surrounding the front and side of the testicle
3. catheter (______)
   a. removal of waste products from blood
   b. tubular, flexible instrument passed through a body channel for withdrawal of fluids
   c. stone found in a body part
   d. tube for insertion into a duct or cavity that allows the escape of fluid
4. infundibulum (______)
   a. triangular area, especially one at the floor of the bladder
   b. one of the layers surrounding the front and side of the testicle
   c. funnel-shaped opening
   d. retaining excessive amounts of urine in the bladder
5. trigone (______)
   a. funnel-shaped opening
   b. stone found in a body part
   c. circular arrangement of muscles controlling the urinary bladder
   d. triangular area, especially one at the floor of the bladder
6. ureterolysis (______)
   a. incision of the ureter
   b. stone in the ureter
   c. paralysis of the ureter
   d. suppurative inflammation within a ureter
7. stricture of ureter (______)
   a. localized narrowing of the tubular ureter, often caused by inflammation
   b. triangular area near the floor of the bladder
   c. layer surrounding the front and side of the testicle
   d. circular arrangement of muscles controlling the urinary bladder

8. tunica vaginalis (____________________)
   a. triangular area near the floor of the bladder
   b. narrowing of the tubular ureter
   c. funnel-shaped opening
   d. one of the layers surrounding the front and side of the testicle
9. urinary retention
   a. albumin in the urine
   b. retaining excessive amounts of urine in the bladder
   c. painful urination
   d. blood in the urine
10. vesicoureteral (____________________)
   a. pertaining to the connection between the ureter and the urinary bladder
   b. pertaining to the area where the ureter leads off from the pelvis of the kidney
   c. pertaining to the triangular area at the floor of the bladder
   d. pertaining to the bladder and ureter

DICTIONARY EXERCISE 3

Pronunciation of the words below is provided. Using your dictionary, find the correct spelling and definition of each word.

	Word	Pronunciation	Definition
1.	__________	sfĭngk'ter	____________________
2.	__________	kăn'ū-lah	____________________
3.	__________	ăn"tĭ-dī-ū-rĕt'ĭk	____________________
4.	__________	băk-tē"rē-ū'rē-ah	____________________
5.	__________	hē'mō-fĭl"tĕr	____________________
6.	__________	pī-ū'rē-ah	____________________
7.	__________	trĭg"ō-nī'tĭs	____________________
8.	__________	pĕrm'căth	____________________
9.	__________	ū-rē'ter-al kŏl'ĭk	____________________
10.	__________	rĕn'ĭn	____________________

DICTIONARY EXERCISE 4

Rewrite each sentence in your own words. Provide the pronunciation for each italicized word.

1. There was evidence of *condyloma acuminatum* (____________________).

   ____

2. The patient suffered from *urodynia* (____________________).

   ____

3. The record indicated "*nocturia* (____________________) × *2*."

   ____

4. The patient indicated that one of the symptoms he experienced was *polydipsia* (____________________).

   ____

5. The condition was marked by *polyuria* (____________________).

   ____

6. He has an *autonomous* (____________________) bladder.

   ____

StudyWARE™ Connection

To take a practice quiz or play interactive games that reinforce the content in this chapter, go to your StudyWARE™ CD-ROM.

Listening Exercise

INSTRUCTIONS

1. Review the spelling, pronunciation, and meaning of the words provided in the preview.
2. Go to your StudyWARE™ CD-ROM and listen to **Listening Exercise 15-1.** Fill in the blank in the report as the word is dictated.
3. At the end of the activity, check your spelling against the preview words. They appear in the preview in the order in which they are encountered in the activity.
4. Review and practice the words you missed.
5. Look up words that are not familiar.

PREVIEW OF WORDS FOR LISTENING EXCERCISE 15-1

Word	Pronunciation	Meaning
tomograms	tō'mō-grăms	x-ray pictures designed to show detailed images of selected structures
creatinine	krē-ăt'ĭn-ĭn	alkaline, nonprotein constituent of urine and blood; increased quantities are found in advanced states of renal disease
angiography	an"jē-ŏg'ră-fē	x-ray of blood vessels after injection of radiopaque substance
nephrectomy	nĕ-frĕk-tō'mē	surgical procedure to remove a kidney voiding evacuating the bowels or bladder
catheterization	kăth"ĕ-tĕr-ĭ-zā'shŭn	use of a catheter or passage into a body cavity to withdraw or drain fluids

Listening Exercise 15-1

*Study*WARE™ Connection

Listen to this report being read on your StudyWARE™ CD-ROM. Fill in each blank as the word is dictated.

Discharge Summary

HISTORY:

This 34-year-old lady was admitted because of a lump in her right side, which had solid echoes and appeared solid on CT. It was associated with the right kidney.

LABORATORY DATA:

The chest ________________________ were negative. The electrocardiogram was normal. Urine pH 5, specific gravity 1.021, negative protein and glucose, 5–8 white cells, 0–2 red cells. White count 6,200, differential normal. Hemoglobin 13.1, hematocrit 38.8. Partial thromboplastin time and prothrombin time normal. Sodium 142, potassium 4.5, chlorides 105. On SMA 1260, all parameters are within normal limits. Postoperative ________________________ is 0.9.

HOSPITAL COURSE:

On 10-19-20—, a selective ________________________ confirmed vascular tumor of the right kidney. Therefore, on 10-20-20—, under general anesthesia, a radical right ________________________ was carried out. A 310-gram specimen revealed a 4.5-centimeter mass in the mid-portion of the right kidney with extensive hemorrhage in it and a cystic pattern was an extremely well differentiated renal cell carcinoma. There was no capsular invasion, no lymphatic invasion, and no venous invasion. She also had a fibrotic appendix removed.

Her postoperative course was benign; she never had significant fever. She did have a little difficulty ________________________, necessitating ________________________ until the fifth postoperative day. Cath was out; she voided all right and was discharged on the sixth postoperative day. On discharge she was given a prescription for Gantanol and Tylenol 3 and I'll see her in the office in about two weeks.

Marcus Sibilsky, MD

d: 10-26-20—

t: 10-29-20—

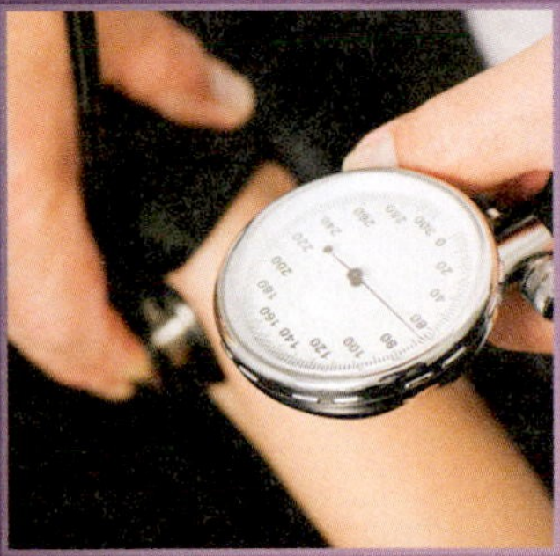
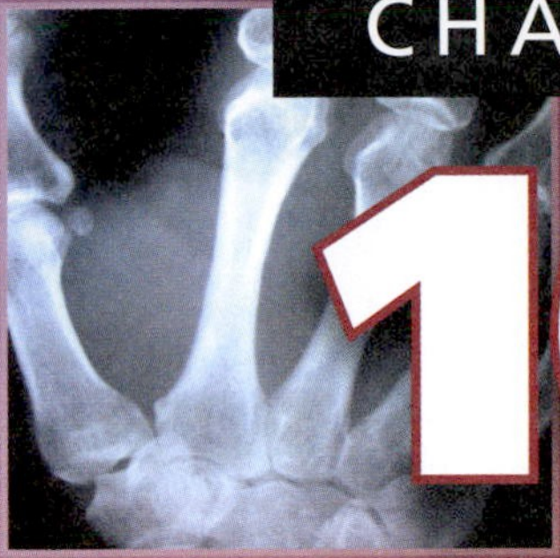

CHAPTER 16

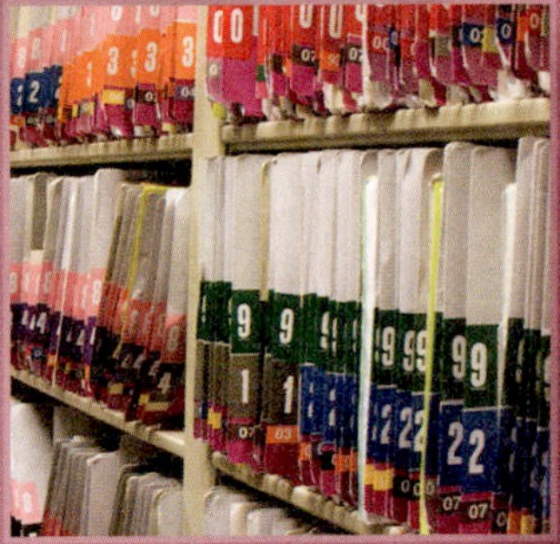

The Female Reproductive System

"Where did you come from, baby dear?
Out of the everywhere into here"

—George MacDonald

OBJECTIVES

When you have completed this chapter on the female reproductive system, you should be able to

1. Spell and define major system components and explain how they operate.
2. Identify the meanings of related word elements.
3. Spell and define diagnostic procedures, diagnoses, treatment procedures, and abbreviations.
4. Spell the names of commonly used medications.
5. Use a dictionary as a tool in processing medical documents.
6. Hear how medical terminology is used in actual medical reports.

INTRODUCTION

Human reproduction is accomplished by a process called fertilization, requiring female ova and male spermatozoa. In addition to reproduction, hormones produced by both genders affect a variety of other bodily functions.

The female reproductive system is studied by a **gynecologist** (gī″nĭ-kŏl′ō-jĭst), who may also manage the childbirth process as an **obstetrician** (ŏb-stĕ-trĭsh′ăn). The female anatomy is discussed in this chapter. The male reproductive system is part of the urologist's specialty and will be discussed in Chapter 17, along with sexually transmitted diseases.

COMPONENTS OF THE FEMALE REPRODUCTIVE SYSTEM

adnex/o	tie, connection
gynec/o	female

The female reproductive system consists of the ovaries, fallopian tubes, uterus, and vagina. These are all internal organs. The external organs, which are called the vulva, include the pubis, labia, clitoris, vestibule, and Bartholin's glands. Breasts are considered a part of the integumentary system, as well as a secondary sex organ. A discussion of each of the components of the female reproductive system follows.

OVARIES

oophor/o	ovary
ovari/o	ovary
ov/i, ov/o, ovul/o	egg

The two **ovaries** (2), illustrated in Figure 16-1, respond to hormones produced by the pituitary gland and are held in position by several ligaments. The largest is a broad ligament that also supports the tubes, uterus, and vagina.

The outer layer of each ovary is made of epithelium, and it is here that the ova are produced. They go through a maturation process of about fourteen days in small sacs called **ovarian follicles**. When an ovum ripens, the follicle literally ruptures, and the ovum is discharged from the surface of the ovary in a process called **ovulation**.

At the time of birth there are 200,000 to 400,000 ova present in each ovary, but only 400 or so will mature. The rest reach various stages of development and then regress and degenerate.

Following ovulation the cells of the follicle increase in size, take on a yellowish color, and become known as a **corpus luteum** (kor'pŭs loo'tē-ŭm). If the ovum is not fertilized, the corpus luteum begins to degenerate after approximately 2 weeks. If the ovum is fertilized, the corpus luteum will remain for several months before it degenerates. During that time it provides the hormone **progesterone** (prō-jĕs'tĕ-rōn). Another hormone, **estrogen** (ĕs'trō-jĕn), is produced by other maturing follicles. Progesterone and estrogen help keep the lining of the uterus in a favorable condition for development of the fertilized egg, or **embryo**.

FALLOPIAN TUBES

salping/o	tube

After the ovum is released at ovulation, it makes its way to the duct connected to the uterus known as the **fallopian** (făl-lō'pē-ăn) **tube** (1), (also called an oviduct). There is no direct connection between the ovary and the fallopian

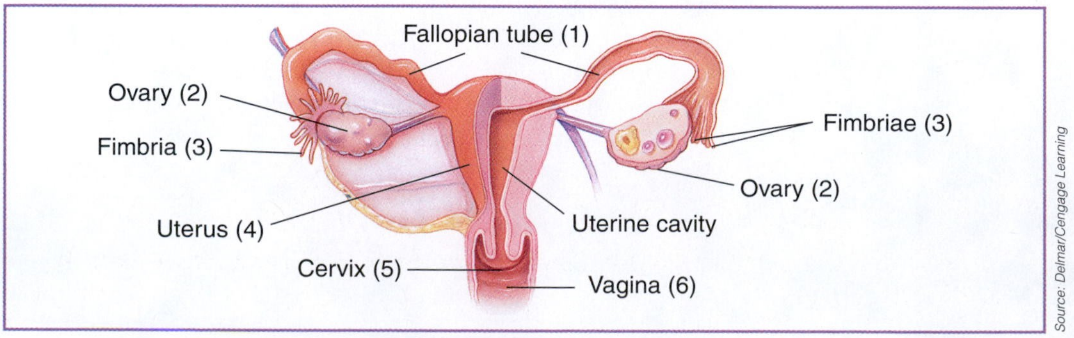

FIGURE 16-1
Female Reproductive System

tubes. Ova are swept into the tubes by a current in the peritoneal fluid produced by small fringelike extensions from the edges of the abdominal opening of the tube. These small extensions are called **fimbriae** (fĭm'brē-ā) (3).

Once inside the tube, the ova are kept moving toward the uterus by the action of cilia in the lining of the tubes, as well as by peristalsis. This journey from the ovary to the uterus takes approximately 5 days.

Fertilization takes place in the first third of the fallopian tube within twenty-four hours of ovulation. If for some reason a fertilized egg does not reach the uterus, a tubal or **ectopic** (ĕk-tŏp'ĭk) **pregnancy** develops.

UTERUS

cervic/o	neck, cervix
hyster/o	uterus
metr/o	uterus
uter/o	uterus

The **uterus** (4) is a muscular, pear-shaped organ located between the urinary bladder and the rectum. The larger upper portion is called the **corpus**. The small, rounded part above the level of the entrance to the fallopian tube is known as the **fundus**. The lower portion of the uterus is called the **cervix** (ser'vĭks) (5). The cervix leads to the vagina, which opens to the outside of the body.

The wall of the uterus has three layers: the endometrium, myometrium, and perimetrium. The innermost layer of the uterus is a specialized epithelium known as **endometrium** (ĕn-dō-mē'trē-ŭm). Each month this layer gradually thickens in preparation for a possible pregnancy. After ovulation, if the ovum is not fertilized while passing through the fallopian tube, it disintegrates upon reaching the uterus. The endometrium also begins to deteriorate. Small hemorrhages appear, producing bleeding known as menstrual flow. Even before the menstrual flow ceases (from 1 to 5 days), the endometrium begins to repair itself through the growth of new cells for the beginning of a new cycle. The muscular or middle layer, the **myometrium**, gives the uterus the ability to contract during the childbirth process. The uterus has an outer layer or membrane called the **uterine serosa** (ŭ'tĕr-ĭn sē-rō'sa) or perimetrium.

VAGINA

colp/o	vagina
vagin/o	vagina

The **vagina** (6) is a muscular tube approximately 3 inches long connecting the uterine cavity to the exterior of the body. The cervix of the uterus dips into the upper vagina, creating circular recesses and areas known as **fornices** (for'nĭ-sēz). The deepest of these spaces is behind the cervix and is called the **posterior fornix**. The lining of the vagina is similar to the mucous membrane found in the stomach. These rugae or folds permit enlargement of the vagina during childbirth. Near the vaginal canal opening to the outside, there is foldlike membrane called the **hymen**.

*Study*WARE™ Connection

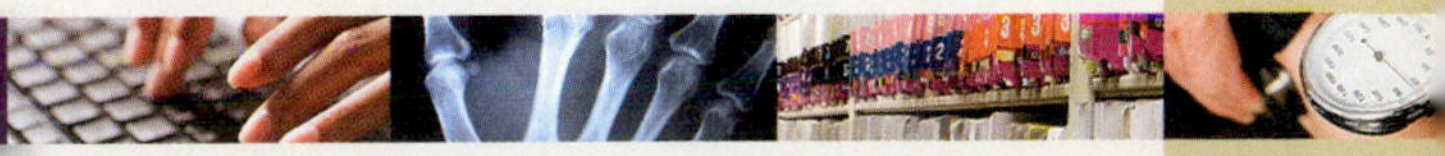

Play an interactive game labeling structures of the **Female Reproductive System** on your StudyWARE™ CD-ROM.

EXTERNAL GENITALIA

episi/o	vulva
vulv/o	vulva

The collective external female genitalia are called the **vulva** (vŭl'vah) and provide protection for the genital area. Uppermost is the area called the **mons pubis** (mŏnz pū'bĭs), which is covered with pubic hair following puberty. Figure 16-2 shows the area below the mons pubis. There are two folds or lips called the **labia majora** (lā'bē-ah mah-jō'rah) (4). Medial to them are two smaller folds of tissue called the **labia minora** (mĭ-no'rah) (3). They surround a space called the vestibule into which the vagina (5) and urethra (2) open.

Just below and to each side of the vaginal opening are two mucous-producing **vulvovaginal** (vŭl"vō-văj'ĭ-năl) or **Bartholin's glands** (6). These glands lubricate the vestibule and facilitate sexual intercourse. The **clitoris** (klĭt'ō-rĭs) (1) is a small structure almost enclosed by the foreskin formed by the labia minora; the exposed portion is the glans. The tissue of the clitoris is similar to the penis in that it, too, is composed of erectile tissue.

Although the entire pelvic floor is properly called the **perineum** (pĕr"ĭ-nē'ŭm) in both men and women, health care specialists who care for pregnant women usually refer to the perineum as the limited area between the vaginal opening and the anus.

StudyWARE™ Connection

Play an interactive game labeling structures of the **Female External Genitalia** on your StudyWARE™ CD-ROM.

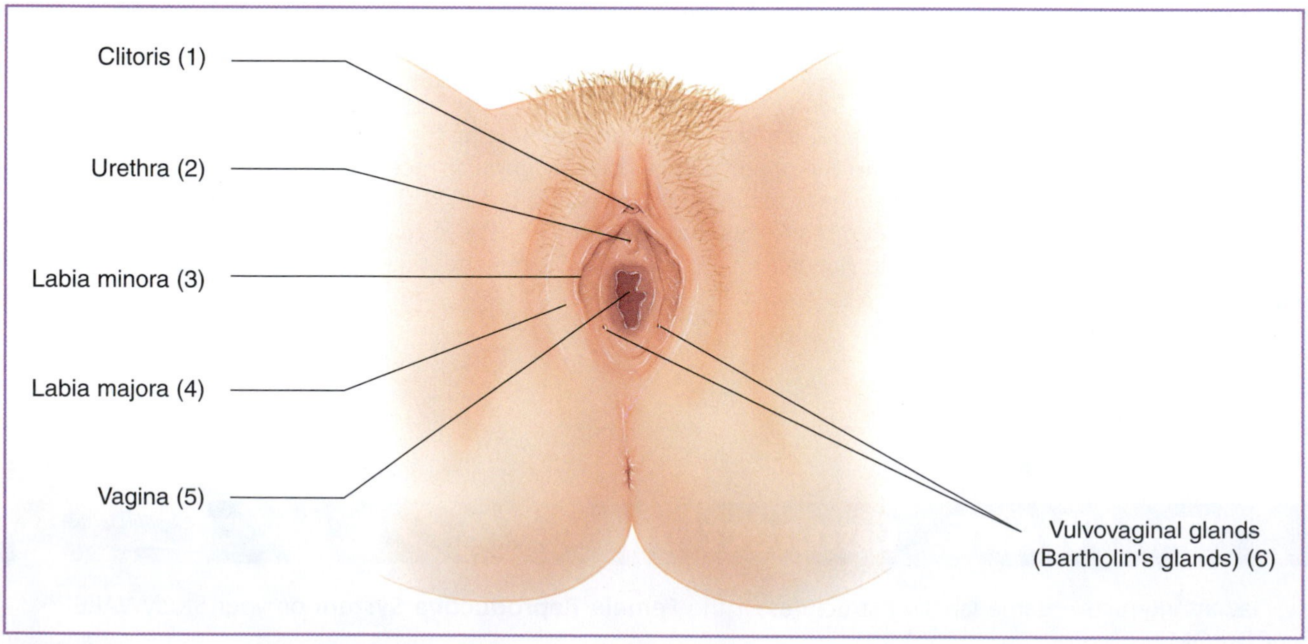

Source: Delmar/Cengage Learning

FIGURE 16-2 Female External Genitalia

BREASTS

lact/o	milk
mamm/o	breast
mast/o	breast
papill/o	nipplelike
pect/o, pector/o	breast, chest
thel/o	nipple

The soft, hemispherical form of the **mamma** (măm'ah) or breast is due to the superficial fascia, which is heavily loaded with fat and surrounds the mammary gland. Technically, breasts are considered an appendage of the skin. In women, breasts are considered a secondary sex organ designed to produce milk after childbirth. In males, it is less common to refer to breasts because they neither function nor develop in the same way.

In a woman, the tiny glands begin gradual development until just before the onset of menstruation (menarche). The mammary gland in the woman then reflects and responds to the ovarian hormones and the pituitary gland, as does the endometrium (uterine lining).

In Figure 16-3, note that the center of the breast is the nipple (3), and its halo is called the **areola** (ah-rē'ō-lah) (2). The glandular tissue (5) of the breast is arranged in fifteen to twenty lobes. The duct (4) of each lobe branches and branches again into smaller ducts called ductules or lobules. The whole internal structure of the breast has been compared to a bunch of tiny grapes.

Milk secretion, which is controlled by the anterior pituitary lobe in humans, is carried to the nipple by sinuses (1). This happens during the lactation period of the birth process.

*Study*WARE™ Connection

View an animation on the **Female Reproductive System** on your StudyWARE™ CD-ROM.

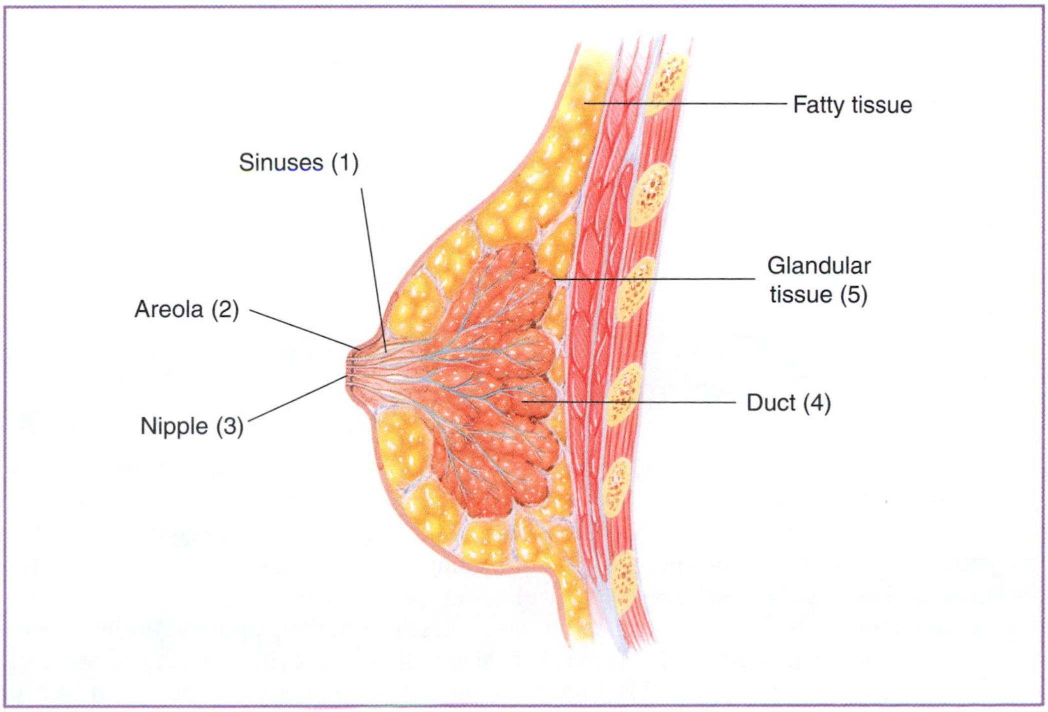

FIGURE 16-3 Structure of the Breast

Source: Delmar/Cengage Learning

MENSTRUAL CYCLE

men/o	menses

The **menstrual cycle** refers to the monthly developmental changes that occur in the endometrium of the uterus. These changes result in a normal flow of blood called the **menses** (mĕn'sēz). The average length of the cycle is 28 days, although this can vary among individuals. Usually the onset of menstrual cycles, or **menarche** (mĕ-năr'kē), occurs between the ages of nine and seventeen; the cessation, or **menopause** (mĕn'ō-pawz), generally occurs between the ages of 45 and 60 years.

Immediately after menstruation the endometrium is very thin; but during the postmenstrual period (from approximately the fifth to fourteenth day of the cycle), the endometrium becomes thicker. This is because of the presence of the hormone estrogen, which is contained in the fluid produced by the follicles on the surface of the ovaries.

Ovulation takes place when the follicle breaks open and the ovum is discharged. Then the cells that form the corpus luteum begin to secrete progesterone. This further develops the endometrium to provide a bed for a fertilized ovum. If the ovum is not fertilized, the corpus luteum ceases production of both hormones, the endometrium begins deterioration, menstrual discharge begins, and the cycle starts again.

The pituitary gland, located in the brain, is extremely important in the function of the reproductive system. It produces two principal gonadotropins that stimulate the ovary. One is the follicle-stimulating hormone (FSH), which stimulates the follicles during the first and second stages of the menstrual cycle. The other is the luteinizing hormone (LH), which is important in the third and fourth stages of the menstrual cycle (ovulation and secretion of progesterone). The release of the gonadotropic hormones by the pituitary is regulated by the hypothalamus, another specialized structure in the brain. If pregnancy occurs, another hormone, human chorionic gonadotropin (HCG), appears and acts on the corpus luteum. Essentially HCG tells the corpus luteum to continue producing estrogen and progesterone, which maintains the endometrium during pregnancy.

StudyWARE™ Connection

Go to your StudyWARE™ CD-ROM to watch an animation on **Ovulation**.

PREGNANCY AND BIRTH

amni/o	amnion
gravid/o	pregnancy
par-, part-	bear
prol-	offspring
umbilic/o	navel

After ovulation, an ovum can be fertilized if sperm are present. When fertilization does occur, it happens in the upper region of the fallopian tube. The egg and the sperm each carry 23 chromosomes containing thousands of genes. When the sperm penetrates to the center of the egg, sperm and egg merge to become a one-cell embryo (**zygote** [zī'gōt]) and fertilization of the ovum is complete. Gender, eye color, and even texture of hair have been determined. Within 12 hours the new cell divides and continues to divide about every 12 hours, reaching about 500 cells within 4 to 5 days. The fertilized ovum then takes several days to travel to the uterus where it will grow.

By the time it reaches the uterus, it is known as a **blastocyst** (blăs'tō-sĭst), another stage in the development of the embryo. One section of the blastocyst contains the cells that will produce an embryo. The outermost layer (**trophoblast** [trŏf'ō-blăst]) will attach itself to the uterine wall and become the **placenta** (plah-sĕn'tah) and the membranes, which will provide nourishment, respiration, and excretion for the developing fetus.

The **umbilical** (ŭm-bĭl'ĭ-kăl) **cord**, which contains two arteries and a vein, connects the fetus to the placenta. The fetus itself is encased in a structure called the **amniotic** (ăm"nē-ŏt'ĭk) **sac**. This sac is filled with a clear liquid called amniotic fluid and serves as a protective cushion for the fetus.

SIGNS AND SYMPTOMS OF PREGNANCY

The signs and symptoms of pregnancy may be presumptive, probable, or positive.

Early symptoms of pregnancy are called *presumptive signs* because they are experienced by the expectant mother. These early symptoms may include amenorrhea, nausea, vomiting, fatigue, urinary disturbances, and/or breast changes. The patient may also feel movement of the fetus, or **quickening**, around the eighteenth to the twentieth week of gestation.

Once the symptoms are observable by the examiner, they are called *probable signs* and are a much stronger indicator of pregnancy. The following chart gives a list of the probable signs and their definitions.

PROBABLE PREGNANCY SIGNS

SIGN	DEFINITION
abdominal stria	stretch marks
ballottement	examiner taps uterus through vagina to cause fetus to bounce within the amniotic fluid
Braxton Hicks contractions	irregular contractions of the uterus
Chadwick's sign	cervix and vagina take on bluish-violet hue
fetal outline	can be palpated at about 24 weeks
Goodell's sign	softening of the cervix and vagina
Hegar's sign	softening of the lower segment of the uterus
hyperpigmentation of the skin	mask of pregnancy
pregnancy tests	based on presence of human chorionic gonadotropin which is secreted during pregnancy
uterine enlargement	presumed presence of growing embryo/fetus

There are only three *positive signs* of pregnancy that indicate a developing fetus with certainty. The first is a fetal heartbeat which can be detected by ultrasound at about 10 weeks' gestation or by use of a fetoscope at 18 to 20 weeks. A **fetoscope** allows detection of the fetal heartbeat through the mother's abdomen. The second positive sign is identification of the fetus by ultrasound as early as 5 to 6 weeks with 100% reliability. The third sign is the fetal movements felt by the physician/examiner by the second trimester of pregnancy.

PRENATAL DEVELOPMENT

The average time from fertilization to delivery is 266 days, which is divided into three trimesters.

First Trimester (Conception to 13 Weeks)

All major organs of the body are formed during the first trimester. Rudiments of a spinal cord are evident almost immediately and the eyes and heart begin to form. By week 5, the placenta and umbilical cord are fully functioning. By week 6, the brain becomes more noticeable and by the end of the second month of the pregnancy, the baby looks like a miniature human with a large head. During week 10, the heart is beating and the embryo is now considered a **fetus** until it is born. At the end of this trimester the baby may be about 3 inches long and weigh about 1 ounce.

Second Trimester (Weeks 14 to 26)

All the organs formed in the first trimester continue to grow and mature. At the end of the fourth month, a heartbeat can be detected with a stethoscope. Soon movements of the fetus may become discernable by the mother. The fetus blinks, grasps, and moves the mouth. By the end of this trimester, the fetus is about 12 inches long and weighs about 1 pound. It has acquired the beginning of eyelashes, eyebrows, hair, and even fat deposits under the skin. Eyes are completely formed and the tongue actually has taste buds.

Third Trimester (Weeks 27 to 40)

During the last trimester, the fetus takes on most of its weight. By 28 weeks the baby's skin is covered with a thick, white protective coating called the **vernix caseosa** (vĕr'nĭks kā"sē-ō'sah). Eyes are open and the baby is capable of crying. At the end of this trimester, the average baby weighs about 7-1/2 pounds. (see Figure 16-4.)

THE STAGES OF LABOR

At the end of the prenatal or pregnancy period (normally about 38 to 40 weeks), the process of giving birth, or **parturition** (pār"tū-rĭsh'ŭn), takes place. It is divided into three stages known as labor.

Stage One

Muscles of the uterus begin contractions, pushing the amniotic sac against the cervix, causing the cervix to dilate until it has opened about 10 centimeters (4 inches). While all women labor differently, there are some basic signposts that indicate progress. This first and longest stage is divided into three phases: early, active, and transition.

The early phase lasts until the cervix has dilated 1–4 centimeters with light contractions about 20 minutes apart. During the active phase, the contractions become more intense, occurring 4–5 minutes apart and lasting

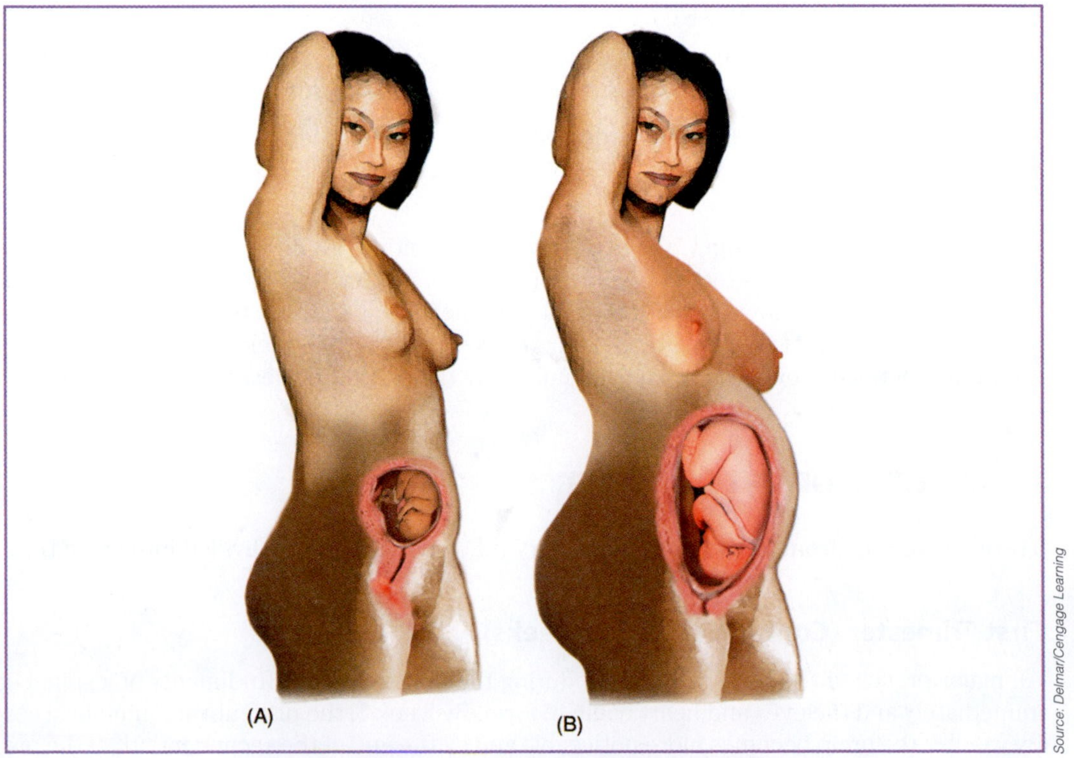

FIGURE 16-4 (A) Woman 20 weeks' pregnant; (B) Woman 36 weeks' pregnant

up to 60 seconds. The cervix dilates to 4–8 centimeters. In the transition phase, contractions can be 2–3 minutes apart and last up to 90 seconds. At this point the cervix is completely dilated. After several hours of labor, the amniotic membranes usually rupture.

Stage Two

If the baby is positioned in the **occiput** (ŏk'sĭ-pŭt) **anterior position** with the head down and its face toward the mother's back (Figure 16-5A), the contractions will propel the baby downward, at which time the mother is instructed to assist by pushing. The vaginal opening becomes dilated and bulges. If the opening does not provide adequate room, the physician makes an incision called an **episiotomy** (ĕ-pĭs"ē-ŏt'ō-mē) at the opening of the vagina. About 96% of babies are born in this head-first, facing-back position.

Unfortunately, some babies are positioned in a way that is dangerous or that may require special measures. The abnormal fetal positions are breech, transverse, and occiput posterior.

The most common abnormal presentation is **breech**, where the baby's buttocks are positioned to emerge first instead of the head (Figure 16-5B). If the infant does not reposition before labor, most physicians will perform a cesarean section (C-section). A **cesarean** (sĭ-zăr'ē-ăn) **delivery** is birth through an incision made in the abdomen and into the uterus. The infant is lifted out, the placenta is removed, and the uterus and abdomen are stitched closed. This is considered major surgery and requires a longer period of recuperation.

The **transverse presentation** (Figure 16-5C) occurs when the baby is at right angles to the birth canal. Vaginal delivery is impossible from this position. Cesarean sections should begin before or just after active labor begins to minimize the risk to mother and child.

The **occiput posterior position** (Figure 16-5D) is when the infant's head is positioned near the cervix, but the baby's face is toward the mother's front. This position makes it difficult to travel down the birth canal and may require use of forceps, and less frequently, a cesarean delivery.

Once the physician clears the baby's airway and the baby is expelled, the baby's umbilical cord, which connects the baby to the placenta, is cut. The depressed scar on the infant's abdomen marks the point of attachment of the cord and is called the **umbilicus** (ŭm-bĭ-lī'kŭs) or navel. The baby is examined, weighed, and cleaned.

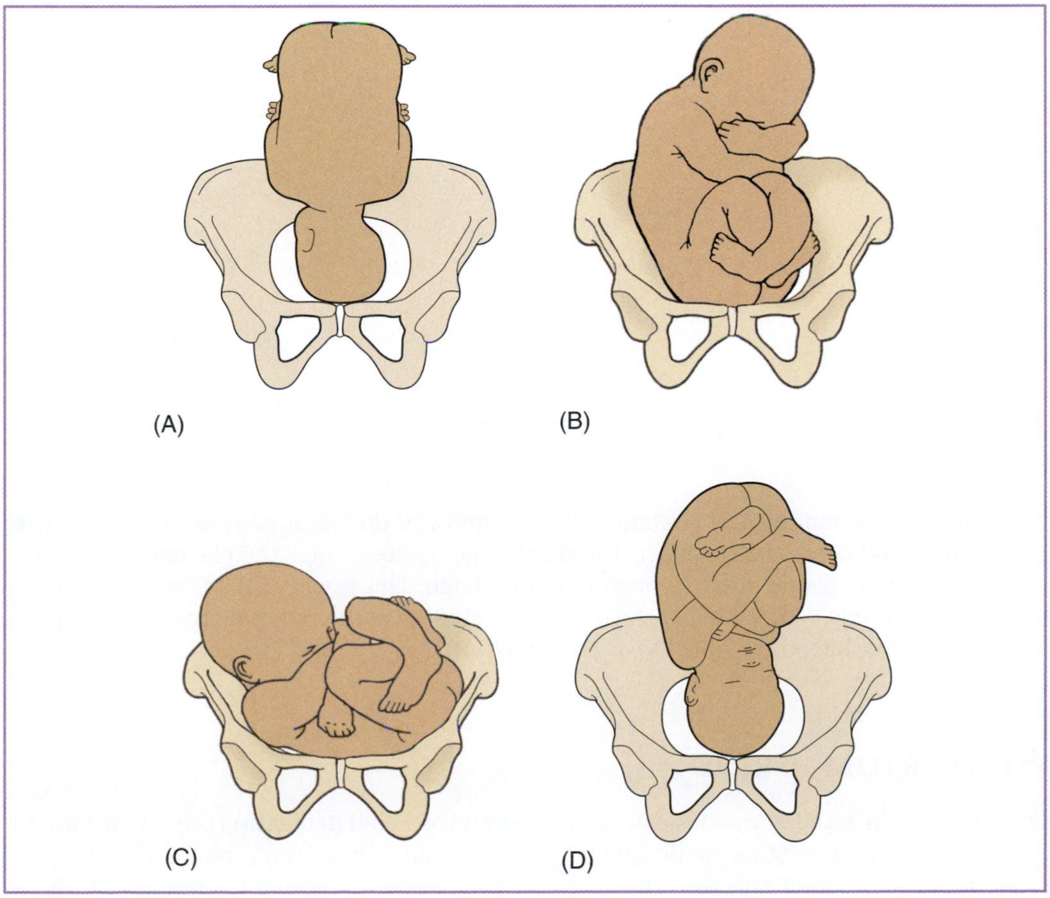

FIGURE 16-5
Delivery Positions: (A) occiput anterior (normal); (B) breech; (C) transverse; (D) occiput posterior

Source: Delmar/Cengage Learning

As soon as the baby is born, the **Apgar score** is taken at 1 and 5 minutes. It is a quick score to determine the physical condition of the newborn. The scale is based on a score of 1 to 10, with 10 indicating the healthiest infant and a score below 5 indicating the newborn needs immediate assistance.

Five categories are assessed: heart rate, respiratory effort, muscle tone, reflex irritability, and color.

APGAR FACTORS	Score 0	Score 1	Score 2
Heart Rate (as evaluated by a stethoscope)			
There is no heartbeat	X		
Heartbeat is less than 100 beats per minute		X	
Heartbeat is greater than 100 beats per minutes			X
Respiratory Effort			
There are no respirations	X		
Respirations are slow or irregular		X	
There is good crying			X
Muscle Tone			
Muscle tone is flaccid	X		
There is some flexion of the extremities	X		
There is active motion			X
Reflex Irritability (the level of newborn irritation in response to stimuli such as a mild pinch)			
There is no reflex irritability	X		
There is grimacing		X	
There is a vigorous cry			X
Color			
The baby is pale blue	X		
The baby is pink and the extremities are blue		X	
The entire body is pink			X

Stage Three

The placenta, membranes of the amniotic sac, and the umbilical cord are expelled as the uterus continues to experience mild contractions during the third stage of labor. Once the placenta and other materials are expelled, the uterus should clamp down to prevent hemorrhage. This is within the first 30 minutes after the birth. Changes in the body include contracting of the uterus and shifting of the internal organs to pre-pregnancy places and sizes. The period after birth is referred to as **postpartum**.

POSTPARTUM PERIOD

During pregnancy the hormones estrogen, progesterone, and **prolactin** (prō-lăk'tĭn) are produced to promote the growth of special breast tissue designed to produce milk. Prolactin, produced by the pituitary gland, also stimulates the production of milk, but this process is suppressed during pregnancy. With the delivery of the placenta, the suppression ends and prolactin begins producing **colostrum** (kō-lŏs'trŭm), a thin, yellowish, milky fluid that fills the breast. The baby's suckling contributes to this process and also stimulates the production of the pituitary hormone oxytocin, which helps the uterus to contract. Colostrum contains a large number of proteins and calories as well as antibodies to resist viruses and bacteria to nourish and protect the baby until true **lactation**, the secretion of milk, begins following the marked decrease of estrogen and progesterone.

The huge hormonal change (by as much as 90% within 48 hours of delivery) and the external stresses that come with having a baby can trigger serious emotional problems. In about approximately 80% of new mothers, a mild depression commonly referred to as the **"baby blues"** occurs within a few days or weeks of birth and typically lasts 2 to 3 weeks. Symptoms are crying, irritability, forgetfulness, insomnia, lethargy, anxiety, and appetite loss. In most cases, with support from family and friends, this remains a normal part of the lifestyle change that occurs with motherhood.

A more severe form of the blues, **postpartum depression**, occurs in 10 to 20% of women, with symptoms more intense and lasting longer than the initial 2 to 3 weeks. Symptoms may include change in mood, sleep patterns, eating, and concentration; body preoccupations or phobias and fear of hurting herself or the baby; loss of interest in activities; and extreme irritability. It can occur anytime during the first year after childbirth and interferes with the mother's ability to function. Professional treatment is advisable. If not treated, the depression can last for years, resulting in long-term or permanent consequences for the child.

An even more severe form, called **postpartum psychosis**, is relatively rare. Symptoms include a break with reality, delusions, hallucinations, a feeling that the baby is either the devil or divine, and development of plans to harm the child. This condition may require others to intervene on behalf of the mother and child or children.

Six weeks after delivery, a postpartum checkup is performed to be sure organs have returned to the correct size and position. This is an opportunity to discuss any issues regarding the mother's health and to consider options for contraception.

Nonsurgical contraception options include the rhythm method or natural family planning that relies on the "safe" days in a woman's menstrual cycle; birth control pills, the most effective method of contraception with 1 pregnancy in 1,000 women per year; **intrauterine devices** (IUD), which are inserted in the uterine cavity by a physician; and **barrier methods**, which block the sperm from access to the egg. Barrier methods include the diaphragm, vaginal sponge, and male or female condoms. Success rates on these devices are 80 to 90% effective but vary considerably. **Contraceptive implants** are similar to progestin-only birth control pills and are implanted under the skin of the upper arm. They last approximately 5 years and are about 95% effective, although the initial cost is high. Another option is birth control shots every 1 to 3 months. Some of these are safe immediately after childbirth and while breast feeding.

Surgical options include tubal ligation, which is accomplished by interrupting the fallopian tubes so that the egg cannot travel down the tubes and the sperm cannot move upward. It is the most common method of female sterilization. A good time for a tubal ligation is immediately after giving birth, shortly thereafter, or at the time of a cesarean section.

FERTILITY

For some women, preventing unwanted pregnancies is a major concern. For others, the inability to become pregnant is devastating. **Infertility** occurs if a couple is unable to achieve pregnancy after a year of unprotected intercourse.

At that point they are advised to seek specialized medical help. Infertility affects 6.1 million couples in the United States alone—approximately 10 to 15% of couples in the reproductive age population. Various factors in both men and women contribute to infertility. The cause may be either male or female, joint, or unexplained. About 40% of couples have more than one cause for infertility.

The first step is a physical examination of both partners to determine their general state of health and to evaluate physical disorders that may be causing infertility. In most infertility cases, about 85 to 90% are treated with conventional therapies such as drug treatment or surgical repair of reproductive organs.

More recent medical advances also enable many couples to have their own biologic child with assisted reproductive technology (ART). The ART team includes physicians, psychologists, embryologists, laboratory technicians, nurses, and allied health professionals who work together to help infertile couples.

The most common ART is **in vitro fertilization** (IVF) where eggs are surgically removed from the ovary and mixed with sperm outside the body in a Petri dish. After 40 hours, the eggs are examined to see if they have become fertilized by the sperm and are dividing into cells. Some or all of the fertilized eggs (now called embryos) are then placed in the women's uterus, thus bypassing the fallopian tubes.

Other forms of ART include zygote intrafallopian transfer (ZIFT), in which an ova is mixed with sperm and the resulting zygote is placed into a fallopian tube the day after removal. With gamete intrafallopian transfer (GIFT), unfertilized ova and sperm are placed directly into a fallopian tube. Other options include electroejaculation, aspiration techniques, and intracytoplasmic sperm injection (ICSI). All options should be discussed thoroughly before embarking on fertility therapy.

INTERNET ASSIGNMENT

The Better Health Channel (BHC) was established by the Australian government and includes reliable, relevant information about a variety of health conditions. It includes a medical dictionary, a medicines guide, and an imagine library, along with other information. They do not accept advertisements or corporate sponsorships. All fact sheets are approved in a rigorous review process, and all links included lead to reputable, quality information.

ACTIVITY

Access the Better Health Channel at **www.betterhealth.vic.gov.au**. At the left edge, select Image Library. On the Image Library Page Content section, select Reproductive System or scroll to Reproductive System. Check the list of Related Fact sheets. Click on one of your choice.

Next, click on Medical Dictionary. Note that you can search a dictionary on line, by abbreviations, or 750 Consumer Medicine Information sheets.

Finally, click on Fact Sheets by category. Scroll to Diseases and Conditions and select Reproductive System. Choose one of the options listed. Summarize your findings about this site for your instructor.

Review *The Female Reproductive System*

- In response to hormones, the ovaries cyclically produce ova, which travel to the fallopian tube where they may or may not be fertilized by male sperm.
- The internal layer of the uterus thickens each month in preparation for a fertilized ovum.
- The uterine lining deteriorates if the ovum has not been fertilized, which causes bleeding known as menstrual flow.
- The vagina leads to the exterior of the body and is surrounded by external genitalia for protection.
- The menstrual cycle is influenced by functions of the pituitary gland.
- When an ovum is fertilized, a pregnancy progresses for approximately 38 to 40 weeks and ends with parturition, or the birth process.
- The female breast produces milk after childbirth.
- The period after birth, postpartum, is marked by hormonal changes that produce the "baby blues" in 80% of new mothers.
- A postpartum checkup is performed 6 weeks after delivery and includes a medical examination as well as discussion of contraceptive options, if desired.

Key Terminology Review

Word	Definition
amniotic sac	sac filled with fluid that encloses the fetus and provides a protective cushion
Apgar score	assessment of baby's heart rate, respiratory effort, muscle tone, reflex irritability, and color at l and 5 minutes after birth
areola	darkened halo surrounding the nipple of the breast
baby blues	a mild form of depression occurring within a few days of childbirth that may last for about 2 weeks
barrier methods	contraceptive measures, including the diaphragm, vaginal sponge, and male and female condoms, that block the sperm from access to the egg
blastocyst	a stage in the development of an embryo
breech birth position	baby's buttocks presents first instead of the head
cervix	lower portion of the uterus
cesarean delivery	birth through an incision made in the abdomen and into the uterus
clitoris	small structure of the vagina made of erectile tissue
colostrum	a thin, yellowish, milky fluid that precedes the secretion of breast milk
contraceptive implant	a device implanted under the skin of the upper arm to prevent conception
corpus	large upper part of the uterus
corpus luteum	cells of the ruptured ovarian follicle that have increased in size and taken on color; they rapidly degenerate if the ovum has not been fertilized
ectopic pregnancy	condition in which a fertilized egg remains in the fallopian tube instead of reaching the uterus
embryo	name of a fertilized ovum from about the second through the tenth week
endometrium	innermost layer of the uterus
episiotomy	incision in the opening of the vagina to widen it for delivery of a baby
estrogen	hormone that aids in the development of female secondary sex characteristics and cyclic changes such as menstruation and pregnancy
fallopian tube	duct connected to the uterus; where fertilization of an ovum occurs
fetoscope	historical name for the stethoscope used to auscultate (or listen to) fetal heart sounds
fetus	developing infant in the uterus after the embryonic period
fimbriae	fringelike extensions of the fallopian tube that help to sweep ova into the tubes
fornix, *pl.* fornices	circular recesses created by the cervix of the uterus dipping into the upper vagina
fundus	small, rounded part of the uterus above the level of the entrance to the fallopian tube
gynecologist	physician who specializes in diseases of the female reproductive system and the breasts
hymen	fold of membrane near the vaginal canal opening to the outside
in vitro fertilization	fertilization procedures whereby eggs are surgically removed from the ovary and mixed with sperm in a Petri dish; fertilized eggs are placed in the woman's uterus

continues

Word	Definition
infertility	inability of a couple to achieve pregnancy after a year of unprotected intercourse
intrauterine device (IUD)	birth control device inserted in the uterine cavity by a physician
labia majora	two folds or lips that are part of the external genitalia
labia minora	two small folds or lips medial to the labia majora
lactation	secretion of milk produced by the breast to nourish the baby
mamma	breast
menarche	onset of the first menstruation cycle
menopause	permanent cessation of menstrual activity
menses	normal flow of blood during the menstrual cycle
menstrual cycle	monthly developmental changes in the endometrium of the uterus resulting in menses
mons pubis	part of the external genitalia that is covered with hair after puberty
myometrium	muscular layer of the uterus that enables the walls to contract during childbirth
obstetrician	physician who treats women during pregnancy and childbirth
occiput anterior presentation	birth position where baby's head is down and facing mother's back; normal position
occiput posterior presentation	birth position where baby's head is down and facing mother's front
ovarian follicles	small sacs on the ovary in which ova mature
ovaries	female glands that produce eggs
ovulation	process that discharges an ovum from the ovarian follicle
parturition	process of giving birth
perineum	entire pelvic floor in both men and women; for pregnant women, health care specialists usually limit the perineum to the area between the vaginal opening and the anus
placenta	organ of nutrition, respiration, and excretion for the fetus during pregnancy
posterior fornix	deepest of the fornices; located behind the cervix
postpartum	after birth
postpartum depression	condition marked by continuation and deepening of symptoms exhibited in the baby blues
postpartum psychosis	serious form of depression that may lead to harm to the child or children
progesterone	hormone that keeps the uterine lining in a favorable condition for a fertilized egg
prolactin	hormone that stimulates the breasts to produce milk and colostrum
quickening	woman's initial awareness of the movement of the fetus within her womb; most commonly first reported between weeks 18 and 20 of gestation
transverse presentation	birth position where baby lies across the abdomen making vaginal delivery impossible
trophoblast	outermost layer of a blastocyst, which will attach itself to the uterine wall and become the placenta

continues

Word	Definition
umbilical cord	structure that connects the fetus to the placenta
umbilicus	navel
uterine serosa	membrane covering the uterus
uterus	pear-shaped organ located between the urinary bladder and the rectum
vagina	muscular tube connecting the uterine cavity to the exterior of the body
vernix caseosa	layer of material that protects the skin of the fetus
vulva	collective female external genitalia
vulvovaginal (Bartholin's) glands	glands that lubricate the vaginal area
zygote	fertilized, one-cell embryo

Key Terminology Practice Exercises

COMPLETION

Complete the following statements.

1. The ova from the female ovary mature in the ________________.
2. After ovulation the cells of the ovarian follicle increase in size, take on a yellowish color, and become known as a ________________.
3. The uterus has three portions: they are the ________________, ________________, and ________________.
4. Circular recesses and areas created by the dip of the uterus into the upper vagina are called ________________; the deepest of the areas is called the ________________.
5. The organ of nutrition, respiration, and excretion for a developing fetus is called the ________________.
6. Until about the tenth week, the fertilized ovum is called a(n) ________________; after that, it is called a(n) ________________.
7. Onset of the first menstrual cycle is referred to as ________________; permanent cessation of menstrual activity is called ________________.
8. After ovulation the ovum is swept into tubes by fringelike extensions on the fallopian tube called ________________.
9. The external female genitalia are called the ________________.
10. A normal pregnancy lasts approximately ________________ weeks.
11. ________________ is the process of giving birth.
12. The three layers of the uterine wall are ________________, ________________, ________________.
13. Depression, ranging from mild ________________ to ________________ to a rare serious form, called ________________, may occur within a few days to a year after a mother gives birth.
14. A one-cell embryo is a ________________; it grows to become a ________________ whose outer layer or ________________ will become the placenta.

15. Two hormones that influence the menstrual cycle in preparation for a possible pregnancy are ________________ and ________________.
16. The ________________ is duct connected to the uterus, where fertilization of an ovum occurs.
17. The ________________ is the fold of membrane near the vaginal canal opening.
18. The secretion of milk produced by the breast to nourish a baby is ________________.
19. The part of external genitalia covered with hair after puberty is the ________________.
20. The female glands that produce eggs are the ________________.

MATCHING

Match the terms to their meanings.

1. halo surrounding the nipple of the breast	a. amniotic sac
2. flow of blood during menstruation	b. Apgar score
3. mucous-producing glands at vaginal opening	c. areola
4. connects fetus and placenta	d. Bartholin's gland
5. structure that encases a fetus	e. breech
6. process of giving birth	f. clitoris
7. baby is positioned to emerge buttocks first	g. colostrum
8. baby is at right angles to the birth canal	h. ectopic pregnancy
9. baby is head down, face to mother's back	i. episiotomy
10. baby is head down, face to mother's front	j. labia majora
11. test taken of infant at 1 and 5 minutes after delivery	k. mamma
12. thin, sticky fluid that initially after birth is secreted by the breast	l. menopause
13. hormone produced by the pituitary that triggers production of colostrum	m. menses
14. after birth	n. menstrual cycle
15. thick, protective coating over fetus' skin	o. obstetrician
16. a fertilized egg that does not reach the uterus	p. occiput anterior
17. small structure of the vagina that is composed of erectile tissue	q. occiput posterior
18. pelvic floor, in gynecology, between vaginal opening and anus	r. ovaries
19. breast	s. ovulation
20. navel	t. parturition
21. glands that lubricate the vaginal area	u. perineum
22. muscular tube connecting uterine cavity to exterior of the body	v. postpartum
23. pear-shaped organ located between urinary bladder and rectum	w. prolactin
24. process that discharges an ovum from the ovarian follicles	x. transverse
25. female glands that produce eggs	y. umbilical cord
26. physician who treats women during pregnancy and childbirth	z. umbilicus
27. permanent cessation of menstrual activity	aa. uterus
28. two folds or lips that are part of external genitalia	bb. vagina
29. incision in opening of vagina to widen it for delivery of a baby	cc. vernix caseosa
30. monthly changes in endometrium resulting in menses	dd. vulvovaginal glands

Word Element Review

Root	Meaning	Example	Definition
adnex/o	tie, connection	**adnexa** (ăd-nĕk'sah)	appendages
amni/o	amnion	**amniocentesis** (ăm"nē-ō-sĕn-tē'sĭs)	puncture of the amniotic sac to remove amniotic fluid for examination
cervic/o	neck, cervix	**cervix uteri** (ser'vĭks ū'ter-ī)	neck of the uterus
colp/o	vagina	**colpoperineorrhaphy** (kŏl"pō-pĕr"ĭn-ē-or'ah-fē)	operation for mending perineal tears in the vagina
episi/o	vulva	**episiotomy** (ĕ-pĭz"ē-ŏt'ō-mē)	incision of the perineum at the end of the second stage of labor to prevent tearing
gravid/o	pregnancy	**gravida** (grăv'ĭ-dah)	pregnant woman
gynec/o	female	**gynecologic** (gī"nĕ-kō-lŏj'ĭk)	pertaining to the female reproductive tract
hyster/o	uterus	**hysterectomy** (his"tĕ-rĕk'tō-mē)	excision of the uterus
lact/o	milk	**lactation** (lăk-tā'shŭn)	period of milk secretion
mamm/o	breast	**mammary** (măm'er-ē)	pertaining to the breast
mast/o	breast	**mastalgia** (măs-tăl-jē-ah)	pain in the breast
men/o	menses	**menorrhagia** (mĕn"ō-rā'jē-ah)	excessive bleeding during menstruation
metr/o	uterus	**metrorrhagia** (mē"trō-rā'jē-ah)	abnormal bleeding from the uterus, especially at a time other than menstruation
oophor/o	ovary	**oophorectomy** (ō"ŏf-ō-rĕk'tō-mē)	excision of one or both ovaries
ovari/o	ovary	**ovarian** (ō-vā'rē-ăn)	pertaining to or resembling an ovary
ov/i, ov/o, ovul/o	egg	**ovum, ova** (ō'vŭm), (ō'vah)	egg, eggs
papill/o	nipplelike	**papilla** (pah-pĭl'ah)	small, nipplelike elevation
pect/o, pector/o	breast, chest	**pectoral** (pĕk'tō-răl)	pertaining to the breast or chest
salping/o	tube	**salpingocele** (săl-pĭng'gō-sēl)	herniation of a fallopian tube
thel/o	nipple	**thelitis** (thē-lī'tĭs)	inflammation of the nipple

continues

Root	Meaning	Example	Definition
umbilic/o	navel	**umbilical** (ŭm-bĭl'ĭ-kăl)	pertaining to the naval (umbilicus)
uter/o	uterus	**uterocervical** (ū"ter-ō-ser'vĭ-kăl)	pertaining to the uterus and cervix
vagin/o	vagina	**vaginitis** (văj"ĭ-nī'tĭs)	inflammation of the vagina
vulv/o	vulva	**vulvovaginal** (vŭl"vō-văj'ĭ-năl)	pertaining to the vulva and vagina
Prefix	**Meaning**	**Example**	**Definition**
par-, part-	bear	**parturition** (păr"tū-rĭsh'ŭn)	process of giving birth
prol-	offspring	**proliferation** (prō-lĭf"ĕ-rā'shŭn)	reproduction of similar forms

Word Element Practice Exercises

WORD ELEMENTS

Provide the correct word element to complete the following words.

1. process of giving birth ____________ turition
2. pertaining to the ovary ____________ an
3. excision of the uterus ____________ ectomy
4. suture of tears in the vagina and perineum ____________ rrhaphy
5. incision of the vulva for obstetric purposes ____________ otomy
6. abnormal bleeding from the uterus ____________ orrhagia
7. puncture of the amniotic sac to remove fluid for examination ____________ centesis
8. pertaining to the female reproductive tract ____________ logic
9. inflammation of the vagina ____________ itis
10. pertaining to the navel ____________ al
11. pain in the breast ____________ algia
12. inflammation of the nipple ____________ itis
13. pregnant woman ____________ a
14. excision of one or both ovaries ____________ ectomy
15. excessive bleeding during menstruation ____________ rrhagia

MATCHING

Match the meanings to their word elements.

1. __________ appendages
2. __________ neck of the uterus
3. __________ pregnant woman
4. __________ pertaining to vulva and vagina
5. __________ small nipplelike elevation
6. __________ reproduction of similar forms
7. __________ excision of one or both ovaries
8. __________ pertaining to the uterus and cervix
9. __________ period of milk secretion
10. __________ egg or eggs
11. __________ herniation of a fallopian tube
12. __________ pertaining to the breast
13. __________ pertaining to the breast or chest
14. __________ excessive bleeding during menstruation
15. __________ inflammation of the vagina

a. adnexa
b. cervix uteri
c. gravida
d. lactation
e. mammary
f. menorrhagia
g. oophorectomy
h. ovum, ova
i. papilla
j. pectoral
k. proliferation
l. salpingocele
m. uterocervical
n. vaginitis
o. vulvovaginal

WORD ELEMENT MEANINGS

Give the meaning of each word element. Then use your dictionary to find a new word that contains each of the word elements. Specify whether the new word is a noun or an adjective by placing N or A in the last column.

Word Element	Meaning	Word	N or A
1. adnex/o	______________	______________	________
2. amni/o	______________	______________	________
3. cervic/o	______________	______________	________
4. colp/o	______________	______________	________
5. episi/o	______________	______________	________
6. gravid/o	______________	______________	________
7. gynec/o	______________	______________	________
8. hyster/o	______________	______________	________
9. lact/o	______________	______________	________
10. mamm/o	______________	______________	________
11. mast/o	______________	______________	________
12. men/o	______________	______________	________
13. metr/o	______________	______________	________
14. oophor/o	______________	______________	________
15. ovari/o	______________	______________	________
16. ov/i	______________	______________	________
17. ov/o	______________	______________	________
18. ovul/o	______________	______________	________

Word Element Practice Exercises continued

19. papill/o ______ ______ ______
20. par- ______ ______ ______
21. part- ______ ______ ______
22. pect/o ______ ______ ______
23. pector/o ______ ______ ______
24. prol- ______ ______ ______
25. salping/o ______ ______ ______
26. thel/o ______ ______ ______
27. umbilic/o ______ ______ ______
28. uter/o ______ ______ ______
29. vagin/o ______ ______ ______
30. vulv/o ______ ______ ______

Working Practice

DIAGNOSTIC PROCEDURES

Word	Pronunciation	Definition
General		
amniocentesis	ăm"nē-ō-sĕn-tē'sĭs	needle puncture of the amniotic sac to withdraw amniotic fluid for analysis in order to detect genetic disorders or maternal-fetal blood incompatibility or to determine fetal maturity (see Figure 16-6)
breast biopsy (aspiration)	bī'ŏp-sē	extraction of suspicious breast tissue to determine the presence of cancer or other conditions; biopsies may be (1) stereotaxic—uses mammograms taken from different angles to locate a suspicious area, aligns a needle with that area, and allows the radiologist to remove a small amount of tissue; (2) needle—withdraws fluid from a fluid-filled lesion; or (3) surgical—physician removes entire lump under local or general anesthesia
cervical biopsy	ser'vĭ-kăl	removal of tissue to evaluate the presence of abnormalities of the cervix; biopsy of tissue at 12, 3, 6, and 9 o'clock positions on the cervix is referred to as a *four-quadrant cervical biopsy*
colposcopy	kōl-pŏs'kō-pē	examination of the cervix with a scope to look for abnormalities
contraction stress test (CST)		test to assess fetal response to the physiological stress of artificially induced uterine contractions
culdocentesis	kŭl"dō-sĕn-tē'sĭs	aspiration or surgical incision through posterior wall of vagina into the cul-de-sac to withdraw intraperitoneal fluid for examination
dilation and curettage (D&C)	dī-lā'shŭn, kū"rĕ-tahzh'	surgical procedure that expands the cervix of the uterus (dilation) so that the uterine wall can be scraped (curettage)

continues

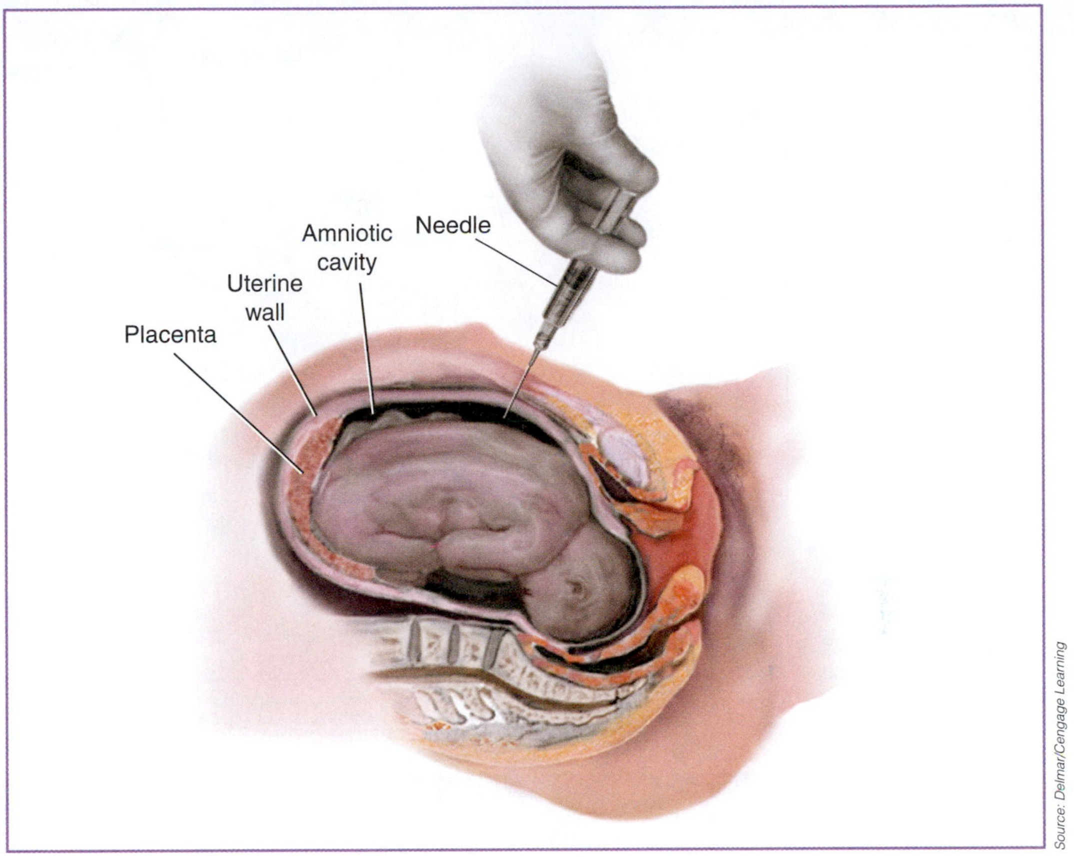

FIGURE 16-6
Amniocentesis

DIAGNOSTIC PROCEDURES		
Word	Pronunciation	Definition
General (*continued*)		
endometrial biopsy	ĕn"dō-mē'trē-ăl	removal of a sample of uterine endometrium for subsequent microscopic study
fetal monitoring	fē'tăl	recording the fetal heart rate by a direct or indirect method
fetoscopy	fē-tŏs'kō-pē	visual examination of the fetus using a lighted instrument inserted through the abdominal and uterine walls into the amniotic sac
hysteroscopy	hĭs"tĕ-r-ŏs'kō-pē	inspection of the uterus by use of a special endoscope
laparoscopy	lăp"ah-rŏs'kō-pē	examination of the interior of the abdomen by inserting a laparascope through the abdominal wall (see Figure 16-7)
laparotomy	lăp-ah-rŏt'ō-mē	surgical incision through the abdominal wall
Nuclear Medicine		
beta human chorionic gonadotrophin (beta-HCG)	bā'tah hū-măn kō"rē-ŏn'ik gŏn"ah-dō-trō'fĭn	pregnancy hormone produced by the placenta; used in the presence of a suspicious adnexal mass to identify the need for surgery and/or further treatment

continues

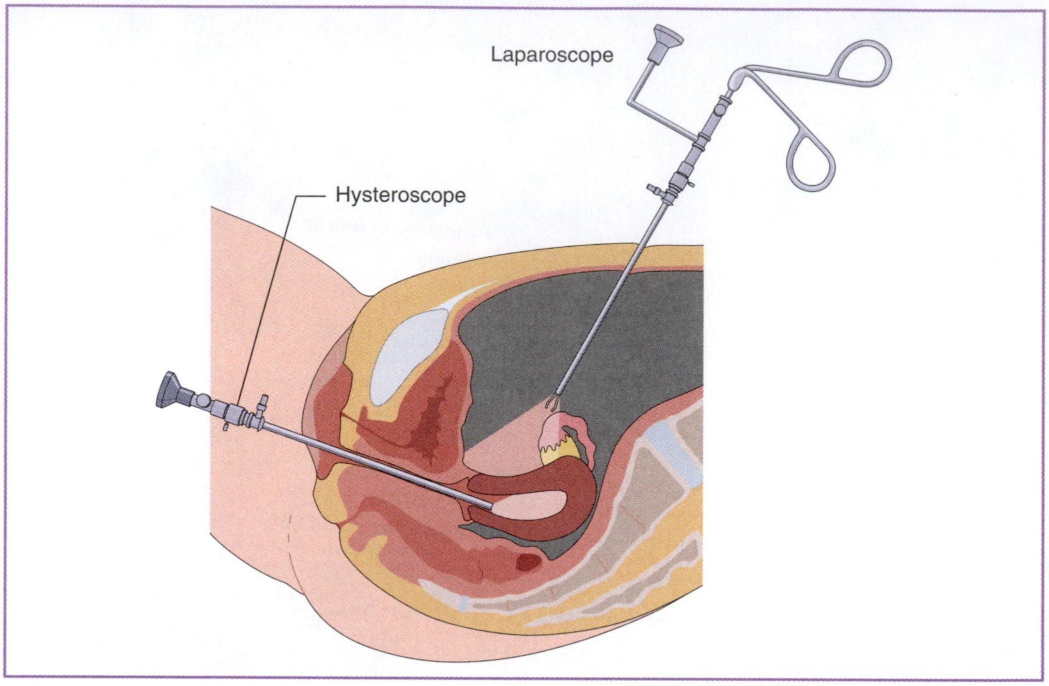

FIGURE 16-7 Laparoscopy Performed with a Hysteroscopy: allows visualizing both the inside and outside of the uterus at the same time

Source: Delmar/Cengage Learning

DIAGNOSTIC PROCEDURES		
Word	Pronunciation	Definition
Radiology		
chorionic villus sampling (CVS)	kō"rē-ŏn'ik vĭl'ŭs	transcervical insertion of a catheter to obtain a sampling of placenta tissue (chorionic villi) to check for fetal abnormalities; procedure is ultrasound guided
endovaginal ultrasound	ĕn"dō-văj'ĭ-nal ŭl-trah-sownd	diagnostic procedure that uses a sound probe placed in the vagina for a closer, sharper look within the pelvis
hysterosalpingography	hĭs"ter-ō-săl"pĭng-gŏg'rah-fē	radiographic procedure using radiopaque material to provide a picture of the uterus and uterine tubes
mammography	ma-mŏg'ră-fē	special breast x-ray used to detect tumors in the breast
pelvimetry	pĕl-vĭm'ĕ-trē	measurement of the proportions of the pelvis using an x-ray to help determine whether normal vaginal delivery is possible
pelvic ultrasonography	pĕl'vĭk ŭl"trah-sŏn-ŏg'rah-fē	use of sound waves to produce a picture of the pelvic area to check on a pregnancy or mass
sonohysterogram (saline-infusion sonography)	sŏn"ō-hĭs-tĕr'ō-grăm	vaginal ultrasound placement of a catheter through the cervix into the uterus to infuse saline into the uterine cavity to look for abnormalities within the uterus

continues

DIAGNOSTIC PROCEDURES		
Word	**Pronunciation**	**Definition**
Laboratory Tests		
estrogen receptor test	es'trō-gĕn	test done on breast tissue from malignant breast tumor to help plan further treatment depending on whether the tumor responds to estrogen
Pap (Papanicolaou)	păp"ah-nĭk"ō-lā'oo	test that uses scrapings from the cervix and smear stain to detect tissue changes that may indicate cancer (see Figure 16-8)
pregnancy test		test performed on maternal urine to determine the presence of human chorionic gonadotropin to confirm pregnancy
Blood Tests		
alpha-fetoprotein analysis		blood test that measures the level of protein produced by the fetus to detect spinal cord abnormalities
FSH and LH		blood test that measures pituitary hormones that stimulate the ovaries; ordered in fertility cases or for detection of menopause (FSH)
glucose	gloo'kōs	test ordered during pregnancy to check for gestational diabetes percutaneous
umbilical	pĕr"kū-tā'nē-ŭs	test to determine oxygen and carbon dioxide cord sampling levels or genetic disorders
prolactin level	prō-lăk'tĭn	test that measures the pituitary hormone, which is responsible for breast milk production

DIAGNOSES		
Word	**Pronunciation**	**Definition**
Menses and Menstrual Disorders		
amenorrhea	ă-mĕn-ō-rē'ă	absence or abnormal cessation of the menses

continues

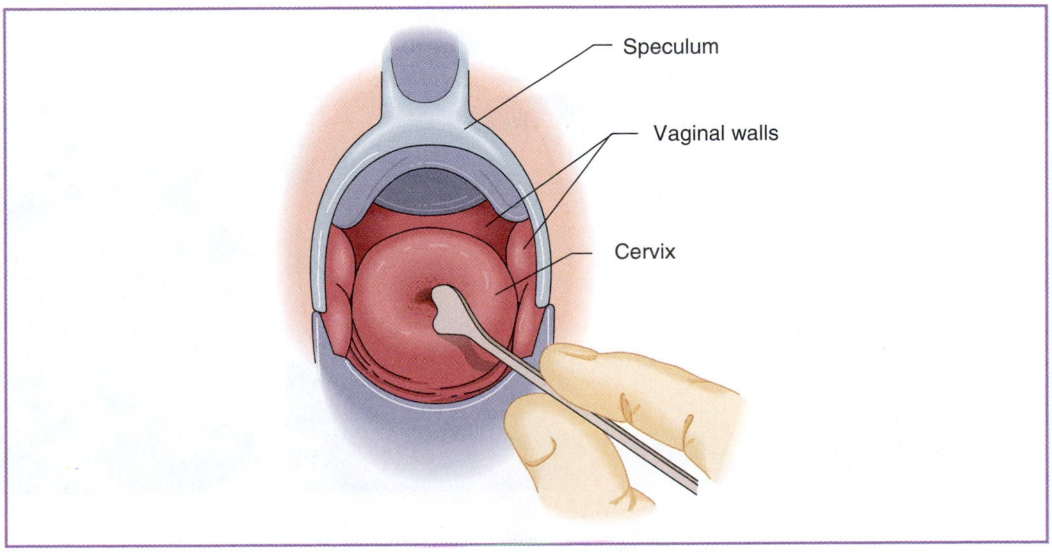

FIGURE 16-8
Papanicolaou (Pap) Smear

DIAGNOSES		
Word	**Pronunciation**	**Definition**
Menses and Menstrual Disorders (*continued*)		
dysmenorrhea	dis"mĕn-ō-rē'ah	painful or difficult menstruation
menopause	mĕn'ō-pawz	permanent cessation of the menses
menorrhagia, hypermenorrhea	mĕn"ō-rā'jē-ah, hī"pĕr-mĕn"ō-rē'ah	heavy menstrual periods
metrorrhagia	mē"trō-rā'jē-ah	uterine bleeding at any time other than during the menstrual period
mittelschmerz	mĭt'ĕl-shmārts	pain that occurs at the time of ovulation
oligomenorrhea	ŏl"ĭ-gō-mĕn"ō-rē'ă	scanty or infrequent menstrual flow
polymenorrhea	pŏl"ē-mĕn"ō-rē'ah	abnormally frequent menstruation
premenstrual syndrome (PMS)	prē-mĕn'stroo-ăl sĭn'drōm	predictable pattern of physical and emotional changes that occur just before menstruation
Problems of the Breast		
breast cancer		malignant tumor in the breast (see Figure 16-9)
fibrocystic disease	fī"brō-sĭs'tĭk	benign condition producing fibroglandular changes; sometimes called chronic cystic mastitis, mammary dysplasia, or benign breast disease
galactorrhea	gă-lăc"tō-rē'ah	condition marked by abnormal discharge of milk from the nipples
intraductal papilloma	ĭn-tră-dŭk'tăl păp-ĭ-lō'mah	tiny benign tumors in the milk ducts of the breast that may result in watery or blood discharge from the nipple
mastitis	măs-tī'tĭs	breast infections caused by bacteria that enter the breast; not uncommon to nursing mothers
Vaginal and Vulvar Disorders		
Bartholin's gland abscess	băr'tō-lĭnz	infection of the vulvovaginal gland (see Figure 16-10)

continues

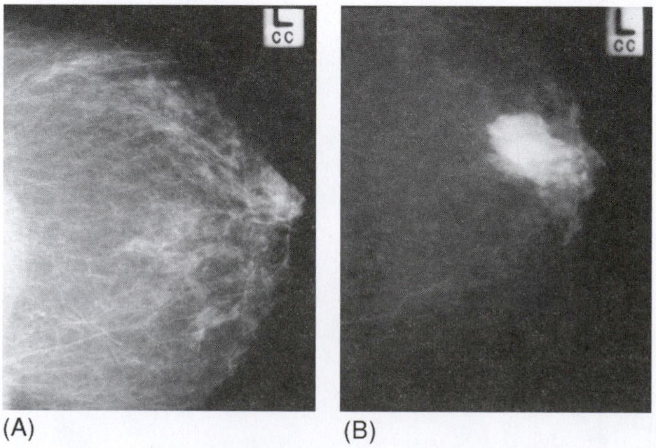

FIGURE 16-9 Mammograms: (A) normal breast; (B) breast with carcinoma

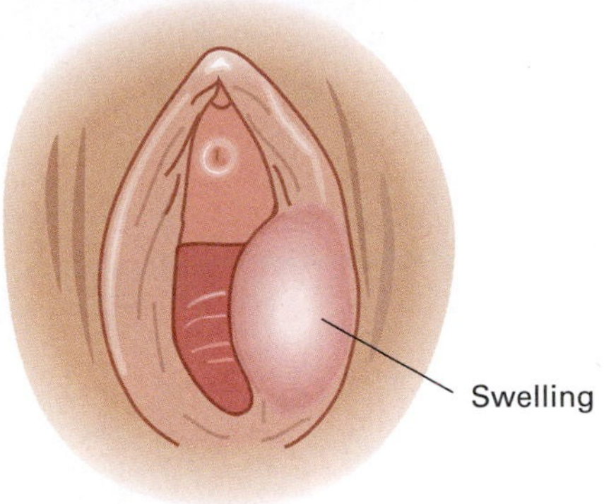

FIGURE 16-10
Bartholin's Gland Infection

DIAGNOSES		
Word	**Pronunciation**	**Definition**
Vaginal and Vulvar Disorders (*continued*)		
cystocele	sĭs'tō-sēl	weakness in the vaginal wall, allowing protrusion of the urinary bladder through the vaginal wall
dyspareunia	dĭs-pă-roo'nē-ah	painful sexual intercourse
enterocele	ĕn'tĕr-ō-sēl	hernia of the intestine through the vagina
bacterial vaginosis (BV)	văj"ĭ-nō'sĭs	inflammation of the vagina caused by a specific genus of bacteria
human papilloma virus	păp-ĭ-lō'mah	any number of strains that cause plantar and genital warts on skin or mucous membrane in humans; transmitted by direct or indirect contact
pruritus vulvae	proo-rī'tŭs vŭl'vā	intense itching, burning, or irritation in the genital area
pubic lice (crabs)	pū'bĭk	parasite that infects pubic and neighboring body parts
rectocele	rĕk'tō-sēl	weakness in the vaginal wall, allowing protrusion of part of the rectum into the vagina
sebaceous cyst	să-bā'shăs	painless, soft, smooth lump in the skin of the vulva
vaginitis	văj"ĭ-nī'tĭs	common treatable inflammation or sexually transmitted disease; may be *trichomoniasis*, *yeast infection* (see Figure 16-11), *nonspecific*, *atrophic* (caused by degeneration of vaginal tissue), or *postmenopausal* (caused by overall decrease in the estrogen level)
vulvitis	vŭl-vī'tĭs	inflammation of the external genitals
Cervix, Uterus, and Fallopian Tube Disorders		
adenomyosis	ăd"ĕ-nō-mī-ō'sĭs	growth of endometrial tissue (uterine lining) within the muscular walls of the uterus
carcinoma in situ	kăr"sĭ-no'mah ĭn si'too	cancer confined to the original site

continues

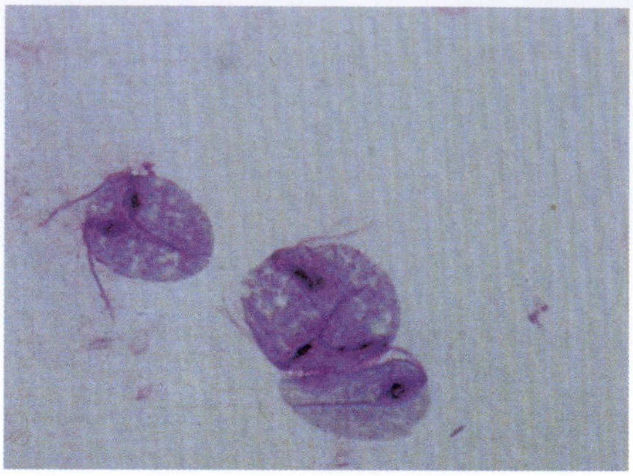

Source: Delmar/Cengage Learning

FIGURE 16-11 Trichomonas Vaginalis: a parasite that causes trichomoniasis, an infection of the genitourinary tract

DIAGNOSES

Word	Pronunciation	Definition
Cervix, Uterus, and Fallopian Tube Disorders (*continued*)		
cervical cancer	sĕr'vĭ-kăl	common cancer affecting female reproductive organs; preceded by *cervical dysplasia* (precancerous) or *carcinoma in situ* (located on the surface of the cervix in the top layers of tissue)
cervical polyps	sĕr'vĭ-kăl pŏl'ĭps	bulging tissue mass on the cervix
cervicitis	sĕr"vĭ-sī'tĭs	inflammation of the cervix; may be caused by a local infection or a symptom of vaginal infections, some sexually transmitted diseases, or pelvic inflammatory disease
choriocarcinoma	kō"rē-ō-kăr-sĭ-nō'mah	highly malignant neoplasm frequently found in the vagina, pelvic organs or other body parts; may follow any type of pregnancy
dysplasia	dĭs-plā'zē-ah	abnormal, pre-cancerous tissue development
endocervicitis	ĕn"dō-sĕr"vĭ-sī'tĭs	inflammation of the inner mucous lining of the cervix
endometrial hyperplasia	ĕn"dō-mē'trē-ăl hī"pĕr-plā'zha	abnormal overgrowth of the endometrium
endometrial polyps	ĕn"dō-mē'trē-ăl pol'ĭps	small, sessile, benign projecting masses on endometrium composed of endometrous stroma containing cystically dilated glands
endometriosis	ĕn"dō-mē'trē-ō'sĭs	escape of endometrial tissue (tissue that lines the uterus) to become attached to other pelvic organs inside the abdomen
fibroids	fī'broids	benign tumors in the uterus (see Figure 16-12)
nabothian cyst	nah-bō'thē-ăn	cyst that occurs when a mucus gland on the cervix is obstructed
pelvic inflammatory disease (PID)	pĕl'vĭk	inflammation and infection of pelvic tissue (uterus, tubes, and ovaries)

continues

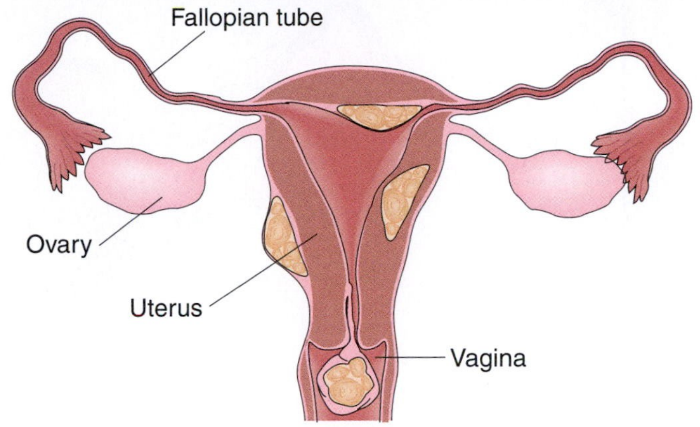

FIGURE 16-12
Fibroid Tumors

Source: Delmar/Cengage Learning

DIAGNOSES

Word	Pronunciation	Definition
Cervix, Uterus, and Fallopian Tube Disorders (*continued*)		
toxic shock syndrome		rare, potentially fatal condition caused by *Staphylococcus aureus* bacteria occurring in women who use tampons
uterine cancer (endometrial cancer)	ū'tĕr-ĭn (ĕn"dō-mē'trē-ăl)	common, slow-growing cancer that starts in the lining of the uterus
uterine leiomyoma	lī"ō-mī-ō'mă	benign, smooth muscle fibrous tumor of the uterus
uterine prolapse	ū'tĕr-ĭn prō'lăps	downward displacement of the uterus so that part or all of it is outside the vaginal orifice
Ovarian Disorders		
ovarian carcinoma	ō-vā'rē-ăn kăr"sĭ-nō'mah	hard-to-diagnose malignant tumor of the ovary
ovarian cyst	ō-vā'rē-ăn	sac filled with fluid on an ovary (see Figure 16-13)
polycystic ovary syndrome	pŏl"ē-sis'tĭk	sclerocystic disease of the ovary
Diseases Related to Pregnancy		
abruptio placentae	ăb-rŭp'shē-ō plă-sĕn'tē	premature detachment of normally situated placenta
choriocarcinoma	kō"rē-ō-kăr"sĭ-nō'mă	rare, very malignant tumor of the uterus
eclampsia	ē-klămp'sē-ah	gravest form of toxemia, characterized by grand mal convulsions, coma hypertension, proteinuria, and edema
ectopic pregnancy	ĕk-tŏp'ĭk	pregnancy in which a fertilized egg is implanted in the wrong place; tubal pregnancy
gestational diabetes	jĕs-tā'shŭn-ăl	diabetes mellitus that begins during pregnancy as a result of changes in glucose metabolism and insulin resistance
hydatidiform mole or hydatid mole	hī"dăh-tĭd'ĭ-form hī'dă-tĭd	rare growth that forms in the uterus at the beginning of pregnancy; molar pregnancy

continues

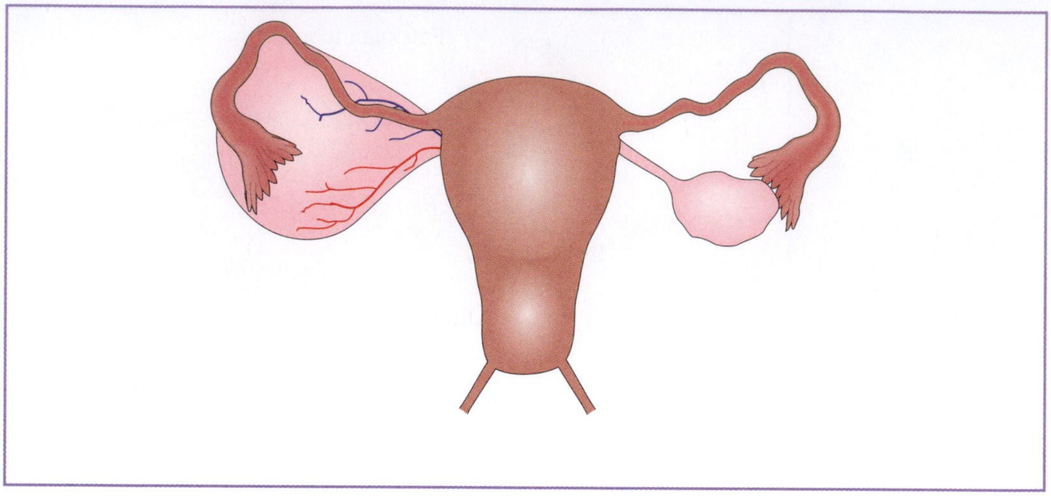

Source: Delmar/Cengage Learning

FIGURE 16-13
Ovarian Cyst

DIAGNOSES		
Word	**Pronunciation**	**Definition**
Diseases Related to Pregnancy (*continued*)		
hyperemesis gravidarum	hī"pĕr-ĕm'ĕ-sĭs grăv-ĭ-dăr'ŭm	persistent, continuous, severe, pregnancy-related nausea and vomiting, often accompanied by dry retching; leads to weight loss
incompetent cervix	sĕr'vĭks	mouth of the uterus opens generally during the second trimester, resulting in miscarriage
intrauterine death	ĭn"tră-ū'tĕr-ĭn	death of a fetus after the fifth month of gestation
placenta previa	plah-sĕn'tah prē'vē-ah	placenta that is implanted in the lower uterine segment so that it precedes a baby in the birth process
preeclampsia	prē"ē-klamp'sē-ah	disorder of pregnancy characterized by hypertension, proteinuria, and edema; also called *toxemia of pregnancy*
spontaneous abortion (miscarriage)		a natural termination of the pregnancy before the fetus leaves on its own
toxemia	tŏk-sē'mē-ah	a condition appearing in the third trimester characterized by hypertension, proteinuria, edema, and sudden weight gain
Neonatal Terms		
Down syndrome		condition marked by mild to moderate mental retardation and certain physical characteristics
erythroblastosis fetalis	ē-rĭth"rō-blăs-tō'sĭs fē-tă'lĭs	hemolytic disease of the fetus and newborn marked by anemia, jaundice, enlargement of liver and spleen, and generalized edema
hydrocephalus	hī-drō-sĕf'ă-lŭs	accumulation of excessive amounts of cerebrospinal fluid within ventricles of the brain

continues

DIAGNOSES		
Word	**Pronunciation**	**Definition**
Neonatal Terms (*continued*)		
kernicterus	kĕr-nĭk'tĕr-ŭs	form of jaundice occurring in a newborn during the second through eighth day after birth
pyloric stenosis	pī-lŏr'ĭk stĕ-nō'sĭs	narrowing of pyloric orifice, which in infants may require surgical division of the muscles of the pylorus
respiratory distress syndrome (RDS)		severe impairment of respiratory function in a preterm newborn, caused by immaturity of the lungs

TREATMENT PROCEDURES		
Word	**Pronunciation**	**Definition**
abortion	ah-bor'shŭn	premature termination of pregnancy, spontaneous or induced
adjuvant therapy	ăd'jŭ-vănt	giving cancer-killing drugs during the early stages of treatment to assist surgery or radiation procedures
breast reconstruction		procedure that uses saline-filled silicone implants in postmastectomy patients to reshape the breast
cauterization	kaw"tĕr-ī-zā'shŭn	destruction of abnormal tissue with chemicals or heat
conization	kŏn"ĭ-zā'shŭn	removal of a cone of tissue from the mouth of the cervix
cryosurgery	krī"ō-sŭr'jĕr-ē	use of cold to destroy tissue; cryocauterization
C-section (cesarean section	sĕ-sā'rē-ăn	birth of an infant by surgical incision into the uterus
endometrial ablation	ĕn"dō-mē'trē-ăl ăb-lā'shŭn	procedure which uses a thermal device or laser to burn the lining of the uterus, usually done with a hysteroscopy, to decrease or eliminate menstrual flow
Essure		hysteroscopic sterilization procedure accomplished by permanently blocking the fallopian tubes
episiotomy	ĕ-pĭs"ē-ŏt'ō-mē	incision made to widen the vagina for delivery of the infant
hormone replacement therapy (HRT)		prescription of estrogen and progestin to replace hormones lost during menopause and to slow down the rate of bone density loss
hysterectomy	hĭs'tĕ-rĕk'tō-mē	surgical removal of the uterus through the abdominal wall or through the vagina (see Figure 16-14), or laparoscopically
Kegel exercises	kē'gŭl	simple exercises for strengthening pubococcygeal muscles

continues

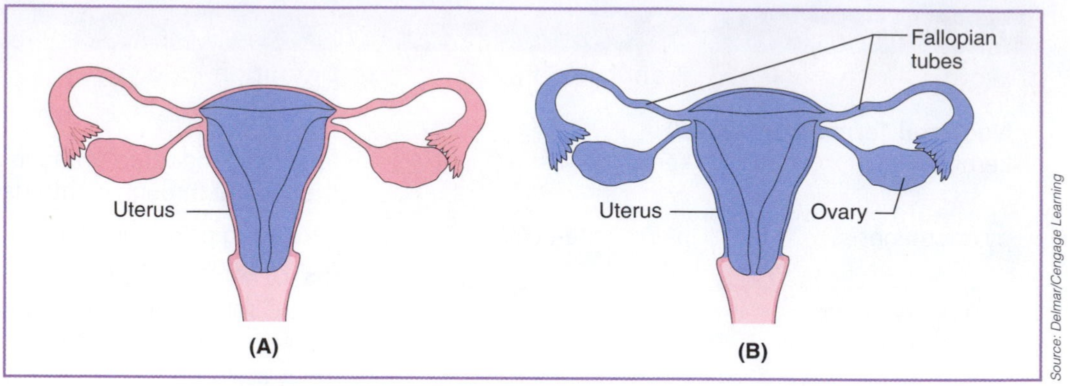

FIGURE 16-14 Hysterectomy: (A) total; (B) total with salpingo-oophorectomy

TREATMENT PROCEDURES		
Word	**Pronunciation**	**Definition**
laparoscopic tubal coagulation and division	lăp"ah-r-ō-skŏp'ĭk	sterilization procedure specifically using cauterization and division of of the fallopian tubes
mastectomy	măs-tĕk'tŏ-mē	Surgical procedure for the treatment of breast cancer may be at any of these levels (see Figure 16-15): • *radical* removes the entire breast including a portion of skin containing the nipple and areola and the underlying chest muscles, as well as extensive removal of lymph nodes underneath the armpit

continues

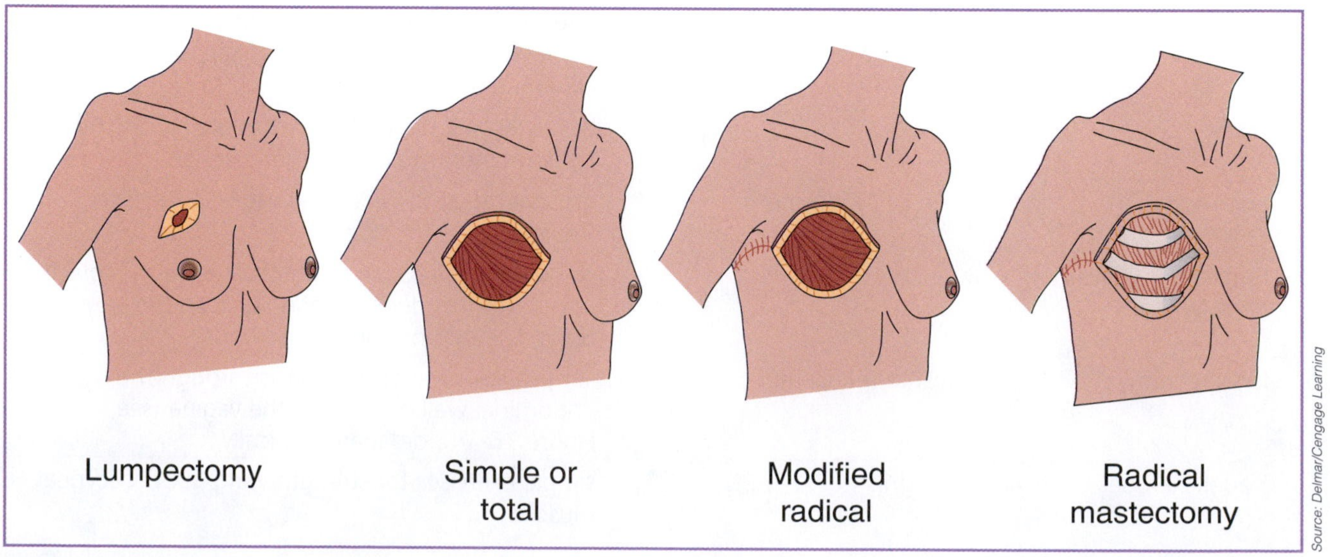

FIGURE 16-15 Types of mastectomy

TREATMENT PROCEDURES		
Word	**Pronunciation**	**Definition**
		• *modified radical* similar to radical, but spares the chest wall muscles and removes fewer lymph nodes • *breast conservation therapy (lumpectomy)* removes the tumor and a small rim of normal breast tissue followed with a 4- to 6-week course of radiation therapy • *simple mastectomy* similar to a modified radical mastectomy, but does not remove the armpit lymph nodes • *subcutaneous mastectomy* removes only breast tissue and spares skin, nipple, areola, chest wall muscles, and lymph nodes
oophorectomy	ō"ŏf-ō-rĕk'tō-mē	excision of an ovary
pelvic exenteration	eks-ĕn"tĕr-ā'shŭn	complete and radical removal of all pelvic organs in treatment of certain cancers
polypectomy	pŏl'ĭ-pĕk'tō-mē	excision of a polyp
salpingo-oophorectomy	săl-pĭng"gō-ō" ŏf-ō-rĕk'tō-mē	excision of a fallopian tube and an ovary
tubal ligation	lī-gā'shŭn	sterilization procedure that involves tying off (ligating) the fallopian tubes (see Figure 16-16)
uterine suspension	ū-ter-īn	surgical reinforcement of the supporting structure of the uterus

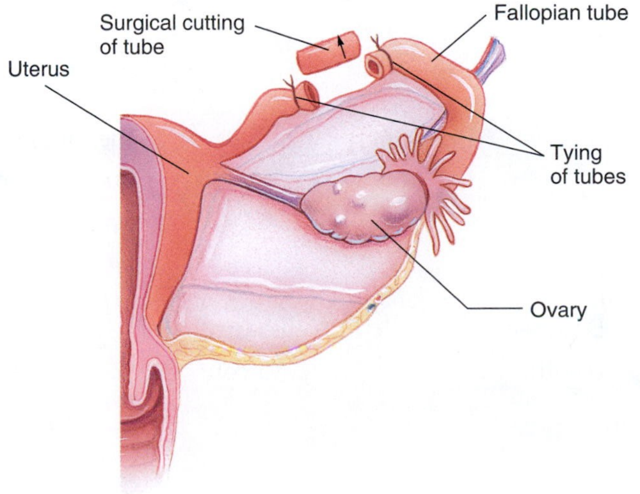

FIGURE 16-16
Tubal Ligation

MEDICATIONS PRESCRIBED		
Trade Name		**Generic Name**
General		
Ampicillin, Polycillin		ampicillin
Anaprox		naproxen sodium
Betadine Vaginal Suppositories		povidone iodine
Cleocin cream		clindamycin
Flagyl		metronidazole
Furadantin, Macrodantin		nitrofurantoin
Gyne-Lotrimin, Mycelex		clotrimazole
Monistat 7 Vaginal Cream		miconazole nitrate
Mycolog-II, Mycostatin, Nilstat		nystatin
Synalar		fluocinolone acetonide
Temovate cream		clobetasol propionate
Terazol Vaginal Cream		terconazole
Vagifem tablets		estradiol
Hormones		
Aygestin		norethindrone acetate
Cenestin		conjugated estrogens
Climara		estradiol transdermal
Depo-Provera, Provera		medroxyprogesterone acetate
Estrace		estradiol
Ogen		estropipate
Premarin		estrogens, conjugated
Vivelle-Dot		estradiol transdermal system
Ovulation Stimulants		
Clomid		clomiphene citrate
Gonadotropins		
Lupron		leuprolide acetate
Pergonal		menotropins
Profasi HP		chorionic gonadotropin
Synarel		nafarelin acetate
Birth Control Pills		
Alesse	Desogen	Lo/Ovral
Demulen	Loestrin	Mircette

continues

MEDICATIONS PRESCRIBED

Trade Name			Generic Name
Birth Control Pills (*continued*)			
Nordette	Ortho-Novum	Tri-Norinyl	
Norinyl	Ortho Tri-Cyclen	Tri-Phasil	
Norlestrin	Ovral	Yaz	
Ortho-Cyclen	Seasonale		
Labor Inducers			
Ergonovine			ergonovine
Methergine			methylergonovine maleate
Pitocin			oxytocin
Vitamin and Iron Supplements			
Ferro-Sequels			
Iberet-Folic-500			
Materna 1-60			
Natabec Rx			
Natalins			
Niferex-PN Forte			
Zenate			

ABBREVIATIONS

AB	abortion
ART	assisted reproductive technology
beta-HCG	beta human chorionic gonadotropin
BV	bacterial vaginosis
CIN	cervical intra-epithelial neoplasia (cervical dysplasia)
CIS	carcinoma in situ
C-section, CS	cesarean section
CST	contraction stress test
CVS	chorionic villus sampling
Cx	cervix
D&C	dilatation (dilation) and curettage
DES	diethylstilbestrol
DUB	dysfunctional uterine bleeding

continues

ABBREVIATIONS	
ECC	endocervical curettage
EDB	expected date of birth
EFM	electronic fetal monitoring
ERT	estrogen replacement therapy
FHR	fetal heart rate
FHT	fetal heart tones
FSH	follicle-stimulating hormone
G	gravida (pregnant)
GIFT	gamete intrafallopian transfer
GPA	gravida, para, abortion
gyn	gynecology
hCG, HCG	human chorionic gonadotropin
HPV	human papillomavirus
HRT	hormone replacement therapy
ICSI	intracytoplasmic sperm injection
IUD	intrauterine device
IVF	in vitro fertilization
L&D, LD	labor and delivery
LMP	last menstrual period
NB	newborn
OB	obstetrics
P	para (number of births)
Pap test	Papanicolaou test
PID	pelvic inflammatory disease
PMS	premenstrual syndrome
RDS	respiratory distress syndrome
SIL	squamous intra-epithelial lesion (cervical dysplasia)
TSS	toxic shock syndrome
ZIFT	zygote intrafallopian transfer

Working Practice Review Exercises

CHOICES

Circle the correct answer in each statement.

1. (Hysterosalpingography/ultrasonography) is a technique that uses sound waves to produce a picture.
2. (Dilation and curettage/cervical biopsy) is the procedure used to scrape the uterine wall.
3. A (laparotomy/laparoscopy) is an incision through the abdominal wall to look for gynecological problems.
4. (Prolactin level/LH) is a test used in fertility cases.
5. (Amniocentesis/pregnancy test) is ordered to determine whether any genetic disorders are present in a pregnancy.
6. (Galactorrhea/mastitis) is a condition marked by abnormal discharge of milk from the nipples.
7. Measurement of the proportions of the pelvis using an x-ray is (pelvimetry/pelvic ultrasonography).
8. A (stereotaxic/needle/surgical) breast biopsy removes an entire lump under anesthesia.
9. Painful or difficult menstruation is (menorrhagia/metrorrhagia/dysmenorrhea).
10. Premature detachment of a normally situated placenta is (abruptio placentae/placenta previa).
11. Escape of endometrial tissue that then becomes attached to other pelvic organs is (adenomyosis/endometriosis).
12. Abnormal tissue development is (dysplasia/choriocarcinoma).
13. Predictable patterns of physical and emotional changes that occur before onset of monthly menstruation is (premenstrual syndrome/polycystic ovary syndrome).
14. A (colposcopy/hysteroscopy) is the examination of the cervix with a scope to look for abnormalities.
15. A (chorionic villus sampling/percutaneous umbilical cord sampling) is the insertion of a catheter, guided by ultrasound, to obtain a sampling of placenta tissue to check for fetal abnormalities.

IDENTIFICATION

Identify the following treatment procedures.

1. surgically reinforcing the supporting structure of the uterus ______________________
2. excision of an ovary ______________________
3. removal of a cone of tissue from the mouth of the cervix ______________________
4. sterilization procedure that involves tying off the fallopian tubes ______________________
5. birth of an infant by a surgical incision into the uterus ______________________
6. procedure that uses saline-filled silicone implants to reshape a breast ______________________
7. surgical treatment of breast cancer that spares the chest wall and takes fewer lymph nodes ______________________
8. complete removal of all pelvic organs ______________________
9. use of cold to destroy tissue ______________________
10. the surgical removal of a polyp ______________________
11. simple exercises for strengthening pubococcygeal muscles ______________________
12. surgical removal of uterus through abdominal wall or vagina ______________________
13. destruction of abnormal tissue with chemicals or heat ______________________
14. incision to widen vagina for delivery of an infant ______________________
15. sterilization procedure using cauterization and division of the fallopian tubes ______________________

16. test to assess fetal response to the physiological stress of artificially induced contractions __________
17. aspiration or surgical incision through posterior wall of the vagina into the cul-de-sac to withdraw intraperitoneal fluid for examination __________
18. procedure to burn the lining of the uterus to decrease or eliminate menstrual flow __________

MATCHING

Match the terms to their meanings.

1. __________ inflammation of the inner mucous lining of the cervix
2. __________ abnormally frequent menstruation
3. __________ gravest form of toxemia
4. __________ benign tumors in the uterus
5. __________ protrusion of the rectum into the vagina
6. __________ inflammation of pelvic tissue
7. __________ protrusion of the bladder through the vaginal wall
8. __________ cancer confined to the original site
9. __________ molar pregnancy
10. __________ test done on malignant tumor for receptivity to estrogen
11. __________ blood test that detects level of protein produced by the fetus
12. __________ test ordered to determine oxygen and CO_2 levels or genetic disease in fetus
13. __________ form of jaundice occurring in a newborn
14. __________ narrowing of pyloric orifice in infants, requiring surgery
15. __________ excessive cerebrospinal fluid within brain ventricles
16. __________ natural termination of a pregnancy
17. __________ tubal pregnancy
18. __________ mouth of uterus opens in 2nd trimester resulting in spontaneous abortion
19. __________ sclerotic disease of the ovary
20. __________ abnormal overgrowth of endometrium

a. alpha-fetoprotein analysis
b. carcinoma in situ
c. cystocele
d. eclampsia
e. ectopic pregnancy
f. endocervicitis
g. endometrial hyperplasia
h. estrogen receptor test
i. fibroids
j. hydatidiform mole
k. hydrocephalus
l. incompetent cervix
m. kernicterus
n. percutaneous umbilical cord sample
o. PID
p. polycystic ovary syndrome
q. polymenorrhea
r. pyloric stenosis
s. rectocele
t. spontaneous abortion

Dictionary Exercises

DICTIONARY EXERCISE 1

Use your dictionary to find the pronunciation and definition of the following words.

	Word	Pronunciation	Definition
1.	adenomatous	________________	________________
2.	anteflexion	________________	________________
3.	caput	________________	________________
4.	climacteric	________________	________________
5.	engagement	________________	________________
6.	forceps	________________	________________
7.	fourchette	________________	________________
8.	hematocele	________________	________________
9.	hematocolpos	________________	________________
10.	hematosalpinx	________________	________________
11.	mesothelioma	________________	________________
12.	oligohydramnios	________________	________________
13.	paraurethral	________________	________________
14.	puerperium	________________	________________
15.	toxic shock syndrome	________________	________________

DICTIONARY EXERCISE 2

Provide the pronunciation and select the correct meaning of each term.

1. canal of Nuck (________________)
   a. structure in the female pelvis containing ovarian vessels and nerves
   b. opening to the vagina
   c. prolongation of peritoneal cavity between anterior surface of the rectum and posterior surface of the uterus
   d. persistent peritoneal pouch that accompanies the round ligament of the uterus through the inguinal canal

2. primigravida (________________)
   a. early weeks of a pregnancy
   b. woman's first pregnancy
   c. abdominal stretch marks during pregnancy
   d. woman who has given birth for the first time

3. cul-de-sac of Douglas (________________)
   a. pouch that accompanies the round ligament of the uterus through the inguinal canal
   b. prolongation of peritoneal cavity between anterior surface of the rectum and posterior surface of the uterus
   c. small cyst at the terminal end of the fallopian tube
   d. structure in the female pelvis containing the ovarian vessels and nerves

4. dystocia (________________)
   a. painful, difficult delivery or birth
   b. painful menses
   c. congenital absence of a normal body opening
   d. menstruation

5. chorion (______________________)
   a. head
   b. menstruation
   c. outer membrane around the fetus
   d. before the onset of labor
6. velamentous insertion (______________________)
   a. umbilical cord attachment to membranes instead of to the placenta
   b. entrance to the vagina
   c. pouch that accompanies the round ligament of the uterus through the inguinal canal
   d. long grasping forceps used in vaginal hysterectomies
7. hydrosalpinx (______________________)
   a. excessive accumulation of amniotic fluid
   b. distention of the fallopian tube by a clear fluid
   c. retained menstrual blood in the vagina
   d. malignant tumor of the ovary
8. uterine serosa (______________________)
   a. near the urethra
   b. menstruation
   c. thin peritoneal covering of the uterus
   d. outer membrane around the fetus
9. antepartum (______________________)
   a. time it takes the uterus to return to normal after delivery
   b. thin peritoneal covering of the uterus
   c. forward flexion of the body of the uterus upon the cervix
   d. before the onset of labor
10. oligomenorrhea (______________________)
   a. painful or difficult menstruation
   b. fewer than normal number of menstrual periods in a year
   c. failure of menstruation
   d. heavy periods
11. amnion (______________________)
   a. before the onset of menstruation
   b. outer membrane around the fetus
   c. bag of water holding the fetus
   d. thin peritoneal covering of the uterus
12. leiomyoma (______________________)
   a. myoma
   b. fibroid tumor
   c. ovarian cancer
   d. cervical cancer

DICTIONARY EXERCISE 3

Provide the pronunciation for the italicized words and then rewrite the sentences in your own words.

1. The patient was *gravida* IV (______________________), para II, and there was concern about *Couvelaire* (______________________) uterus.

   ____

2. During her first delivery, *version* (______________________) was necessary.

   ____

3. The physician saw that the patient had presented with a *prolapse* (______________________) of the umbilical cord during labor.

   ____

4. The danger of *hyaline* (______________________) membrane disease is present in many premature deliveries.

   ____

5. The patient was relieved that she had a *Brenner's* (______________________) tumor rather than a malignant tumor.

   ____

6. The physician suspected *hydatid of Morgagni* (________________________).

____

7. The nurse checked the baby's *fontanelles* (________________________).

____

8. The final diagnosis was *dysgerminoma* (________________________).

____

9. Her problem was caused by an *arrhenoblastoma* (________________________).

____

10. On Friday, the patient will undergo *colpoperineoplasty* (________________________).

____

11. The obstetrician administered a *pudendal block* (________________________).

____

12. Sometimes delivery requires a *vacuum extractor* (________________________).

____

13. Dr. Ahmad prescribed a *Depo-Provera* (________________________) injection once every 12 weeks.

____

14. Their only birth control was a *spermicidal* (________________________) jelly.

____

15. There was evidence of *leucorrhea* (________________________) in the cervical area.

____

DICTIONARY EXERCISE 4

Pronunciation of the words below is provided. Using your dictionary, find the correct spelling and definition of each word.

	Word	Pronunciation	Definition
1.	____________	ah-trē'zē-ah	____________
2.	____________	kăt"ah-mē'nē-ah	____________
3.	____________	kō'ĭ-tŭs	____________
4.	____________	hĕm"ah-tō-mē'trah	____________
5.	____________	hī-drăm'nē-ŏs	____________
6.	____________	ĭn"fŭn-dĭb"ū-lō-pĕl'vĭk	____________
7.	____________	ĭn-trō'ĭ-tŭs	____________
8.	____________	pī"ō-mē'trah	____________
9.	____________	vă'sah prē'vē-ah	____________
10.	____________	mŭl-tĭp'ah-rus	____________

*Study*WARE™ Connection

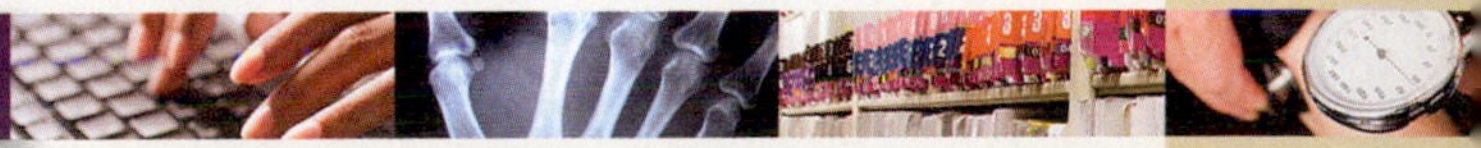

To take a practice quiz or play interactive games that reinforce the content in this chapter, go to your StudyWARE™ CD-ROM.

Listening Exercise

INSTRUCTIONS

1. Review the spelling, pronunciation, and meaning of the words provided in the preview.
2. Go to your StudyWARE™ CD-ROM and listen to **Listening Exercise 16-1**. Fill in the blank in the report as the word is dictated.
3. At the end of the exercise, check your spelling against the preview words. They appear in the preview in the order in which they are encountered in the activity.
4. Review and practice the words you missed.
5. Look up words that are not familiar.

PREVIEW OF WORDS FOR LISTENING EXERCISE 16-1

Word	Pronunciation	Meaning
hysteroscopy	hĭs"tĕr-ŏs'kō-pē	inspection of the uterus by use of a special endoscope
menorrhagia	mĕn"ō-rā'jē-ă	heavy menstrual periods
endometriosis	ĕn"dō-mē"trē-ō'sĭs	escape of endometrial tissue to become attached to other pelvic organs
peritoneal	pĕr"ĭ-tō-nē'ăl	pertaining to the membrane lining of the abdominal and pelvic cavities
cervix	sĕr'vĭks	lower portion of the uterus
endometrium	ĕn-dō-mē'trē-ŭm	innermost layer of the uterus
insufflated	ĭn'sū-flā'tĕd	body part filled with vapor or gas

Listening Exercise 16-1

StudyWARE™ Connection

Listen to this report being read on your StudyWARE™ CD-ROM. Fill in each blank as the word is dictated.

Operative Report

Preoperative Diagnoses

1. Cyclic pelvic pain.
2. Menorrhagia.
3. Endometriosis.

Postoperative Diagnoses

1. Cyclic pelvic pain.
2. Menorrhagia.
3. Endometriosis.

Name of Operation

Diagnostic laparoscopy with biopsy, ________________ with endometrial sampling.

Indications

Increasing right-sided pelvic pain, perimenstrual, with _________________ .

Findings

There was a prior appendectomy, some adhesions to the cecum down to the right lower quadrant. The liver edge was normal. Gallbladder was not visualized. Both tubes and ovaries were normal. Anterior bladder flap was normal other than prior caesarean section scarring. No _______________________. The uterine serosa had a mosaic pattern and vesicular pattern consistent with serosal endometriosis. Down in the cul-de-sac was a blue powder-burn cluster of endometriosis along the right uterosacral ligament consistent with the patient's pain and a few vesicular __________ changes also consistent with endometriosis scattered about.

Procedure

The patient was brought to the operating room where she was anesthetized by general endotracheal tube technique, placed in the dorsal lithotomy position, and prepped and draped for a laparoscopic and hysteroscopic procedure. The bladder was emptied with a catheter. The ______ was grasped with a tenaculum and tested with a #4

continues

Operative Report (*continued*)

Hegar dilator, and a hysteroscope was placed inside the uterus under direct vision with findings of a normal endometrial cavity. There were no polyps, no fibroids, and no obvious areas of adenomyosis. The cervix was dilated to an 8 Hegar and a small curet was used to produce normal ____________________. Uterine elevator was placed on the uterus. An umbilical incision was made and through this a Veress needle placed. Intra-abdominal placement was verified by the saline technique, and the abdomen ______________________ with carbon dioxide. A 5-mm expandable sleeve trocar was placed umbilically, and suprapubically, a 5-mm port was placed. Pelvic inspection was done with the above findings. The biopsy forceps were not working well but attempts at biopsying the uterosacral ligament were made, excising some tissue for sampling. The pelvis was then irrigated and gas was suctioned and expressed under direct vision. Instruments were removed and incisions closed with 4–0 rapidly absorbable Vicryl and injected with 0.5% Marcaine. The patient was awakened and transferred to the recovery room in good condition.

Estimated Blood Loss

Minimal.

Complications

None.

Plan

The patient will return to the office in one week for review of operative findings and further planning. The patient would be a candidate for further laparoscopic surgery if necessary. The patient was given a prescription for Toradol 10 mg tablets for postoperative pain.

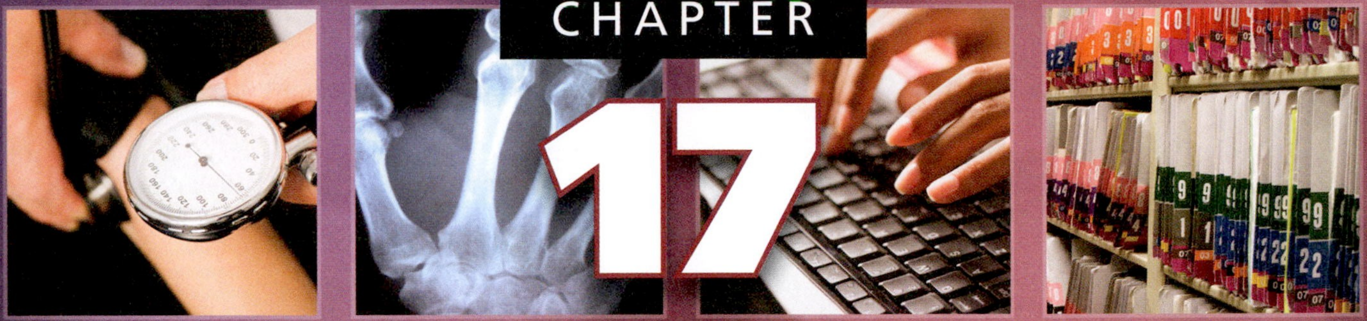

CHAPTER 17

The Male Reproductive System

"Man is a piece of the universe made alive"

—Ralph Waldo Emerson

OBJECTIVES

When you have completed this chapter on the male reproductive system, you should be able to

1. Spell and define major system components and explain how they operate.
2. Identify the meanings of related word elements.
3. Spell and define diagnostic procedures, diagnoses, treatment procedures, and abbreviations.
4. Spell and define laboratory tests, diagnoses, and abbreviations of male and female sexually transmitted diseases.
5. Spell the names of commonly used medications.
6. Use a dictionary as a tool in processing medical documents.
7. Hear how medical terminology is used in actual medical reports.

INTRODUCTION

Reproduction is accomplished by a process called **fertilization**. The female component of the reproduction process was discussed in Chapter 16, which included the role of male and female **gonads** (gō'nădz) (a generic name for reproductive organs). In the male, specialized cells called spermatozoa are produced by the testes. Their counterparts, the ova, originate in the female ovaries. The male reproductive system is generally part of the **urologist's** (ū-rŏl'ō-jĭst) specialty.

COMPONENTS OF THE MALE REPRODUCTIVE SYSTEM

The male reproductive system consists of several organs—the testes, epididymis, vas deferens (all of which are paired), the ejaculatory duct, urethra, and penis. The accessory organs are the seminal vesicles, prostate gland, and Cowper's or bulbourethral glands. Note each of the organs in Figure 17-1.

TESTES (TESTICLES)

orch/o, orchi/o, orchid/o	testis	sperm/o, spermat/o	spermatozoa
scrot/o	scrotum	test/o	testes, testicles

The male **testes** (tĕs'tēz) (8) are located outside the body in a sac of skin called the **scrotum** (skrō'tŭm) (7). The testes begin their development in the abdominopelvic cavity and later move or descend into the scrotum. This places the testes in an environment where the optimum temperature can be maintained for sperm production and maturation. **Spermatozoa** (sper"mah-tō-zō'ah) (sperm) development occurs in highly convoluted structures in the testes called **seminiferous tubules** (sĕ"mĭ-nĭf'er-ŭs too'būles) (13). A single sperm has a body and tail and is about one six hundredth of an inch long. The tail enables the sperm to move (see Figure 17-2).

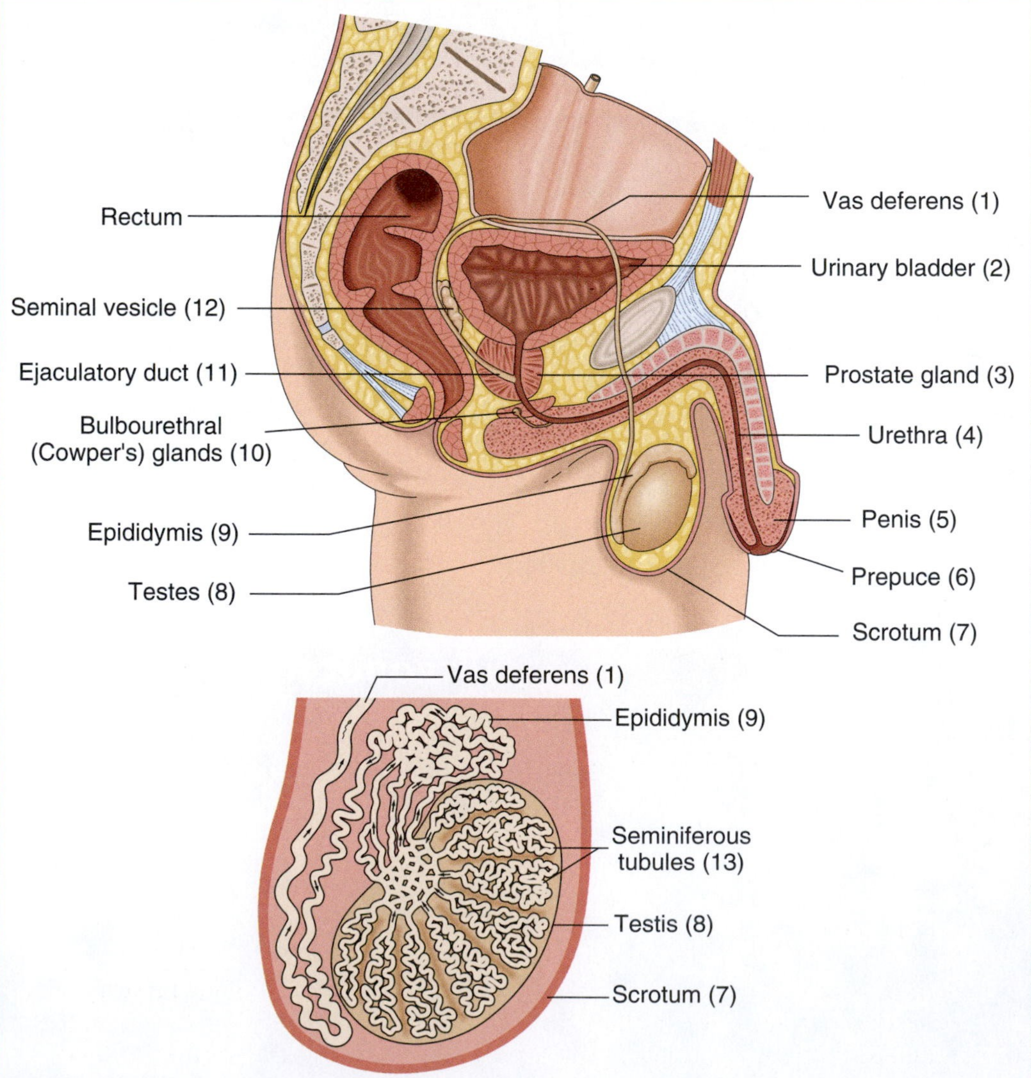

FIGURE 17-1 Male Reproductive System with Inset of Scrotum Seminiferous tubules (13) Vas deferens (1) Epididymis (9) Scrotum (7) Testis (8)

Source: Delmar/Cengage Learning

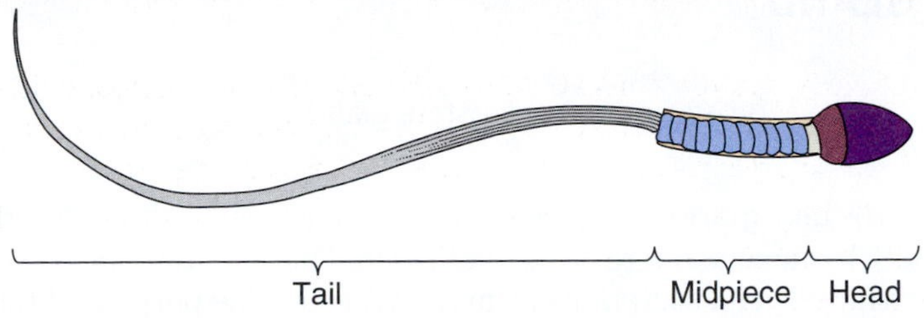

FIGURE 17-2 Anatomy of a Sperm Cell

Also produced in the testes is the male sex hormone **testosterone** (tĕs-tŏs'tĕ-rōn). This hormone is responsible for the growth of facial and body hair and for the deepening of the male voice, sexual drive, and the ability to have an erection.

EPIDIDYMIS

epididym/o	epididymis

Sperm need to mature after they are produced. Maturation begins to take place in the **epididymis** (ĕp"ĭ-dĭd'ĭ-mĭs) (9) as shown in Figure 17-1. Sperm continue to mature as they move through the epididymis, which is a coiled tube 20 feet long. Eventually the spermatozoa reach the vas deferens.

VAS DEFERENS

vas/o	vessel, duct

The **vas deferens** (văs dĕf'er-ĕnz) (1) is a tube or duct that is a continuation of the epididymis. There is one on each side of the midline. Its path is upward from the epididymis to the inferior portion of the urinary bladder (2). Here, it is joined by ducts of the seminal vesicles.

SEMINAL VESICLES

semen, semin/o	seed	vesicul/o	seminal vesicles

There are two **seminal vesicles** (sĕm'ĭ-năl vĕs'ĭ-k'ls) (12), or membranous pouches. The duct of each joins with a vas deferens to form the ejaculatory duct. The seminal vesicles produce a secretion that enhances sperm motility and nourishes the sperm. It also provides protection to the spermatozoa at the time of ejaculation.

EJACULATORY DUCT

The union of both vas deferens and the seminal vesicle is called the **ejaculatory** (ē-jăk'ū-lah-tō"rē) **duct** (11). This duct passes through the prostate and enters the urethra just below where the urethra exits from the urinary bladder. Spermatozoa are propelled from the vas deferens into the urethra (4) by contraction of the ejaculatory duct. This occurs at the culmination of sexual arousal.

PROSTATE GLAND

prostat/o	prostate gland

The **prostate** (prŏs'tāt) **gland** (3) surrounds the first section of the urethra. It is a single organ and can be assessed manually by means of a rectal examination. During intercourse the prostate gland secretes a fluid that precedes the sperm cells and secretions from the vesicles. The purpose of that fluid is to reduce the acidity of the vaginal secretions in order to provide a suitable environment for survival of the sperm cells.

BULBOURETHRAL OR COWPER'S GLANDS

Two small glands on either side of the urethra are called the **bulbourethral** (bul"bō-ū-rē-thrăl), or **Cowper's, glands** (10). Their function is to secrete a clear lubricant that is an additional protective substance for the spermatozoa during ejaculation.

URETHRA

The **urethra** (ŭ-rē'thră) (4) is a canal extending from the urinary bladder to the external opening of the penis. Its function is to carry semen during ejaculation and urine at other times.

PENIS

balan/o	glans penis

The **penis** (5) is made up of three masses of spongy tissue and attached skin as well as an expanded tip called the **glans**. During sexual arousal this tissue becomes swollen with blood, which causes the penis to enlarge and become firm. At birth the glans penis is covered with a fold of skin called the **prepuce** (prē'pūs) (6), or foreskin. Surgical removal of this skin (an elective procedure) is called **circumcision**.

StudyWARE™ Connection

Label structures and watch an animation of the **Male Reproductive System** on your StudyWARE™ CD-ROM.

SEMEN

Semen is composed of spermatozoa from the testes and fluids from the seminal vesicles, prostate, and Cowper's or bulbourethral glands. Each ejaculation of semen contains about 300 million sperm. A sperm count of less than 60 million per cubic centimeter (cc) usually indicates an inability to fertilize the ovum, but this is not a hard-and-fast rule.

StudyWARE™ Connection

View an animation on **Sperm Production** on your StudyWARE™ CD-ROM.

INTERNET ASSIGNMENT

The American Academy of Family Physicians (**www.familydoctor.org**) is an excellent source of information. The site content is authored and reviewed by individuals with acknowledged expertise. Choices on the top, horizontal bar of the home page include, among others, conditions A-Z, specialized sections for women, men, parents and kids, senior, and an OTC drug guide as well.

ACTIVITY

Access **www.familydoctor.org**. From the horizontal bar at the top of the home page, select Men. Scroll to STDs (sexually transmitted diseases) and click on one of the options.

Next, go to the Reproductive Health section and click on one of the options. Finally, go to the bar at the top of the page and select OTC. From the lists provided, click on a topic of interest.

Summarize your findings about this site for your instructor.

Review *The Male Reproductive System*

- The male reproductive system consists of the testes, epididymis, vas deferens (all three of which are paired), ejaculatory duct, urethra, and penis.
- Spermatozoa are produced in the testes and mature in the epididymis.
- The seminal vesicles, prostate gland, and Cowper's glands are accessory organs that protect the sperm cells by adding protective secretions to the seminal fluid during intercourse.
- Mature sperm are transported through the vas deferens and the seminal vesicles and finally passed through the ejaculatory duct, where they are propelled into the urethra and out of the body during ejaculation.
- The penis is made up of three masses of spongy tissue, attached skin, and an expanded tip called the glans.
- The infusion of blood in the penis during sexual arousal causes an erection and ultimately an ejaculation of semen.

Key Terminology Review

Word	Definition
bulbourethral (Cowper's) gland	gland or organ that secretes an additional protective substance for spermatozoa during ejaculation
circumcision	surgical removal of the prepuce or foreskin from the penis
ejaculatory duct	duct where the vas deferens and seminal vesicle join
epididymis	coiled, 20-foot tube where spermatozoa mature
fertilization	condition in which the male sperm joins the female ovum in the fallopian tube, which results in pregnancy
glans	expanded tip of the penis
gonads	generic name for the male and female reproductive organs
penis	external male organ that enlarges and becomes firm during sexual arousal
prepuce	fold of skin covering the glans penis; foreskin
prostate gland	gland that secretes a fluid that precedes the sperm cells and vesicular secretions during ejaculation
scrotum	sac of skin outside the male body that houses the testes
semen	spermatozoa and fluids from the vesicles, prostate, and bulbourethral glands
seminal vesicles	two saclike glands that produce a secretion that enhances sperm motility, nourishes the sperm, and protects the spermatozoa at the time of ejaculation
seminiferous tubules	structures in the testes that produce spermatozoa
spermatozoa	male sex cells that develop in the seminiferous tubules of the testes; sperm
testes	male reproductive organs that produce spermatozoa and testosterone
testosterone	male sex hormone
urethra	canal extending from the urinary bladder to the external opening of the penis; carries semen during ejaculation and urine at other times
urologist	physician who specializes in the male reproductive system
vas deferens	tube or duct that is a continuation of the epididymis

Key Terminology Practice Exercises

COMPLETION

Complete the following statements.

1. Spermatozoa are produced in the seminiferous tubules in the male glands called the ____________________.
2. Male testes are located in the ____________________.
3. The testes are where ____________________ are produced and mature.

4. Spermatozoa mature in a coiled tube called the ____________________.
5. Fluid secreted from the ____________________ protects sperm at the time of ejaculation.
6. Additional protective substances are added during ejaculation by the ____________________ gland and ____________________ glands.
7. The ____________________ carries semen during ejaculation to the external opening of the penis.
8. The ____________________ becomes swollen with blood, which causes enlargement during sexual arousal.
9. ____________________ is composed of spermatozoa and fluids from the seminal vesicles, prostate, and bulbourethral glands.
10. The ____________________ is referred to as the foreskin.
11. The continuation of the upper portion of the epididymis is the ____________________.
12. The ____________________ are the male reproductive organs that produce spermatozoa and testosterone.
13. ____________________ results when a male sperm joins the female ovum in the fallopian tube
14. The generic name for the male and female reproductive organs is ____________________.
15. The surgical removal of the prepuce or foreskin from the penis is ____________________.

MATCHING

Match the meaning to the term. Terms may be used more than once.

1. __________ convoluted structures within the testes
2. __________ male sex hormone
3. __________ propels spermatozoa from vas deferens into the urethra by contractions at the culmination of sexual arousal
4. __________ expanded tip of the penis
5. __________ elective surgical removal of prepuce
6. __________ specialist in the male reproductive system
7. __________ sac of skin located outside the body
8. __________ maturation of sperm begins here
9. __________ leads from epididymis to urinary bladder
10. __________ formed by union of ducts of seminal vesicles and vas deferens

a. circumcision
b. ejaculatory duct
c. epididymis
d. glans
e. scrotum
f. seminiferous tubules
g. testosterone
h. urologist
i. vas deferens

Word Element Review

Root	Meaning	Example	Definition
balan/o	glans penis	**balanitis** (băl"ah-nī'tĭs)	inflammation of the glans penis and mucous membrane beneath it
epididym/o	epididymis	**epididymotomy** (ĕp"ĭ-dĭd-ĭ-mŏt'ō-mē)	incision into the epididymis
orch/o, orchi/o orchid/o	testis	**orchiopathy** (ŏr"kē-ŏp'ah-thē)	any disease or condition of the testes
prostat/o	prostate gland	**prostatism** (prŏs'tah-tĭzm)	any condition of the prostate gland that causes retention of urine in the bladder
scrot/o	bag, pouch	**scrotum** (skrō'tŭm)	pouch containing the testes
semen, semin/o	seed	**seminal** (sĕm'ĭ-năl)	pertaining to the semen or to seed
sperm/o, spermat/o	spermatozoa	**spermatic** (spĕr-măt'ĭk)	pertaining to semen or spermatozoa
test/o	testes, testicles	**testicle** (tĕs'tĭ-k'l)	the testis; the male gonad
		testicular (tĕs'tĭk'ū-lăr)	pertaining to the male testes
vas/o	vessel, duct	**vasorrhaphy** (văs-ŏr'ah-fē)	suture of the vas deferens
vesicul/o	seminal vessels	**vesiculitis** (vĕ-sĭk"ū-lī'tĭs)	inflammation of a vessel, particularly the seminal vesicle

Word Element Practice Exercises

WORD ELEMENTS

Provide the correct word element to complete the following words.

1. any disease of the testes ________________ pathy
2. incision into the epididymis ________________ otomy
3. the male gonad ________________ icle
4. inflammation of the seminal vesicle ________________ itis
5. any condition of the prostate gland that causes retention of urine in the bladder ________________ ism
6. pertaining to semen or sperm ________________ ic
7. suture of the vas deferens ________________ rrhaphy
8. inflammation of glans penis and mucous membrane beneath it ________________ itis
9. pouch containing testicles ________________ um
10. pertaining to semen ________________ al

MATCHING

Match the word elements to their meanings.

1. __________ spermatozoa
2. __________ testes, testicles
3. __________ epididymis
4. __________ prostate gland
5. __________ vessel
6. __________ glans penis
7. __________ seminal vessels
8. __________ bag, pouch
9. __________ seed
10. __________ testis

a. orch/o, orchi/o, orchid/o
b. spermat/o
c. vas/o
d. vesicul/o
e. epididym/o
f. prostat/o
g. balan/o
h. scrot/o
i. semin/o
j. test/o

CLASSIFICATION

Classify each of the following words using A for adjective, D for diagnosis, P for procedure, and N for noun.

1. balanitis __________
2. epididymotomy __________
3. orchiopathy __________
4. prostatism __________
5. scrotum __________
6. seminal __________
7. spermatic __________
8. testicle __________
9. testicular __________
10. vasorrhaphy __________
11. vesiculitis __________

WORD ELEMENT MEANINGS

Give the meaning of each word element. Then use your dictionary to find a new word that contains each of the word elements. Specify whether the new word is a noun or an adjective by placing N or A in the last column.

Word Element	Meaning	Word	N or A
1. balan/o	__________	__________	__________
2. epididym/o	__________	__________	__________
3. orch/o	__________	__________	__________
4. orchi/o	__________	__________	__________
5. orchid/o	__________	__________	__________
6. prostat/o	__________	__________	__________
7. scrot/o	__________	__________	__________
8. semen	__________	__________	__________

9. semin/o ______ ______ ______
10. sperm/o ______ ______ ______
11. spermat/o ______ ______ ______
12. test/o ______ ______ ______
13. vas/o ______ ______ ______
14. vesicul/o ______ ______ ______

Working Practice

DIAGNOSTIC PROCEDURES		
Word	**Pronunciation**	**Definition**
General		
cystoscopy	sĭs-tŏs'kō-pē	insertion of a cystoscope through the urethra to examine the urinary tract
digital rectal examination (DRE)		examination of the prostate gland using finger palpation through the rectum
semen analysis		procedure in which sperm cells are counted and examined for motility and shape
Laboratory Tests		
prostate specific antigen (PSA)		blood test used to help identify prostrate carcinoma and monitor effectiveness of therapy for prostate cancer
prostatic acid phosphatase (PAP)	prŏs-tat'-ĭk as'ĭd fŏs'fah-tās"	blood test used to help identify prostate carcinomas or other conditions such as benign prostatic hypertrophy
wet mount		microscopic examination of fresh male urethral secretions to test for presence of living organisms

DIAGNOSES		
Word	**Pronunciation**	**Definition**
Testicles and Scrotum		
anorchidism	ăn-or'kĭ-dĭzm"	congenital absence of one or both testes
carcinoma of testes	kăr"sĭ-nō'mah, tĕs'tēz	malignant tumor of the testicles: seminoma is most common (see Figure 17-3)
cryptorchidism, cryptorchism	krĭpt-or'kĭ-dĭzm, krĭpt-or'kĭzm	failure of the testicle(s) to descend into the scrotum one month before birth; undescended testicle (see Figure 17-4)
epididymitis	ĕp"ĭ-dĭd"ĭ-mĭ'tĭs	inflammation of the epididymis (see Figure 17-5)

continues

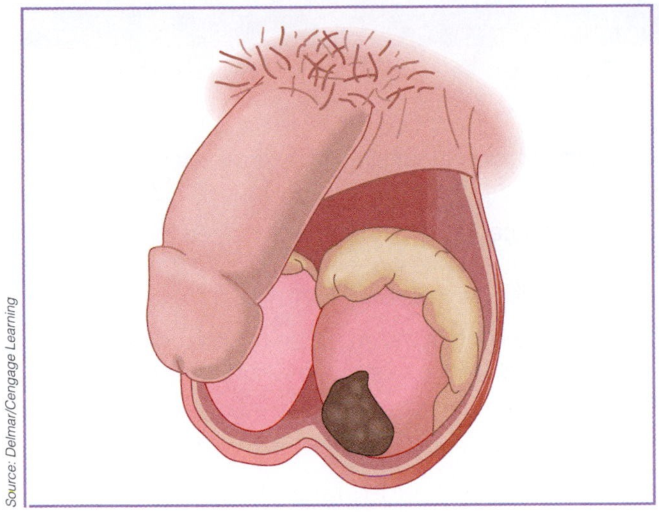

FIGURE 17-3 Carcinoma of the Testes

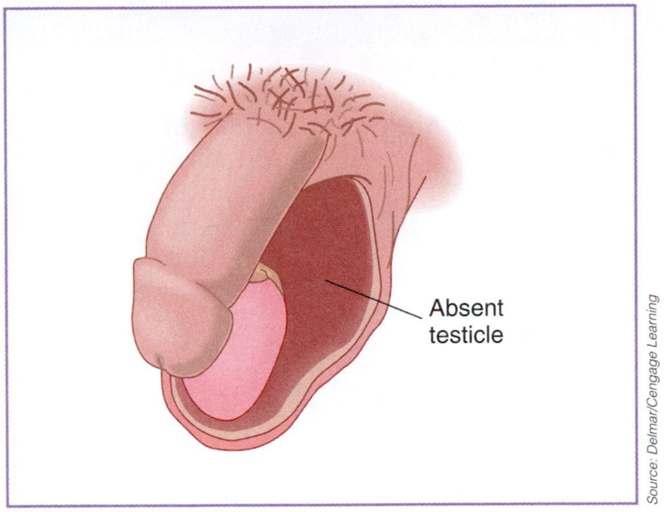

FIGURE 17-4 Cryptorchidism

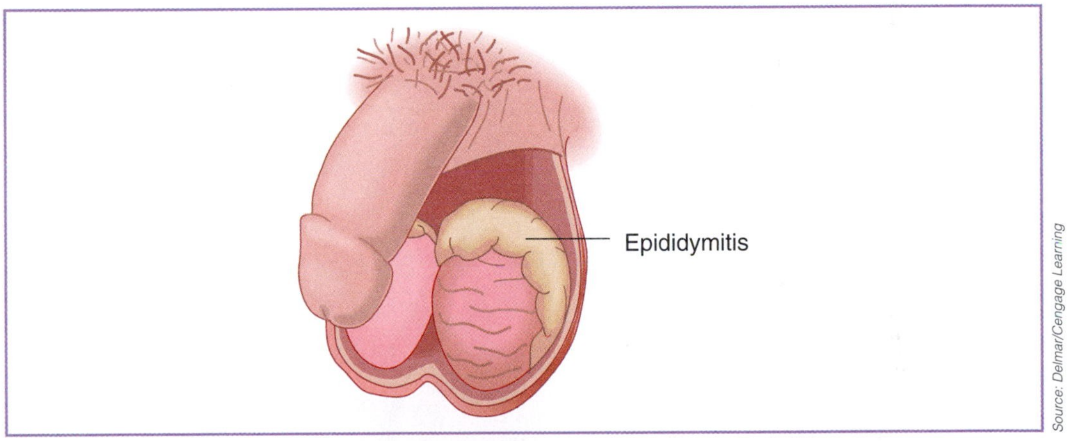

FIGURE 17-5 Epididymitis

DIAGNOSES		
Word	**Pronunciation**	**Definition**
Testicles and Scrotum (*continued*)		
hydrocele	hī'drō-sēl	collection of fluid in the scrotum surrounding the testes (see Figure 17-6B)
orchitis	ōr-kī'tĭs	inflammation of a testicle
spermatocele	spĕr-măt'ō-sēl	cyst of the epididymis containing sperm
testicular torsion	tĕs-tĭk'ū-lăr tŏr'shŭn	rotation producing ischemia of the testes
varicocele	văr'ĭ-kō-sēl	enlargement of the spermatic cord veins, commonly occurring above the left testicle (see Figure 17-6C)
Penis, Urethra, Bladder		
balanitis	băl-ă-nī'tĭs	inflammation of the glans penis or glans clitoris
cystitis	sĭs-tī'tĭs	inflammation of the bladder

continues

DIAGNOSES		
Word	**Pronunciation**	**Definition**
Penis, Urethra, Bladder (*continued*)		
epispadias	ĕp-ĭ-spā'dē-ăs	malformation in which the urethra opens on the dorsum of the penis (see Figure 17-7)
hypospadia, hypospadias	hī"pō-spā'dē-ah	developmental anomaly characterized by an abnormal urethral opening on the ventral side of the penis (see Figure 17-8)
paraphimosis	păr"ă-fī-mō'sĭs	painful swelling at the end of an uncircumcised penis due to failure to reduce (pull forward) the prepuce
phimosis	fī-mō'sĭs	narrowness of the opening of the prepuce preventing its retraction (see Figure 17-9)
urethral stricture	ū-rē'thral	narrowing lesion of the urethra
urethritis	ū"rē-thrī'tĭs	inflammation of the urethra
urinary incontinence	ū'rĭ-năr"ē	inability to control urination some of the time

continues

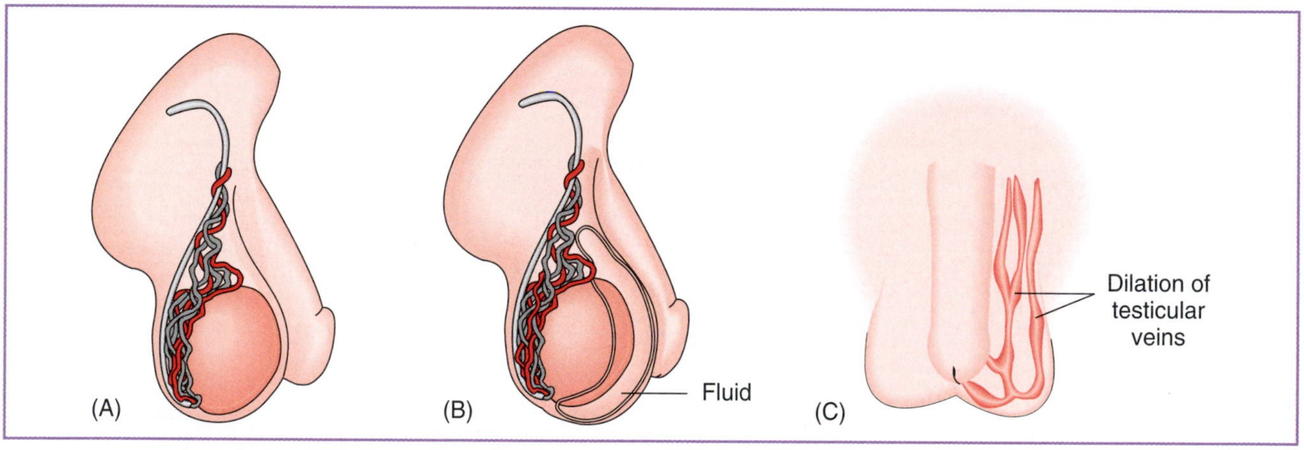

Source: Delmar/Cengage Learning

FIGURE 17-6 Hydrocele and Varicocele: (A) normal; (B) hydrocele; (C) varicocele

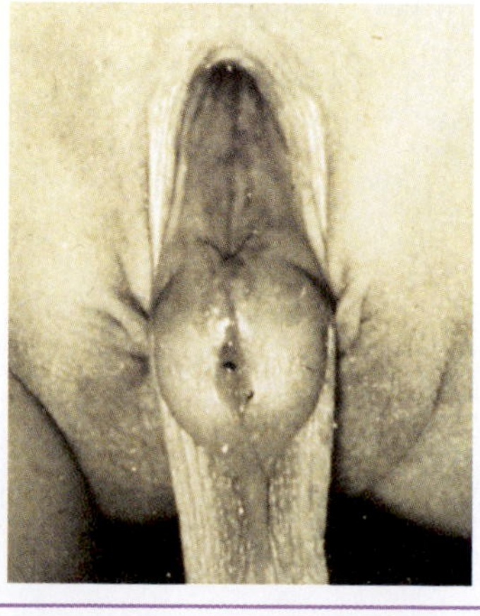

Courtesy of Dr. James Mandell, Children's Hospital, Boston

FIGURE 17-7 Epispadias

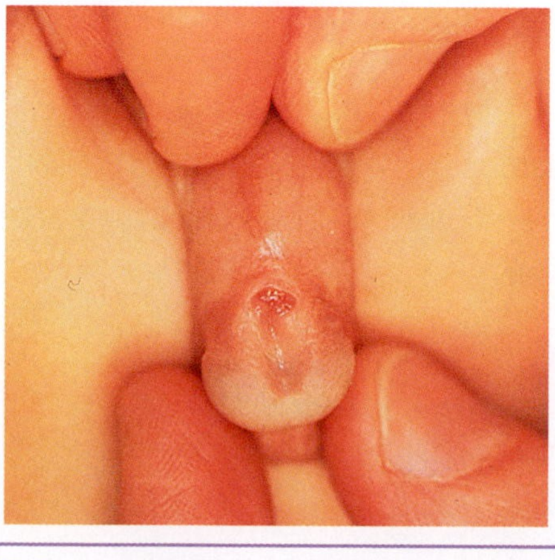

Courtesy of Dr. James Mandell, Children's Hospital, Boston

FIGURE 17-8 Hypospadias

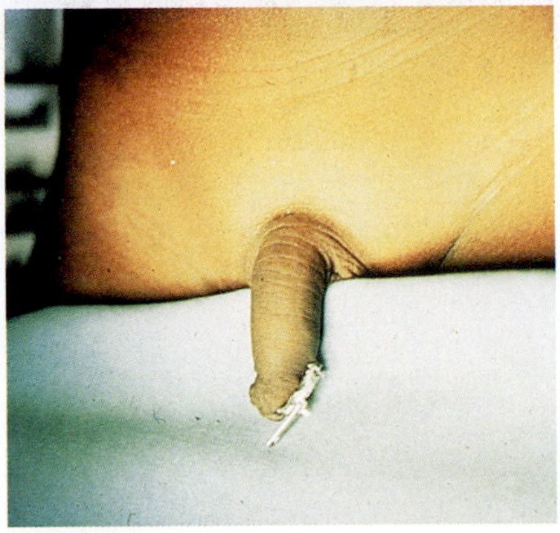

Courtesy of Dr. James Mandell, Children's Hospital, Boston

FIGURE 17-9
Phimosis

DIAGNOSES

Word	Pronunciation	Definition
Prostate Gland		
benign prostatic hypertrophy (BPH)	bē-nīn' prŏs-tăt'ĭk hī-per'trō-fē	benign overgrowth of the prostate gland; hyperplasia of the prostate
carcinoma of the prostate	kăr"sĭ-nō'mah; prŏs'tāt	malignant tumor of the prostate
prostatitis	prŏs"tah-tī'tĭs	inflammation of the prostate gland; may be acute or chronic
Sexual Dysfunction		
condyloma (genital warts)	kon"di-lo'mah	warts caused by papilloma virus
impotence	ĭm'pō-tĕnse	inability of male to achieve or maintain a penile erection
Peyronie's disease	pā-rōn-ēz'	induration (hardening) of part of the penis
premature ejaculation	ē-jăk"ū-lā'shŭn	ejaculation too soon to satisfy the sexual partner
priapism	prī'ă-pĭzm	prolonged, painful erection of penis with no associated sexual excitement
retrograde ejaculation	rĕt'rō-grād ē-jăk"ū-lā'shŭn	little or no semen is ejaculated from the penis during sexual climax

TREATMENT PROCEDURES

Word	Pronunciation	Definition
circumcision	ser"kŭm-sĭzh'ŭn	removal of the end of the prepuce; usually performed on infant males in this culture as a hygienic measure; religious rite in the Hebrew culture
hydrocelectomy	hī"drō-sē-lĕk'tō-mē	excision of a hydrocele (sac containing watery fluid)
orchiectomy (castration)	or"kē-ĕk'tō-mē	excision of one or both testes

continues

TREATMENT PROCEDURES		
Word	**Pronunciation**	**Definition**
orchiopexy; orchidopexy	or"kē-ō-pěk'sē; or'kĭd-ō-pěk'sē	surgical fixation of an undescended testis in the scrotum; brings testes into the scrotum
prostatectomy (perineal, suprapubic/ transvesical, or retropubic)	prŏs"tah-těk'tō-mē	removal of the prostate
transurethral incision of the prostate (TUIP)	trăns"ū-rē'thrăl; prŏs'tāt	surgical procedure that makes small cuts in the bladder neck to widen the urethra
transurethral microwave thermotherapy (TUMT)	trăns"ū-rē'thrăl thĕr"mō-thĕr'ă-pē	nonsurgical treatment for destruction of prostate tissue
transurethral needle ablation (TUNA)	trăns"ū-rē'thrăl; ăb-lā'shŭn	treatment using low-level radiofrequency energy through needles to burn away a defined region of an enlarged prostate
transurethral resection of the prostate (TURP)	trăns"ū-rē'thrăl	procedure in which an endoscope is passed through the urethra, and prostate tissue is removed by electrocautery, cryogenic, laser, or hyperthermia techniques (see Figure 17-10)
vasectomy	vah-sěk'tō-mē	removal of all or a segment of the vas deferens to produce sterility in the male (see Figure 17–11)

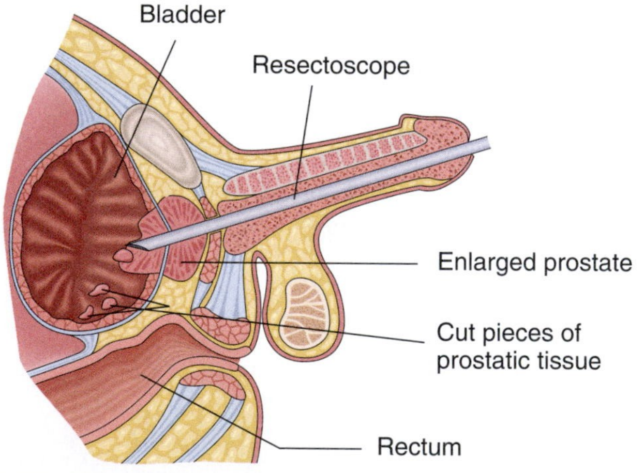

FIGURE 17-10 Transurethral Resection of Prostate (TURP)

Source: Delmar/Cengage Learning

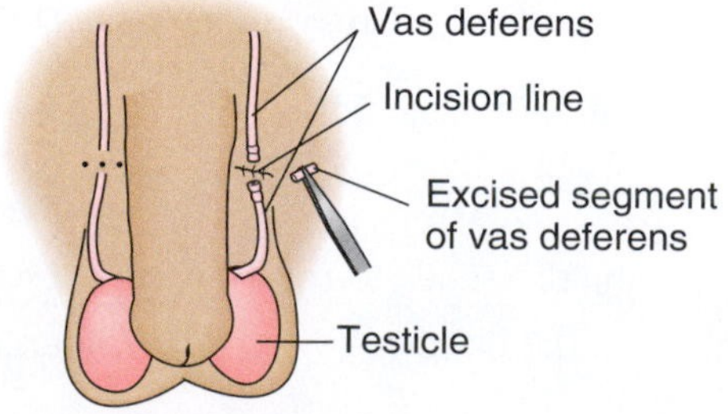

FIGURE 17-11 Vasectomy

Source: Delmar/Cengage Learning

MEDICATIONS PRESCRIBED	
Trade Name	Generic Name
Antibiotics	
Bactrim, Septra	sulfamethoxazole and trimethoprim
Cipro	ciprofloxacin
Noroxin	norfloxacin
Gonadotropins	
Pergonal	menotropins
For Impotence	
Viagra	sildenafil
Yocon	yohimbine

ABBREVIATIONS	
BPH	benign prostatic hypertrophy
DRE	digital rectal examination
GU	genitourinary
NGU	nongonococcal urethritis
PAP	prostatic acid phosphatase
PSA	prostate-specific antigen
TRUS	transrectal ultrasound
TUIP	transurethral incision of the prostate
TUMT	transurethral microwave thermotherapy
TUNA	transurethral needle ablation
TURP	transurethral resection of the prostate

MALE AND FEMALE SEXUALLY TRANSMITTED DISEASES (VENEREAL DISEASES)		
Word	Pronunciation	Definition
Laboratory Tests		
cytomegalovirus test (CMV)	sī"tō-mĕg"ah-lo-vi'rus	test for the presence of cytomeaglic inclusion disease
enzyme immunoassay (EIA)	ĭm"ū-nō-ăs'sā	enzyme immunochemical test for determining the presence of antigens or antibodies in the blood; one of the primary diagnostic tests for many infectious diseases, including the human immunodeficiency virus (HIV); after a second test that is also HIV positive, the Western blot test is perform to verify HIV

continues

MALE AND FEMALE SEXUALLY TRANSMITTED DISEASES (VENEREAL DISEASES)		
Word	Pronunciation	Definition
Laboratory Tests (*continued*)		
FTA-ABS test		test for syphilis
Gram stain/culture		test for gonorrhea or other bacterial infections
rapid plasma reagin (RPR)	rē'ah-jĭn	test for syphilis
TORCH test (toxoplasma, other infections, rubella, cytomegalovirus, and herpes simplex virus)		test performed on the mother and newborn to determine exposure to any of the diseases caused by specific viruses
VDRL (Venereal Disease Research Laboratory) test		one of the screening tests for syphilis
Western blot		test to confirm the presence of the human immunodeficiency virus (HIV)
Diagnoses		
acquired immune deficiency syndrome (AIDS)*		advanced stage of HIV infection, which is characterized by opportunistic infections, malignancies, and other disorders
Chlamydia	klah-mĭd'ē-ah	genital infection in men and women caused by the bacteria *Chlamydia*; known as the "silent STD" because its symptoms may be mild
cytomegalic inclusion disease (CID)	sī"tō-mĕg"ăl'ĭk	viral infection that is transmitted in the uterus from the mother to the fetus
cytomegalovirus (CMV)	sī"tō-mĕg"ah-lo-vi'rus	herpes-type virus with a wide variety of disease effects
genital herpes, herpes genitalis	jĕn'ĭ-tăl hĕr'pēz; hĕr'pēz jĕn'ĭ-tăl-ĭs	infection of the skin and the mucosa of the genitals; caused by the herpes simplex virus (HSV; see Figure 17-12)
gonorrhea	gŏn"ō-rē'ah	inflammation of the genital tract mucosa membrane caused by gonococcus

continues

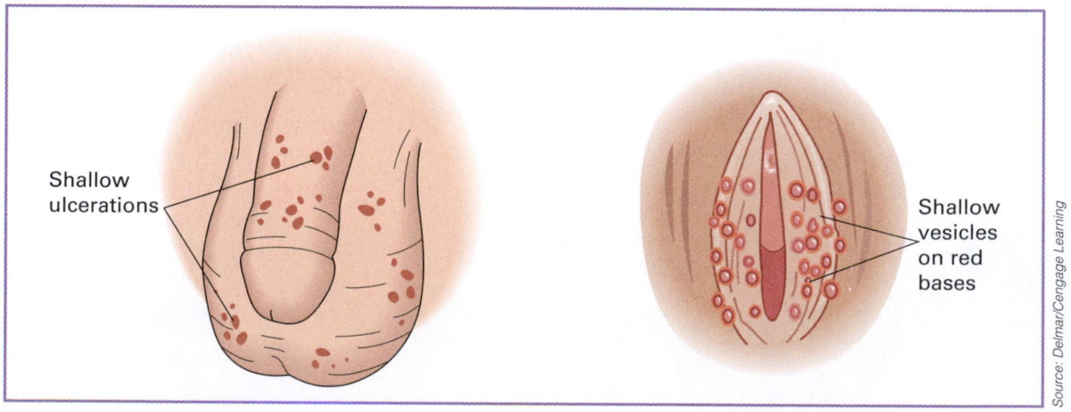

FIGURE 17-12 Genital Herpes (A) in the male; (B) in the female

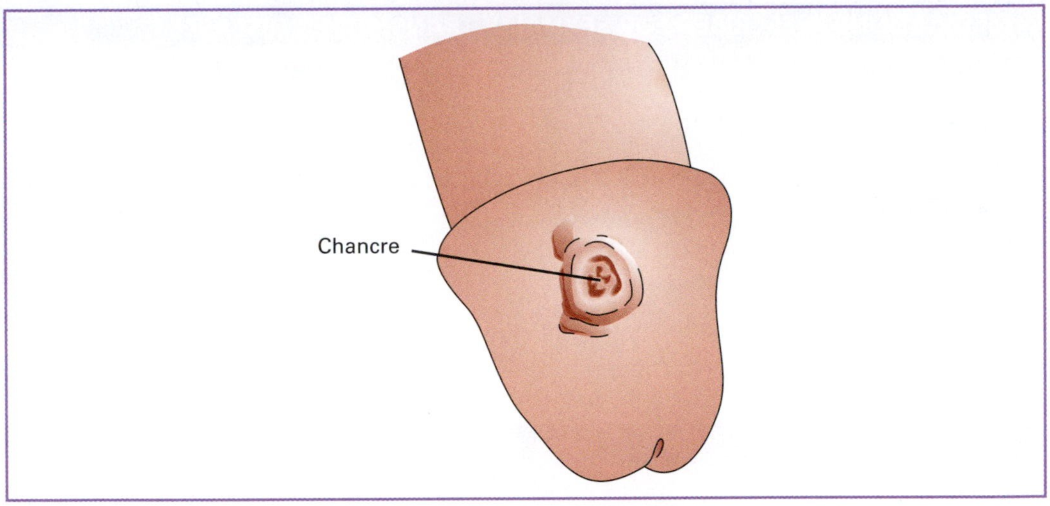

FIGURE 17-13
Primary Syphilis: Male

MALE AND FEMALE SEXUALLY TRANSMITTED DISEASES (VENEREAL DISEASES)

Word	Pronunciation	Definition
Diagnoses (*continued*)		
human immunodeficiency virus (HIV)*		viral infection that damages the body's natural immune defenses against disease; an infected individual may transmit the virus to another through the exchange of body fluids; this can be from sexual activity, sharing of contaminated needles and syringes, untested blood transfusion, or from mother to child during pregnancy or birth
syphilis	sĭf'ĭ-lĭs	chronic, infectious disease caused by spirochete bacterium, affecting any organ of the body (see Figure 17-13)
trichomoniasis	trĭk"ō-mō-nī'ah-sĭs	infection of the genitourinary tract caused by Trichomonas
venereal warts (genital warts)	vĕ-nē'rē-ăl	sexually transmitted condition caused by the human papillomavirus (HPV) that affects both men and women; may appear in men on the shaft or near the end of the penis or on the scrotum, and in women on the vaginal lips, inside the vagina, on the cervix, or around the anus

MEDICATIONS PRESCRIBED FOR SEXUALLY TRANSMITTED DISEASES

Trade Name	Generic Name
Achromycin V	tetracycline
Ampicill, Ampicillin	ampicillin
Benemid	probenecid
Bicillin, Wycillin, Beepen-VK, Pen-Vee-K, Betapen-VK	penicillin

continues

MEDICATIONS PRESCRIBED FOR SEXUALLY TRANSMITTED DISEASES	
Trade Name	**Generic Name**
Flagyl	metronidazole
Gyne-Lotrimin, Mycelex	clotrimazole
Rocephin	ceftriaxone
Vibramycin	doxycycline
Zovirax	acyclovir

ABBREVIATIONS	
CID	cytomegalic inclusion disease
CMV	cytomegalovirus
EIA	enzyme immunoassay
HIV	human immunodeficiency virus
HSV	herpes simplex virus
RPR	rapid plasma reagin
STD	sexually transmitted disease
STI	sexually transmitted infection
VD	venereal disease
VDRL	Venereal Disease Research Laboratories

Working Practice Review Exercises

MATCHING

Match the terms to their meanings.

1. __________ a count and examination of spermatozoa
2. __________ excision of one or both testes
3. __________ inflammation of the prostate
4. __________ removal of prostate tissue by electrocautery or cryogenic techniques
5. __________ male sterilization procedure
6. __________ removal of the end of the prepuce
7. __________ surgical fixation of a testis
8. __________ an enlarged, swollen vein near the spermatic cord
9. __________ excision of the prostate gland
10. __________ testicle that has failed to drop into the scrotum

a. circumcision
b. cryptorchidism
c. cystitis
d. hydrocele
e. hypospadia
f. orchiectomy
g. orchiopexy
h. orchitis
i. Peyronie's disease
j. prostatectomy

11. __________ rotation producing ischemia of the testes		k. prostatitis
12. __________ inflammation of the urinary bladder		l. semen analysis
13. __________ fluid in the scrotum or tubes leading from the testes		m. testicular torsion
		n. transurethral needle ablation
14. __________ abnormal urethral opening on the penis		o. transurethral resection of the prostate
15. __________ induration of part of the penis		p. urethritis
16. __________ narrowing lesion of the urethra		q. urethral stricture
17. __________ inflammation of the testicle		r. urinary incontinence
18. __________ inflammation of the urethra		s. varicocele
19. __________ inability to control urination some of the time		t. vasectomy
20. __________ treatment using low-level radiofrequency energy through needles to burn away defined region of enlarged prostate		

MATCH ABBREVIATIONS

Match the meanings with their abbreviations.

1. __________ test for syphilis	a. AIDS
2. __________ acquired immune deficiency syndrome	b. CID
3. __________ venereal disease	c. CMV
4. __________ herpes simplex virus	d. EIA
5. __________ cytomegalovirus	e. HIV
6. __________ human immunodeficiency virus	f. HSV
7. __________ enzyme immunoassay	g. RPR
8. __________ rapid plasma reagin/test of syphilis	h. STD
9. __________ cytomegalic inclusion disease	i. VD
10. __________ sexually transmitted disease	j. VDRL

COMPLETION

Complete the following statements about sexually transmitted diseases.

1. An infection of the genitourinary tract is ____________________.
2. A test for gonorrhea is ____________________.
3. A test used to confirm the presence of HIV is the ____________________.
4. ____________________ is a bacterial infection found in both men and women and known as the "silent STD."
5. Infection of the skin and the mucosa of the genitals is called ____________________.
6. A ____________________ is performed on mother and newborn to determine exposure to any of several viral diseases.
7. Viral infection that is transmitted in the uterus from mother to fetus is called ____________________.
8. A test for syphilis is ____________________.
9. The advanced stage of HIV infection is known as ____________________.
10. ____________________ are a sexually transmitted condition caused by the human papillomavirus that affects both men and women.
11. A chronic, infectious disease caused by spirochete bacterium affecting any organ of the body is ____________________.

12. ____________________ is an inflammation of the genital tract mucosa membrane caused by gonococcus.
13. A blood test for the presence of cytomegalic inclusion disease is a ____________________test.
14. A blood test to detect for the presence of HIV antibodies is ____________________.
15. A viral infection that damages the body's natural immune defenses against disease is ____________________.

ABBREVIATION MEANINGS

Identify the following abbreviations. Specify whether it is a diagnosis (D), test (T), or procedure (P).

Abbreviation	Meaning	D, T, or P
1. BPH	____________________	________
2. DRE	____________________	________
3. PAP	____________________	________
4. TURP	____________________	________
5. PSA	____________________	________
6. TUIP	____________________	________
7. EIA	____________________	________
8. CID	____________________	________
9. RPR	____________________	________
10. TUNA	____________________	________

Dictionary Exercises

DICTIONARY EXERCISE 1

Provide the pronunciation and select the meaning of each term.

1. anorchism (____________________)
   a. narrowing of the opening of the prepuce
   b. congenital absence of one or both testes
   c. male deprived of testes or external genitals
   d. absence of sperm in semen
2. ejaculation (____________________)
   a. ejection of sperm and fluid from the male urethra
   b. a tube formed by union of vas deferens and duct of seminal vesicles
   c. secretion responsible for male sex characteristics
   d. formation of sperm
3. corpora cavernosa (____________________)
   a. abnormal congenital opening on the underside of the penis
   b. deficient amount of sperm in the seminal fluid
   c. narrowing of the opening of the prepuce
   d. two columns of erectile tissue lying side by side that form the bulk of the penis
4. perineum (____________________)
   a. pelvic floor
   b. area between anus and scrotum in the male
   c. tissue composed of the essential cells of any organ
   d. skin covering the tip of the penis

5. vasovasostomy (____________________)
   a. removal of all or a segment of the vas deferens to produce
   b. excision of one or both testes
   c. surgical fixation of undescended testes in the scrotum
   d. reversal of a vasectomy by rejoining the cut ends of vas deferens
6. oligospermia (____________________)
   a. deficient amount of sperm in the seminal fluid
   b. malignant tumor of the testes
   c. absence of sperm in the semen
   d. failure of testes to ejaculate semen
7. masturbation (____________________)
   a. stimulation of the genital organs by some means other than sexual intercourse
   b. deficiency of the testes or their secretion with impaired sexual power and eunuchoid symptoms
   c. inability of the male to achieve an erection to perform sexual intercourse successfully
   d. sensitive tip of the penis
8. eunuchoidism (____________________)
   a. male deprived of testes or external genitals
   b. inability of the male to achieve a sufficient erection
   c. stimulation of the genital organs by some means other than intercourse
   d. deficiency of the testes or their secretion with impaired sexual power and eunuchoid symptoms
9. chancre (____________________)
   a. skin lesion
   b. discharged pus
   c. tightness of foreskin
   d. cauliflower-like, fleshy growths
10. castration (____________________)
   a. deficient amount of sperm
   b. sterilization
   c. removal of damaged tissue
   d. weak muscle tone

DICTIONARY EXERCISE 2

Pronunciation of the words below is provided. Using your dictionary, find the correct spelling and definition for each of these words.

	Word	Pronunciation	Definition
1.	__________	spĕr"măt-ō-jĕn'ĕ-sĭs	__________
2.	__________	ah-spĕr'mē-ah	__________
3.	__________	shăng'kĕr	__________
4.	__________	spĕr"măt-ō-zō'ŏn	__________
5.	__________	tĕr-ă-tō'mah	__________
6.	__________	ū'nŭk	__________
7.	__________	sĕm"ē-nō'mah	__________
8.	__________	băl'ă-nō-plăs"tē	__________
9.	__________	ă-zō"ō-spĕr'mē-ah	__________
10.	__________	ăn'drō-jen	__________
11.	__________	tĕs-tĭk'ū-lăr	__________
12.	__________	ĭn"tĕr-stĭsh'ăl	__________
13.	__________	kō'ĭ-tŭs ĭn-tĕr-rŭp'tŭs	__________
14.	__________	ăn-ŏr'kĭz-ĕm	__________
15.	__________	pō'tĕn-sē	__________
16.	__________	spĕr-mō-lĭt'ĭk	__________

17.	______________	flă-jĕl'ŭm	______________________________
18.	______________	vĕ-nĕ'rē-ăl	______________________________
19.	______________	stĕr"ĭl-ĭ-zā'shŭn	______________________________
20.	______________	tĕs-tŏp'ă-thē	______________________________
21.	______________	ā"sĭmp-tō-măt'ĭk	______________________________
22.	______________	flăk'sĭd	______________________________
23.	______________	mă-lāz'	______________________________
24.	______________	mō-tĭl'ĭ-tē	______________________________
25.	______________	mū-kō-pūr'ū-lĕnt	______________________________
26.	______________	pūr'ū-lĕnt	______________________________
27.	______________	trŭs	______________________________
28.	______________	ĭng'gwĭ-năl hĕr'nē-ă	______________________________
29.	______________	jĕn'ĭ-tăl wortz	______________________________
30.	______________	spĕr"mă-tī'tĭs	______________________________

StudyWARE™ Connection

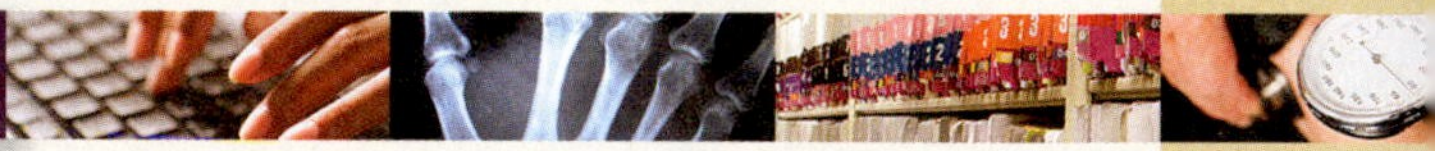

Play more interactive games and take a practice quiz for this chapter on your StudyWARE™ CD-ROM.

Listening Exercise

INSTRUCTIONS

1. Review the spelling, pronunciation, and meaning of the words provided in the preview.
2. Go to your StudyWARE™ CD-ROM and listen to **Listening Exercise 17-1**. Fill in the blank in the report as the word is dictated.
3. At the end of the activity, check your spelling against the preview words. They appear in the preview in the order in which they are encountered in the activity.
4. Review and practice the words you missed.
5. Look up words that are not familiar.

PREVIEW OF WORDS FOR LISTENING EXERCISE 17-1		
Word	**Pronunciation**	**Meaning**
nocturia	nŏk-tū'rē-ah	urination during the night
hematuria	hĕm"ah-tū'rē-ah	blood in the urine
pyelogram	pī'ĕ-lō-grăm	picture of the renal pelvis and ureter after the injection of a contrast material
meatus	mē-ā'tŭs	passage or opening on body surface through which urine is discharged
spermatocele	spĕr-măt'ō-sēl	cyst of the epididymis containing sperm
testicle	tĕs'tĭ-k'l	male sex gland located in the scrotum
benign prostatic hypertrophy	bē-nīn' prŏs-tăt'ĭk hī-pĕr'trō-fē	benign overgrowth of the prostate gland

StudyWARE™ Connection

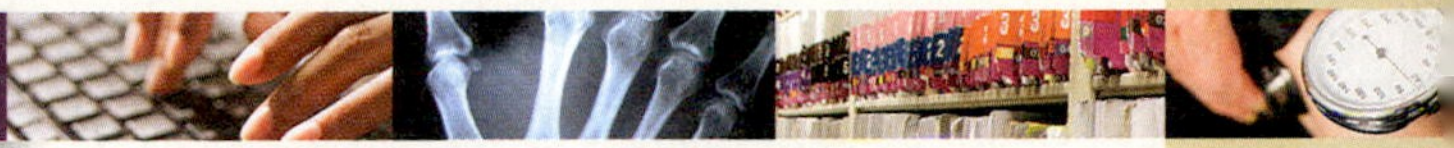

Listen to the report on the next page being read on your StudyWARE™ CD-ROM. Fill in each blank as the word is dictated.

Listening Exercise 17-1

History and Physical Examination

HISTORY: This is an 81-year-old male referred by Dr. George with progressive symptoms of bladder outlet obstruction of approximately six to eight months' duration. He has experienced a decrease in the size of force of stream, strains to void, ________________ × 2, and has some slight precipitant urgency. No history of urinary tract infection. About a month ago he noted on several occasions with burning on urination and urgency. It cleared by forcing fluids. There is no history of calculus disease or previous retention. An intravenous ________________ is being done on the day of admission.

PAST HISTORY: Surgery: He had an appendectomy in 1967 and a left inguinal hernia in 1942. He has never had cardiac symptoms, hypertension, myocardial infarction, or angina. He has not used cardiac medications. Allergies: No known drug allergies. No asthma or hay fever.

Review of Systems

RESPIRATORY: No hemoptysis or TB.

CARDIAC: Noncontributory at this time.

GASTROINTESTINAL: Denies ulcer, hematemesis, melena, jaundice, infectious mononucleosis, hepatitis, or diabetes.

GENITOURINARY: Symptoms and problems as described. No gross abnormalities present.

Physical Examination

GENERAL: This 81-year-old male is well developed, well nourished, alert, cooperative, and in no acute distress. Blood pressure is 160/80.

HEENT: Essentially negative. Mouth is clear.

NECK: Supple. Thyroid not enlarged.

CHEST: Symmetrical. Lungs are clear to auscultation and percussion.

HEART: No megaly, no murmurs.

ABDOMEN: Flat, no masses, with no flank pain or CVA pain. Bladder not distended.

GENITALIA: Penis has normal ________________. Adequate scrotum and contents. He does seem to have a loculated or hydrocele of the cord on the left. ________________ itself is normal. Right scrotum and contents are normal.

RECTAL: About a 50-mm benign-feeling prostate. No other rectal masses.

EXTREMITIES: Negative.

IMPRESSION: 1. ________________ with bladder outlet obstruction.

PLAN: Medical treatment will be initiated and tried for two weeks. Depending on progress, the patient will be advised as to the need for more aggressive intervention.

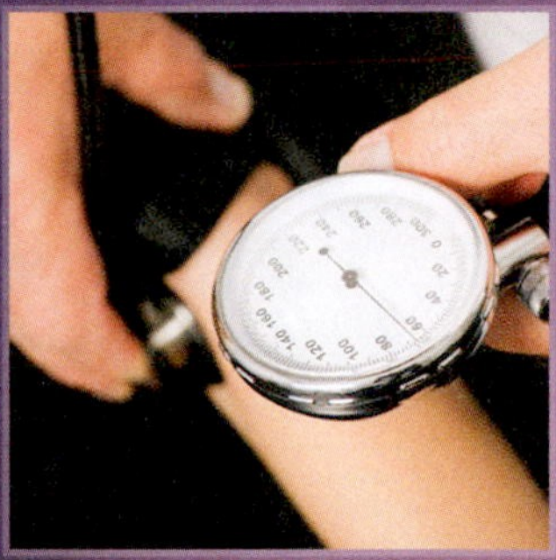
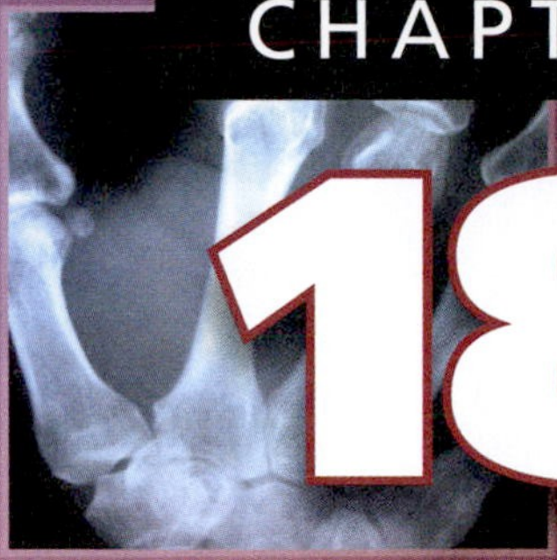
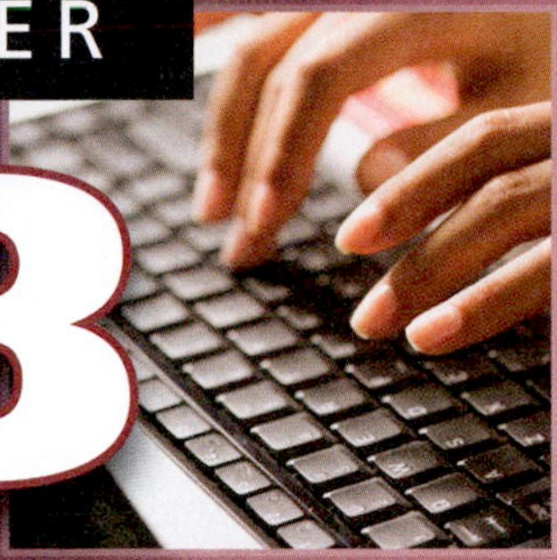
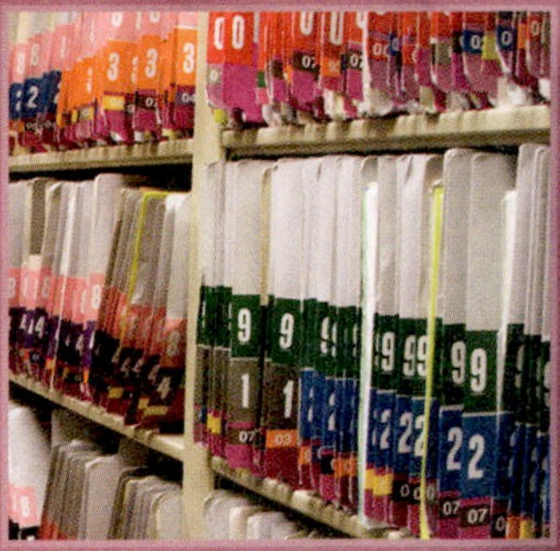

CHAPTER

18

Pathology and Autopsies

"Death should be distinguished from dying, with which it is often confounded."

—Sydney Smith

OBJECTIVES

When you have completed this chapter on pathology and autopsies, you should be able to

1. Identify and define clinical pathology, anatomic pathology and surgical pathology.
2. Identify and define components of surgical pathology and autopsy reports.
3. Identify and spell the names of chemicals, instruments, and stains used.
4. Identify abbreviations related to pathology and autopsy reports.
5. Identify the meanings of related word elements.
6. Hear how medical terminology is used in actual medical reports.

INTRODUCTION

Pathology (pă-thŏl'ō-jē) is a specialized branch of medicine that is concerned with disease-related deviations from normal anatomy and physiology. A **disease** usually refers to a condition marked by the occurrence of abnormal symptoms and the presence of a pathological state. A normal body is extraordinary in its ability to maintain **homeostasis** (hō"mē-ō-stā'sĭs), the state of normalcy; but when normalcy is not maintained, the body is said to be diseased. Two other terms are used interchangeably with disease, but they do not have exactly the same meaning. A **disorder** is often defined as an abnormality of function. A **syndrome** (sĭn'drōm) usually refers to a group of symptoms that may be caused by a specific disease or by several interrelated problems (e.g., Down syndrome).

Pathologists (pă-thŏl'ō-jĭsts), who may be certified in clinical and/or anatomic pathology, are physicians who study disease. **Clinical pathology** is the study of blood and body fluids. Blood, urine, feces, and sputum are used in certain functional tests to determine the general working order of the body. These tests have been included with each system of the body.

Anatomic (ăn"ă-tōm'ĭk) **pathology** is the study of the effect of disease on the body structure as applied to both surgical pathology and autopsies. In either case, they take into account factors that are the cause or **etiology** (ē"tē-ŏl'ō-jē) of the disease; action of the disease; changes brought about in cells, tissues, organs, and the organism as a whole; any destructive forces; and the end result—healing.

In the study of disease, the pathologist uses a variety of terms to describe the disease or disease processes. Bacteria, viruses, fungi, protozoans, and helminth (worms) are **pathogens** (păth'ō-jĕnz) or agents that cause disease. **Pathogenesis** (păth"ō-jĕn'ĕ-sĭs) is a description of how a disease progresses. An acute disease is short term and includes problems such as pneumonia or a fracture. A chronic condition, such as hypertension or asthma, lasts for an extended period of time. If the cause or etiology is unknown, the term **idiopathic** (ĭd"ē-ō-păth'ĭk) is often used.

Surgical pathology is the study of body tissue removed by surgical means and seeks to identify and confirm the patient's disease or problem before, during, or after surgery. In doing so, prognosis and treatment will reflect the findings. Such tissue is placed in fixatives and chemical preparations to preserve it as close to its original state as possible. Samples are then sectioned, stained, placed upon a glass slide, and examined by means of a microscope.

Causes of disease are often divided into six categories.

1. *Hereditary diseases*, or congenital disorders, are caused by a genetic error and may be or may not be present at birth. They may also include problems during a pregnancy or a difficult delivery. Examples of hereditary diseases are cystic fibrosis, congenital heart anomalies, and Down syndrome.
2. *Traumatic diseases* are caused by physical injury from an external source. Motor vehicle accidents, falls, drowning, burns, ingesting or inhaling objects, poisoning, penetrating wounds, or physical abuse are responsible for most serious injury.
3. *Inflammation/infection* is the result of a protective immune response.
4. *Hyperplasias/neoplasms* are overgrowths of cells leading to an increase in tissue size. Hyperplasia is an overgrowth in response to a stimulus, while neoplasms are new growths (benign or malignant).
5. *Nutritional imbalance* may cause problems with physical growth, mental and intellectual retardation, and may even cause death. Malnutrition, obesity, and excessive or deficient vitamins or minerals are specific problems.
6. *Impaired immunity* occurs when part of the immune system breaks down, as in cases of allergy, autoimmunity, and immunodeficiency.

Certain factors predispose individuals to be more susceptible to disease—age, sex, environment, lifestyle, and heredity. Some factors cannot be controlled, such as age, but others, such as lifestyle, can be influenced by the individual.

Pathology specialists also generate autopsy reports. An **autopsy** (aw'tŏp-sē) is performed after the death of a patient. Chemical, bacteriologic, and analytic studies are performed on any part of the body. Tissue samples from all organs are eventually analyzed by microscope.

This chapter presents information about both surgical pathology and autopsy reports that will be encountered in the allied health field.

SURGICAL PATHOLOGY REPORT

During the course of an operation, a surgeon must determine whether an inflammatory process or a malignancy is involved. This decision will often affect the extent of the surgery.

One method used to make the determination is to examine a quick-frozen tissue section. The procedure is simple. During surgery a small piece of tissue is given to the pathologist, who places it in an instrument that uses a quick-freezing technique. Freezing permits slicing thin sections of the sample for analysis under a microscope.

Other tests are applied to tissue samples that may require several days to complete. Therefore, the final report could be delayed until the additional information is made available.

All of these data is gathered in the Surgical Pathology Report. This report may be examined by any number of physicians and will guide follow-up care for the patient, often determining requirements for subsequent surgery, hospitalization, chemotherapy, or other treatment. Because of this impact, a pathology report should be designed to facilitate accurate interpretation of the information provided. To that end, these four formatting standards are helpful.

- use diagnostic headings
- maintain layout continuity from report-to-report, between departments, and between institutions
- prepare the report text so that the information density is appropriate for the reader
- eliminate clutter that can distract attention and create confusion

The Association of Directors of Anatomic and Surgical Pathology has recommended that all demographic information should be placed in the top portion of the report. This should include the patient's name, location, gender, age and/or date of birth, and race; the requesting physician's name; the attending physician's name (if different from the requesting physician); and medical record or unit number.

The complete name and address of the laboratory should be presented at the top of the report, and the Surgical Pathology number should be in an easily identifiable location at the top of every page. A summary of pertinent Clinical History is also recommended.

Regardless of variations in reporting practices in individual institutions, a Surgical Pathology Report generally consists of three sections: the Gross Description, the Microscopic Description, and the Pathologic Diagnoses.

GROSS DESCRIPTION

The **Gross Description** of a specimen submitted for analysis includes the size, color, location, and any other descriptive data that are apparent to the naked eye. The following is an example of the Gross Description of a gallbladder removed from a patient.

EXAMPLE

GROSS: The specimen is a gallbladder weighing 46 gm and measuring 8.5 cm in length and 3.5 cm in diameter. It has been opened before this examination. The lumen contains numerous small stones, and the wall measures up to 7 mm in thickness. The cystic duct at the proximal portion measures 2 cm in length. The surface is dull and red and appears inflamed. The stones measure from 0.5 mm to 6 mm in diameter. Approximately 80 stones are present.

MICROSCOPIC DESCRIPTION

The second portion of the report, the **Microscopic Description**, details the microscopic examination of the specimen. Sometimes it is also referred to as either the *Micro* or the *Histology*. Listing each stain used and the results of that staining is recommended. When immunohistochemical stains are included, each antibody tested and the results of that testing should be included, as well as grading of tumors. This example continues describing the gallbladder being examined.

EXAMPLE

MICRO: The gallbladder mucosa has tall branching strands of connective tissue covered with a tall columnar epithelium. In focal areas, the connective tissue of the mucosa has collections of foam-filled macrophages. There are numerous acute and chronic inflammatory cells within the stroma. The muscle layer is thickened. The perimuscular layer has a marked increase in connective tissue and is infiltrated with numerous round cells and many eosinophils. Areas of erosion of the mucosa are present. There is no evidence of malignancy.

PATHOLOGIC DIAGNOSES

The final section of the pathology report is the **Pathologic Diagnoses**. The Diagnoses and Conclusions from the examination procedures are indicated in the same way as they are listed and/or numbered in a Physical and History or a Discharge Summary Report. This last example shows the diagnoses for the gallbladder being examined.

EXAMPLE

DIAGNOSES:
1. Cholelithiasis.
2. Chronic cholecystitis.

Standard practices vary from institution to institution, but all include gross microscopic descriptions and final diagnoses. See the web site (**www.panix.com**) of the Association of Directors of Anatomic and Surgical Pathology for the current recommendations. An example of a completed Pathology Report is presented in Figure 18-1.

AUTOPSY REPORT

A test performed on the body after death is called an autopsy or postmortem examination. The purpose of this examination, which requires written permission from the next of kin, is to ascertain the exact cause of death. The tests used may be chemical, bacteriologic, or analytical studies. Sections of tissues are taken from all representative organs, and apparent lesions are then analyzed. The branch of medicine that deals with criminal situations is called **forensic** (fo-rĕn'zĭk) **medicine**.

The Autopsy Committee of the College of American Pathologists (**www.autopsydb.org**) has the responsibility for setting guidelines for autopsy reporting. While they recognize that protocols will vary among institutions, they have identified common components that will appear in all reports: Autopsy Face Sheet, Clinical Summary, Objective Description of Gross Autopsy Observation, a Slide and Block Catalog, reports of Ancillary Studies, and a Clinicopathologic Interpretive Summary.

The Autopsy Face Sheet should include information arranged in two subsections: the public information and the private information. This provides a balance between patient confidentiality and the need for public investigation. Information provided should include

1. Name and address of the institution
2. Patient name, hospital number, or social security for verification of identity
3. Patient date of birth and date and time of death
4. Gender and race/ethnicity as indicated by patient in the medical record
5. Final admission date from hospital record
6. Place of death
7. Date and time of autopsy
8. If pertinent, designation as a forensic case, including permissions, restrictions, and responsible party
9. Prosecutor's name
10. Patient's address, occupation, list of ancillary studies, and patient's physicians of record
11. Cause of death statement

Model Report Form 4

PATHOLOGY REPORT

Patient Name: Sumio Yukimura

Hospital No.: 11449

Pathology Report No.: 03-S-942

Admitting Physician: Donna Yates, MD

Preoperative Diagnosis: Cholelithiasis.

Postoperative Diagnosis: Cholelithiasis.

Specimen Submitted: Gallbladder and stone.

Date Received: 06/05/- - - -

Date Reported: 06/06/- - - -

GROSS DESCRIPTION: Specimen received in one container labeled "gallbladder." Specimen consists of a 9-cm gallbladder measuring 2 cm in average diameter. The serosal surface demonstrates diffuse fibrous adhesion. The wall is thickened and hemorrhagic. The mucosa is eroded, and there is a single large stone measuring 2 cm in diameter within the lumen. Representative sections are submitted in one cassette.

GROSS DIAGNOSIS: Gallstone.

KM:xx
D:06/05/- - - -
T:06/05/- - - -

MICROSCOPIC DIAGNOSIS: Gallbladder, hemorrhagic chronic cholecystitis with cholelithiasis.

____
Robert Thompson, MD

RT:xx
D:06/06/- - - -
T:06/06/- - - -

C: Donna Yates, MD

HILLCREST Medical Center

FIGURE 18-1 A Pathology Report

The autopsy procedure is similar to the procedure applied to surgically removed tissue. It is first examined by the naked eye (macroscopically) and then by the microscope. However, the autopsy is more extensive in scope, and the Autopsy Report includes some additional information. The sections of an Autopsy Report are: a History Summary (or Clinical History); a Gross (or Macroscopic) Examination and a Gross Diagnosis; a Microscopic Examination and a Final Diagnosis; and a Discussion or Summary Statement specifying the cause of death.

The examples used in the rest of this chapter represent each section of an Autopsy Report. Words commonly found in such reports are in bold and are pronounced and defined in the Review of Terminology Presented.

HISTORY SUMMARY

The first part of an autopsy report, the **History Summary** or Clinical History, *briefly* describes the patient's hospital stay or the circumstances of his or her death.

EXAMPLE

HISTORY SUMMARY: This patient had an apparent cardiac arrest at home where CPR was attempted by a daughter. An ambulance arrived at the scene to find the patient with constricted pupils and a pulse that was questionably present. On arrival at the emergency room, pupils were dilated and fixed, and there was no response. The patient had repeated defibrillation attempts with no response. Provisional diagnosis was cardiac arrest. The family requested an autopsy.

MACROSCOPIC (GROSS) EXAMINATION

The second part of the report is the **Macroscopic**, or **Gross**, **Examination**, which is examination by the *naked* eye. It usually contains the results of an external and internal examination and includes every major section of the body.

EXAMPLE

GROSS EXAMINATION:

EXTERNAL EXAMINATION: The body is that of a 78-year-old white male measuring 64.5 inches in length and weighing approximately 145 pounds. The scalp is balding, and hair is light gray in color. There is a laceration with crusted blood present over the left midnose. This measures 10 mm in length and is horizontal. There is an **abrasion** (ah-brā'zhŭn) present over the left mideyebrow that also measures approximately 10 mm in length. The entire left eye, including both upper and lower lids and onto the cheek, is deep purple in color from **ecchymoses** (ĕk"ĭ-mō'sēz) and measures 5 cm from top to bottom and 7.5 cm from medial to lateral. A bluish-black raised firm lesion is present over the right cheek 23 mm below the outer portion over the right eye. The lesion measures 6 mm in diameter, is elevated 1.5 mm, and has a pearly border. The ears and mouth are not remarkable. A 5-cm incision in the right lower neck was for introduction of embalming fluid. The chest is not unusual. Breasts are flat. Abdomen is **scaphoid** (skăf'oid). Several needle marks are present in the anterior left chest. The external genitalia are male. The testicles are small. Extremities are well developed, and there is no peripheral edema. There is a grade 2 **lividity** (lĭ-vĭd'ĭ-tē) of the dependent portions of the back.

INTERNAL EXAMINATION: There is hemorrhage into the tissues of the interior chest bilaterally with fractured ribs secondary to CPR. On opening the abdominal cavity, the right lobe of the liver is 6 cm above the right **costal** (kŏs'tal) margin in the midclavicular line. The left lobe of the liver is at the base of the **xiphoid** (zĭf'oid) **process**. The right diaphragm is in the region of the third interspace. The left diaphragm stands in the region of the fourth rib.

Musculature (mŭs'kŭ-lah-chur) of the anterior chest is pink in color and somewhat thin. Bone marrow is a deep red-brown in color and juicy. The appendix is present in the right lower quadrant and **retrocecal** (rĕt"rō-sē'kăl) in position. Small and large bowels are not remarkable. Pleural spaces are moist, and there is no free fluid. The pericardial space contains approximately 10 cc of bloody fluid. The transpericardial diameter is 14 cm. Milk patches are noted over the anterior left ventricle. These areas measure up to 6 × 5 cm.

HEART: The heart weighs 550 gm. Four centimeters from its origin, the right coronary artery has a marked calcification of its wall, and the **lumen** (loo'mĕn) is narrowed to approximately 60%. The left anterior descending coronary artery also has **calcification** (kăl"sĭ-fī-kā'shŭn) of the wall with some thickening and a narrowing of the lumen of approximately 50%. There is some arteriosclerotic change also noted in the left circumflex coronary artery. All four chambers of the heart are dilated. The valve measurements are as follows: tricuspid 12 cm, pulmonary 8.5 cm, mitral 7 cm, aortic 6.5 cm. The valve edges are thin and not remarkable. The **chordae tendineae** (kor'dē tĕn-dĭn'ē-ē) are thin and delicate. The **trabeculae carneae** (trah-bĕk'ū-lē kăr'nē-ē) are flattened. The **foramen ovale** (fō-rā'mĕn ō-vāl'ē) is closed. The myocardium is red-brown in color. The left ventricle measures 17 mm in thickness, and the right ventricle measures 4 mm in thickness.

LUNGS: The left lung weighs 350 gm. The right lung weighs 450 gm. The trachea and bronchi have a light pink-tan mucosa, which is moist. There is a small amount of foamy white material present. The lungs collapse readily on removal from the chest. Sections are **crepitant** (krĕp'ĭ-tănt). The lower lobes are **atelectatic** (ăt"ĕ-lĕk-tăt'-ĭk). The upper lobes are **emphysematous** (ĕm"fĭ-sĕm'ah-tŭs).

GI TRACT: The esophagus is in its usual position and of equal caliber throughout. The mucosa is blue-gray in color, and longitudinal **striations** (strī-ā'shūnz) are present. The stomach contains approximately 50 cm of watery fluid and mucous material. The mucosa is gray-tan in color; rugal folds are present and not remarkable. The duodenum contains greenish semifluid material; its muscle walls, mucosa, and serosa are not remarkable. On compression of the gallbladder, a green bile **exudes** (ĕks-ūdz') from the ampulla of Vater. The gallbladder contains approximately 20 cc of a green bile. The mucosa is soft and velvety. The extrahepatic bile ducts are patent, and the common duct measures 10 mm in circumference.

LIVER: The liver weighs 1530 gm. The surface is smooth and edges are sharp. On sectioning, the **parenchyma** (pah-rĕng'kĭ-mah) is light brown in color, and consistency is somewhat increased.

PANCREAS: The pancreas is light pink in color and coarsely lobular. It is of usual size, shape, and position. On sectioning, the duct is patent and not unusual. It has an appearance of **autolysis** (aw-tŏl'ĭ-sĭs).

SPLEEN: The spleen weighs 125 gm. Its surface is purple-gray in color and dull. On sectioning, the parenchyma is deep purple in color, and pulp scrapes with difficulty from the surface.

ADRENAL GLANDS: The adrenal glands are the usual size, shape, and position. On sectioning, the cortex is light yellow in color, and the medulla is light gray.

KIDNEYS: The left kidney weighs 157 gm; the right kidney weighs 160 gm. The capsules strip with ease. Surfaces are relatively smooth. On sectioning, the cortex measures 9 mm in thickness, and the **corticomedullary** (kŏr"tĭ-kō-mĕd'ū-lār"ē) **junction** is distinct. The pyramids stand out as dark purple, while the cortex is light tan. Ureters are of their usual position and size. The bladder is not remarkable. The prostate measures 3 × 2.5 × 3 cm. On sectioning, the parenchyma is firm and gray in color. The seminal vesicles contain their usual yellow gelatinous material. The rectum is not remarkable.

SPINE: The spine has a grade 1 bridging of the bodies of the vertebrae in the lower portion.

AORTA: The aorta has a minimal plaquing in the upper portion. In the lower portion there is calcium deposition within the wall. The superior mesenteric, celiac, and renal arteries are not remarkable.

HEAD: The scalp is not remarkable. The **calvarium** (kăl-vā'rē-ŭm) measures up to 6 mm in thickness. The dura is tough and not unusual. The cerebral spinal fluid is clear and colorless. The brain weighs 1,180 gm. The vessels at the base of the brain have their usual configuration. The **gyri** (jī'rī) and **sulci** (sŭl'sī) are not remarkable. Multiple sections through the cerebrum, midbrain, pons, medulla, and cerebellum are not remarkable.

GROSS DIAGNOSIS

The gross examination concludes with the **Gross Diagnoses** made on the basis of changes visible to the naked eye.

EXAMPLE

GROSS DIAGNOSES:

I. Hypertrophy and dilatation of heart, consistent with hypertensive cardiovascular disease.
   A. Cardiac arrest with status after CPR.

II. Coronary arteriosclerosis, grade 1.

III. Osteoarthrosis of spine, grade 1.

MICROSCOPIC EXAMINATION

The **Microscopic Examination** is the next section of an autopsy report. Specimens from representative sections of the body are closely examined with the use of a microscope, as the following example shows.

EXAMPLE

MICROSCOPIC EXAMINATION:

CORONARY ARTERIES: The coronary arteries reveal severe arteriosclerosis with **atheroma** (ăth"er-ō'mah) showing **hyalinization** (hī"ah-lĭn"ĭ-zā'shŭn) and calcification. The lumena are narrowed up to 70%.

HEART: The myocardial fibers are hypertrophied. Cross striations are present. A few scattered inflammatory cells are seen.

LUNGS: The lungs have a grade 2 to 3 chronic passive congestion with pigmented macrophages in alveolar spaces and thickened alveolar walls. A pulmonary edema is present. Sections reveal grade 3 pulmonary emphysema. Focal areas of atelectasis are noted. There is a congestion of large vessels.

LIVER: The liver has a grade 3 fatty **metamorphosis** (mĕt"ah-mor'fō-sĭs). An early portal cirrhosis is present. Pigment is present within **canaliculi** (kăn"ah-lĭk'ū-lī).

PANCREAS: The pancreas has a grade 4 autolysis with loss of nuclear staining. This includes islets of Langerhans.

SPLEEN: The splenic sinusoids are dilated and contain few red blood cells. Cords of bill-roth are prominent. Scattered neutrophils are seen within the parenchyma. **Malpighian corpuscles** (măl-pĭg'ĭ-ăn kor'pŭs'lz) are not remarkable.

ADRENAL GLANDS: There is a tubular formation of the cortex that is consistent with a loss of lipoid content. The medullae are not remarkable.

KIDNEYS: Glomerular capillaries contain few red blood cells. Subcapsular spaces contain small amounts of **amorphous** (ah-mor'fŭs) eosinophilic material. Convoluted tubules contain large amounts of eosinophilic material; they are dilated. Bowman's capsules of the glomeruli are thin. Small vessels through the kidney are not remarkable. A few hyalinized glomeruli are noted.

PROSTATE: Many **corpora amylacea** (kor'pō-rah ăm"ĭ-lā'sē-ah) are present within the lumens of the glands.

BRAIN: Neuron and glial cells are orderly. There is no evidence of congestion.

FINAL DIAGNOSES

The **Final Diagnoses** section lists the findings of the microscopic examination.

EXAMPLE

FINAL DIAGNOSES:

I. Cardiomegaly consistent with hypertensive cardiovascular disease (550 gm).
   A. Dilatation of heart.
      1. Grade 3 chronic passive congestion of lungs.
      2. Pulmonary edema.
      3. Laceration of left midforehead and ecchymoses of left eye.

II. Grade 2 coronary arteriosclerosis.

III. Grade 3 pulmonary emphysema.

IV. Grade 3 fatty metamorphosis of liver.

V. Early portal cirrhosis of liver.

VI. Autolysis of pancreas (postmortem).

VII. Basal cell carcinoma of right cheek.

VIII. Grade 1 osteoarthrosis of spine.

DISCUSSION

The **Discussion**, or Clinicopathological Correlative Summary and Comments, is the final section of an autopsy report. It summarizes the cause of death in three parts. First is the *underlying cause*, which refers to the disease or injury that initiated events leading directly to death. Second, the *intermediate cause* presents the important diseases, complications, or conditions that occur sometime between the underlying and immediate cause of death. And finally, the *immediate cause* provides the final disease or complications leading to death.

EXAMPLE

DISCUSSION: This patient had an apparent cardiac arrest at home, and CPR was given. When the ambulance arrived, the pupils were constricted; however, when the patient arrived at the emergency room, the pupils were dilated and fixed, and there was no response. Defibrillation attempts had no response, and a medical examiner's autopsy was performed. The autopsy examination revealed a cardiomegaly, which is consistent with hypertensive cardiovascular disease. There was also a coronary arteriosclerosis present. Secondary to the myocardial **decompensation** (dē"kŏm-pĕn-sā'shŭn), a grade 3 chronic passive congestion of lungs was noted, and there was a pulmonary edema present. The body had already been embalmed; therefore, blood levels for alcohol could not be determined. A grade 3 fatty metamorphosis of the liver was present, and an early portal cirrhosis was noted. The cause of death was due to the hypertensive cardiovascular disease with cardiac arrest.

THE PATHOLOGIST'S PRACTICE

Chemicals, instruments, and stains used in the study of body tissues, as well as commonly used abbreviations, are listed in the following sections.

CHEMICALS

Word	Pronunciation	Definition
acetone	ăs'ĕ-tōn	dimethyl ketone, a colorless liquid that is a fat solvent
Bouin's solution	boo-ăns'	fixation solution for tissue using picric acid, formalin, and acetic acid
formaldehyde	fōr-mal'dĕ-hīd	colorless, water-soluble gas
formalin	fōr'mah-lĭn	aqueous solution of 37% formaldehyde in distilled water used to fix tissues in preparation for sectioning and making microscopic slides
Zenker's fixative	zĕng'kerz	solution for fixing tissue

INSTRUMENTS

Word	Pronunciation	Definition
cryostat	krī'ō-stăt	microtome (instrument that is used to cut tissue in very thin slices) that is contained in a refrigerated chamber
tissue processor		instrument in which selected tissue sections are successively passed into different solutions by a timed mechanism in preparation for sectioning, staining, and mounting on microscopic slides

continues

STAINS		
Word	**Pronunciation**	**Definition**
acid fast stain		used to test a specimen for presence of microorganisms
eosin	ē'ō-sĭn	fluorescent red stain used with hematoxylin for cytoplasmic staining
Giemsa's stain	gēm'sah	deep blue dye that stains bacteria and cellular details
Gomori's methenamine	gō-mor'ēz mĕth-ĕn'ah-mēn	stain specifically for melanin, iron, or urate crystals
Gram's stain	gramz	stain to differentiate gram-positive and gram-negative bacteria
hematoxylin stain	hēm"ah-tŏk'sĭ-lĭn	intense blue stain used for nuclear staining
iron stain		stain for hemosiderin
luxol fast blue	lŭk'sōl	special stain for myelin in nerve cells
mucicarmine stain	mū"sĭ-kăr'mĭn	reddish stain designed to show selectively the presence of mucinous material

COMMONLY USED ABBREVIATIONS	
ASCP	American Society of Clinical Pathologists
MT	medical technologist
MT (ASCP)	Registered Medical Technologist
Path	pathology
spec	specimen
stat	immediately
cc (cm^3)	cubic centimeter
cm	centimeter
mm	millimeter
mg	milligram
mL or ml.	milliliter

INTERNET ASSIGNMENT

The Doctor's Doctor is a site that provides information about laboratory tests and diagnoses and is dedicated to patient empowerment. It is a commercial site that has five areas identified at the bottom of the home page. Two that may be helpful to you are Your Laboratory Report in Everyday Language and What's Your Diagnosis? Examples of a surgical pathology report and one that is translated for you are provided in Your Laboratory Report in Everyday Language. The examples are found in What's Your Diagnosis?

ACTIVITY

Visit the Doctor's Doctor at **www.thedoctorsdoctor.com**. First select Who We Are and then Translating the Report. Check each of the options.

Return to the home page and select Diseases and Medical Information. Check any of those listed.

Now check Search This Site and enter one of the terms presented in Chapter 18. Summarize your findings for your instructor.

Review *Pathology and Autopsies*

- Pathology deals with deviations from normal anatomy or physiology.
- Pathogens are agents that cause disease. Pathogenesis is a description of how a disease progresses.
- Samples submitted to the pathologist during surgery can be quick-frozen for a rapid determination of the presence of malignancy or inflammation and/or submitted for a more detailed analysis taking several hours or days.
- The Surgical Pathology Report made by the pathologist includes a Gross Description (apparent to the naked eye), a Microscopic Description (made after examination with a microscope), and a Diagnosis based on this examination.
- An autopsy is a thorough pathological examination of the body after death.
- The sections of an Autopsy Report are: a History Summary (or Clinical History); a Macroscopic (or gross) Examination and a Gross Diagnosis; a Microscopic Examination and a Final Diagnosis; and a Discussion or Summary Statement specifying the cause of death.

Key Terminology Review

Word	Definition
abrasion	injury resulting in the scraping away of a portion of the skin or mucous membrane
amorphous	without definite structure
anatomic pathology	study of the effect of disease on the body structure as applied in both surgical pathology and autopsies
atelectatic	pertaining to incomplete expansion or collapse of the lung
atheroma	fatty degeneration or thickening of the walls of the larger arteries
autolysis	self-digestion in tissues by enzymes from the cells, such as occurs after death

continues

Word	Definition
autopsy	tests performed on the body after death
calcification	process in which organic tissue becomes hardened by the deposit of lime salts in the tissue
calvarium	domelike superior portion of the cranium composed of the top portion of the frontal, parietal, and occipital bones; also called the skull cap
canaliculi	small channels or canals
chordae tendineae	small tendinous cords that connect the free edges of the atrioventricular valves to the papillary muscles
clinical pathology	study of blood and body fluids and fragments using laboratory methods
corpora amylacea	small masses of degenerate cells found in the prostate
corticomedullary junction	junction of the cortex and medulla of the kidneys
costal	pertaining to a rib
crepitant	crackling
decompensation	failure of the heart to maintain adequate circulation
Discussion	last part of the Autopsy Report where causes of death are summarized
disease	condition marked by the occurrence of abnormal symptoms and the presence of a pathological state
disorder	function that is abnormal
ecchymoses	bruises; large purplish patches
emphysematous	affected with chronic pulmonary disease, characterized by larger than normal air sacs in the lungs
etiology	science dealing with the causes of disease
exude	to pass off slowly through the tissues
Final Diagnoses	part of the Autopsy Report that lists the findings of the microscopic examination
foramen ovale	opening between the two atria of the heart in the fetus
forensic medicine	branch of medicine dealing with criminal situations
Gross Description	part of the Surgical Pathology Report that provides a physical description of the specimen as determined by the naked eye
Gross Diagnoses	part of the Autopsy Report that lists the findings of the macroscopic examination by the naked eye
gyri (*sing.*, gyrus)	convolutions of the cerebral hemispheres of the brain
History Summary	first part of an Autopsy Report briefly describing the patient's hospital stay or circumstances of death; also called *Clinical History*
homeostasis	body's normal state
hyalinization	conversion of tissue into a glasslike substance
idiopathic	describes a situation where the cause or etiology of a disease is unknown
lividity	skin discoloration, as from a bruise
lumen	space within an artery, vein, intestine, or tube

continues

Word	Definition
Macroscopic or Gross Examination	part of an autopsy reporting the results of the examination of the internal and external parts of the body by the naked eye
malpighian corpuscles	renal corpuscles that consist of a glomerulus and Bowman's capsule
metamorphosis	change in form or structure
Microscopic Description	part of a Surgical Pathology Report that reports results of microscopic examination of specimens from representative sections of the body
Microscopic Examination	part of an Autopsy Report that indicates the result of microscope examination of representative sections of the body
musculature	arrangement of the muscles in a body part
parenchyma	essential part of an organ concerned with its function rather than its framework
pathogenesis	description of how a disease progresses
pathogens	agents that cause disease
Pathologic Diagnoses	part of a Surgical Pathology Report listing the various diagnoses or conclusions from the examination procedures
pathologist	physician who studies disease
pathology	specialized branch of medicine dealing with diseases causing deviations from normal anatomy or physiology
retrocecal	pertaining to the area in back of the cecum
scaphoid	boat-shaped
striations	series of streaks
sulci	depressions or grooves that separate convolutions of the brain
surgical pathology	study of body tissues removed by surgical means
syndrome	group of symptoms caused by several interrelated problems
trabeculae carneae	thick, muscular tissue bands attached to the inner walls of the ventricles of the heart
xiphoid process	lowest portion of the sternum

Key Terminology Practice Exercises

COMPLETION

Complete the following statements.

1. The two areas classified under anatomic pathology are ______________ and ______________.
2. A ______________ provides information about whether tissue is cancerous or inflammatory.
3. A brief description of the circumstances of a patient's hospital stay or death is the ______________.

4. Diagnoses based on the macroscopic observation are called ________________.
5. Descriptions of specimens examined under a microscope for an autopsy are found in the ________________.
6. An instrument that prepares tissues for sectioning, staining, and mounting on microscopic slides is a ________________.
7. Two solutions for fixing tissue are ________________ and ________________.
8. A function that is abnormal is a ________________.
9. The body's normal state is ________________.
10. A description of how a disease progresses is ________________.
11. ________________ describes a situation where cause or etiology of a disease is unknown.
12. A physician who studies disease is a ________________.
13. The study of the effect of disease on body structure is ________________ pathology.
14. The study of blood and body fluids and fragments is ________________ pathology.
15. The cause of a disease is referred as its ________________.
16. Part of the autopsy that lists the findings of the microscopic examination is the ________________.
17. A description based on what is seen with the naked eye is a ________________ description.
18. The branch of medicine dealing with criminal situations is ________________ medicine.
19. The essential part of an organ concerned with its function rather than its framework is the ________________.
20. One afflicted with ________________ has a chronic pulmonary disease which is characterized by larger than normal air sacs in the lung.

MATCHING

Match the terms to their meanings.

1. ________ report section that details the examination by the naked eye
2. ________ very cold microtome used to cut very thin slices
3. ________ 37% formaldehyde in distilled water used to fix tissue in preparation for sectioning and making slides
4. ________ a colorless liquid that is a fat solvent
5. ________ report section summarizing the cause of death that follows the final diagnoses
6. ________ a group of symptoms caused by several interrelated problems
7. ________ agents that cause disease
8. ________ lowest portion of the sternum
9. ________ boat-shaped
10. ________ series of streaks
11. ________ change in form or structure
12. ________ skin discoloration
13. ________ conversion into a glasslike substance

a. acetone
b. amorphous
c. atelectatic
d. autolysis
e. canaliculi
f. costal
g. crepitant
h. cryostat
i. Discussion
j. ecchymoses
k. formalin
l. hyalinization
m. lividity
n. Macroscopic or Gross Examination
o. metamorphosis

14. ________ bruises
15. ________ without a definite structure
16. ________ pertaining to collapse of the lung
17. ________ small channels or canals
18. ________ pertaining to a rib
19. ________ crackling
20. ________ self-digestion in tissues by enzymes from cells

p. pathogens
q. scaphoid
r. striations
s. syndrome
t. xiphoid process

IDENTIFICATION

Identify the following abbreviations.

1. ml or mL ________________________
2. cm ________________________
3. stat ________________________
4. Path ________________________
5. MT ________________________
6. mg ________________________
7. mm ________________________
8. spec ________________________
9. MT(ASCP) ________________________
10. ASCP ________________________

Word Element Review

Root	Meaning	Example	Definition
alg/o	pain, cold	**algor** (ăl'gor)	chill, coldness
ameb/o	change	**ameba, amoeba** (ah-mē'bah)	one-celled animal that moves by constantly changing its shape; causes infection
antr/o	chamber, cavity	**antrum** (ăn'trŭm)	cavity or sinus
astr/o	star-shaped	**astroblast** (ăs'trō-blăst)	star-shaped cell
		asteroid (ăs'troid)	star-shaped

continues

Root	Meaning	Example	Definition
coll/o	gluelike	**collagen** (kŏl'ah-jĕn)	gelatin or sticky substance of skin, bone, cartilage, and connective tissue
		colloid (kŏl'oid)	gluelike substance
cry/o	cold	**cryobank** (krī'ō-bănk")	facility for storage of biological tissues at very low temperatures
dendr/o	branching	**dendroid** (dĕn'droid)	branching like a tree
ependym/o	wrapping	**ependyma** (ĕ-pĕn'dĭ-mah)	membrane lining the cavities of the brain and the canal in the spinal column
fibr/o	fiber	**fibrosarcoma** (fī"brō-săr-kō'mah)	spindle-cell sarcoma containing much connective tissue
hist/o	tissue	**histology** (hĭs-tŏl'ō-jē)	microscopic study of the structure, composition, and function of tissues
		histoma (hĭs-tō'mah)	tumor formed from fully developed tissue
hydr/o	water	**hydremia** (hī-drē'mē-ah)	excess of watery fluid in the blood
		hydrocyst (hī'drō-sĭst)	cyst filled with water
lei/o	smooth	**leiomyoma** (lī"ō-mī-ō'mah)	tumor composed of smooth muscle fibers
lip/o	fat	**lipoid** (lĭp'oid)	resembling fat
lob/o	section	**lobe** (lōb)	well-defined portion of an organ separated by boundaries
micr/o	small size, microscopic	**microsurgery** (mī'krō-ser"jer-ē)	dissection of small structures under a microscope
necr/o	death	**necrosis** (nĕ-krō'sĭs)	death of individual or groups of cells or localized areas of tissue
		radiculoneuritis (rah-dĭk"ū-lō-nū-rī'tĭs)	disease of nerve roots and nerves
oment/o	covering	**omentum** (ō-mĕn'tŭm)	fold of peritoneum extending from the stomach to adjacent abdominal organs
pariet/o	wall of an organ, cavity	**parietal** (pah-rī'ĕ-tăl)	pertaining to or forming the walls of a cavity
radic/o	root	**radical** (răd'ĭ-kăl)	directed to the cause, origin, or root

continues

Root	Meaning	Example	Definition
scirrh/o, scirr/o	hard	**scirrhous** (skĭr'rŭs)	hard, like a scirrhus
		scirrhus (skĭr'ŭs)	hard cancerous tumor due to an overgrowth of fibrous tissue
sphen/o	wedge	**sphenoid** (sfē-noid)	resembling a wedge
		sphenoid bone	wedge-shaped bone at the base of the cranium
spir/o	coil	**Spirillum** (spī-rĭl'ŭm)	spiral-shaped bacterium
		spiroid (spī'roid)	resembling a coil
strept/o	twisted	**strep throat**	abbreviation for streptococcal infection of the throat
		streptococcus (strĕp"tō-kŏk'ŭs)	infectious, twisted-shaped microorganism
turbin/o	shaped like a top	**turbinal** (tur'bĭ-năl)	shaped like a top; one of the turbinates
vestibul/o	entrance	**vestibular** (vĕs-tĭb'ū-lăr)	pertaining to the entrance or beginning of a canal

Prefix	Meaning	Example	Definition
meta-	change	**metabolism** (mĕ-tăb'ō-lĭzm)	sum of all physical and chemical processes by which a living organized substance is produced and maintained
neo-	new, recent	**neonatal** (nē"ō-nā'tăl)	newborn
		neoplasm (nē'ō-plăzm)	any new, abnormal growth, such as a tumor

Word Element Practice Exercises

IDENTIFY

Provide the term for the following definitions.

1. resembling fat ____________
2. dissection of small structures with a microscope ____________
3. shaped like a top ____________
4. gluelike substance ____________
5. spiral-shaped bacterium ____________
6. directed to the cause ____________
7. tumor of smooth muscle fibers ____________
8. resembling a wedge ____________
9. newborn ____________
10. star-shaped ____________
11. one-celled animal ____________
12. resembling a coil ____________
13. wedge shaped bone ____________
14. hard, cancerous tumor ____________
15. death of individual or groups of cells or tissues ____________
16. cyst filled with water ____________
17. gelatin or sticky substance ____________
18. abbreviation for streptococcal throat infection ____________
19. sum of all chemical and physical processes by which a living substance is produced and maintained ____________
20. microscopic study of tissues ____________

MATCHING

Match the word elements to their meanings.

1. ________ excess fluid in the blood
2. ________ branching like a tree
3. ________ disease of nerve roots and nerves
4. ________ forming the walls of a cavity
5. ________ hard, cancerous tumor
6. ________ infectious, twisted-shaped microorganisms
7. ________ any new, abnormal growth
8. ________ chill, coldness
9. ________ cavity or sinus
10. ________ star-shaped cell
11. ________ membrane lining the cavities of the brain and the canal in the spinal column
12. ________ spindle-cell sarcoma containing much connective tissue

a. algor
b. antrum
c. astroblast
d. cryobank
e. dendroid
f. ependyma
g. fibrosarcoma
h. histoma
i. hydremia
j. lobe
k. neoplasm
l. omentum
m. parietal

13. ________ tumor formed from fully developed tissue
14. ________ fold of peritoneum extending from stomach to adjacent abdominal organs
15. ________ facility for storage of biological tissues at very low temperatures
16. ________ well-defined portion of an organ separated by boundaries
17. ________ pertaining to the beginning of a canal
18. ________ resembling a coil
19. ________ resembling a wedge
20. ________ shaped like a top

n. radiculoneuritis
o. scirrhus
p. sphenoid
q. spiroid
r. streptococcus
s. turbinal
t. vestibular

CIRCLE

Circle the word element and define the following words

1. astroblast ________________________________
2. colloid ________________________________
3. dendroid ________________________________
4. hydremia ________________________________
5. lipoid ________________________________
6. necrosis ________________________________
7. parietal ________________________________
8. scirrhus ________________________________
9. spirillum ________________________________
10. vestibular ________________________________

WORD ELEMENT MEANINGS

Give the meaning of each word element. Then use your dictionary to find a new word that contains each of the word elements. Specify whether the new word is a noun or an adjective by placing N or A in the last column.

Word Element	Meaning	Word	N or A
1. alg/o	________	________	________
2. ameb/o	________	________	________
3. antr/o	________	________	________
4. astr/o	________	________	________
5. coll/o	________	________	________
6. cry/o	________	________	________
7. dendr/o	________	________	________
8. ependym/o	________	________	________
9. fibr/o	________	________	________
10. hist/o	________	________	________
11. hydr/o	________	________	________

Word Element Practice Exercises continued

12. lei/o	________	________	________
13. lip/o	________	________	________
14. lob/o	________	________	________
15. meta-	________	________	________
16. micr/o	________	________	________
17. necr/o	________	________	________
18. neo-	________	________	________
19. oment/o	________	________	________
20. pariet/o	________	________	________
21. radic/o	________	________	________
22. scirr/o	________	________	________
23. scirrh/o	________	________	________
24. sphen/o	________	________	________
25. spir/o	________	________	________
26. strept/o	________	________	________
27. turbin/o	________	________	________
28. vestibul/o	________	________	________

Dictionary Exercises

DICTIONARY EXERCISE 1

Use your dictionary to find the pronunciation and definition of the following words.

Word	Pronunciation	Definition
1. rigor mortis	________	________
2. livor mortis	________	________
3. putrefaction	________	________
4. patent	________	________
5. imperforate	________	________
6. incarcerated	________	________
7. pathognomonic	________	________
8. stroma	________	________
9. granulation	________	________
10. keloid	________	________
11. exudation	________	________
12. fibrosis	________	________
13. sloughing	________	________

14. chromatin ______________ ______________________________
15. caseation ______________ ______________________________
16. concretion ______________ ______________________________
17. fasciculus ______________ ______________________________
18. focus ______________ ______________________________
19. syncytial ______________ ______________________________
20. hyaline ______________ ______________________________
21. mitosis ______________ ______________________________
22. pyknosis ______________ ______________________________

DICTIONARY EXERCISE 2

Select the correct meaning and provide the pronunciation of each term.

1. cavitation (________________)
   a. becoming like cheese
   b. a calculus or an inorganic mass
   c. to surround with a capsule
   d. formation of a cavity or an empty space
2. postmortem lividity (________________)
   a. cooling of the body after death
   b. rigidity of skeletal muscles developing 2–4 hours after death and lasting 3–4 days
   c. discoloration of dependent parts of the body after death
   d. degeneration of cells or tissues by endogenous enzymes
3. desquamation (________________)
   a. process of removing calcium and other elements from bone
   b. shedding of the epidermis
   c. broken-down cellular material
   d. to remove a natural surface
4. frond (________________)
   a. base of an organ
   b. point from which disease arises
   c. oval opening
   d. movable, branchlike structure
5. glairy (________________)
   a. smooth, glassy substance
   b. benign overgrowth of normal cellular elements
   c. sticky, gummy, gelatinlike
   d. like a fish scale
6. hyperemia (________________)
   a. presence of bacterial poisons in the blood
   b. unusual amount of blood in any part of the body
   c. benign overgrowth of normal cellular elements
   d. containing blood
7. panniculus (________________)
   a. clothlike layer of tissue
   b. fine net or network
   c. little beam or crossbar
   d. a covering membrane
8. stippling (________________)
   a. shedding
   b. surrounding a capsule
   c. like cheese
   d. a speckled condition
9. whorl (________________)
   a. fine net or network
   b. spiral arrangement of cells or tissues
   c. pear-shaped
   d. movable, branchlike structure
10. serosanguineous (________________)
    a. pertaining to blood
    b. presence of bacterial poisons in the blood
    c. containing serum and blood
    d. fibrous tissue left after healing of a wound

11. theca (____________________)
    a. enclosing case or sheath
    b. covering membrane
    c. cellular structure lining major body cavities
    d. scar
12. proliferation (____________________)
    a. physical makeup of a substance
    b. multiplication of similar forms
    c. conversion into a liquid form
    d. conversion of tissues into a dry, amorphous mass
13. trabecula (____________________)
    a. a supporting structure
    b. tissue forming the supporting framework of an organ
    c. base of an organ
    d. small pit or hollow cavity
14. autolysis (____________________)
    a. process of removing calcium and other elements from bone
    b. degeneration of cells or tissues by endogenous enzymes
    c. series of changes through which the muscles of a cell go in the course of division
    d. condensation and increased basophilic staining of a cell nucleus
15. vacuole (____________________)
    a. fine net or network
    b. outgrowth from the surface of a part
    c. structure with open spaces that may be filled with fluid or the remains of ingested materials
    d. points from which a disease arises

DICTIONARY EXERCISE 3

Match the terms to their meanings. Provide the pronunciation for words where indicated.

1. ________ caseous (____________________)
2. ________ denude
3. ________ exfoliation (____________________)
4. ________ globoid (____________________)
5. ________ hydatid (____________________)
6. ________ infiltrate
7. ________ lacuna (____________________)
8. ________ foramen ovale (____________________)
9. ________ reticulum (____________________)
10. ________ section
11. ________ stellate (____________________)
12. ________ tenacious (____________________)
13. ________ tunica (____________________)
14. ________ daughter cyst
15. ________ parent cyst
16. ________ bulla (____________________)
17. ________ fundus (____________________)
18. ________ translucent (____________________)
19. ________ septicemia (____________________)
20. ________ serrated (____________________)

a. scaling off dead tissue
b. to invade an area
c. thin slice of tissue
d. like cheese
e. covering membrane
f. fetal heart opening
g. arising from preexisting cyst
h. to remove a natural surface
i. fine net or network
j. primary cyst
k. cyst formed in the tissues
l. clinging or adhering to
m. small pit or hollow cavity
n. shaped like a star
o. resembling a globe
p. blister
q. base of an organ
r. bacterial poisons in blood
s. sawtoothlike borders
t. permitting passage of light

DICTIONARY EXERCISE 4

Pronunciation of the words below is provided. Using your dictionary, find the correct spelling and definition of each word.

	Word	Pronunciation	Definition
1.	____________	kō"lē-sĭs-tī'tĭs	____________
2.	____________	dĕs'ĭ-kāt-ĕd	____________
3.	____________	ĕks-krĕs'ĕns	____________
4.	____________	flō'rah	____________
5.	____________	jĕm-ĭs"tō-sī'tĭk	____________
6.	____________	hē"mō-sĭd'er-ĭn	____________
7.	____________	kĕr'ah-tĭn-īzed	____________
8.	____________	loo'tē-ĭn	____________
9.	____________	pō"dō-rahnj'	____________
10.	____________	săng-gwĭn'ē-ŭs	____________
11.	____________	skwā'mŭs	____________
12.	____________	trah-bĕk'ū-lah	____________
13.	____________	lĭk"wē-făk'shŭn	____________
14.	____________	āb'sēs	____________
15.	____________	lŏb'ūl	____________
16.	____________	mĕs'en-kīm	____________
17.	____________	mĕs"ō-thē'lē-ŭm	____________
18.	____________	ŏs'tē-ŭm	____________
19.	____________	pah-rĕng'kĭ-mah	____________
20.	____________	prī-mor'dē-ăl	____________

*Study*WARE™ Connection

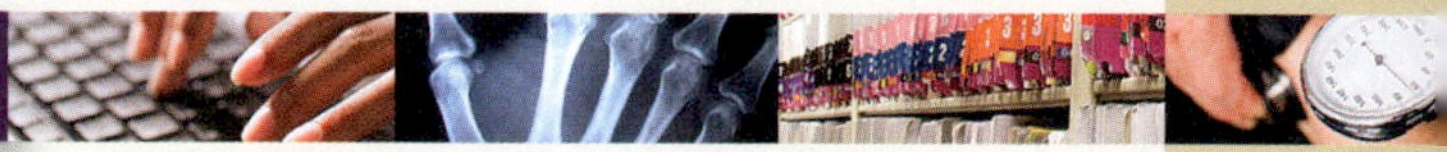

To take a practice quiz or play interactive games that reinforce the content in this chapter, go to your StudyWARE™ CD-ROM.

Listening Exercise

INSTRUCTIONS

1. Review the spelling, pronunciation, and meaning of the words provided in the preview.
2. Go to your StudyWARE™ CD-ROM and listen to **Listening Exercise 18-1**. Fill in the blank in the report as the word is dictated.
3. At the end of the activity, check your spelling against the preview words. They appear in the preview in the order in which they are encountered in the activity.
4. Review and practice the words you missed.
5. Look up words that are not familiar.

PREVIEW OF WORDS FOR LISTENING EXERCISE 18-1

Word	Pronunciation	Meaning
foci	fō'sī	chief centers of a morbid process (*sing*., focus)
paravesical	păr"ă-vĕs'ĭk-ăl	beside the bladder
endometrioid	ĕn"dō-mē'trē-oid	similar to the endometrium
perisigmoidal	pĕr"ĭ-sĭg"moy'dăl	pertaining to the peritoneum of the sigmoid curvature
cystadenoma	sĭst"ăd-ĕn-ō'mă	cystic tumor blended with an adenoma (benign epithelial tumor)
subserosal	sŭb-sē-rō'săl	pertaining to the area below membrane-producing or containing serum

Listening Exercise 18-1

StudyWARE™ Connection

Listen to this report being read on your StudyWARE™ CD-ROM. Fill in each blank as the word is dictated.

Letter of Consultation

Dear Dr. Barton:

Mrs. Casandra Petaja was evaluated for increasing pelvic discomfort with a history of endometriosis. At exploration she was noted to have pelvic endometriosis, but in addition, had carcinoma which had arisen in ____________________ of endometriosis. Total abdominal hysterectomy, bilateral salpingo-oophorectomy, and cytoreductive surgery were performed. At the end of the procedure, there was no evidence of visible or palpable residual tumor.

The pathology was as follows: "Uterus (135 grams), left tube and ovary (95 grams), tissue from ____________________ cul-de-sac, and peritoneal regions, 25 cm of sigmoid colon and portion of omentum (12 × 7 × 2 cm). Grade 3 adenocarcinoma compatible with gynecologic origin is identified forming a mass, 1 × 1 × 0.9 cm, on the surface of the resected sigmoid colon. The tumor shows an ____________________ histologic pattern and is present forming a tumor mass in the cul-de-sac as well. Metastatic carcinoma is present in one of the eight ____________________ lymph nodes removed with the resected bowel. Foci of endometriosis are present in the peritoneum and paravesical tissues. Microscopic foci of carcinoma are also present in tissue submitted from paravesical region. A benign ____________________ (9 × 5.5 × 2 cm) is identified in the left ovary. The hysterectomy specimen shows inactive endometrium, mild chronic cervicitis, and multiple (12) intramural, ____________________, and submucosal leiomyomas ranging in size from 0.5 to 2 cm in greatest dimension. Right and left fallopian tube and omentum are negative for tumor. 07-13-20—ADDENDUM: Permanent sections show a microscopic foci of endometrioid adenocarcinoma in the left ovary."

I will send further plans for postoperative chemotherapy at her dismissal from Grandview Hospital. Thank you for the opportunity to share in her care.

Sincerely yours,

Duane Crookston, MD

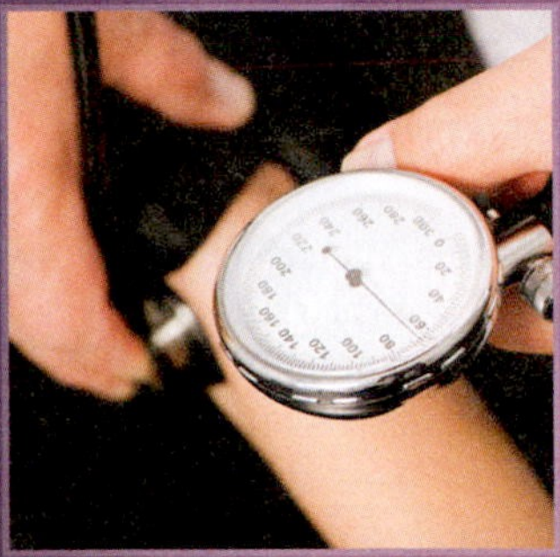

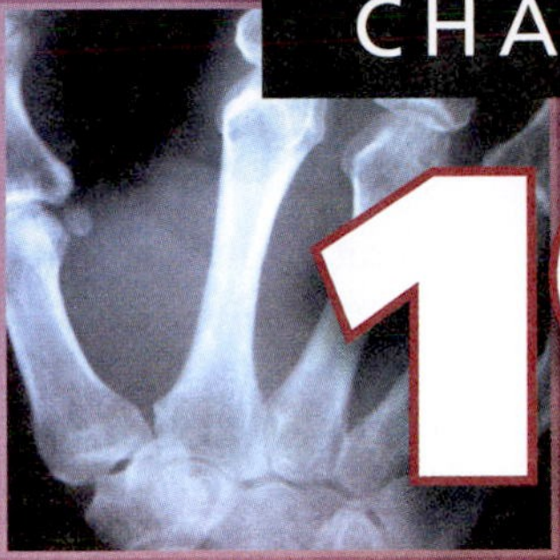

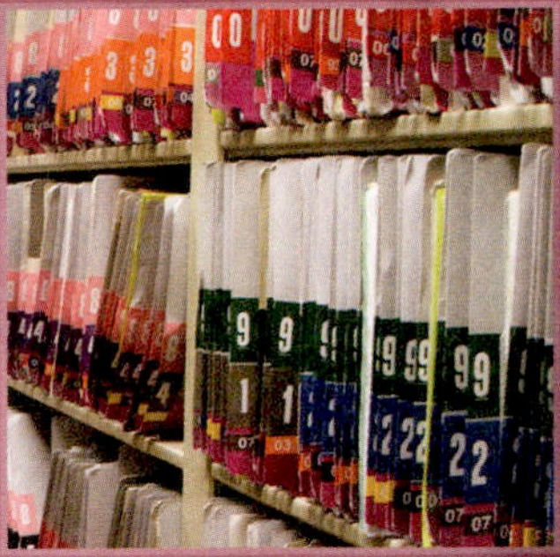

CHAPTER

19

The Endocrine System

"It would indeed be rash for a mere pathologist to venture forth on the uncharted sea of the endocrines, strewn as it is with the wrecks of shattered hypotheses, where even the most wary mariner may easily lose his way as he seeks to steer his bark amid the glandular temptations whose siren voices have proved the downfall of many who have gone before."

— William Boyd

OBJECTIVES

When you have completed this chapter on the endocrine system, you should be able to

1. Spell and define major system components and explain how they operate.
2. Identify the meanings of related word elements.
3. Spell and define diagnostic procedures, diagnoses, treatment procedures, and abbreviations.
4. Spell the names of commonly used medications.
5. Use a dictionary as a tool in processing medical documents.
6. Hear how medical terminology is used in actual medical reports.

INTRODUCTION

Endocrinology (ĕn"dō-krĭ-nŏl'ō-jē) is a science concerned with the function of glands that secrete chemical compounds known as hormones into the bloodstream. Physicians who are trained to diagnose and treat endocrine disorders are called **endocrinologists**. Probably no other system of the anatomy has experienced so many shifts and changes in theory and thinking as has the endocrine system. Although the anatomy of the system is fairly well known, all of its functions are not.

COMPONENTS OF THE ENDOCRINE SYSTEM

The glands that make up the endocrine system are the thyroid, parathyroids, pituitary, adrenals, pancreas, testes or ovaries, and the pineal gland. (Although the thymus is included here and in other texts as part of the endocrine system, its function is usually attributed to the immune system.) Each of these glands has one or more specific functions, but they are all dependent upon other glands in the system for maintenance of a normal hormonal balance.

The glands of the endocrine system affect the activity of every cell in the body. Some of their specific effects are mental alertness, physical agility, body build and stature, bodily hair growth, voice pitch, and sexual behavior. They constantly modify the way we feel, think, behave, and react to all sorts of stimuli. For this reason, the endocrine system is closely linked to the nervous system.

Specifically, a **gland** is any organ that produces a secretion. This secretion is manufactured from blood constituents by specialized cells within the gland. Glandular secretions may be divided into two main groups. The first is secretions carried through a duct from glandular cells to a nearby organ or body surface. Examples are digestive juices and tears. These secretions come from **exocrine** (ĕk'sō-krĭn) **glands**. The second group of glands produces internal secretions, which are carried to all parts of the body by blood or lymph systems. These are called hormones and originate in the **endocrine glands**. These endocrine glands, which are ductless, make up the endocrine system. Note in the following table how many hormones there are.

MAJOR ENDOCRINE GLANDS AND THE HORMONES THEY PRODUCE

Endocrine Gland	Hormones Produced	Function
Adrenals		
cortex	aldosterone (mineralocorticoid)	regulates the amount of salts in the body and the body fluid volume, and helps to control blood pressure
	cortisol (glucocorticoid)	regulates the quantities of sugars, fats, and proteins in cells, and helps the body respond to stresses like illness and injury
	androgens, estrogens, and progestins	maintains secondary sex characteristics
medulla	epinephrine (adrenaline)	sympathomimetic; constriction or dilation of arterioles depending on type of vascular tissue involved; accelerates the heart rate; opens airways; helps the body respond to stress and excitement
	norepinephrine (noradrenaline)	sympathomimetic; constriction of arterioles; neurotransmitter; increases blood pressure
Ovaries	estrogen	development and maintenance of secondary sex characteristics in the female
	progesterone	prepares the uterus for pregnancy and maintenance of pregnancy
Pancreas islets of Langerhans	insulin	regulates the transport and storage of glucose in the body
	glucagon	increases blood sugar by causing the conversion of glycogen to glucose
Parathyroids	parathyroid hormone (PTH)	regulates calcium and phosphorus levels in the blood

continues

MAJOR ENDOCRINE GLANDS AND THE HORMONES THEY PRODUCE		
Endocrine Gland	**Hormones Produced**	**Function**
Pituitary (hypophysis)		
anterior lobe (adenohypophysis)	adrenocorticotropin (ACTH) (corticotropin)	stimulates the adrenal cortex to secrete cortisol and weak androgens, which control adrenal cortex development and functioning
	gonadotropins	
	• *follicle-stimulating hormone (FSH)*	stimulates ovarian follicles to grow and produce estrogen; stimulates the ovaries to release eggs (ovulate) in women; stimulates spermatozoa development in men
	• *luteinizing hormone (LH)*	increases synthesis of testosterone in males; stimulates the synthesis of androgens, estrogen, and progestin in the ovaries and the hormone-releasing development of the corpus luteum in females
	• *melanocyte-stimulating hormone (MSH)*	causes pigmentation of the skin
	• *prolactin*	stimulates breast development during pregnancy and milk secretion after delivery of the baby; can affect sex hormone levels from the ovaries in women and the testes in men
	• *growth hormone (GH), (somatotropin), human growth hormone (HGH)*	stimulates growth in bone and other tissues; important in maintaining muscle mass and bone mass
	• *thyroid-stimulating hormone (TSH) (thyrotropin)*	regulates the structure and function of the thyroid gland and stimulates synthesis and release of the thyroid hormones thyroxine and triiodothyronine
posterior lobe (neurohypophysis)	antidiuretic hormone (ADH) (vasopressin)	produced by hypothalamus and stored here for release to stimulate the reabsorption of water by kidney tubules; also stimulates muscles of blood vessels to cause vasoconstriction
	oxytocin	produced by hypothalamus and stored here for release to stimulate contraction of the uterus during labor and childbirth; necessary for milk letdown during lactation
Testes	testosterone	promotes growth and maintenance of secondary sex characteristics in the male
Thymus	humoral factors	aids in the development of the lymphoid system
Thyroid	calcitonin	secreted by the thyroid C cells; participates in calcium and phosphorous metabolism
	thyroxine (T_4), triiodothyronine (T_3)	increases the rate of metabolism in body cells

PITUITARY GLAND

The **pituitary** (pĭ-tū'ĭ-tăr"ē) **gland**, or **hypophysis** (hī-pŏf'ĭ-sĭs) (1), as shown in Figure 19-1, is a small gland about the size of a raisin located behind the optic nerve crossing. It is surrounded by bone except for the area where it connects with the brain. The gland consists of two parts: the anterior lobe (or adenohypophysis) and the posterior lobe (or neurohypophysis). The anterior lobe is glandlike in nature whereas the posterior lobe is composed of neural tissue.

The pituitary gland is called the *master gland* because it regulates the functions of the other endocrine glands. In turn, the pituitary gets its direction from the hypothalamus region of the brain. These directions may be in the form of neurons to stimulate or inhibit hormone secretion by the anterior lobe or may be neurohormones sent to the posterior lobe for storage and later release. See the following list of hypothalamic neurohormones and their function.

Hypothalamic Neurohormone	Function
corticotropin-releasing hormone (CRH)	stimulates ACTH secretion
dopamine	inhibits prolactin, LH, FSH, and TSH secretion
gonadotropin-releasing hormone (GnRH) (luteinizing hormone-releasing hormone [LHRH])	stimulates LH and FSH secretion
growth hormone-releasing hormone (GHRH)	stimulates GH secretion
prolactin-releasing factors	stimulate prolactin release
somatostatin	inhibits GH and TSH secretion
thyrotropin-releasing hormone (TRH)	stimulates prolactin and TSH secretion

THYROID GLAND

parathyroid/o	parathyroid glands	thyr/o, thyroid/o	thyroid gland

The **thyroid gland** (see Figure 19-2) is located in the neck just below the larynx. It has left (2) and right (4) lateral lobes located on either side of the trachea and are connected by a narrow band called the isthmus (1). The hormones **thyroxine** (thī-rŏk'sĭn) **(T_4)** and **triiodothyronine** (trī"ī-ō"dō-thī'rō-nēn) **(T_3)** are produced by the thyroid gland. They regulate the production of heat and energy in the body tissues and are necessary to maintain a normal level of metabolism. The blood must have an adequate amount of iodine in order to produce the proper supply of these hormones.

PARATHYROID GLANDS

On the back of the thyroid gland are four tiny epithelial bodies called **parathyroid** (păr-ă-thī'royd) **glands** (7) (see Figure 19-1), which produce parathyroid hormone (PTH). PTH regulates the levels of calcium and phosphorus in the circulating blood and the amount of calcium retained in storage areas such as bones and teeth.

PANCREAS

gluc/o	sugar	pancreat/o	pancreas
glyc/o	sugar		

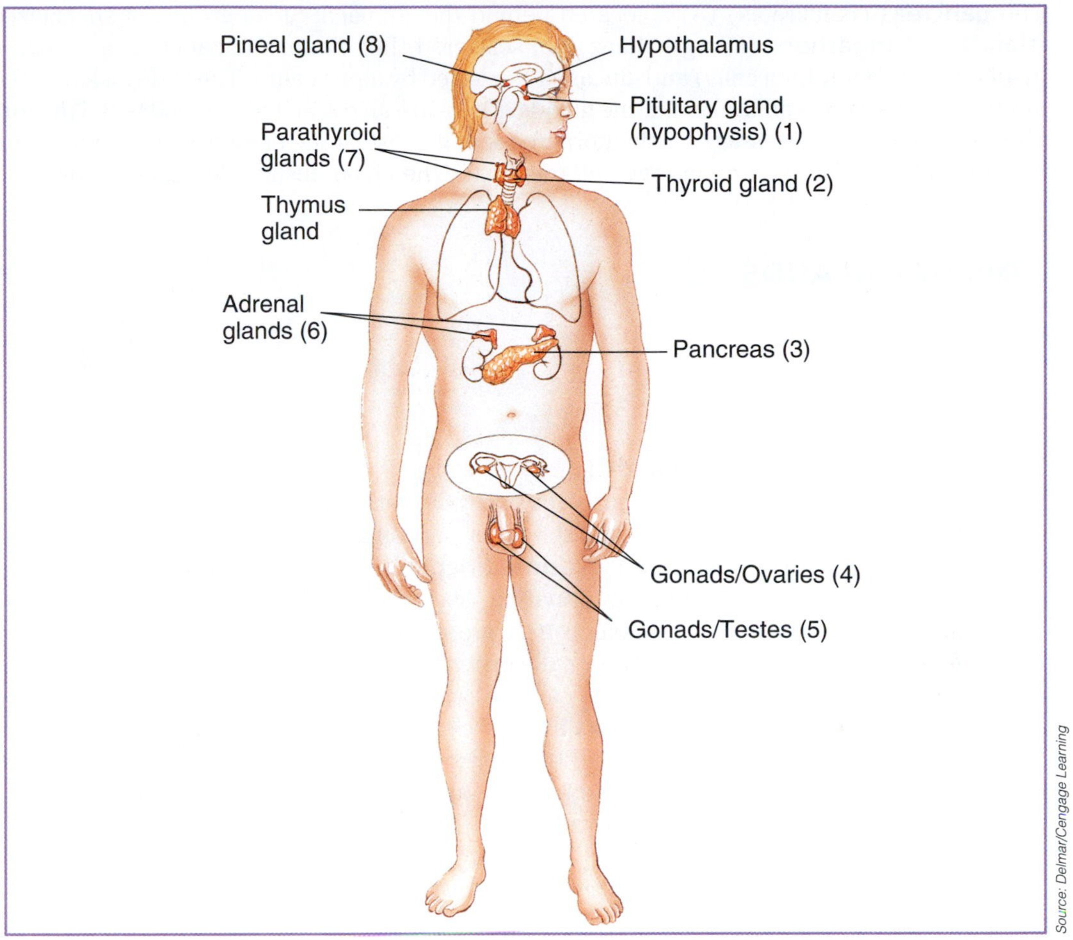

FIGURE 19-1
Endocrine System

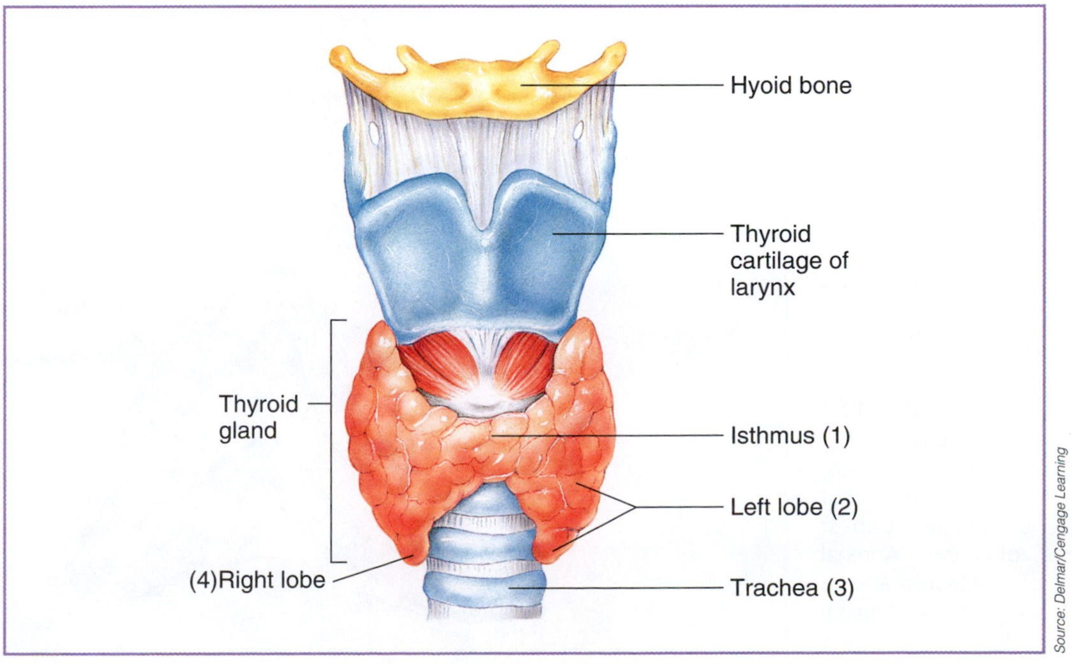

FIGURE 19-2
Thyroid Gland

The **pancreas** (păn'krē-ăs) (3) is located behind the stomach. Small groups of specialized cells called **islets** or **islands of Langerhans** (lăhng'er-hănz) are scattered throughout the pancreas and manufacture the hormones insulin (secreted by beta cells) and glucagon (secreted by alpha cells). These tiny islands of insulin-producing cells are the best hidden of all the endocrine glands. There are an estimated 250,000 to 2.5 million of these islands in the pancreas. Insulin is necessary for the normal use of glucose in the body tissues. If not enough insulin is produced, sugar is not transformed into energy and remains in the blood. Insulin deficiency causes diabetes mellitus.

ADRENAL GLANDS

adrenal/o	adrenal gland	adren/o	adrenal gland

The two **adrenal** (ah-drē'năl) **glands** (1) (see Figure 19-3) (also called simply the adrenals) are located above each kidney (2). The glands each consist of two different parts, each part acting as a separate gland. The inner area is the medulla (mĕ-dul'ah) (4), and the outer portion is the cortex (3). Hormones from the medulla are **epinephrine** (ĕp"ĭ-nĕf'rĭn) (adrenaline) and **norepinephrine** (nor"ĕp-ĭ-nĕf'rĭn) (noradrenaline). These are helpful when the body responds to emergency situations and in maintaining blood pressure.

The hormones from the adrenal cortex are called **steroids** (stē'roids) and have three main functions. **Aldosterone** (ăl'dŏs'-tĕr-ōn") controls reabsorption of sodium in the kidney tubules and excretion of potassium. **Cortisol** (kor'tĭ-sŏl) maintains the carbohydrate reserve of the body and helps the body respond to stress. **Androgens**, **estrogens**, and **progestins** influence secondary sexual characteristics.

At least 26 hormones are produced by the adrenal glands. The production of these hormones is stimulated by ACTH from the pituitary gland. Adrenal hormones are essential to life because they aid the body in adapting itself to the constant changes in the environment.

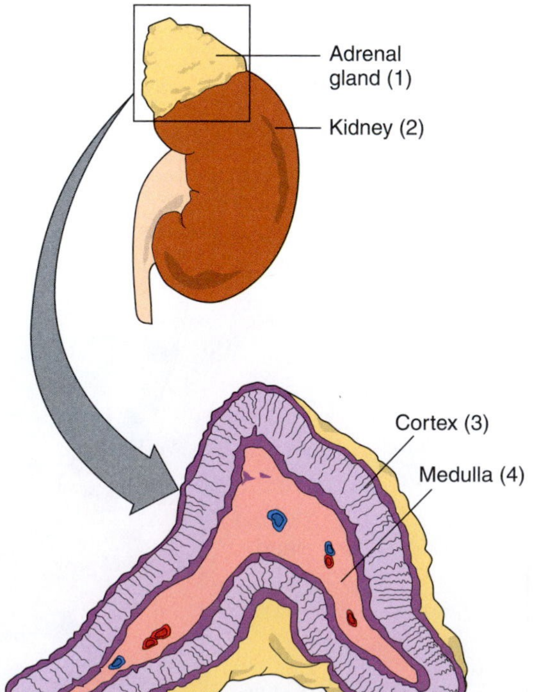

FIGURE 19-3 The Adrenal or Suprarenal Glands, Found on Top of Each Kidney, Consist of an Inner Adrenal Medulla and an Outer Adrenal Cortex

GONADS

The sex glands in males and females are **gonads** (gō'năds) (5 and 4). Hormones produced by the sex glands are important in the development of sexual characteristics and in their maintenance once full development has been attained. Testosterone is the hormone produced by the male sex glands. The female hormone is estrogen. Another hormone is produced by the female sex glands to prepare the uterus for pregnancy and to maintain the pregnancy; it is called progesterone. These glands and their function were described in greater detail in Chapter 16.

PINEAL GLAND

The **pineal** (pĭn'ē-ăl) **gland** (see Figure 19-4) lies above the roof of the third ventricle of the brain, to which it is attached by the pineal stalk. The pineal gland secretes the hormone **melatonin** (mĕl"ah-tō'nĭn) into the blood. Melatonin is linked to circadian (daily) rhythm and is normally released at night. Melatonin may also affect the development of the ovaries and testes.

StudyWARE™ Connection

Watch an animation and label structures of the **Endocrine System** on your StudyWARE™ CD-ROM.

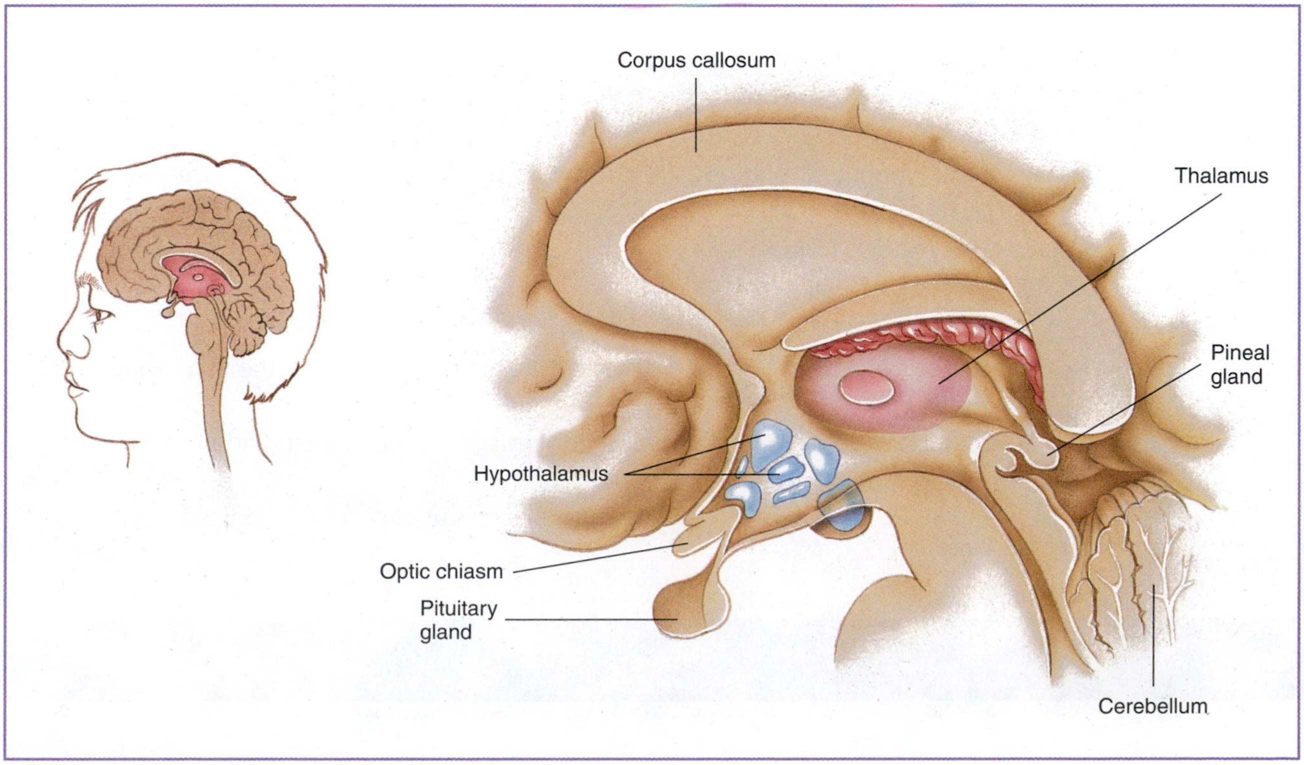

Source: Delmar/Cengage Learning

FIGURE 19-4 The Location of the Pineal Gland

INTERNET ASSIGNMENT

The Hormone Foundation at **www.hormone.org**, an independent organization established by The Endocrine Society (**www.endo-society.org**), is a leading source for consumer information about hormones made available free of charge to the public. It is dedicated to improving the quality of life of patients by promoting the prevention, diagnosis, and treatment of human disease in which hormones play a role.

Endocrinology includes many problems, but diabetes, reproductive endocrinology, growth hormone therapy, thyroid disease, hormone replacement therapy, and osteoporosis are some of the most frequent conditions encountered. To see an index of hormone-related disorders and diseases, click the Fact Sheets button in the list on the left of the Hormone Foundation homepage.

ACTIVITY

Access the Hormone Foundation at **www.hormone.org**. Select one of the conditions listed on the left side of the screen. That will take you to specific links for that condition as well as a list of other useful and related links. Select one of the specific sites, review it, and then visit one of the Useful Links and report on both sites. Submit your report to your instructor.

Review *The Endocrine System*

- Exocrine and endocrine glands produce secretions: exocrine gland secretions pass through ducts to nearby organs; endocrine gland secretions (called hormones) are carried to all parts of the body by the blood and lymph systems.
- The pituitary gland, or hypophysis, is the master gland that regulates the functions of the other endocrine glands.
- The largest gland, the thyroid, secretes hormones that regulate the production of heat and energy in body tissue and maintains normal metabolism.
- The pancreas produces insulin, which transforms glucose into energy for the body.
- The adrenals help the body respond to emergency situations and generally help the body adapt to constant changes in the environment.
- Gonads, the sex glands in males and females, are important in the development and maintenance of sexual characteristics.
- Parathyroid glands regulate the amount of calcium and phosphorus circulating and the amount of calcium retained in storage.

Key Terminology Review

Word	Definition
adrenal glands	two glands each composed of a medulla and a cortex
aldosterone	hormone from the adrenal cortex that controls reabsorption of sodium in kidney tubules and excretion of potassium
androgens	hormones from the testes that influence male characteristics
cortisol	hormone from the adrenal cortex that maintains carbohydrate reserves of the body and helps the body respond to stresses
endocrine glands	ductless glands that produce hormones that are carried to all parts of the body by blood or lymph systems
endocrinologist	physician who is trained to diagnose and treat endocrine disorders
endocrinology	science concerned with the function of glands that secrete hormones into the bloodstream
epinephrine (adrenaline)	hormone produced in the adrenal medulla that helps the body to respond to emergency situations
estrogens	hormones from the adrenal cortex and ovaries that influence secondary female sex characteristics
exocrine glands	glands that produce external secretions that are carried through a duct from glandular cells to a nearby organ or body surface
gland	any organ that produces a secretion
gonads	sex glands in males and females; produce the hormones testosterone in the male and estrogen and progesterone in the female
hypothalamus	part of the diencephalon that contains centers for control of various body functions; produces neurons and neurohormones that act on or are stored by the pituitary gland
islets or islands of Langerhans	small specialized collections of cells in the pancreas that manufacture insulin, glucagon, and other hormones
melatonin	hormone produced by the pineal gland; affects circadian rhythm
norepinephrine (nonadrenaline)	hormone produced in the adrenal medulla that helps the body to respond to emergency situations and maintain blood pressure
pancreas	a large gland that produces insulin, which controls the normal use of glucose in the body
parathyroid glands	four tiny glands that regulate the amount of calcium and phosphorous stored and circulated in the body
pineal gland	gland that secretes melatonin
pituitary gland (hypophysis)	small gland composed of two lobes located in the brain; master gland
progestins	hormones from the adrenal cortex and ovaries that influence secondary sexual characteristics and prepare the uterus for pregnancy
steroids	hormones that are produced in the adrenal cortex
thyroid gland	gland that produces the hormones thyroxine (T_4) and triiodothyronine (T_3)
thyroxine (T_4)	one of two forms of the principal hormone secreted by the thyroid gland that maintains metabolic rate and growth and development of all tissues
triiodothyronine (T_3)	one of two forms of the principal hormone secreted by the thyroid gland that maintains metabolic rate and growth and development of all tissues

Key Terminology Practice Exercises

SELECTION

Select the correct word from the list below to complete each of the following statements.

adrenals gonads pancreas parathyroids pituitary thyroid

1. The ______________ gland is located in the neck just below the larynx.
2. The master gland is the ______________.
3. Calcium is regulated by the ______________.
4. The islets of Langerhans are located in the ______________ and produce insulin and glucagon.
5. The ______________ is composed of two lobes called the adenohypophysis and neurohypophysis.
6. Another name for the sex glands is ______________.
7. The ______________ gland produces thyroxine and triiodothyronine.
8. Two glands made up of two parts called the medulla and cortex are the ______________.
9. GH or HGH, TSH, ACTH, FSH, and LH are produced by the anterior lobe of the ______________.
10. Oxytocin is produced by the hypothalamus and stored in the posterior lobe of the ______________.
11. Estrogen, progesterone, and testosterone are produced by the ______________.
12. Epinephrine and norepinephrine are produced by the medulla of the ______________.
13. Aldosterone and cortisol are produced by the cortex of the ______________.
14. Insulin and glucagons are produced in specialized cells in the ______________.
15. Hypophysis is another name for the ______________ gland.

SHORT ANSWER

Supply a short answer to the following.

1. Explain the overall function of hormones.

____
____
____
____
____

2. State the difference between endocrine and exocrine glands.

____
____
____
____
____

3. Identify the three main functions of the steroids produced by the adrenal cortex.

____
____
____
____
____

MATCHING

Match the terms with their meanings.

1. hormone that affects circadian rhythm
2. hormones produced in the adrenal cortex
3. hormone that controls reabsorption of sodium
4. two organs each composed of a medulla and a cortex
5. any organ that produces a secretion
6. small specialized cells in pancreas that manufacture insulin, glucagons, and other hormones
7. gland that secretes melatonin
8. hormone that prepares the uterus for pregnancy
9. part of diencephalons that contains centers for control of various body functions
10. glands that produce hormones that are carried to all parts of the body by blood or lymph stream
11. glands producing external secretions
12. hormone that regulates production of body heat and energy
13. hormone that maintains carbohydrate reserves of body
14. science concerned with secretions of hormones
15. narrow band connecting the two lobes of the thyroid gland

a. adrenal glands
b. aldosterone
c. cortisol
d. endocrine
e. endocrinology
f. exocrine
g. gland
h. hypothalamus
i. islands of Langerhans
j. isthmus
k. melatonin
l. pineal
m. progestin
n. steroids
o. thyroxine

Word Element Review

Root	Meaning	Example	Definition
adrenal/o, adren/o	adrenal gland	**adrenopathy** (ăd"rĕn-ŏp'ah-thē)	any disease of the adrenal glands (also called adrenalopathy)
duct/o	carry	**ductule** (dŭkt'ūl)	very small duct
ect/o	outside	**ectopic** (ĕk-tŏp'ĭk)	located away from the normal position
gluc/o	sugar	**glucose** (gloo'kōs)	sugar
glyc/o	sugar	**glycosuria** (glī"kō-sū'rē-ah)	presence of glucose in urine (also called glucosuria)
pancreat/o	pancreas	**pancreatitis** (păn'krē-ah-tī'tĭs)	inflammation of the pancreas

continues

Root	Meaning	Example	Definition
parathyroid/o	parathyroid glands	**parathyroidectomy** (păr"ă-thī-royd-ĕk'tō-mē)	excision of one or more of the parathyroid glands
thyr/o, thyroid/o	thyroid gland	**hypothyroidism** (hī"pō-thī'roy-dĭzm)	deficiency of thyroid activity
		hyperthyroidism (hī"per-thī'roy-dĭzm)	excess activity of the thyroid gland
Prefix	**Meaning**	**Example**	**Definition**
crin-	secrete	**crinogenic** (krĭ"nō-jĕn'ĭk)	stimulating secretion
Suffix	**Meaning**	**Example**	**Definition**
-fusion	pour	**transfusion** (trăns-fū'zhŭn)	introduction of blood directly into the bloodstream
		effusion (ĕ-fū'zhŭn)	escape of fluid into a material

Word Element Practice Exercises

WORD ELEMENTS

Provide the correct word element to complete the following words.

1. deficiency of thyroid activity hyp( ) ______________ ism
2. stimulating secretion ______________ genic
3. a very small duct ______________ ule
4. escape of fluid into a material ef ______________
5. presence of glucose in urine ______________ uria
6. any disease of the adrenal glands ______________ opathy
7. excess activity of the thyroid hyp( ) ______________ ism
8. sugar ______________ ose
9. introduction of blood direction into the blood stream trans ______________
10. inflammation of the pancreas ______________ itis
11. located away from the normal position ______________ topic
12. excision of one or more of the parathyroid glands ______________ ectomy

MATCHING

Match the word elements to their meanings.

1. ________ thyroid gland	a. adrenal/o, adren/o
2. ________ sugar	b. crin-
3. ________ secrete	c. duct/o
4. ________ adrenal gland	d. ect/o
5. ________ carry	e. –fusion
6. ________ outside	f. gluc/o, glyc/o
7. ________ pour	g. pancreat/o
8. ________ pancreas	h. parathyroid/o
9. ________ parathyroid glands	i. thyr/o, thyroid/o

SPELLING

Correct the words that are misspelled.

1. ductule ________________
2. gleucose ________________
3. adrenopathy ________________
4. ectoppic ________________
5. glycosuria ________________
6. crynogenic ________________
7. effussion ________________
8. transfusion ________________
9. hyperthyroidism ________________
10. pancretitis ________________

WORD ELEMENT MEANINGS

Give the meaning of each word element. Then use your dictionary to find a new word that contains each of the word elements. Specify whether the new word is a noun or an adjective by placing N or A in the last column.

Word Element	Meaning	Word	N or A
1. adrenal/o	________	________	________
2. adren/o	________	________	________
3. crin-	________	________	________
4. duct/o	________	________	________
5. ect/o	________	________	________
6. -fusion	________	________	________
7. gluc/o	________	________	________
8. glyc/o	________	________	________
9. pancreat/o	________	________	________
10. parathyroid/o	________	________	________
11. thyr/o	________	________	________
12. thyroid/o	________	________	________

DIAGNOSTIC PROCEDURES		
Word	Pronunciation	Definition
General		
exophthalmometry	ĕk"sŏf-thăl-mŏm'ĕ-trē	measures the extent of eyeball protrusion
fine-needle aspiration biopsy		uses a thin needle to remove cells and/or fluid samples for evaluation
needle biopsy		used to remove tissue samples from endocrine glands to establish a diagnosis; often done under CT or ultrasound guidance
thyroid biopsy	thī'royd bī'ŏp-sē	removal of representative tissue for microscopic examination to establish a diagnosis
Nuclear Medicine		
positron emission tomography (PET) scan	pŏz'ĭ-trŏn ē-mĭsh'ŭn tō-mŏg'ră-fē	type of nuclear medicine imaging used to evaluate how well organs and tissues are functioning and to evaluate the extent of cancer
radioactive iodine uptake (RAIU)		measures the uptake of a dose of radioactive iodine by the thyroid gland
radioimmunoassay (RIA)	rā'dē-ō-ĭm"ū-nō-ăs'ā	measures hormone levels in plasma (estrogen, FSH, insulin, and others) by using radioactively labeled molecules
thyroid scintiscan,	thī'royd skĭn'tĭ-skăn	procedure that uses images from radioactive emissions to thyroid scan visualize the size, shape, position, and function of the thyroid gland
X-ray or Radiological Procedures		
adrenal arteriography, adrenal angiography	ă-drē'năl ăr-tĕr-ē-ŏg'ră-fē, ăn"jē-ŏg'ră-fē	procedure where radiopaque contrast is injected into an artery to obtain information about the adrenal gland and arterial system
adrenal vein catheterization	ă-drē'năl vān kăth"ĕ-tĭr-ĭ-zā'shŭn	procedure that uses a catheter inserted through the femoral vein into the adrenal vein to withdraw a blood specimen to detect the function of each adrenal gland
computerized tomography (CT) scan, computerized axial tomography (CAT)	tō-mŏg'ră-fē	procedure that provides a three-dimensional cross-sectional view of tissues in order to define normal or abnormal anatomy; may be done with or without contrast dye
long bone x-rays		series of x-rays of long bones to determine bone growth
Magnetic Imaging		
magnetic resonance imaging (MRI)		procedure that uses magnetic fields to define normal or abnormal anatomy; may be done with or without gadolinium dye
Ultrasonography or Ultrasound Procedures		
ultrasonography (ultrasound)	ŭl"tră-sŏn-ŏg'ră-fē (ŭl'tră-sownd")	uses sound waves to obtain images of the size, shape, and position of glands

continues

DIAGNOSTIC PROCEDURES

Laboratory Tests
The following measurements are made on blood samples to help diagnose and manage endocrine disorders. They are listed by the endocrine gland that produces or regulates them.

Pancreas

- blood glucose, fasting blood sugar (FBS)
- C-peptide level
- glucagon, plasma
- glucose tolerance test (GTT)
- glycosylated hemoglobin (Hb A_{1C} or A_{1C})
- insulin, plasma
- ketones (in diabetic ketoacidosis)
- proinsulin, plasma
- 2-hour postprandial glucose (2hPPG)

Pituitary Gland

- adrenocorticotropic hormone (ACTH), corticotropin
- antidiuretic hormone (ADH), vasopressin
- follicle-stimulating hormone (FSH)
- growth hormone (GH), human growth hormone (HGH), somatotropin
- growth hormone (GH) stimulation test, GH provocation test, insulin tolerance test (ITT), arginine test
- insulinlike growth factor I (IGF-I)
- luteinizing hormone (LH) assay
- prolactin level (PRL)
- thyrotropin-releasing hormone (TRH) test, thyrotropic-releasing factor (TRF) test

Thyroid Gland

- antithyroglobulin antibodies (anti-Tg antibodies)
- antithyroid peroxide antibodies (anti-TPO)
- calcitonin, thyrocalcitonin
- triiodothyronine serum (T_3), triiodothyronine serum free (FT_3, Free T_3)
- thyroglobulin
- thyroid-releasing hormone (TRH) stimulation test
- thyroid-stimulating antibodies
- thyroid-stimulating hormone (TSH), thyrotropin, sensitive TSH, ultrasensitive TSH
- thyroid-stimulating hormone (TSH) stimulation test
- thyroid-stimulating immunoglobulins
- thyroxine (T_4) screen
- thyroxine index free (FTI, FT_4 Index)
- thyroxine serum (T_4), thyroxine serum free (FT_4, Free T_4)

continues

DIAGNOSTIC PROCEDURES

Laboratory Tests *(continued)*

Parathyroid Gland

- parathyroid hormone (PTH), parathormone
- calcium, total/ionized Ca^{++}
- phosphorus

Adrenal Gland

- adrenocorticotropic hormone (ACTH) stimulation test, cortisol stimulation test, cosyntropin test
- corticotrophin
- cortisol
- dehydroepiandrosterone (DHEA)
- dexamethasone suppression test (DST), prolonged/rapid DST, cortisol suppression test, ACTH suppression test
- plasma aldosterone to renin ratio (PAC/PRA)
- plasma renin assay, plasma renin activity (PRA)
- progesterone assay (17-hydroxyprogesterone)

Other Blood Tests

- serum thyroglobulin

The following tests are done on urine samples.

- 17-hydroxycorticosteroids (17-OHCS)
- 17-ketosteroids (17-KS)
- aldosterone assay
- calcium
- catecholamines: epinephrine, free catecholamines, metanephrines (fractionates and total), norepinephrine, vanillylmandelic acid (VMA)
- cortisol, free cortisol
- creatinine clearance
- ketones
- potassium
- sodium
- specific gravity

DIAGNOSES

Word	Pronunciation	Definition
General		
multiple endocrine (MEN) or multiple endocrine adenomatosis (MEA)	ĕn'dō-krīn nē"ō-plā'zē-ah ăd"ĕ-nō-mă-tō'sĭs	associated endocrine disorders that neoplasia tend to run in families
Adrenal Glands		
congenital adrenal hyperplasia	kŏn-jĕn'ĭ-tăl ăd-rē'năl hī"pĕr-plā'zē-ah	genetic abnormality causing adrenal glands to produce a distorted pattern of steroid hormones
hypoadrenalism (Addison's disease)	hī"pō-ăd-rē'năl-ĭzm	decreased functioning of the adrenal cortex
hyperadrenalism	hī"pĕr-ăd-rē'năl-ĭzm	oversecretion of hormones; the hormone determines the specific form of the problem
• *Conn's syndrome (primary aldosteronism)*		overproduction of aldosterone
• *Cushing's disease*		hypercortisolemia due to an ACTH-secreting pituitary tumor
• *Cushing's syndrome*		abnormalities due to chronic exposure to excessive cortisol
• *gynecomastia*	jī"nĕ-kō-măs'tēah	excessive breast development in males
• *hirsutism*	hŭr'sūt'ĭzm	presence of an adult male pattern of hair distribution in women
• *precocious puberty*	prē-ko'shŭs pū'bĕr-tē	early development of secondary sex characteristics in children
• *virilism*	vĭr'ĭl-ĭzm	development of male secondary sex characteristics in a female
pheochromocytoma	fē-ō-krō"mō-sī-tō'mah	tumor of the adrenal medulla that secretes catech-lamines
Pancreas		
diabetes mellitus	dī-ă-bē'tēz mĕ-lī'tŭs	inability to oxidize and utilize carbohydrates because of a lack of insulin secretion or insulin resistance
• *Type 1 (IDDM)*		insulin-dependent
• *Type 2 (NIDDM)*		noninsulin-dependent
• *secondary diabetes*		diabetes secondary to medicines or other conditions such as gestational diabetes as a result of a pregnancy
diabetic ketoacidosis (DKA)	dī-ă-bĕt'ĭk kē"tō-ă"sĭ-dō'sĭs	acute complication of Type1 diabetes
diabetic nephropathy	nĕ-frŏp'ă-thē	secondary complication of diabetes; renal insufficiency

continues

DIAGNOSES		
Word	**Pronunciation**	**Definition**
Pancreas *(continued)*		
diabetic retinopathy	rĕt"ĭ-nŏp'ă-thē	secondary complication of diabetes that can result in visual loss and blindness
hypoglycemia	hī"pō-glī-sē'mē-ah	low blood sugar that may be the result of excessive insulin production by the islet cells or excessive diabetic treatment
hyperglycemic-hyperosmolar coma (syndrome) or non-ketotic hyperglycemic hyperosmolar coma (syndrome) (NKHHC)	hī"pĕr-glī-sē'mē-ĭk hī"pĕr-ŏz'mō-lăr nŏn-kē-tō'tĭk	condition that occurs when there is insufficient insulin to prevent hyperglycemia
hyperinsulinism	hī"pĕr-ĭn'sū-lĭn-ĭzm	excess secretion of insulin causing hypoglycemia
impaired glucose tolerance		abnormally high glucose level after carbohydrate ingestion
metabolic syndrome (syndrome X)		syndrome which includes insulin resistance (along with three other interrelated atherosclerotic risk factors: hypertension, hyperlipidemia, and obesity)
pancreatic cancer	păn"krē-ăt'ĭk	life-threatening primary malignant neoplasm of the pancreas
pancreatitis	păn"krē-ă-tī'tĭs	acute or chronic inflammation of the pancreas
prediabetes	prē-dī"ă-bē'tēz	insulin resistance leading to elevated blood sugars between the normal and diabetic ranges; diabetes often develops in the future
Parathyroid		
hyperparathyroidism	hī"per-păr"ah-thī'royd-ĭzm	excessive production of the parathyroid hormone, resulting in hypercalcemia and osteoporosis
hypoparathyroidism	hī"pō-păr"ah-thī'royd-ĭzm	underactivity of the parathyroid gland, which may result in hypocalcemia
Pituitary		
acromegaly	ăk"rō-mĕg'ah-lē	disorder characterized by enlargement of facial and extremity bones; caused by excessive growth hormone secretion in adults
diabetes insipidus	ĭn-sĭp'ĭ-dŭs	congenital disorder resulting from insufficient secretion of the antidiuretic hormone (ADH) from the posterior pituitary gland; should not be confused with diabetes mellitus
dwarfism		disorder characterized by extreme shortness of stature; caused by growth hormone deficiency
gigantism	jī-găn'tĭzm	disorder resulting in excessive size and stature; caused by excessive secretion of growth hormone during childhood or adolescence

continues

DIAGNOSES		
Word	**Pronunciation**	**Definition**
Pituitary *(continued)*		
hypopituitarism	hī"pō-pĭ-tū'ĭ-tă-rĭzm	disorder resulting from a deficiency of anterior pituitary hormones
panhypopituitarism	păn-hī"pŏ-pĭ-tū'ĭ-tăr-ĭzm	disorder resulting from the deficiency of all pituitary hormones
pituitary incidentaloma	ĭn"sĭ-den"tă-lō'mă	nonfunctioning pituitary tumor discovered by chance
syndrome of inappropriate ADH secretion (SIADH)		disorder caused by excessive secretion of the antidiuretic hormone, resulting in excess water retention in the body and low serum sodium
Reproductive Gland Diseases		
erectile dysfunction		may be caused by testosterone deficiency
hypergonadism	hī"pĕr-gō'năd-ĭzm	increased sex hormone production
hypogonadism	hī"pō-gō'năd-ĭzm	decreased sex hormone production
Thyroid		
euthyroid sick syndrome	ū-thī'royd	syndrome where abnormal thyroid function tests occur in patients with severe nonthyroid illness
goiter (endemic, colloid, nodular, adenomatous, Hashimoto's, simple)	goi'tĕr	enlargement of the thyroid gland (see Figure 19-5)
Hashimoto's thyroiditis (autoimmune or chronic lymphocytic thyroiditis)	hăsh"ĭ-mō'tōz thī"royd-ī'tĭs	chronic inflammation of the thyroid; often a cause of hypothyroidism
Hürthle cell tumor	hĕr'tĕl	benign or malignant thyroid tumor
hyperthyroidism (Graves' disease)	hī"pĕr-thī"roy-dĭzm	overactivity of the thyroid gland; also called *thyrotoxicosis* (thī"rō-tŏks"ĭ-kō'sĭs); the crisis state of Graves' disease

continues

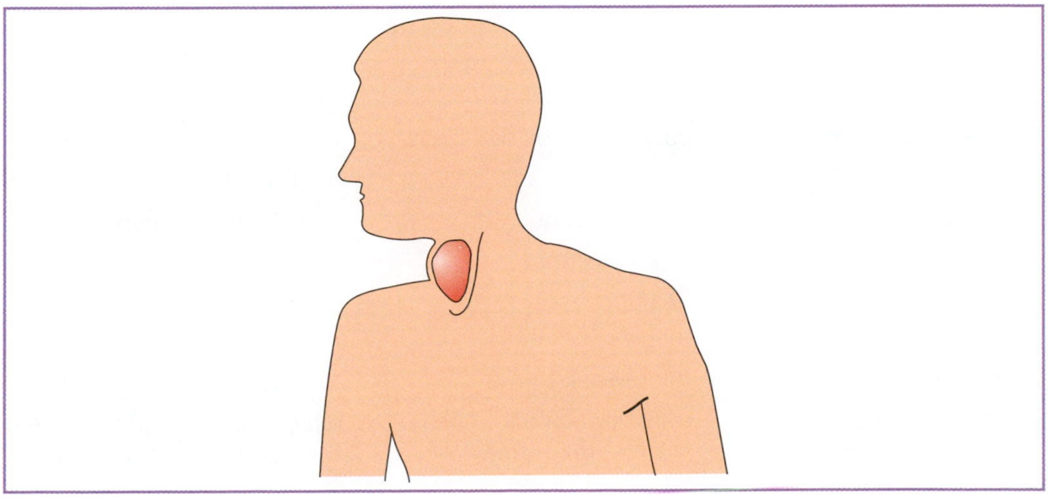

FIGURE 19-5
Goiter

DIAGNOSES		
Word	**Pronunciation**	**Definition**
hypothyroidism	hī"pō-thī'roy-dĭzm	underactivity of the thyroid gland
• *myxedema*	mĭks-ĕ-dē'mah	severe form of hypothyroidism
• *cretinism*	krē'tĭn-ĭzm	form of hypothyroidism found in youngsters
iodine-induced hyperthyroidism (Jod-Basedow phenomenon)		overactivity of the thyroid gland caused by excessive iodine intake
thyroid cancer		type of cancer; common varieties are papillary, follicular, and medullary
thyroid storm (thyrotoxic crisis)		rare but often life-threatening medical situation induced by excessive release of thyroid hormones in individuals with thyrotoxicosis
thyroiditis	thī-roy-dī'tĭs	inflammation of the thyroid gland, acute, subacute (de Quervain's) or chronic
thyrotoxicosis	thī"rō-tŏks"ĭ-kō'sĭs	acute overactivity of the thyroid gland resulting in excessive thyroid hormone; may be fatal

TREATMENT PROCEDURES		
Word	**Pronunciation**	**Definition**
adrenalectomy	ah-drē"năl-ĕk'tō-mē	surgical removal of the adrenal gland
CyberKnife system		noninvasive, frameless stereotactic radiosurgery system for use anywhere in the body
gamma knife		stereotactic radiosurgical device used in brain surgery
linear accelerator (LINAC)		stereotactic radiosurgical device targeting the brain (and other areas) with cancer-destroying x-rays
oophorectomy	ō"ŏf-ō-rĕk'tō-mē	surgical removal of the female gonads
orchiectomy	or"kē-ĕk'tō-mē	surgical removal of the male gonads
pancreas transplantation		surgical procedure performed primarily on patients with Type 1 diabetes who also need kidney or other organ transplants
pancreatectomy	păn"krē-ah-tĕk'tō-mē	surgical removal of the pancreas
parathyroidectomy	par"ah-thi"roy-dek'tō-me	total or partial removal of the parathyroid glands
pituitary irradiation		method of treating pituitary tumors
radioiodine	rā"dē-ō-ī'ō-dīn	uses ^{131}I to treat hyperthyroidism and thyroid cancer
stereotactic radiosurgery (SRS)	stĕr"ē-ō-tăk'tĭk rā"dē-ō-sŭr'jĕr-ē	method of delivering radiation therapy to a small lesion
thymectomy	thī-mĕk'tō-mē	surgical removal of the thymus
thyroidectomy	thī"roy-dĕk'tō-mē	total or partial removal of the thyroid gland
transsphenoidal hypophysectomy	trăns"sfē-noi'dăl hī-pŏf"ĭ-sĕk'tō-mē	removal of all or part of the pituitary gland through the sphenoid sinus

MEDICATIONS PRESCRIBED	
Trade Name	**Generic Name**
Adrenal	
Acthar	corticotropin
Aldactone	spironolactone
Cortrosyn	cosyntropin (synthetic corticotropin)
Adrenocortical Steroids	
Aristocort, Kenalog	triamcinolone acetonide
Celestone	betamethasone
Cortef, Solu-cortef, Hydrocortone	hydrocortisone
Decadron	dexamethasone
Deltasone, Orasone	prednisone
Florinef	fludrocortisone
Medrol, Solu-Medrol	methylprednisolone
Pediapred, Prelone, Orapred	rednisolone
Androgens	
Halotestin	fluoxymesterone
Diabetes	
Actos	pioglitazone
Amaryl	glimepiride
Avandia	rosiglitazone
Byetta	exenatide
DiaBeta, Micronase, Glynase	glyburide
Diabinese	chlorpropamide
Glucagon, GlucaGen	glucagon
Glucophage	metformin
Glucotrol	glipizide
Glucovance	glyburide/metformin hydrochloride
Glyset	miglitol
Januvia	sitagliptin
Orinase	tolbutamide
Prandin	repaglinide
Precose	acarbose
Starlix	nateglinide
Tolinase	tolazamide
Insulins	
Humalog	insulin lispro
Humulin (L, N, R, U)	human insulin

continues

MEDICATIONS PRESCRIBED	
Trade Name	Generic Name
Insulins *(continued)*	
Lantus	insulin glargine
Novolin (N, L or R)	human insulin
Novolog	insulin aspart
Pituitary Hormones	
Growth Hormones	
• Genotropin, Humatrope, Nutropin, Norditropin	somatropin
Antidiuretic Hormones	
• DDAVP, Desmopressin AC, Stimate	desmopressin acetate
• Pitressin	vasopressin
Labor Inducers	
• Ergotrate	ergonovine
• Methergine	methylergonovine
• Pitocin	oxytocin
Uterine Relaxants	
• Yutopar	ritodrine
Other	
• Parlodel bromocriptine mesylate	
• Sandostatin octreotide acetate	
Thyroid	
Armour Thyroid	desiccated thyroid, thyroid extract
Cytomel	liothyronine sodium
Levothroid, Synthroid, Levoxyl	levothyroxine sodium
Lugol's Solution	iodine and potassium iodide
P.T.U.	propylthiouracil
S.S.K.I.	potassium iodide saturated solution
Tapazole	methimazole
Thyrogen	thyrotropin alfa
Thyrolar	liotrix
Treatment of Hyperlipidemia	
Atromid-S	clofibrate
Colestid	colestipol
Crestor	rosuvastatin
Lescol	fluvastatin
Lipitor	atorvastatin
Lopid	gemfibrozil

continues

MEDICATIONS PRESCRIBED	
Trade Name	**Generic Name**
Treatment of Hyperlipidemia *(continued)*	
Lorelco	probucol
Mevacor	lovastatin
Niaspan, Nicobid, Slo-Niacin, Nicolar	nicotinic acid
Pravachol	pravastatin sodium
Questran, Prevalite	cholestyramine
Tricor	fenofibrate
Welchol	colesevelam
Zeita	ezetimibe
Zocor	simvastatin
Treatment of Osteoporosis	
Actonel	risedronate sodium
Boniva	ibandronate
Calciferol	ergocalciferol
Caltrate, OSCal	oyster shell calcium
Citracal	calcium citrate
Climera, Estrace, Estraderm, Vivelle	estradiol
Evista	raloxifene hydrochloride
Fosamax	alendronate
Forteo	teriparatide
Dht	dihydrotachysterol
Miacalcin Nasal Spray	calcitonin salmon
Ogen, Ortho-Est	estropipate
Premarin, Cenestin	conjugated estrogens
Prempro, Premphase	conjugated estrogen *and* medroxyprogesterone
Reclast	zoledronic acid
Rocaltrol	calcitrol

ABBREVIATIONS	
17-KS	17-ketosteroids
17-OHCS	17-hydroxycorticosteroids
2hPPG	2-hour postprandial glucose
ACTH	adrenocorticotropic hormone
ADH	antidiuretic hormone
anti-TPO	thyroid peroxide antibodies
CRH	corticotropin-releasing hormone

continues

ABBREVIATIONS	
DHEA	dehydroepiandrosterone
DI	diabetes insipidus
DM	diabetes mellitus
DST	dexamethasone suppression test
FBS	fasting blood sugar
FSH	follicle-stimulating hormone
FT_3, Free T_3	free triiodothyronine serum
FT_I, FT_4 Index	free thyroxine index
FT_4, Free T_4	free thyroxine serum
GH	growth hormone
GnRH	gonadotropin-releasing hormone
GTT	glucose tolerance test
Hb A_{1C}. A_{1C}	glycosylated hemoglobin
HGH	human growth hormone
IDDM	insulin-dependent diabetes mellitus
IGF-I	insulin-like growth factor I
ITT	insulin tolerance test
K	potassium
LH	luteinizing hormone
LHRH	luteinizing hormone-releasing hormone
MEA	multiple endocrine adenomatosis
MEN	multiple endocrine neoplasia
MSH	melanocyte-stimulating hormone
Na	sodium
NIDDM	noninsulin-dependent diabetes mellitus, Type II DM
NKHHC	nonketotic hyperglycemia-hyperosmolar coma (syndrome)
OCT	oxytocin challenge test
PRA	plasma renin activity
PRL	prolactin level
PTH	parathyroid hormone
RAIU	radioactive iodine uptake
RIA	radioimmunoassay
SRS	stereotactoc radiosurgery
T_3	triiodothyronine
T_4	thyroxine
TBG	thyroid-binding globulin
TFT	thyroid function test
TRF	thyrotropic-releasing factor
TRH	thyrotropin-releasing hormone
TSH	thyroid-stimulating hormone
VMA	vanillylmandelic acid

Working Practice Review Exercises

IDENTIFICATION

Identify the following procedures, diagnoses, and treatments.

1. measures the uptake of a dose of iodine by the thyroid gland ____________
2. measures the extent of eyeball protrusion ____________
3. measures hormone levels in plasma by using radioactively labeled molecules ____________
4. removal of all or part of the pituitary gland through the sphenoid sinus ____________
5. surgical removal of male gonads ____________
6. total or partial removal of parathyroid glands ____________
7. surgical removal of the thymus ____________
8. partial or total removal of the thyroid gland ____________
9. form of hypothyroidism found in youngsters ____________
10. congenital disorder resulting from insufficient secretions of antidiuretic hormone ____________
11. surgical removal of the pancreas ____________
12. overactivity of thyroid gland caused by excessive iodine intake (Jod-Basedow phenomenon) ____________
13. excessive production of the parathyroid hormone resulting in hypercalcemia and osteoporosis ____________
14. nonfunctioning pituitary tumor discovered by chance ____________
15. associated endocrine disorders that tend to run in families ____________

MATCHING

Match the terms to their meanings.

1. ________ overactivity of the thyroid		a. acromegaly
2. ________ enlargement of the thyroid gland		b. Addison's disease
3. ________ chronic exposure to excessive cortisol		c. Conn's syndrome
4. ________ lack of insulin secretion		d. Cushing's syndrome
5. ________ inflammation of the thyroid gland		e. diabetes mellitus
6. ________ deficiency of all anterior pituitary hormones		f. diabetic ketoacidosis
7. ________ abnormal growth of hair		g. goiter
8. ________ severe underactivity of the thyroid gland		h. hirsutism
9. ________ enlargement of facial and extremity bones		i. hyperthyroidism
10. ________ tumor of the adrenal medulla		j. hypoglycemia
11. ________ acute complication of Type I diabetes		k. myxedema
12. ________ low blood sugar or excessive diabetic treatment		l. panhypopituitarism
13. ________ development of male secondary sex characteristics in a female		m. pheochromocytoma
14. ________ overproduction of aldosterone		n. thyroiditis
15. ________ decreased functioning of the adrenal cortex		o. virilism

ABBREVIATIONS

Identify the following abbreviations.

1. ACTH ______
2. FSH ______
3. LH ______
4. ADH ______
5. TSH ______
6. RIA ______
7. T_3 ______
8. T_4 ______
9. DM ______
10. GTT ______

IDENTIFICATION

Indicate which measurements can be collected from a specific endocrine gland.

adrenal pancreas parathyroid pituitary thyroid

1. fasting blood sugar ______
2. thyroglobulin ______
3. prolactin level ______
4. calcium ______
5. plasma rennin assay ______
6. phosphorus ______
7. cortisol ______
8. calcitonin ______
9. follicle-stimulating hormone ______
10. ketones ______

Dictionary Exercises

DICTIONARY EXERCISE 1

Use your dictionary to find the pronunciation and definition of the following words.

	Word	Pronunciation	Definition
1.	metabolism	______	______
2.	tophus	______	______
3.	osmolarity	______	______
4.	osmolality	______	______
5.	aldosteronism	______	______

6. alkalosis	____________	____________
7. hypoplasia	____________	____________
8. thyroglossal duct	____________	____________
9. pressor effect	____________	____________

DICTIONARY EXERCISE 2

Pronunciation of the words below is provided. Using your dictionary, find the correct spelling and definition of each word.

	Word	Pronunciation	Definition
1.	____________	ăs"ĭ-dō'sĭs	____________
2.	____________	ĭk'ter-ŭs	____________
3.	____________	tĕt'ah-nŭē	____________
4.	____________	gloo'kă-gŏn	____________
5.	____________	hĭ"pĕr-plā'zē-ah	____________
6.	____________	kă"tĕ-kŏl-ah-mēns	____________

DICTIONARY EXERCISE 3

Rewrite each sentence in your own words. Provide the pronunciation for each italicized word.

1. One of the patient's problems was *polyphagia* (____________).

   ____

2. The diagnosis included *thymoma* (____________).

   ____

3. She reported *polydipsia* (____________).

   ____

4. Blood tests revealed *hyperuricemia* (____________).

   ____

StudyWARE™ Connection

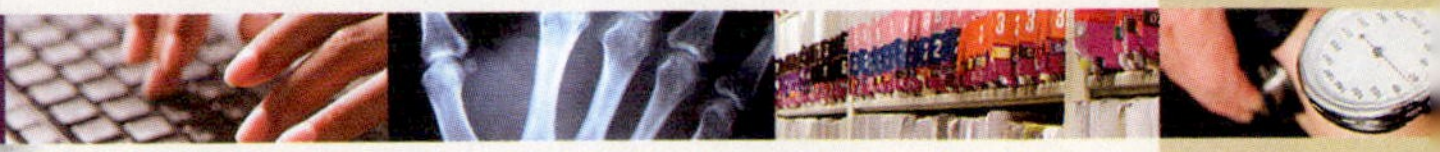

Take a practice quiz and play interactive games that reinforce the content in this chapter on your StudyWARE™ CD-ROM

Listening Exercise

INSTRUCTIONS

1. Review the spelling, pronunciation, and meaning of the words provided in the preview.
2. Go to your StudyWARE™ CD-ROM and listen to **Listening Exercise 19-1**. Fill in the blank in the report as the word is dictated.
3. At the end of the activity, check your spelling against the preview words. They appear in the preview in the order in which they are encountered in the activity.
4. Review and practice the words you missed.
5. Look up words that are not familiar.

PREVIEW OF WORDS FOR LISTENING EXERCISE 19-1

Word	Pronunciation	Meaning
hyperparathyroidism	hī"pĕr-păr"ă-thī'roy-dĭzm	excessive production of the parathyroid hormone, resulting in hypercalcemia
hypercalcemia	hī"pĕr-kăl-sē'mē-ah	excessive amount of calcium in the blood
triglycerides	trī-glĭs'ĕr-īds	combination of glycerol with three of five different fatty acids
hypertrophy	hī-pĕr'trō-fē	increase in the size of a body part that does not involve tumor formation
xerosis	zē-rō'sĭs	abnormal dryness of skin
hyperglycemia	hī"pĕr-glī-sē'mē-ah	increase of blood sugar

StudyWARE™ Connection

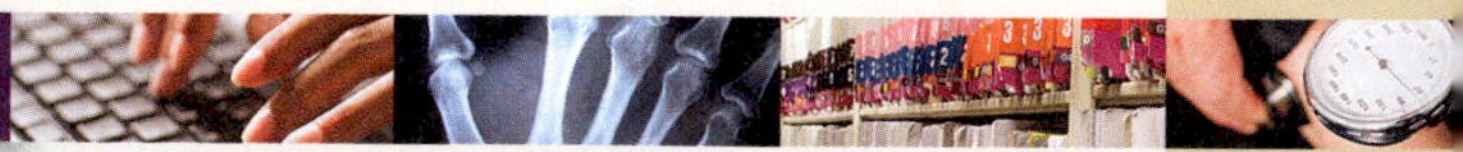

Listen to the report on the next page being read on your StudyWARE™ CD-ROM. Fill in each blank as the word is dictated.

Listening Exercise 19-1

Discharge Summary

DISCHARGE SUMMARY

ADMITTED: 6/12/20— DISCHARGED: 6/17/20—

CONSULTATIONS: Dr. Andres SanMiguel, cataract surgery

Dr. Herman Brunner, dermatology

SURGICAL PROCEDURES: Intracapsular cataract extraction of the left eye with peripheral iridectomy.

ADMITTING DIAGNOSIS: Rule out ______________________.

HISTORY: This 55-year-old woman exhibited symptoms of endocrine disturbance and other health problems during her office visit and consequently was admitted for further testing. A complete history and physical is in the patient's record.

LABORATORY DATA: Uric acid excretion was 296 mg/24 hours (normal from 400 to 800), calcium 61 mg/24 hours (30 to 150), phosphorus 278 mg/24 hours (340 to 1,000).

SMA–12 showed these abnormalities: at ______________________ 11.4, hyperglycemia at 112, hyperuricemia at 8.4, and total protein 8.2 with an albumin of 4.6. Several calcium determinations were elevated. Fasting glucose was 110.

Fasting cholesterol was 291 mg%, and ______________________ were 152. Elevated parathyroid hormone levels have been found × 2 in the past when compared with calcium levels.

Hand x-rays showed degenerative arthritis. Chest, spine, and skull x-rays were normal. Electrocardiogram showed a possible left ventricular ______________________.

HOSPITAL COURSE: The patient was admitted at 182½ lb. and discharged at 178 lb. She was seen in consultation with Dr. Andres SanMiguel for cataract surgery and Dr. Herman Brunner, dermatologist. She was placed on a low-calcium diet and tolerated the above tests and procedures very well.

DISCHARGE DISPOSITION AND PLAN: Patient was improved at discharge. Instructions were to follow up with Dr. SanMiguel for her eyes, with me at the office in four to six weeks, and with Dr. Brunner in six to eight weeks. For her ______________________, she was given a dermatological ointment. She should follow a low-sodium, low-calcium diet for weight reduction.

DISCHARGE DIAGNOSES:

1. Hypercalcemia, probably primary hyperparathyroidism.
2. Intracapsular cataract, left eye.
3. Hypertension.
4. Hyperuricemia.
5. ____________.
6. Xerosis.
7. Seborrheic dermatitis of the scalp.

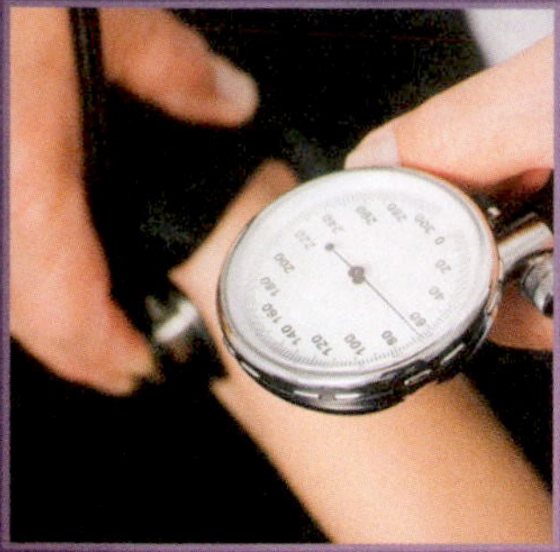
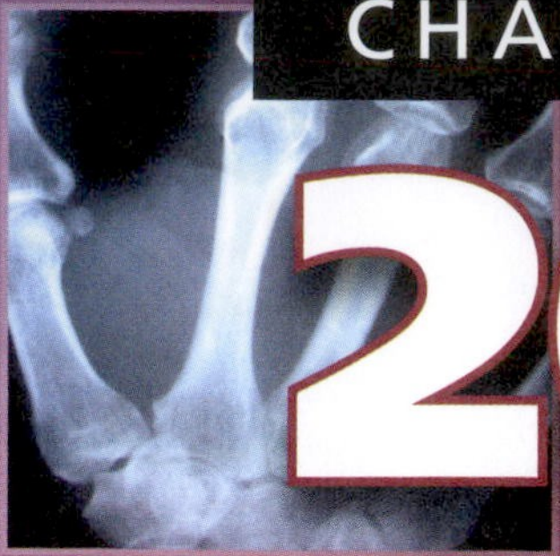

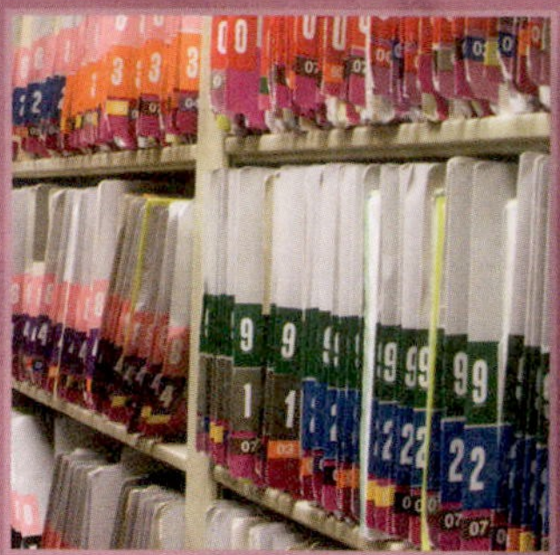

CHAPTER

20

The Nervous System

"The human brain is a world consisting of explored continents and great stretches of unknown territory."

—Santiago Ramón y Cajal

OBJECTIVES

When you have completed this chapter on the nervous system, you should be able to

1. Spell and define major system components and explain how they operate.
2. Identify the meanings of related word elements.
3. Spell and define diagnostic procedures, diagnoses, treatment procedures, and abbreviations.
4. Spell the names of commonly used medications.
5. Use a dictionary as a tool in processing medical documents.
6. Hear how medical terminology is used in actual medical reports.

INTRODUCTION

The nervous system can most readily be described as the body's communication network. From the moment we are born to the moment we die, our every thought, emotion, movement, and impression is controlled by this communication network. Specialized communication cells create a network so intricate that nothing in the world can approach its complexity. A physician who specializes in the study of the nervous system is a **neurologist** (nū-rŏl'ō-jĭst). A surgeon who specializes in the surgical treatment of diseases of the nervous system is called a **neurosurgeon** (nū"-rō-sŭr'jŭn).

COMPONENTS OF THE NERVOUS SYSTEM

neur/o	nerve, nervous system

The entire nervous system is composed of tissue made up of neurons interspersed with **neuroglia** (nū-rŏg'lē-ah), which are the supportive and connective cells of the nervous system. The basic unit of the nervous system, the **neuron** (nū'rŏn), is illustrated in Figure 20-1. It has the appearance of a drop of liquid that has splattered on the floor. The length of a neuron can be anywhere from a fraction of an inch to three or four feet, depending on its location.

The large part of the cell is referred to as the **cell body** (3), which is made up of cytoplasm and the nucleus. The **nucleus** (2) is the central controlling structure essential to the cell's life. Spraying out from the cell body are short, threadlike receptive fibers called **dendrites** (dĕn'drīts) (1). An **axon** (ăk'sŏn) (4), a long, straight fiber ending in a brushlike tip, conducts impulses away from the cell body. Many axons are covered by a sheath of white, fatty material called **myelin** (mī'ĕ-lĭn) (5).

Three general classes of neurons comprise more than 99% of the approximately 12 billion neurons in the nervous system. They are grouped according to their function. **Sensory**, or **afferent** (ăf'ĕr-ĕnt), **neurons** carry signals or directives to the brain and spinal cord. **Motor**, or **efferent** (ĕf'ĕr-ĕnt), **neurons** stimulate the contraction or relaxation of muscles and spur the activity of glands. Finally, **interneurons** shuttle messages back and forth through the central nervous system pathways.

These neurons form a network for communicating messages through the body. For example, an axon transmits a signal to an adjacent neuron across a junction called a **synapse** (sĭn'ăps), where it is received by a dendrite. This transmission of neural impulses is chemical in nature, as there is no direct contact between the axon of one neuron and the dendrites of another.

Injury to neurons may result in temporary or permanent loss of function. If a neuron's nucleus is destroyed, it will not regenerate. On the other hand, if the nerve fiber is cut, it can eventually regrow. If enough related neurons are permanently destroyed, an entire bodily function may be impaired or lost.

The protection of the nervous system is very important because its continued operation is critical to so many body functions. For protection, major portions are located within the skull and the strong, flexible spinal column. Both the brain and spinal cord are also surrounded by cerebrospinal fluid, which acts as a shock absorber. Most of the other nerve trunks are protected by being buried deep in the body.

The parts of the nervous system are grouped according to structure and function: the **central nervous system**, which includes the brain and spinal cord as the two bases of operation; the **peripheral nervous system**, which is made up of cranial and spinal nerves; and the **autonomic** (aw"tō-nŏm'ĭk) nervous system, which applies to activities conducted automatically by certain peripheral nerves. A discussion of each subsystem follows.

StudyWARE™ Connection

Play an interactive game labeling structures of a **Neuron** on your StudyWARE™ CD-ROM.

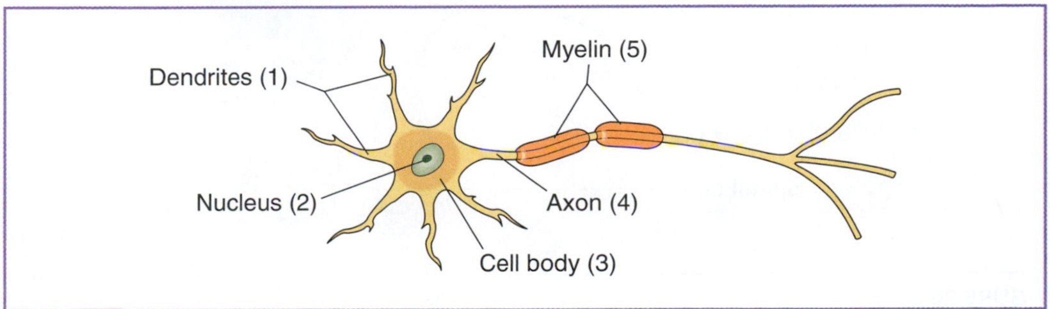

FIGURE 20-1
A Neuron

Source: Delmar/Cengage Learning

CENTRAL NERVOUS SYSTEM

The central nervous system includes the brain and the spinal cord.

cephal/o	head	dur/o	dura mater
cerebell/o	cerebellum	encephal/o	brain
cerebr/o	brain	mening/o	meninges
cornu	horn-shaped	pont/o	pons
crani/o	head, skull	thalam/o	thalamus

THE BRAIN

A physical description of the brain is unimpressive. It is pinkish-gray, furrowed, and weighs about three pounds. An estimated 12 billion nerve cells are present, each potentially linked to countless others.

The brain and its major components are illustrated in Figure 20-2. Both the brain and the spinal cord are covered by membranes called **meninges** (mĕ-nĭn'jĕz) (2). The outer membrane is called the **dura mater** (dū'rah mā'ter) (3), which is tough connective tissue underlain by a web of **arachnoid** (ah-răk'noid) **membrane** (4). The inner membrane follows the convolutions of the brain and is called the **pia mater** (pī'ah mā'ter) (5).

The largest part of the brain is the **cerebrum** (sĕr-ĕ'brŭm) (12). It has an outer surface of gray matter called the **cerebral cortex** (sĕ-rē'brŭl kor'tĕks), which is responsible for the generation of impulses. Figure 20-3 shows the location of some of the centers of the cerebral cortex.

Beneath the cerebral cortex is a white tissue that is responsible for the conduction of messages. As shown in Figure 20-2, the gray cortex is arranged in folds, forming elevated ridges known as **gyri** (jī'rī) or **convolutions** (1). These are separated by depressions or grooves called **sulci** (sŭl'kī) or **fissures**. A deep vertical fissure divides the cerebrum into halves called hemispheres. Other fissures divide each hemisphere into lobes.

Although individual brains vary somewhat, the larger fissures in each hemisphere do remain constant enough to serve as surface landmarks by which each hemisphere can be divided. These lobes are the frontal (13), parietal (16), temporal (14), and occipital (15).

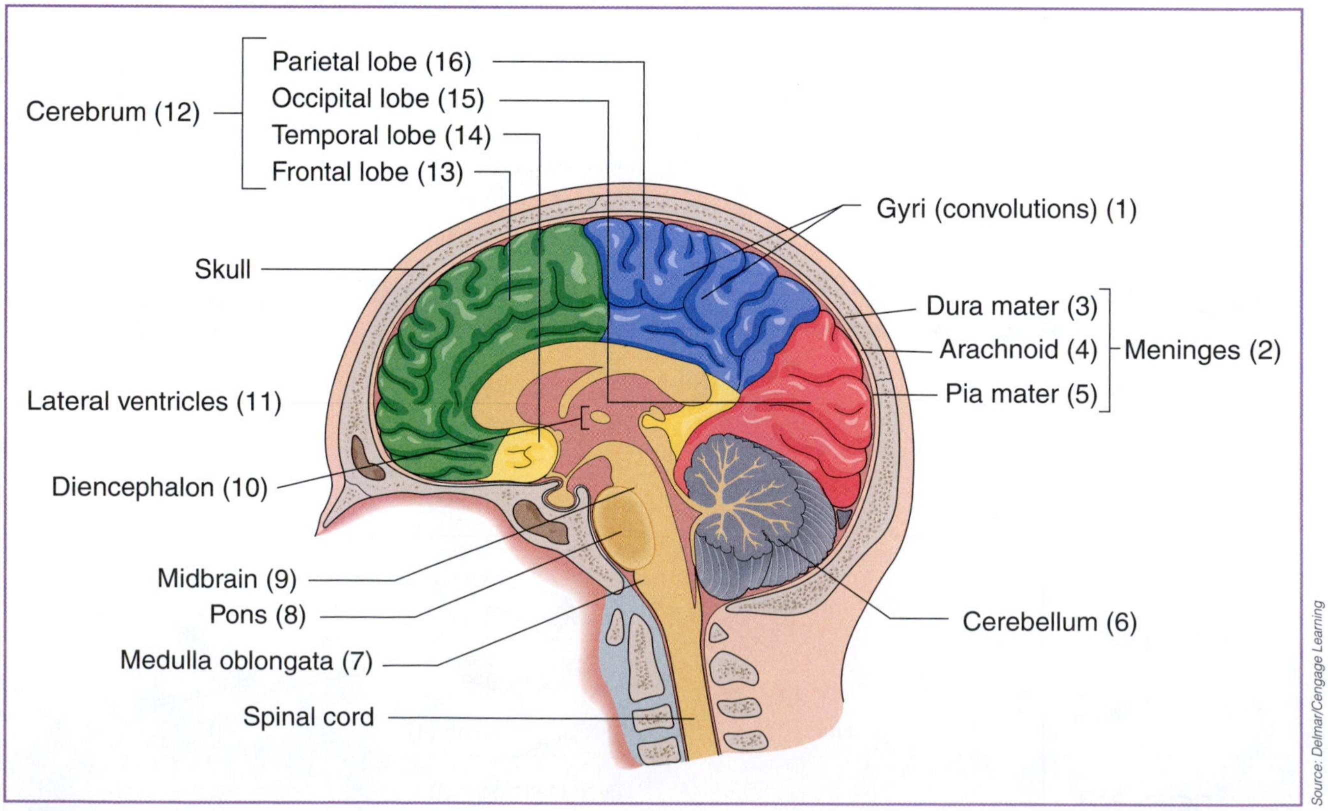

FIGURE 20-2 The Brain

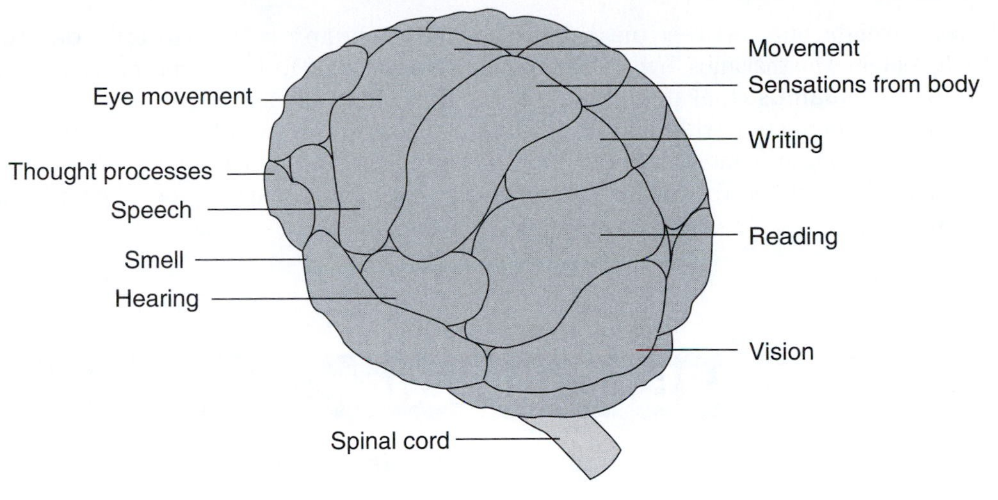

FIGURE 20-3 Centers of the Cerebral Cortex

The **frontal lobe**, also known as the **somatic** (sō-măt'ĭk) **motor area**, controls voluntary muscles. The left side of the frontal lobe governs the right side of the body and the muscles involved in speech. The right side of the frontal lobe governs the left side of the body. The frontal lobe influences personality and is associated with mental activities such as planning, judgment, and conceptualizing.

The **parietal** (pah-rī'ĕ-tăl) **lobe** is the primary sensory area or **somatic sensory area**. It determines distance, size, shape, and taste, as well as the sensory aspects of speech.

The **temporal lobe** contains the auditory center for hearing impulses and determines the sense of smell. It also is involved with memory and learning. Choices about which thoughts to express are made here.

The **occipital** (ŏk-sĭp'ĭ-tăl) **lobe** occupies a small area in the posterior portion of the cerebrum. Vision, one of the special senses, is governed by this lobe.

There are four ventricles, or cavities, in the brain. The two **lateral ventricles** (vĕn'trĭ-k'lz) (11), one located in each hemisphere, are the largest, extending from the frontal portion of the cerebral hemisphere to the posterior lobe. They have a hornlike projection, or **cornu** (kor'nū), that reaches into the frontal, occipital, and temporal lobes.

The third ventricle—the smallest of the four—communicates with the lateral ventricles. The fourth ventricle is the one that communicates with the central canal of the spinal cord and subarachnoid space.

The cerebrospinal fluid is a watery substance contained in the ventricles of the brain. It flows throughout the brain and around the spinal cord, serving to cushion shocks that would otherwise injure delicate organs.

Brainstem

The brainstem is one of the major divisions of the brain and is composed of several parts—the medulla oblongata (7), the pons (8), and the **midbrain** (9). At the upper part of the brainstem above the pons is the midbrain, which connects the lower brain centers to the higher centers, contains optic reflex centers, and serves to correlate optic and tactile (touch) impulses.

The **pons**, or bridge, is located between the midbrain and the medulla oblongata. It contains the nerve tracts from the right and left halves of the cerebellum. These nerve tracts coordinate the muscles on the two sides of the body. The pons also contains four pairs of cranial nerve centers.

The **medulla oblongata** (mĕ-dul'ah ŏb"lŏng-gā'tah) is continuous with the spinal cord and regulates heart action, breathing, and circulation. Nerve fibers establish communication between the higher parts of the brain and the spinal cord. As these nerve fibers pass through this area, some cross over from one side of the spinal cord to the other. Thus the right side of the brain controls the left side of the body, and the left side controls the right side. Eight pairs of cranial nerves are associated with the medulla oblongata.

Cerebellum

The "little brain," or **cerebellum** (sĕr"ĕ-bĕl'ŭm) (6), is the second largest division of the brain. It consists of a central body called the **vermis** (vĕr'mĭs) and two lateral masses called the right and left cerebellar hemispheres. The chief function of the cerebellum is to bring balance, harmony, and coordination to motions of the body started by the cerebrum.

Diencephalon

The section of the brain between the midbrain and the cerebrum is referred to as the **diencephalon** (dī"ĕn-sĕf'ah-lŏn) (10). It contains the thalamus, hypothalamus, and epithalamus. The third ventricle is also located in the diencephalon.

In the **thalamus** (thăl'ah-mŭs), the nerve fibers from the spinal cord and the lower part of the brain provide synaptic connection with neurons leading to the sensory areas of the cerebrum. The **hypothalamus** (hī'pō-thăl'ah-mŭs) contains centers for the control of body temperature, carbohydrate metabolism, fat metabolism, and emotions that affect heartbeat, blood pressure, appetite, and sexual reflexes. The **epithalamus** (ĕp"ĭ-thăl'ah-mŭs) contains the pineal body, which was discussed in Chapter 19.

StudyWARE™ Connection

Play an interactive game labeling structures of the **Nervous System** on your StudyWARE™ CD-ROM.

THE SPINAL CORD

gangli/o	swelling	spondyl/o	vertebra
myel/o	marrow, spinal cord		

Below the medulla oblongata, the nervous system continues as the spinal cord. The cord performs the following two functions.

1. Reflex activities. This involves the translation of a sensory message entering the cord into a motor message as it leaves.
2. Pathway. The spinal cord serves as a pathway for conducting sensory impulses from the sensory nerve upward through the ascending tracts to the brain. It also serves as a pathway for motor impulses to move through the descending tracts from the brain to the nerve that will supply messages to muscles or glands.

Except for the 12 pairs of cranial nerves that connect directly with the brain, all spinal nerves enter or leave the spinal cord through openings in the vertebrae.

The spinal cord, as depicted in Figure 20-4, is divided into four parts: **cervical** (1), **thoracic** (2), **lumbar** (3), and **sacral** (4). It is comprised of an inner core of gray matter and an outer covering of white matter. The gray matter is composed of neuroglia and neuron networks of nerve fibers. The cord is covered with the meninges, the same three layers that cover the brain (dura mater, arachnoid, and pia mater). Injury of the spinal cord in any segment can endanger any or all of its functions.

PERIPHERAL NERVOUS SYSTEM

The peripheral nervous system is composed of spinal nerves and cranial nerves.

THE SPINAL NERVES

The 31 pairs of spinal nerves carry both voluntary and involuntary impulses, and all emerge from the spinal cord. At different levels of the cord, these spinal nerves regulate activities of different parts of the body. Each is named after its corresponding vertebra.

Figure 20-5 illustrates how each nerve is made up of all types of **sensory** (3) and **motor fibers** (4) of both the autonomic and voluntary nervous systems. Each spinal nerve divides into **dorsal** (7) and **ventral roots** (5), which enter the cord at different points.

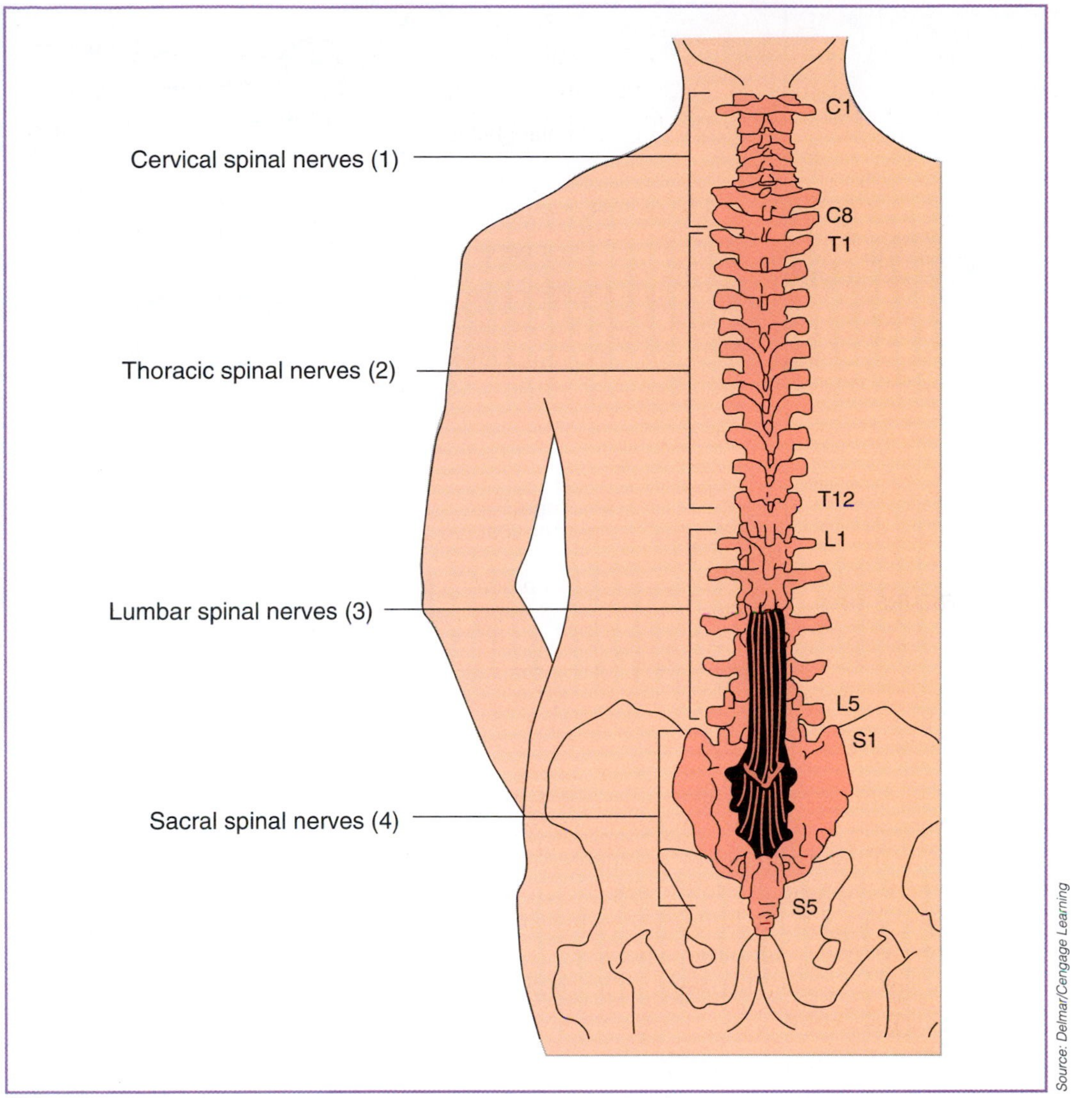

FIGURE 20-4
The Spinal Cord

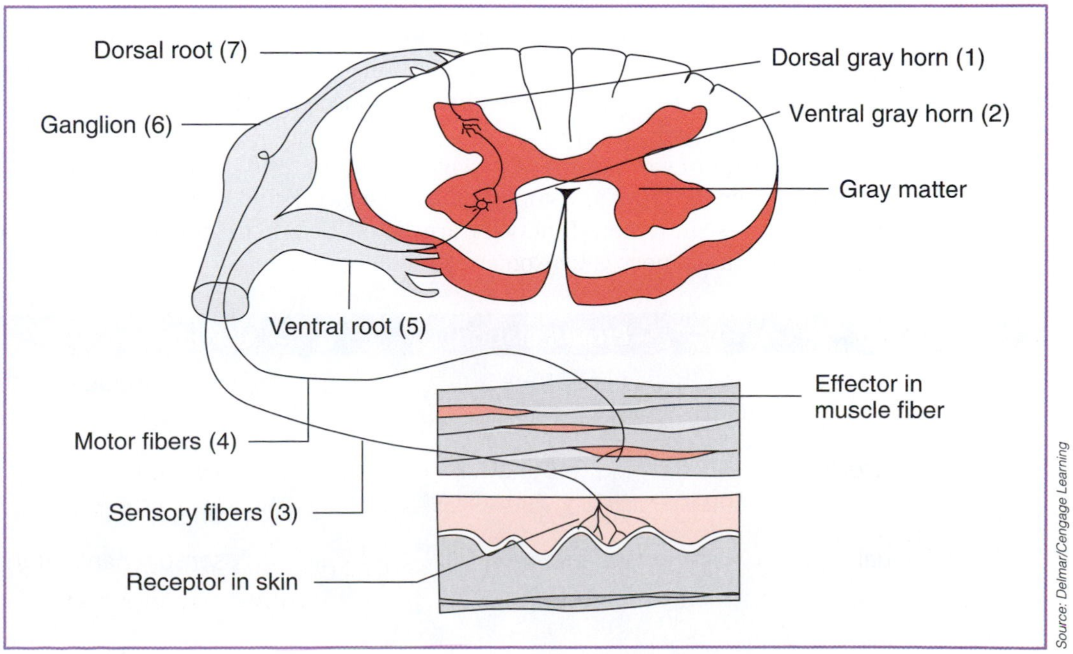

FIGURE 20-5
A Spinal Nerve

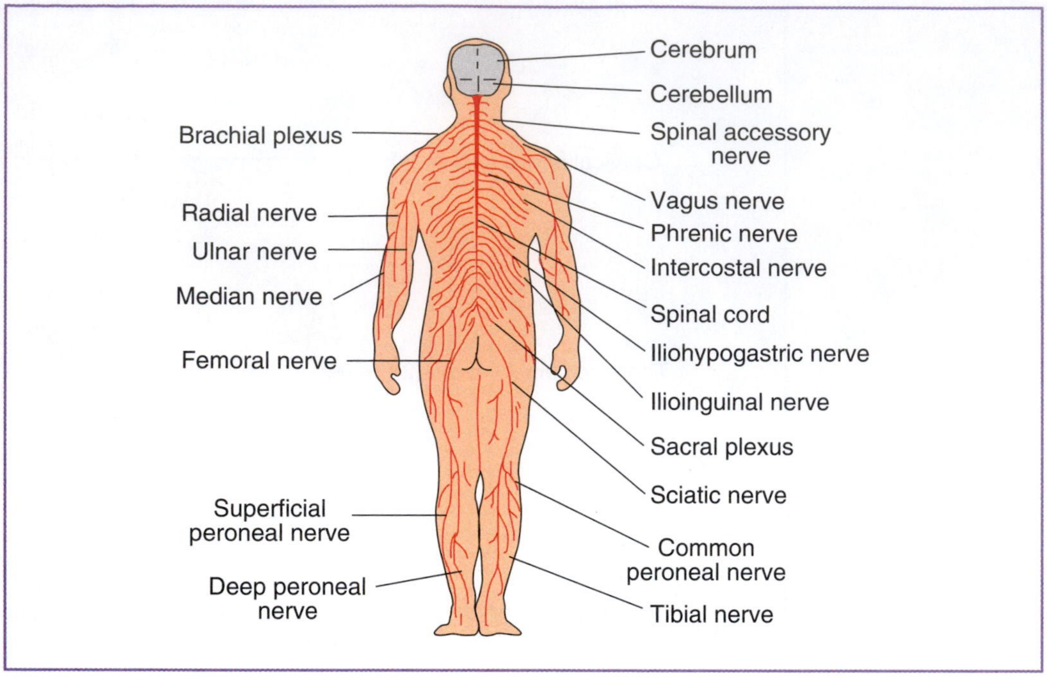

FIGURE 20-6 Peripheral Nervous System

The incoming nerve bulges into a **ganglion** (găng'glē-ŏn) (6) (a cluster of nerve cell bodies), enters the posterior section of the cord, and connects with one of the dorsal gray horns (1) of the H-shaped gray matter of the cord. Outgoing motor fibers connect with the corresponding ventral gray horn (2) at the front of the cord and send a direction or impulse to the effector in the muscle fiber.

In some areas of the body, these fibers form an interlocking network called a **plexus** (plĕk'sŭs), such as the brachial plexus in the shoulder. There is a cervical plexus (in the neck), a sacral plexus, a lumbar plexus, and a coccygeal plexus. As can be seen in Figure 20-6, many nerves are named after bones, organs, or the body regions in which they are located.

THE CRANIAL NERVES

There are 12 pairs of cranial nerves. The first four are located in the front of the brain, the next four are related to the pons, and the last four are attached to the medulla. Ten of these pairs of nerves supply nerve fibers to structures of the head. Of the other two pairs, one extends to muscles in the neck and the other sends branches into the thoracic and abdominal organs.

From a functional point of view, these nerves handle messages of four types: special sense impulses; general sense impulses, such as pain and touch; voluntary muscle control; and involuntary control.

The 12 cranial nerves and their functions are listed below, including their Roman numeral reference. Physicians often refer to cranial nerves by Roman numeral reference.

Nerve	Pronunciation	Function
I olfactory	ŏl-făk'tō-rē	smell impulses to the brain
II optic	ŏp'tĭk	vision
III oculomotor	ŏk"ū-lō-mō'tor	eye muscles and the pupil
IV trochlear	trŏk'lē-ăr	one eyeball muscle on each side
V trigeminal	trī-jĕm'ĭ-năl	sensory nerve of the face and head

continues

Nerve		Pronunciation	Function
VI	abducens	ăb-dū'sĕnz	eyeball muscle
VII	facial	fă'shāl	largely motor to the face
VIII	acoustic	ah-kōōs'tĭk	balance and hearing
IX	glossopharyngeal	glŏs"ō-fah-rĭn'jē-ăl	taste, saliva secretion, swallowing
X	vagus	vā'gŭs	most organs in the thoracic and abdominal cavities
XI	accessory		two muscles of the neck
XII	hypoglossal	hī"pō-glŏs'ăl	muscles of the tongue

AUTONOMIC NERVOUS SYSTEM

The autonomic nervous system automatically controls various involuntary body functions and activities based on feedback from sensory nerves. Some of these are shown in Figure 20-7; they include the action of the glands, the smooth muscles of the hollow organs, and the heart.

This system has two divisions—the sympathetic and parasympathetic—both controlled by the hypothalamus, cerebral cortex, and medulla oblongata.

Essentially, the sympathetic system increases activity, whereas the parasympathetic system decreases activity. For instance, action of the heart would be quickened by the sympathetic system, whereas the parasympathetic

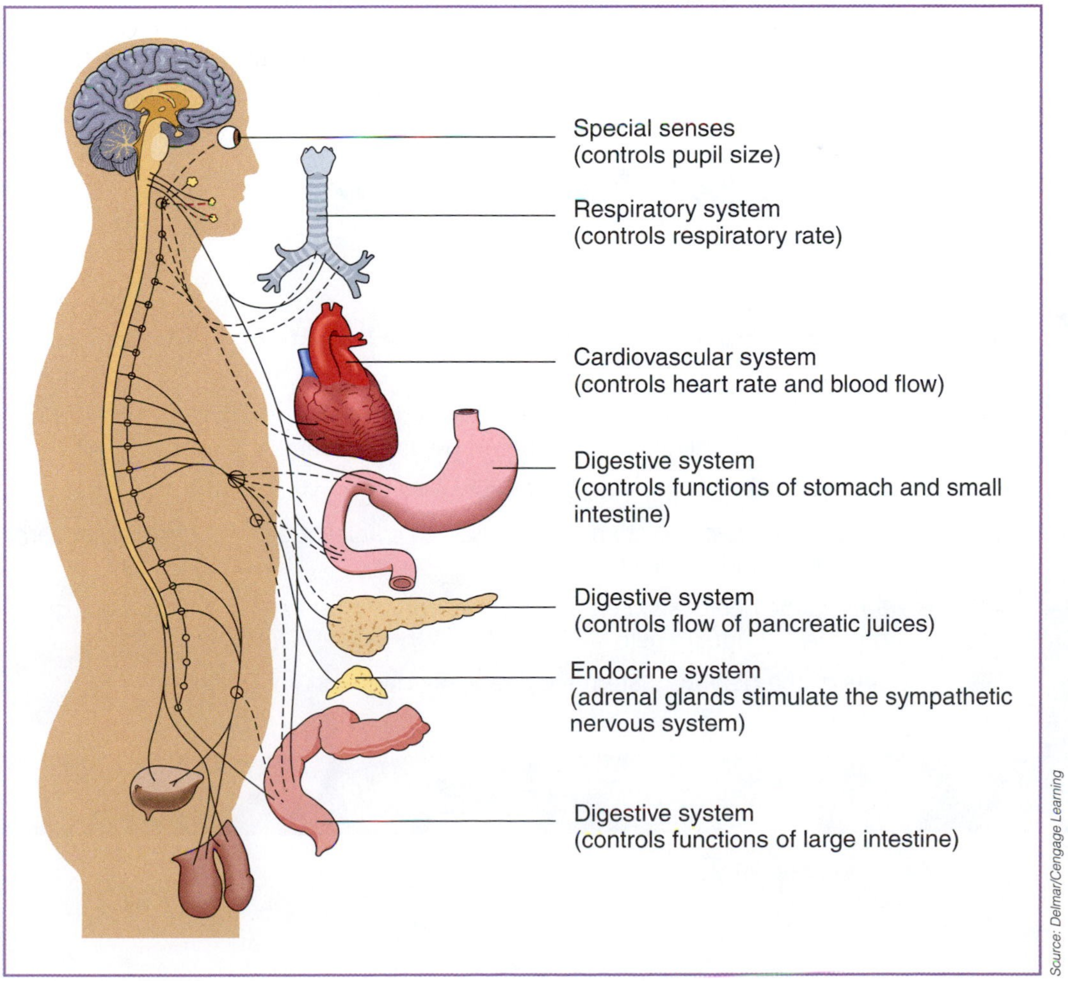

FIGURE 20-7 Autonomic Nervous System with Examples of Major Body Systems Involved

system would slow it down. Interaction of these two systems normally keeps the body processes at a steady state of activity.

INTERNET ASSIGNMENT

The National Institute of Neurological Disorders and Stroke (NINDS) is part of the National Institutes of Health and is accessible at **www.ninds.nih.gov.** The mission of the NINDS is to reduce the burden of neurological disease in people all over the world. To accomplish this goal, the NINDS supports and conducts research, both basic and clinical, on the normal and diseased nervous systems; fosters the training of investigators in the basic and clinical neurosciences; and seeks better understanding, diagnosis, treatment, and prevention of neurological disorders.

This site covers a wide variety of neurological disorders that can be accessed by clicking on Disorders in the banner of the homepage. News and Events highlight current NINDS press releases.

ACTIVITY

Visit the National Institute of Neurological Disorders and Stroke (NINDS) at **www.ninds.nih.gov**. Check your text to find a condition about which you would like more information. Click on Disorders and either select the first letter of the condition in the A to Z choices or scroll through the links. Select the condition and submit a report to your instructor on the results of your investigation.

Review *The Nervous System*

- Neurons interspersed with neuroglia cells are the basic structural and functional components of the nervous system.
- The three parts of the nervous system, grouped according to structure and function, are referred to as the central, peripheral, and autonomic nervous systems.
- The central nervous system includes the brain and spinal cord, the two bases of operation.
- The peripheral nervous system is composed of cranial and spinal nerves that carry messages to and from the brain and spinal column.
- The autonomic nervous system functions automatically, responding and adjusting as necessary without the individual's help.
- All parts of the nervous system are interdependent and interconnected.

Key Terminology Review

Word	Definition
arachnoid membrane	weblike membrane between the dura mater and the pia mater of the meninges
autonomic nervous system	system concerned with activities conducted automatically by certain peripheral nerves
axon	a long, straight fiber originating from a cell body and ending in a brushlike tip; its purpose is to conduct impulses away from the cell body
cell body	part of a cell that contains the nucleus and surrounding cytoplasm
central nervous system	brain and spinal cord
cerebellum	second largest division of the brain; "little brain"
cerebral cortex	outer surface of the cerebrum that is responsible for the generation of impulses
cerebrum	largest part of the brain
cervical, thoracic, lumbar, sacral	four sections of the spinal cord
cornu	hornlike projection of the lateral ventricle reaching into the frontal, occipital, and temporal lobes
dendrites	short fibers that branch out from a cell body
diencephalon	section of the brain between the midbrain and cerebrum
dorsal and ventral roots	divisions of the spinal nerve that enter the spinal cord at different points
dura mater	outer membrane of meninges
epithalamus	part of the diencephalon that contains the pineal body
frontal lobe	anterior lobe of the brain that controls voluntary muscles
ganglion	cluster of nerve cell bodies
gyri (convolutions)	folds of the cerebral cortex forming elevated ridges
hypothalamus	part of the diencephalon that contains centers for the control of body temperature, carbohydrate metabolism, fat metabolism, and emotions that affect heartbeat, blood pressure, appetite, and sexual reflexes
interneurons	neurons that shuttle messages back and forth through the neural pathways
lateral ventricle	cavity of the brain extending from the frontal portion of the cerebral hemisphere to the posterior lobe
medulla oblongata	one part of the brainstem that regulates heart action, breathing, and circulation
meninges	membranes that cover the brain and spinal cord
midbrain	upper part of the brainstem
motor (efferent) neurons	neurons that stimulate the contraction or relaxation of muscles and spur the activities of glands
myelin	white, fatty material that forms a sheath around most axons

continues

Word	Definition
neuroglia cells	supporting and connecting cells of the nervous system
neurologist	physician who specializes in the study of the nervous system
neuron	basic unit of the nervous system
neurosurgeon	surgeon who specializes in the surgical treatment of diseases of the nervous system
nucleus	central controlling structure within a living cell
occipital lobe	posterior lobe of the brain that governs vision
parietal lobe	lobe of the brain that contains the sensory areas and determines distance, size, shape, taste, and the sensory aspects of speech
peripheral nervous system	cranial and spinal nerves
pia mater	inner membrane of meninges
plexus	interlocking network of nerves
pons	part of the brainstem located between the midbrain and medulla oblongata
sensory and motor fibers	part of the composition of spinal nerves of both the autonomic and voluntary nervous systems
sensory (afferent) neurons	neurons that carry signals to the brain and spinal cord
somatic sensory area	parietal lobe
somatic motor area	frontal lobe
sulci (fissures)	depressions or grooves that separate gyri (convolutions)
synapse	junction between neurons
temporal lobe	lobe of the brain that contains the auditory center for hearing impulses and determines the sense of smell
thalamus	part of the diencephalon where nerve fibers from the spinal cord and lower part of the brain synapse with neurons leading to the cerebrum
vermis	central portion of the cerebellum

Key Terminology Practice Exercises

MATCHING

Match the cranial nerves to the functions they control.

1. __________ taste		a. abducens
2. __________ one eyeball muscle on each side		b. accessory
3. __________ smell impulses to the brain		c. acoustic
4. __________ muscles of the tongue		d. facial
5. __________ sensory nerve of the face and head		e. glossopharyngeal
6. __________ largely motor to the face		f. hypoglossal
7. __________ most organs in the thoracic and abdominal cavities		g. oculomotor
8. __________ two muscles of the neck		h. olfactory
9. __________ vision		i. optic
10. __________ balance and hearing		j. trigeminal
11. __________ eyeball muscle		k. trochlear
12. __________ eye muscles controlling the pupil		l. vagus

COMPLETION

Complete the following statements.

1. The basic unit of the nervous system is the __________________.
2. A __________________ is a junction between one neuron and another.
3. There are more than __________________ billion neurons in the nervous system.
4. The nervous system is made up of nerve cells interspersed with __________________.
5. The hornlike projection of the lateral ventricle reaching into the frontal, occipital, and temporal lobes is called the __________________.
6. The part of a cell that contains the nucleus and surrounding cytoplasm is a/n __________________.
7. Short fibers that branch out from a cell body are __________________.
8. The __________________ is the central portion of the cerebellum.
9. A/n __________________ conducts impulses away from the cell body.
10. The central controlling structure within a living cell is the __________________.
11. The white, fatty material that forms a sheath around most axons is __________________.
12. The upper part of the brainstem is the __________________.
13. Neurons that shuttle messages back and forth through neural pathways are __________________.
14. A cluster of nerve cell bodies is a/n __________________.
15. The section of the brain between the midbrain and cerebrum is the __________________.
16. The pineal body is part of the __________________ in the diencephalons.
17. Neurons that carry signals to brain and spinal cord are __________________.
18. Neurons that stimulate contraction or relaxation of muscles are __________________.
19. The __________________ is part of the brainstem located between the midbrain and medulla oblongata.
20. The somatic sensory area is in the __________________ lobe.

SELECTION

From the list at the right, select in which portion of the brain each of the following is located.

1. __________ vermis
2. __________ medulla oblongata
3. __________ cerebral cortex
4. __________ parietal lobe
5. __________ pons

a. cerebrum
b. brainstem
c. cerebellum

DEFINITIONS

Define the following terms.

1. sulci
   ____
2. gyri
   ____
3. peripheral nervous system
   ____
4. central nervous system
   ____
5. meninges
   ____
6. dura mater
   ____
7. arachnoid membrane
   ____
8. plexus
   ____

SHORT ANSWERS

Supply a short answer to the following.

1. Name the four divisions of the spinal cord.
   ____
2. Name the four lobes of the cerebrum.
   ____
3. Describe the function of the spinal cord.
   ____
4. Identify the number of spinal and cranial nerves.
   ____
5. Define the autonomic nervous system, and name its two divisions.
   ____

Word Element Review

Root	Meaning	Example	Definition
cephal/o	head	**cephalic** (sĕ-făl'ĭk)	pertaining to the head
cerebell/o	cerebellum	**cerebellitis** (sĕr"ĕ-bĕl-ī'tĭs)	inflammation of the cerebellum
cerebr/o	brain	**cerebrospinal** (sĕr"ĕ-brō-spī'năl)	pertaining to the brain and spinal cord
crani/o	head, skull	**craniotomy** (krā"nē-ŏt'ō-mē)	incision through the cranium
		cranium (krā'nē-ŭm)	that portion of the skull that encloses the brain
dur/o	dura mater	**duraplasty** (dŭ'ră-plăs"tē)	plastic repair of the dura mater
encephal/o	brain	**encephalon** (ĕn-sĕf'ah-lŏn)	the brain
		encephalopathy (ĕn-sĕf"ah-lŏp'ah-thē)	any disease of the brain
gangli/o	swelling	**ganglion** (găng'glē-ŏn)	mass of nerve tissue composed principally of nerve bodies and lying outside the brain or spinal cord
mening/o	meninges	**meningeal** (mĕ-nĭn'jē-ăl)	pertaining to the meninges
		meningitis (mĕn"ĭn-jī'tĭs)	inflammation of the membranes covering the brain and spinal cord
myel/o	marrow, spinal cord	**osteomyelitis** (ŏs"tē-ō-mī"ĕ-lī'tĭs)	inflammation of bone and bone marrow
neur/o	nerve, nervous	**neuralgia** (nū-răl'jē-ah)	severe, sharp pain along the course of a nerve system
pont/o	pons	**pontocerebellar** (pŏn"tō-sĕr"ĕ-bĕl-ăr)	pertaining to the pons and the cerebellum
spondyl/o	vertebra	**spondylosis** (spŏn"dĭ-lō'sĭs)	immobility or fixation of vertebrae
		spondylous (spŏn'dĭ-lŭs)	pertaining to the spinal column
thalam/o	thalamus	**thalamocele** (thăl'ăm-ō-sēl")	third ventricle of the brain

Word Element Practice Exercise

IDENTIFICATION

Identify each of the following definitions.

1. pertaining to the brain and spinal column ______________________
2. concerning the spinal column ______________________
3. any disease of the brain ______________________
4. inflammation of the membranes covering the brain and spinal column ______________________
5. severe, sharp pain along the course of a nerve ______________________
6. plastic repair of dura mater ______________________
7. pertaining to the pons and cerebellum ______________________
8. third ventricle of the brain ______________________
9. pertaining to the meninges ______________________
10. the brain ______________________
11. incision trough the cranium ______________________
12. pertaining to the head ______________________
13. immobility or fixation of vertebrae ______________________
14. inflammation of the cerebellum ______________________
15. portion of the skull that encloses the brain ______________________
16. inflammation of bone or bone marrow ______________________
17. mass of nerve tissue composed principally of nerve bodies lying outside the brain or spinal column ______________________

MATCHING

Match the following meanings with the correct root.

1. __________ head, skull		a. cephal/o
2. __________ brain		b. cerebell/o
3. __________ pons		c. cerebr/o
4. __________ head		d. crani/o
5. __________ swelling		e. dur/o
6. __________ marrow, spinal cord		f. encephal/o
7. __________ vertebra		g. gangli/o
8. __________ meninges		h. mening/o
9. __________ dura mater		i. myel/o
10. __________ nerve, nervous system		j. neur/o
11. __________ thalamus		k. pont/o
12. __________ brain		l. spondyl/o
13. __________ cerebellum		m. thalam/o

WORD ELEMENT MEANINGS

Give the meaning of each word element. Then use your dictionary to find a new word that contains each of the word elements. Specify whether the new word is a noun or an adjective by placing N or A in the last column.

Word Element	Meaning	Word	N or A
1. cephal/o	________	________	________
2. cerebell/o	________	________	________
3. cerebr/o	________	________	________
4. crani/o	________	________	________
5. dur/o	________	________	________
6. encephal/o	________	________	________
7. gangli/o	________	________	________
8. mening/o	________	________	________
9. myel/o	________	________	________
10. neur/o	________	________	________
11. pont/o	________	________	________
12. spondyl/o	________	________	________
13. thalam/o	________	________	________

Working Practice

DIAGNOSTIC PROCEDURES

Word	Pronunciation	Definition
General		
cisternal puncture	sĭs-tĕr'năl	insertion of short, beveled spinal needle into cisterna magna at the base of the brain to drain cerebrospinal fluid (CSF) or obtain a CSF specimen
electroencephalography	ē-lĕk"trō-ĕn-sĕf"ah-lŏg'rah-fē	study of the electrical activity of the brain using electrodes attached to the scalp; produces an electroencephalogram (EEG)
electromyography	ĕ-lĕk"trō-mī'ŏg'rah-fē	study of the contraction of a muscle as a result of electrical stimulation; produces an electromyogram (EMG)
Glasgow Coma Scale		assessment tool that evaluates eye movement, verbal response, and motor response to describe the level of consciousness: may be semicomatose, stupor, lethargic, or comatose
lumbar puncture for cerebrospinal fluid (CSF) analysis	sĕr"ĕ-brō-spī'năl	procedure that detects abnormal substances and variations in the cerebrospinal fluid through extraction of fluid for examination, pressure recording, or injection

continues

DIAGNOSTIC PROCEDURES		
Word	**Pronunciation**	**Definition**
Nuclear Medicine		
brain scan		procedure using radioactive chemicals and special machines to record their passage and absorption into any brain lesions; brain barrier will not allow the radioactive chemical in normal brain tissue
positron emission tomography (PET scan)	pŏz'ĭ-trŏn, tō-mŏg'rah-fē	an agent is mixed with a radioactive substance and is injected into the blood to record and measure images of the target site
single-photon emission computer tomography (SPECT)	fō'tŏn, tō-mŏg'rah-fē	method for reconstructing sectional images of radiotracer distributions
Radiology		
angiography	ăn"jē-ŏg'rah-fē	x-ray study using contrast material injected into blood vessels to diagnose blockages, tumors, and the like
cervical spine, thoracic spine, lumbosacral spine		x-ray of specific sections of the spinal column
computerized axial tomography (CAT)	tō-mŏg'rah-fē	computer-assisted x-ray technique used to distinguish pathological conditions such as tumors, abscesses, and hematomas
echoencephalography	ĕk"ō-ĕn-sĕf"ă-lŏg'ră-fē	ultrasound used to analyze the intracranial structure of the brain
magnetic resonance		technique used to distinguish imaging (MRI) pathological lesions of the brain and spinal cord (see Figure 20-8)
myelography	mī"ē-lŏg'rah-fē	x-ray study of the spinal canal and cord after an injection of contrast material into the subarachnoid space
routine skull series		standard x-ray views of the skull

continues

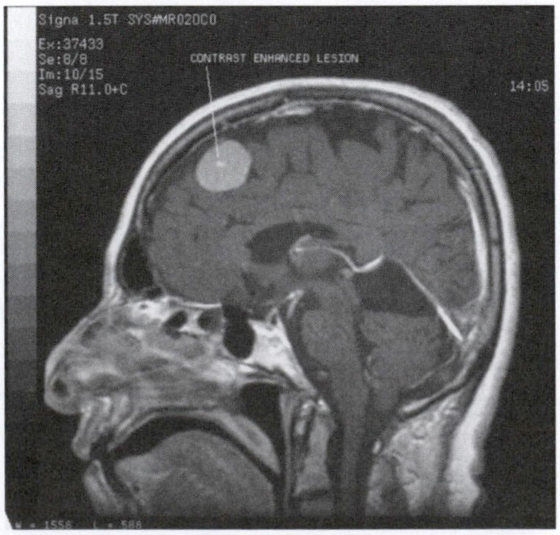

FIGURE 20-8 Tumor of the Brain Visualized Through Magnetic Resonance Imaging (MRI)

Source: Delmar/Cengage Learning

DIAGNOSTIC PROCEDURES		
Word	**Pronunciation**	**Definition**
Radiology (*continued*)		
ultrasound		use of ultrasonic sound waves to outline the shape of various tissues and organs in the body

DIAGNOSES		
Word	**Pronunciation**	**Definition**
Infections		
brain abscess		accumulation of pus located anywhere in the brain tissue due to an infectious process, either a primary or secondary infection
encephalitis	ĕn-sĕf"ă-lī'tĭs	inflammation of brain tissue
human immunodeficiency virus encephalopathy		brain disease and dementia occurring with AIDS
meningitis	mĕn-ĭn'jī'tĭs	inflammation of the meninges (membranes of the spinal cord or brain)
peripheral neuritis	nū-rī'tĭs	inflammation of one or more peripheral nerves
poliomyelitis	pōl"ē-ō-mī"ĕl-ī'tĭs	viral infection affecting brain and spinal cord
rabies	rā'bēz	often fatal encephalomyelitis caused by a virus transmitted to humans by an animal bite
Reye's syndrome	rīz	acute brain encephalopathy following acute viral infections in children under age 18
shingles (herpes zoster)	shĭng'lz	viral disease affecting peripheral nerves (see Figure 20-9)
tetanus	tĕt'ă-nŭs	acute, often fatal infection of nerve tissue caused by the bacteria *Colstridium tetani*

continues

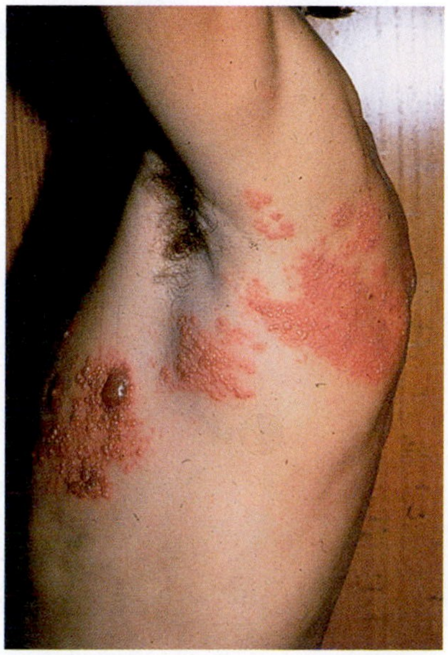

FIGURE 20-9 Shingles: vesicles follow a nerve pathway

Courtesy of Robert A. Silverman, M.D., Clinical Associate Professor, Department of Pediatrics, Georgetown University

DIAGNOSES		
Word	**Pronunciation**	**Definition**
Vascular Disorders		
aneurysm	ăn'ū'rĭzm	sac formed by localized dilation of the walls of an artery or a vein
cerebrovascular accident (CVA)	sĕr-ĕ"brō-văs'kū-lăr	damage to the brain caused by a disorder of the blood vessels of the brain; also known as a stroke; may be caused by a thrombus (a blood clot), an embolus (a clot that breaks off), or a *hemorrhage* (see Figure 20-10)

continues

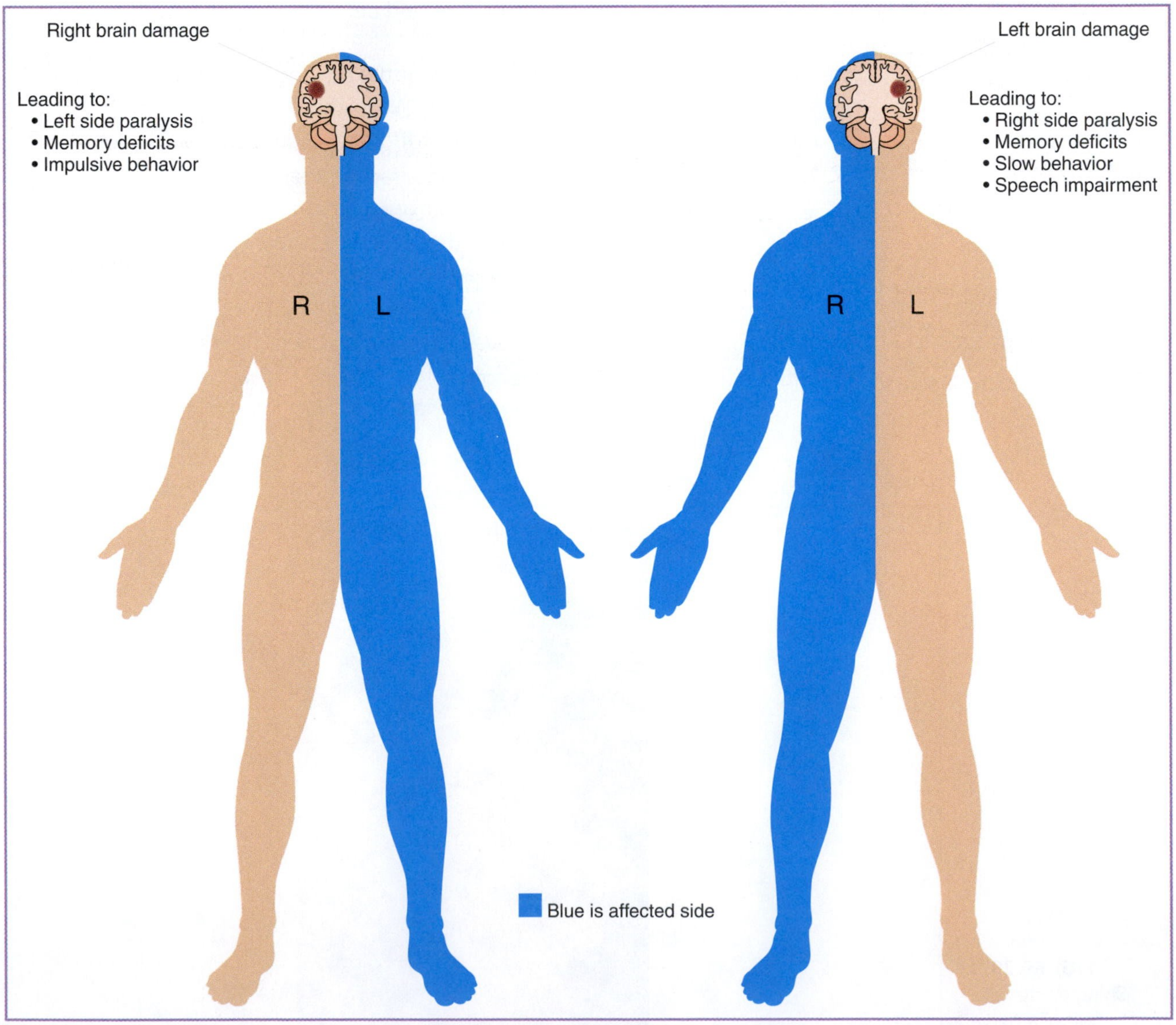

FIGURE 20-10 Symptoms of right and left CVA vary to some degree

DIAGNOSES		
Word	**Pronunciation**	**Definition**
Vascular Disorders (*continued*)		
transient ischemic attack (TIA)	trăns'ē-ĕnt ĭs-kē'mĭk	sudden episode of temporary symptoms due to diminished blood flow through the brain; early warning symptom of stroke (see Figure 20-11)
Functional Disorders		
Bell's palsy	pawl'ze	disease causing paralysis of one side of the face (see Figure 20-12)
cephalalgia (headache)	sĕf-ă-lăl"jē-ah	pain in various locations in the head or neck
• *cluster*		series of intense, short-term recurring headaches felt near one eye; occur at night after falling asleep
• *migraine*	mī'grān	severe headache accompanied by nausea, vomiting, and vision problems; may be limited to one side
• *postlumbar puncture*	pōst-lŭm'băr	follows a lumbar puncture in forty percent of the cases
• *stress*		caused by stress, strain, tension of the face, neck, and scalp muscles
cerebral palsy	sĕr'ĕ-brăl pawl'ze	disorder discovered after birth, involving the brain
degenerative disk disease	dĭ-jĕ-nĕ-ră"tĭv	condition marked by wearing away of intervertebral disk causing spinal stenosis
dementia	dē-mĕn'shē-ah	decreased mental functioning
• *Alzheimer's disease*	ălts'hī-mĕrs	irreversible senile dementia characterized by deteriorating intellectual capacities
• *head trauma*	trăw'mah	death of brain cells related to head trauma
• *substance induced*		death of brain cells caused by toxicity of drugs and toxins
• *vascular*	văs'cū-lăr	atrophy and death of brain cells due to decreased blood flow

continues

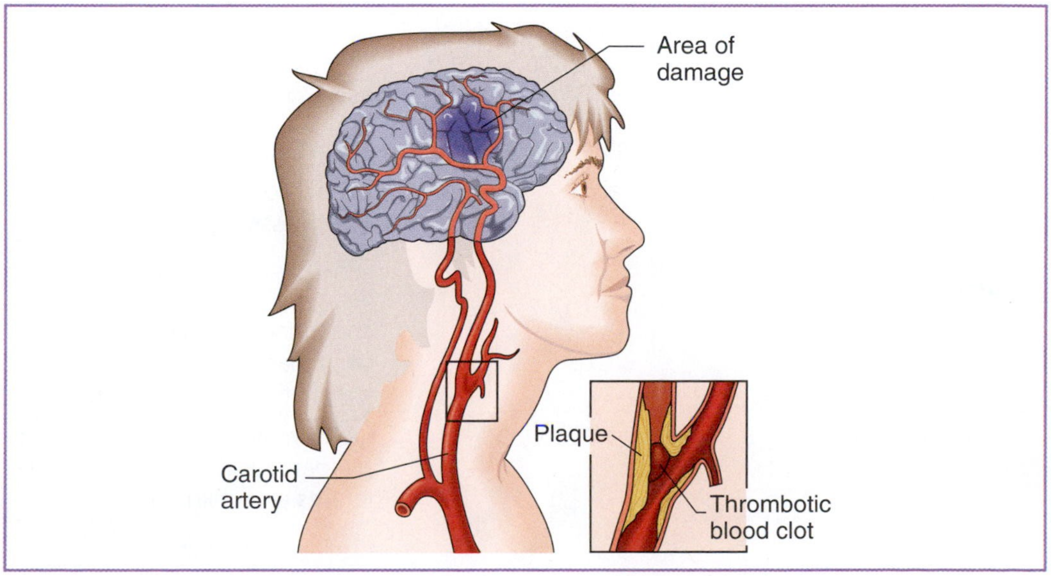

FIGURE 20-11 Transient Ischemic Attack (TIA)

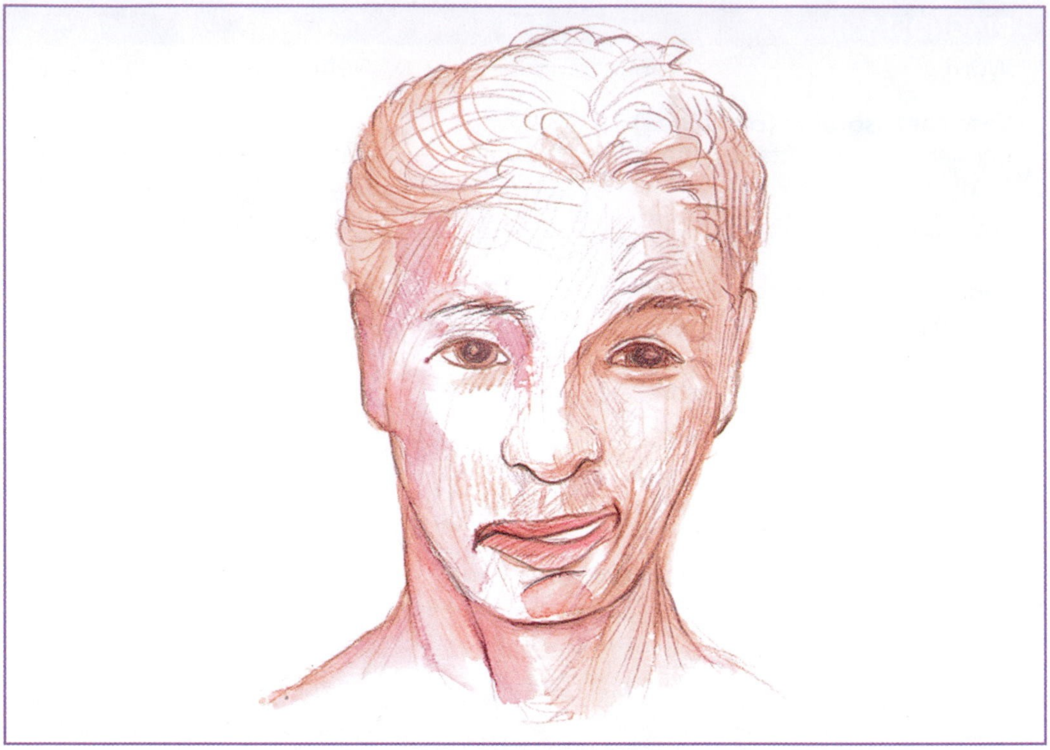

FIGURE 20-12
Facial appearance of Bell's palsy

DIAGNOSES

Word	Pronunciation	Definition
Functional Disorders (*continued*)		
epilepsy	ĕp'ĭ-lĕp"sē	recurrent disorder of neuronal function manifested by a variety of seizure types
hydrocephalus	hī-drō-sĕf'ah-lŭs	abnormal accumulation of spinal fluid within the ventricles of the brain
Tourette's syndrome, Tourette's disorder	tŭr-ĕts'	disorder marked by involuntary, spasmodic, twitching movements; uncontrollable vocal sounds; and inappropriate words
trigeminal neuralgia	trī-jĕm'ĭn-ăl nū-răl'jē-ah	severe, sharp pain along the fifth cranial nerve
Sleep Disorders		
insomnia	ĭn-sŏm'nē-ah	inability to fall or stay asleep
sleep apnea	ăp'nē-ah	sleep disorder characterized by periods of apnea or breathlessness
Tumors		
brain tumor		abnormal growth of brain tissue and meninges; may be primary (originating in brain tissue) or secondary (originating elsewhere and metastasizing to the brain)
neuroblastoma	nū"rō-blăs-tō'mă	highly malignant hemorrhagic tumor of the sympathetic nervous system occurring chiefly in infants and children

continues

DIAGNOSES		
Word	**Pronunciation**	**Definition**
Trauma		
concussion	kŏn-kŭsh'ŭn	posttraumatic syndrome, which can include severe headaches, memory loss, dizziness, and extreme breathing rates
carpal tunnel syndrome	kăr'păl	pain or numbness caused by the pinching or compression of the median nerve distribution of the hand due to inflammation or swelling of the tendons of the wrist; may radiate into the arm
contusion	kŏn-too'shŭn	injury to the brain causing bruising of the brain
hematoma		localized collection of blood within the cranium
• *subdural*	sŭb-dū'răl	blood collecting below the dura caused by a break in a blood vessel and often the result of a head injury
• epidural	ĕp"ĭ-dū'răl	blood collecting between the cranium and the dura mater
• *intracerebral*	ĭn"tră-sĕ-rē'brăl	blood collecting within the brain tissue itself (see Figure 20-13)
skull fractures		trauma causing bone fractures that may lead to permanent or temporary brain tissue damage
spinal cord injury		injury to spinal cord at any level; site, type, and degree of injury determine whether temporary or permanent paralysis will occur
• *hemiplegia*	hĕm-ē-plē'jē-ah	injury or paralysis to one side of the body

continues

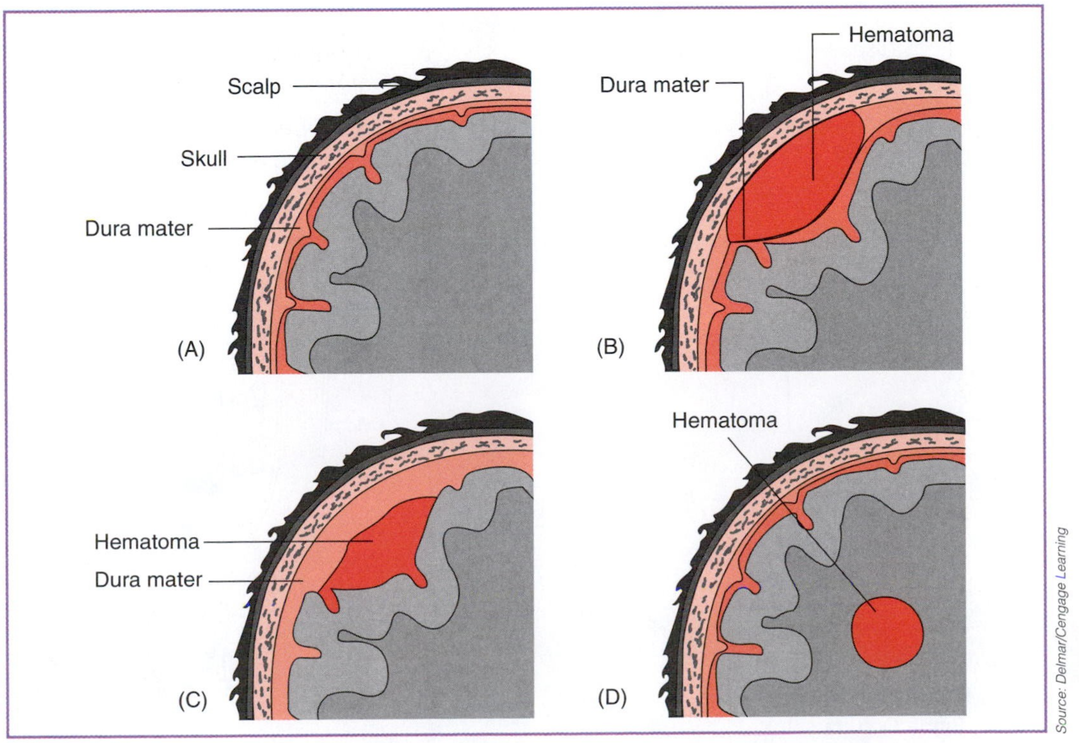

FIGURE 20-13
Cranial Hematomas: (A) normal; (B) epidural; (C) subdural; (D) intracerebral

DIAGNOSES

Word	Pronunciation	Definition
Trauma (*continued*)		
• *paraplegia*	păr-ă-plē'jē-ah	injury to thoracic or lumbar section of spinal cord, which leads to loss of movement and feeling either in both legs or both arms
• *quadriplegia*	kwod"rĭ-plē'jē-ah	injuries to cervical spine or neck area, C1 to C6; leads to loss of movement and feeling in all four extremities
Other Diseases		
amyotrophic lateral sclerosis (ALS)	ă-mī"ō-trōf'ĭk lăt'ĕr-ăl sklē-rō'sĭs	destructive disease of motor or movement neurons; Lou Gehrig's disease
Guillain-Barré Syndrome	gē-yăn'băr-rā'	acute, progressive disease affecting the peripheral and spinal nerves
Huntington's chorea, Huntington's disease	kō-rē'ah	inherited disease that appears in middle age and is marked by progressive degeneration of the brain
multiple sclerosis (MS)	mŭl'tĭ-pl sklē-rō'sĭs	disease that causes demyelination of nerves of the central nervous system
myasthenia gravis	mī-ăs-thē'nē-ă gră'vĭs	neuromuscular disorder characterized by weakness of voluntary muscles from repetitive use
Parkinson's disease		slow, progressive brain degeneration with a deficiency of dopamine in the brain
spina bifida cystica	spī'nah bĭf'ĭ'dah sĭs'tĭ-kah	congenital defect in the walls of the spinal canal caused by a lack of union between the laminae of the vertebrae
spina bifida occulta	spī'nah bĭ-fă'dah ō-kŭl'tah	failure of the vertebrae to close, without protrusion of neural tissues (see Figure 20-14)
Tay-Sachs disease	tā'săks	congenital disorder caused by altered lipid metabolism resulting from an enzyme deficiency
trigeminal neuralgia (tic douloureux)	trī-jĕm'ĭn-ăl nū-răl'jē-ă (tĭc doo"lă-roo')	short periods of severe pain radiating along the fifth cranial (trigeminus) nerve

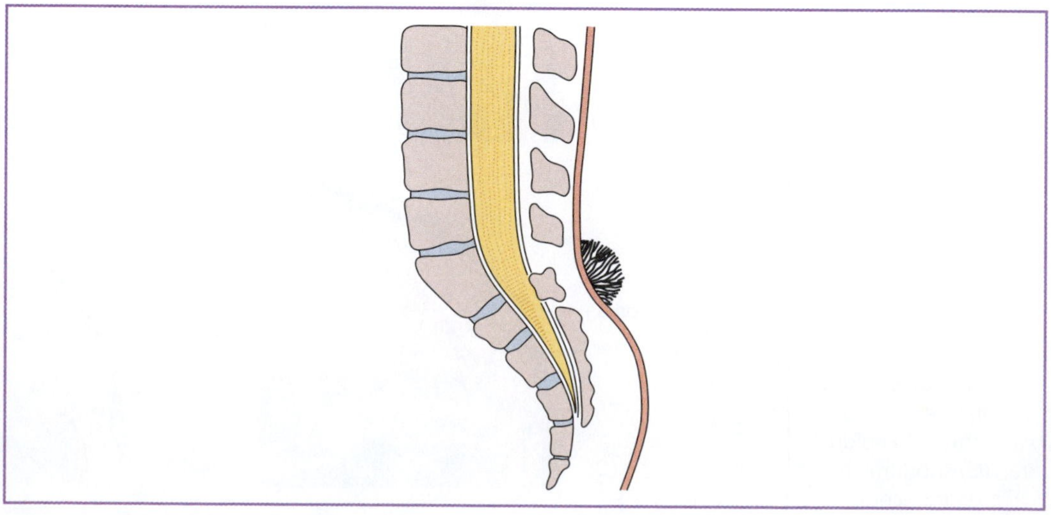

FIGURE 20-14
Spina Bifida Occulta

TREATMENT PROCEDURES		
Word	**Pronunciation**	**Definition**
carotid endarterectomy	kah-rŏt'ĭd ĕnd"ăr-tĕr-ĕk'tō-mē	removal of plaque or thickened lining of a carotid artery to unclog the artery
cerebrospinal fluid shunts	sĕr"ĕ-brō-spī'năl	creation of channels to detour accumulated cerebrospinal fluid in the brain; the two most common are ventriculoatrial and entriculoperitoneal
cordotomy (chordotomy)	kor-dŏt'ō-mē (kor-dŏt'ō-mē)	procedure which interferes with pathways within the spinal cord that control pain
craniotomy	krā"nē-ŏt'ō-mē	any operation to open the cranium
decompression		surgical procedure to relieve intracranial pressure
halo traction		traction device for connecting the head and cervical area for neck stability
laminectomy	lăm"ĭ-nĕk'tō-mē	removal of a vertebral lesion or herniated disk
myelocele repair	mī'ĕ-ō-lŏ-sēl	repair of an open spine or the cord components, which is usually congenital
neurectomy	nū-rĕk'tō-mē	procedure to relieve pain in a localized area by partial or total excision or resection of cranial or peripheral nerves
percutaneous electrocoagulation	pĕr"kū-tā'nē-ŭs ē-lĕk"trō-kō-ăg"ū'lā'shŭn	procedure for longer-term pain relief affecting pain-sensory fibers
stereotactic radiosurgery (stereotaxic neurosurgery)	stĕr"ē-ō-tăk'tĭk (stĕr"ē-ō-tăks'sĭk)	use of a specialized instrument to precisely find, cut, or remove targets in the brain
stereotaxic thalamotomy	stĕ"rē-ō-tăk'sĭk thăl-ă-mŏt'ō-mē	use of a stereotaxic instrument to locate a target and disrupt the transmission of motor impulses (tremors)
sympathectomy	sĭm"pă-thĕk'tō-mē	procedure used to excise a portion of the sympathetic nerve pathway to relieve chronic pain
tractotomy	trăk-tŏt'ō-mē	procedure that involves a craniotomy through which the anterolateral pathway in the brain stem is surgically divided in an attempt to relieve intractable pain
transcutaneous electrical nerve stimulation (TENS)	trăns"kū-tā'nē-ŭs	application of mild electrical stimulation to the skin by electrodes placed over a painful area to alleviate pain
trephination	trĕf"ĭ-nā'shŭn	cutting a circular incision into the skull to make brain surgery possible
ulnar nerve transposition	ul'năr	transfer and decompression of the ulnar nerve at the elbow to relieve trauma to the nerve

MEDICATIONS PRESCRIBED	
Trade Name	Generic Name
Anticonvulsants	
Depakene, Depakote	valproic acid
Diamox	acetazolamide
Dilantin	phenytoin
Klonopin	clonazepam
Mysoline	primidone
Phenobarbital	phenobarbital
Tegretol	carbamazepine
Tranxene	clorazepate dipotassium
Zarontin	ethosuximide
Antiemetic and Antivertigo	
Antivert, Bonine	meclizine
Compazine	prochlorperazine maleate
Dramamine	dimenhydrinate
Tigan	trimethobenzamide
Torecan	thiethylperazine maleate
Antiparkinson's Agents	
Artane	trihexyphenidyl
Cogentin	benztropine
Elavil	amitriptyline HCl
Eldepryl	selegiline
Pagitane	cycrimine HCl
Parisdol	ethopropagine HCl
Parlodel	bromocriptine mesylate
Permax	pergolide mesylate
Sinemet	carbidopa, levodopa
Symmetrel	amantadine
Tofranil	imipramine HCl
CNS Stimulants	
Dexedrine	dextroamphetamine sulfate
Ritalin	methylphenidate
Edema control	
Decadron	dexamethasone
Mannitol	mannitol
Solu-Medrol	methylprednisolone

continues

MEDICATIONS PRESCRIBED	
Trade Name	**Generic Name**
MS Agents	
ACTH	adrenocorticotropic steroid
Avonex, Betaseron	interferon beta
Capaxone	glatiramer acetate
Cytoxan	cyclophosphamide
Dantrium	dantrolene sodium
Deltasone	prednisone
Glatiramer acetate	copaxone
Imuran	azathioprine
Lioresal	baclofen
Pro-Banthine	propantheline bromide
Sandimmune	cyclosporine
Headache Agents	
Cafergot	ergotamine and caffeine
Catapres	clonidine HCl
Ergostat	ergotamine tartrate
Inderal	propranolol HCl
Phenergan	promethazine HCl
Sansert	methysergide maleate

ABBREVIATIONS	
CAT	computerized axial tomography
CNS	central nervous system
CP	cerebral palsy
CSF	cerebrospinal fluid
CVA	cerebrovascular accident
EEG	electroencephalogram
EMG	electromyogram
LP	lumbar puncture
MRI	magnetic resonance imaging
MS	multiple sclerosis
TENS	transcutaneous electrical nerve stimulation
TIA	transient ischemic attack

Working Practice Review Exercises

IDENTIFICATION

Identify the following diagnostic procedures.

1. measures muscle contractions as a result of electrical stimulation ____________________
2. extraction of cerebrospinal fluid for examination ____________________
3. radioactive chemicals are given, and special machines record whether brain lesions are present ____________________
4. injection of contrast material into arteries to diagnose blockages and tumors ____________________
5. studies electrical activity of the brain by means of electrodes attached to the scalp ____________________
6. x-ray study of spinal canal and cord after contrast material is injected into subarachnoid space ____________________
7. method for reconstructing sectional images of radiotracer distributions ____________________
8. standard x-ray views of the skull ____________________
9. test to evaluate level of consciousness ____________________
10. technique used to distinguish pathological lesions of the brain and spinal cord ____________________

MEANINGS

Give the meaning of the italicized words.

1. There is an *aneurysm* on the right middle cerebral artery.

   ____

2. The damage to the brainstem was caused by *hydrocephalus*.

   ____

3. The patient sustained a *subdural hematoma* as a result of the boating accident.

   ____

4. Miss Chenevey has *Parkinson's disease*.

   ____

5. Their son has a *contusion*.

   ____

6. After-surgery recovery was complicated by *meningitis*.

   ____

7. The patient suffered a *CVA* last year.

   ____

8. The doctor's report indicated she suffers frequently from *cephalalgia*.

   ____

9. She explained the difference between a *concussion* and contusion.

   ____

10. Dr. Jarrod finally concluded that Mathew's problem was *Huntington's chorea*.

   ____

MATCHING

Match the terms to their meanings.

1. __________ repair of an open spine or the cord components
2. __________ disc surgery
3. __________ removal of thickened lining of an artery
4. __________ an operation on the cranium
5. __________ creation of a channel to detour cerebrospinal fluid in the brain
6. __________ surgical procedure to relieve intracranial pressure
7. __________ locate a target and disrupt transmission of motor impulses resulting in tremors
8. __________ traction device for connecting head and cervical area for neck stability
9. __________ cutting a circular incision into skull to make brain surgery possible
10. __________ procedure for longer-term pain relief affecting pain-sensory fibers

a. carotid endarterectomy
b. cerebrospinal fluid shunts
c. craniotomy
d. decompression
e. halo traction
f. laminectomy
g. mycocele repair
h. percutaneous electrocoagulation
i. stereotactic thalamotomy
j. trephination

COMPLETION

Complete the following statements.

1. A viral disease affecting peripheral nerves is ____________________.
2. A hematoma where blood collects between the cranium and dura mater is referred to as ____________________.
3. A severe, sharp pain along the fifth cranial nerve is ____________________.
4. The death of brain cells related to head trauma is ____________________.
5. A series of intense, short-term, recurring headaches felt near one eye is a ____________________ headache.
6. An early symptom of a stroke is a(n) ____________________.
7. A recurrent disorder of neuronal function manifested by a variety of seizure types is ____________________.
8. The inability to fall or stay asleep is ____________________.
9. An injury or paralysis to one side of the body is ____________________.
10. Lou Gehrig's disease is more technically known as ____________________.
11. An acute, progressive disease affecting peripheral and spinal nerves is ____________________.
12. A congenital defect in the walls of the spinal canal is ____________________.
13. A disease that causes demyelination of nerves of the central nervous system is ____________________.
14. The failure of the vertebrae to close without protrusion is ____________________.
15. Blood collecting within the brain tissue is a(n) ____________________.

Dictionary Exercises

DICTIONARY EXERCISE 1

Use your dictionary to find the pronunciation and definition of the following words.

Word	Pronunciation	Definition
1. disorientation	____________	____________
2. compression	____________	____________
3. neurotomy	____________	____________
4. polyneuritis	____________	____________
5. radiculoneuritis	____________	____________
6. Babinski's reflex	____________	____________
7. Ménière's disease	____________	____________
8. meningoencephalomyelitis	____________	____________
9. meningomyelitis	____________	____________
10. microcephaly	____________	____________
11. glioma	____________	____________
12. Hoffmann's reflex	____________	____________
13. jacksonian epilepsy	____________	____________
14. radiculitis	____________	____________
15. Romberg's sign	____________	____________

DICTIONARY EXERCISE 2

Select the correct definition and provide the pronunciation where indicated.

1. anarthria (____________)
   a. inability to read
   b. inability to remember
   c. inability to speak
   d. inability to speak remembered words properly
2. anencephalus (____________)
   a. congenital absence of the brain and cranial space
   b. lack of memory
   c. loss of the power to recognize sensory stimuli even though sensory facilities are intact
   d. loss of sensation
3. astrocytoma (____________)
   a. tumor composed of neuroglial cells (astrocytes)
   b. tumor arising from specialized tissue found in the brain and spinal cord
   c. soft, infiltrating malignant tumor of the roof of the fourth ventricle and cerebellum
   d. rapidly growing malignant tumor composed of primitive glial cells
4. agnosia (____________)
   a. inability to read
   b. inability to fix the range of movement in muscular activity
   c. severe sharp pain
   d. loss of the power to recognize sensory stimuli even though sensory facilities are intact
5. dysmetria (____________)
   a. inability to read despite normal vision
   b. impairment of intellectual ability
   c. inability to fix the range of movement in muscular activity
   d. severe pain along the course of a nerve
6. paresthesia (____________)
   a. severe pain along the course of a nerve
   b. sensation of numbness, pricking, burning, crawling, or tingling
   c. disease marked by tingling, itching, and disturbing sensations
   d. impairment or lessening of sensitivity to touch

7. tabes dorsalis (____________)
   a. terminal portion of the spinal cord and roots of spinal nerves below first lumbar nerve
   b. proliferation of neuroglial tissue in CNS
   c. disease of CNS, usually caused by syphilis
   d. rare disease of nervous system; Guillain-Barré syndrome
8. encephalocele (____________)
   a. rapidly growing malignant tumor
   b. congenital hernia in which meninges protrude through an opening in the skull or spinal column
   c. abnormal smallness of the head
   d. protrusion of the brain through any opening in the skull
9. gliosis (____________)
   a. proliferation of neuroglial tissue in CNS
   b. impairment of sensitivity to touch
   c. inflammation of the spinal cord
   d. to and fro movement of the eyeballs as seen in brain damage
10. meralgia paresthetica (____________)
    a. sensitivity to pain
    b. severe pain along the course of a nerve
    c. disease marked by tingling, itching, and disturbing sensations in the thigh
    d. sharp pain along a nerve
11. medulloblastoma (____________)
    a. soft, infiltrating malignant tumor of the roof of the fourth ventricle and cerebellum
    b. star-shaped tumor
    c. tumor arising from specialized tissue found in the brain and spinal cord
    d. tumor composed of glial cells in the cerebral hemisphere
12. retrogasserian neurotomy (____________)
    a. interruption of a nerve fiber tract within the spinal cord for relief of pain
    b. dissection of the posterior root of the trigeminal ganglion
    c. excision of a nerve
    d. suture of a nerve
13. convulsion (____________)
    a. injury resulting from a blow
    b. tremor
    c. violent involuntary muscular contractions and relaxations
    d. involuntary and quick repetitious spasms of a muscle
14. glioblastoma multiforme (____________)
    a. rapidly growing malignant tumor composed of primitive glial cells
    b. tumor arising from specialized tissue found in the brain and spinal cord
    c. tumor composed of glial cells in the cerebral hemisphere
    d. inflammation of the brain and spinal cord and their membranes
15. hypesthesia (____________)
    a. sensation of numbness, tingling, prickling, etc.
    b. lessening of sensitivity to touch
    c. decreased sensitivity to pain
    d. consciousness

DICTIONARY EXERCISE 3

Pronunciation of the words below is provided. Using your dictionary, find the spelling and definition of each word.

	Word	Pronunciation	Definition
1.	______	dĕr'mă-tōm	______
2.	______	ă-grăf-ē-ah	______
3.	______	ă-lĕks'ē-ah	______
4.	______	ah-fă'zē-ah	______
5.	______	ăs-thē'nē-ah	______
6.	______	ah-tăk'sē-ah	______
7.	______	dĭs-lĕk'sē-ah	______
8.	______	ĕn-sĕf"ah-lŏp'ah-thē	______
9.	______	glī-ō'mah	______
10.	______	hĕm"ē-păr'ē-sĭs	______
11.	______	mī"ĕ-lī'tĭs	______
12.	______	năr'kō-lĕp"sē	______
13.	______	nĭs-tăg'mŭs	______
14.	______	sī-ăt'ĭ-kah	______
15.	______	tĭk	______

DICTIONARY EXERCISE 4

Rewrite each sentence in your own words.

1. The patient displayed an *intention tremor* when attempting to remove the jar lid.

______

2. The first evidence of meningitis was *Brudzinski's sign*.

______

3. His wife experienced a *subarachnoid hemorrhage*.

______

4. On physical exam, there was no evidence of *neuropathy*.

______

5. The surgeon performed *neurorrhaphy* after his accident.

______

6. Cerebral *dysrhythmia* was evident.

______

7. Part of the reason for her problems in school was that she has *dyslexia*.

______

8. Her mother was confined to a wheelchair as a result of contracting *poliomyelitis* as a child.

______

DICTIONARY EXERCISE 5

Match the terms to their meanings.

1. __________ encephalitis
2. __________ encephalomalacia
3. __________ lethargy
4. __________ insomnia
5. __________ myelopathy
6. __________ neurectomy
7. __________ paresis
8. __________ sensorium
9. __________ tentorium
10. __________ tremor
11. __________ agraphia
12. __________ bulbar
13. __________ syncope
14. __________ polyneuropathy
15. __________ nuchal rigidity

a. softening of the brain
b. tentlike structure
c. any disease of the spinal cord
d. slight paralysis
e. loss of the ability to write
f. pertaining to the brainstem
g. excision of a nerve
h. inability to sleep
i. inflammation of the brain
j. shaking
k. fainting
l. roughly approximates consciousness
m. neck is resistant to flexion
n. state of being sluggish
o. disease involving many nerves at once

StudyWARE™ Connection

To help you learn the content of this chapter, take a practice quiz or play interactive games on your StudyWARE™ CD-ROM.

Listening Exercise

INSTRUCTIONS

1. Review the spelling, pronunciation, and meaning of the words provided in the preview.
2. Go to your StudyWARE™ CD-ROM and listen to **Listening Exercise 20-1**. Fill in the blank in the report as the word is dictated.
3. At the end of the activity, check your spelling against the preview words. They appear in the preview in the order in which they are encountered in the activity.
4. Review and practice the words you missed.
5. Look up words that are not familiar.

PREVIEW OF WORDS FOR LISTENING EXERCISE 20-1

Word	Pronunciation	Meaning
bradykinesia	brăd"ē-kĭ-nē'sē-ah	abnormal slowness of movement
facies	fā'shē-ēz	expression or appearance of the face
dysarthria	dĭs-ăr'thrē-ă	imperfect articulation of speech due to damage of the nervous system
pseudobulbar	sū"dō-bŭl'bĕr	apparently, but not really, due to a bulbar lesion
palsy	pawl'ze	paralysis
extrapyramidal disorder	ĕks"tră-pĭ-răm'ĭ-dăl	disorder marked by abnormal involuntary movements such as Parkinsonism

Listening Exercise 20-1

StudyWARE™ Connection

Listen to this report being read on your StudyWARE™ CD-ROM. Fill in each blank as the word is dictated.

Letter of Consultation

Dear Doctor Grimes:

Mr. Morton Herkimer recently returned for a recheck neurologic evaluation. Since leaving the hospital on the 7th of February, he has made considerable progress and has shown much improvement in his overall clinical condition. Of increasing concern has been tremor primarily involving the right upper extremity and _______________.

On neurological examination at this time I found Morton to be alert, bright, and communicative. The major findings were a prominent rest tremor involving the right upper extremity as well as bradykinesia with masked ________________, a mild hypokinetic ____________ and associated postural change. In addition, he had signs of a ______________ with positive jaw jerk, suck and snout reflexes, brisk deep tendon reflexes, and bilateral extensor plantar responses. His tone was increased bilaterally. The clinical findings are, thus, those of a parkinsonian-like picture with superimposed pseudobulbar palsy.

The question of antiparkinson therapy was quite appropriately raised by yourself, and I believe this to be quite reasonable. On discussing this with him, I, however, felt that we might be able to hold off on this therapy in view of the way his clinical picture seems to be changing and perhaps improving. Therapy at this point, therefore, seems optional.

As I review his overall clinical picture, one wonders if his progressive dysfunction beginning in January was not an initial manifestation of what will subsequently become more typical of an ___________________ of the parkinsonian type.

I suggested a recheck neurologic examination in approximately two to three months.

Sincerely yours,

J. Michael Sandok, MD

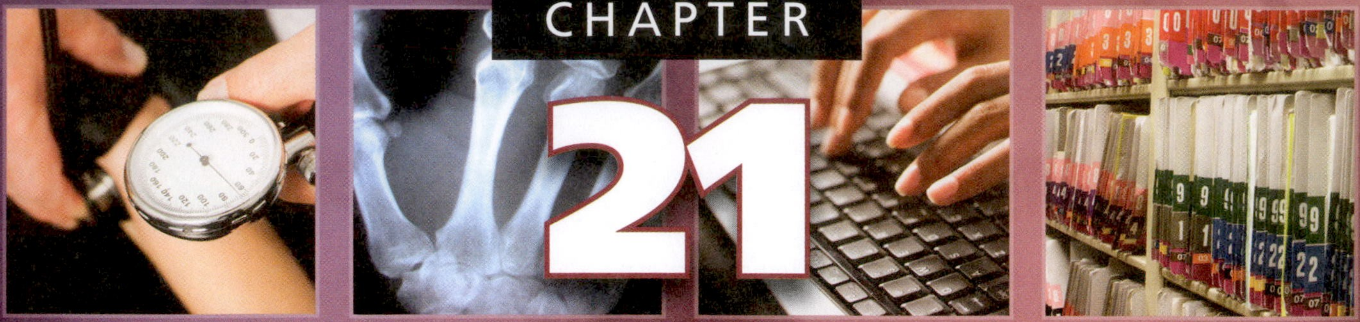

CHAPTER 21

Mental Health

"The Brain—is wider than the sky—for—put them side by side—
The one the other will contain with ease—and you—beside—"

—Emily Dickinson

OBJECTIVES

When you have completed this chapter on mental health, you should be able to

1. Define classifications of mental disorders.
2. Define the treatment process including the diagnostic interview, clinical tests, and psychotherapeutic techniques.
3. Spell the names of commonly used medications.
4. Identify abbreviations related to the mental health field.
5. Identify the names of related word elements.
6. Hear how medical terminology is used in actual medical reports.

INTRODUCTION

iatr/o	treatment, physician
ment/o	mind
psych/o	mind

Mental health describes a relative state of mind in which individuals who are healthy are able to cope with and adjust to the events of life, good or bad, in a way that allows their personalities to remain intact and even to grow emotionally. **Psychiatry** (sī-kī'ă-trē) is the medical specialty that deals with the development and maintenance of good mental health by dealing with causes, treatment, and prevention of mental, emotional, and behavioral disorders.

Understanding the relationship of the body, including the brain and nervous system, and psychological factors requires the expertise of a **psychiatrist** (sī-kī'ă-trĭst), who is a medical doctor with several additional years of training in methods of psychotherapy, neurology, and pharmacology. A psychiatrist may also specialize. For instance, forensic psychiatrists deal with legal situations such as determining mental competence in criminal cases, while child psychiatrists treat children. Geropsychiatrists specialize in the treatment of older adults.

In addition to the psychiatrist, there are nonmedical persons trained in psychology. A **psychologist** (sī-kŏl'ō-jĭst) has a doctorate in psychology, is qualified to use many of the same treatments as a psychiatrist, but may not use such techniques as electroconvulsive or drug therapies. A psychologist has training in psychotherapy and psychodiagnostic assessment through the use of various tests. Another position coming into prominence is the **Advanced Practice Nurse** (APN). This person is a registered nurse who has a Masters Degree or Doctorate Degree with a specific specialty—in this case, mental health. This specialist is qualified to prescribe medications under the supervision of a licensed physician. In some states this position may also be filled by a Nurse Practitioner or a Clinical Nurse Specialist (CNS).

Because psychiatry is not an anatomy-based specialty, this chapter will use a different format. It will look at the definition and classification of mental disorders, the types of treatment, the psychotherapeutic techniques used, including the psychiatric interview, the clinical tests administered, and abbreviations commonly used.

MULTIAXIAL CLASSIFICATION OF MENTAL DISORDERS

The *Diagnostic and Statistical Manual of Mental Disorders* (DSM-IV-TR) (2000) is the principal guide for mental health professionals. This edition incorporates information found when a literature review was conducted of research published since the 1994 version was printed. The term used in the DSM-IV-TR for a mental disturbance is **mental disorder**, but the term historically has not had one distinct definition. In fact, the DSM-IV-TR conceptualizes each mental disorder as

> a clinically significant behavioral or psychological syndrome or pattern that occurs in an individual and is associated with present distress or disability or with significantly increased risk of suffering death, pain, disability, or important loss of freedom. (p. xxii)

From the manual's perspective, categories of mental disorders are not limited by absolute boundaries dividing them from other mental disorders or, for that matter, from no mental disorder.

To help a mental health professional plan treatment for and predict outcomes of mental disorders, information from several domains, or axes, is useful. There are five axes included in the DSM-IV-TR. They are collectively referred to as the multiaxial assessment classification and are viewed as an efficient, effective way to organize and communicate information (see Table 21-1). These axes also closely coordinate with the *International Statistical Classification of Diseases and Related Health Problems* (ICD-9). The next version, ICD-10, expands the number of categories and will be available in the near future.

These five axes and some of their subcategories are discussed in the sections that follow.

TABLE 21-1 MULTIAXIAL ASSESSMENT CLASSIFICATIONS

Axis	Classification	Description
I	Clinical Disorders Other Conditions That May Be a Focus of Clinical Attention	Reports all various conditions or disorders in the classification except for personality disorders and mental retardation.
II	Personality Disorders Mental Retardation	Reports personality disorders and mental retardation.

continues

TABLE 21-1 MULTIAXIAL ASSESSMENT CLASSIFICATIONS

Axis	Classification	Description
III	General Medical Conditions	Reports current medical conditions that are potentially relevant to understanding or managing an individual's mental disorders.
IV	Psychosocial and Reports Environmental Problems	Psychosocial and environmental problems that may affect the diagnosis, treatment, and prognosis of mental disorder(s).
V	Global Assessment of Functioning	Reports the clinician's judgment of the individual's overall level of functioning and is useful in planning treatment, measuring its impact, and predicting its outcome.

AXIS I: CLINICAL DISORDERS AND OTHER CONSIDERATIONS THAT MAY BE A FOCUS OF CLINICAL ATTENTION

To follow is a list of some of the Axis I disorders included in the DSM-IV-TR.

Disorders first diagnosed in infancy, childhood, and adolescence
Delirium, dementia, and amnestic and other cognitive disorders
Substance-related disorders
Schizophrenia and other psychotic disorders
Mood disorders
Anxiety disorders
Somatoform disorders
Sexual and gender identity disorders
Sleep disorders
Impulse-control disorders

Disorders First Diagnosed in Infancy, Childhood, and Adolescence

Disorders First Diagnosed in Infancy, Childhood, and Adolescence include, among others, learning disorders, motor skills disorders, communication disorders, pervasive development disorders, and attention-deficit and disruptive behavior disorders.

Learning disorders may occur in children with normal health and intelligence but who have problems with the *ability* to learn. Usually such difficulties are limited to one particular academic skill such as reading, mathematics, or written expression. **Motor skills disorders** are characterized by motor coordination that is substantially below that expected for a person of a given age and intellectual level and includes developmental coordination disorder. **Communication disorders** are often characterized by failure to use speech sounds correctly, stuttering, or by slow speech development. **Pervasive development disorders** relate most specifically to social interaction with others as well as with family members. Behavior may include unreasonable insistence on routines, repetition of previously heard speech, or difficulty in naming objects. **Attention-deficit** and **disruptive behaviors** are separate problems despite the similarity of their names. An attention-deficit hyperactivity disorder (ADHD) is defined as the habitual inability of a child to pay attention for more than a minute or two. Medications can be used to help focus the child's attention and reduce overactivity. Disruptive behavior disorders violate the basic rights of others and include negative, hostile, and age-inappropriate behaviors.

Dementia, Delirium, and Amnestic and Other Cognitive Disorders

A significant decrease in memory capacity is one prominent symptom shared by dementia, delirium, and amnestic and other cognitive disorders. The cause may be either a general medical condition, an injury, or a substance.

Dementia (dē-mĕn'shē-ă) is a progressive, generally irreversible decline in mental function characterized by multiple cognitive deficits that include memory impairment. **Delirium** (dē-lĭr'ē-ŭm) is characterized by a disturbance in consciousness and a change in cognition that develops over a short period of time. An amnestic disorder is also a memory disturbance, but with the absence of other significant cognitive impairments.

Dementia, the more common of these conditions, is caused by the destruction of brain cells and refers to a group of illnesses that involve memory, behavior, learning, and communicating problems. The symptoms are progressive and may involve language, memory, perception, emotional behavior or personality, and cognitive skills (such as calculation, abstract thinking, or judgment). Dementia may be diagnosed when a patient has two or more problems in brain function. Higher mental functions are affected first in the process. The disorder is rare in those under 60 but has been diagnosed in 20 to 40 percent of those over 85, more frequently so in women than men.

Two major causes of degenerative (irreversible) dementia are Alzheimer's disease and vascular dementia. Treatment for degenerative dementia involves the use of acetylcholinestercase inhibitors (AChE) such as Aricept, Exelon, Reminyl, and Cognex and N-methyl-D-aspartate Blockers (NMDA) such as Namenda. Although these drugs do not halt the disease or reverse existing brain damage, they can improve symptoms and slow the progression of the disease.

But dementia may also be reversible, such as normal pressure hydrocephalus, brain tumors, and dementia due to metabolic causes, thyroid conditions, low vitamin B12 levels, and infections. If properly diagnosed, these conditions have been treated with favorable results.

Substance-Related Disorders

Long-term use of alcohol and drugs can result in a state of psychological and/or physical dependence, referred to as **substance-related disorders**. Psychological dependence occurs when a person compulsively takes a drug or alcohol in spite of dire consequences. Physical dependence produces serious and uncomfortable conditions, which are most apparent when withdrawal from a substance is being attempted. Substances known to be associated with dependency are: alcohol, which when used regularly and excessively, results in **alcoholism**, a chronic and often progressive disease; aerosol products, various aromatic glues and inhalants, and over-the-counter drugs such as barbiturates and benzodiazepines; marijuana and cannabis compounds; amphetamines (uppers) and cocaine; opioids painkillers such as Vicodin, hydrocodone, and OxyContin; hallucinogens such as LSD (lysergic acid diethylamide) and PCP (phencyclidine); and other substances such as caffeine and nicotine.

Detoxification (dē-tŏk"sĭ-fĭ-kā'shŭn), a medically supervised treatment program to counteract or destroy toxic properties, may be necessary if the patient becomes intoxicated with alcohol or any other drug. Regardless of the agent, withdrawal takes several days and may require a week or more of treatment, often in a hospital. Some individuals experience delirium tremens (DTs), which occur in withdrawal from alcohol. After detoxification, the patient should attend drug therapy sessions to learn the steps necessary to remain free of abusive substances.

Schizophrenia and Other Psychotic Disorders

phren/o	mind	schiz/o	split

The defining feature of the disorders in this classification is a group of psychotic symptoms that includes delusions, hallucinations, and disorganized thinking. The most frequent and most destructive form of the psychoses is **schizophrenia** (skĭz"ō-frē'nē-ă), which is characterized by withdrawal from reality into a fantasy world. The brain scan of a schizophrenic individual is shown in Figure 21.1. Individuals with these psychoses are unable to sustain self-initiated, goal-directed activity. Hallucinations are common, including the likelihood of hearing voices. If a patient exhibits symptoms for any of the types for just a few weeks and then fully recovers, the diagnosis is brief-reaction psychosis. However, should the symptoms endure for more than a month or two, full return to the previous level of functioning is unlikely. The consumption of large amounts of alcohol or drugs have been known to precipitate a substance-induced psychotic disorder.

Mood Disorders

-phoria	feeling

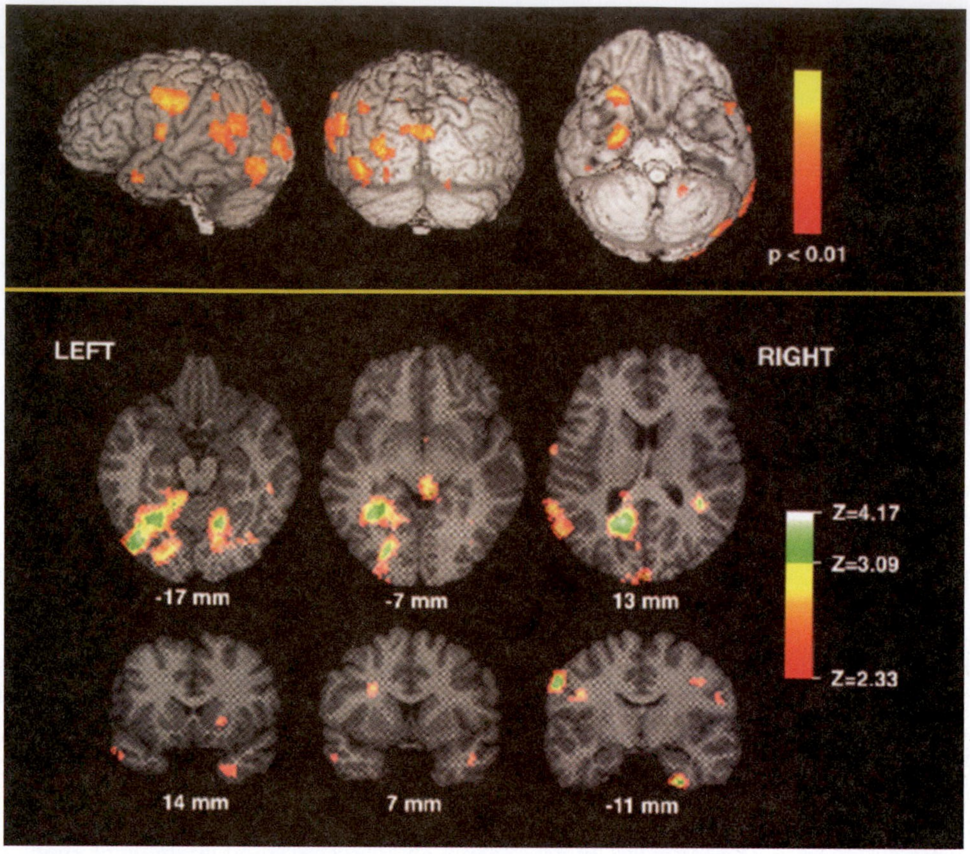

FIGURE 21-1 Surface and Slice Images of the Brain of a Patient With Schizophrenia

Courtesy of D. Silbersweig, M.D., and E. Stern, M.D. Functional Neuroimaging Laboratory, The New York Hospital-Cornell Medical Center

A prolonged emotion pervading an individual's entire mental life is referred to as a **mood disorder**. The DSM-IV-TR identifies two subcategories: depressive and bipolar.

Depressive disorders, whether mild or severe, have several common symptoms: withdrawal from activities, disturbed sleep, reduced appetite, inability to concentrate or make decisions, low energy levels, lack of self-esteem, and thoughts of suicide and death. A major depressive disorder (endogenous depression) is a genuine psychiatric illness affecting both body and mind. It can be so severe that the individual cannot function personally, socially, nor in the workplace. A situational depression is a midlife disappointment or loss followed by prolonged episodes of "the blues." A seasonal affective disorder (SAD) is a temporary condition generally occurring in the winter months when the days are shorter and grayer.

Bipolar disorder is sometimes referred to as manic-depressive illness. Primary symptoms are extreme and unpredictable mood swings from emotional highs (euphoria) to emotional lows (despair), which are not in response to circumstances as they could be for a normal person.

Anxiety Disorders

anxi/o	uneasy, anxious	phobia	fear

In the mental health field, an **anxiety disorder** refers to tension about an unidentified anger or fear relating to a specific cause. Both are normal reactions to the presence of danger, but if the symptoms persist for a month or more, treatment may be needed. Some specific examples follow.

A **panic attack** occurs when the individual displays normal physical reaction to life-threatening situations although there is no such situation present. It is a fairly common disorder that may be confused with cardiac or respiratory problems by the individual involved.

A **phobia** is a persistent, irrational fear triggered by a specific type of stimulus. Some common examples are *claustrophobia* (fear of being enclosed), *acrophobia* (fear of high places), and *agoraphobia* (fear of open public places).

An **obsessive-compulsive disorder** is a condition characterized by persistent thoughts (obsessions) and persistent behaviors (compulsions). The patient believes the obsessions are unrealistic and the compulsions are inappropriate, but is unable to resist the behavior.

Post-traumatic stress disorder occurs among survivors of traumatic events such as severe physical danger, harm, injury, and natural catastrophes. Individuals may experience vivid flashbacks resulting in a sense of detachment, estrangement from others, and a loss of all hope.

Somatoform Disorders

somat/o	body

Somatoform (sō-măt'ō-form) **disorders** are a group of disorders that suggest a general medical condition when no general medical condition fully accounts for the physical symptoms. These disorders are often referred to as psychosomatic illnesses. They usually begin at a time of crisis and clear up when the situation changes for the better or the individual learns to adapt.

A variety of conditions are included in this classification, some of which are:

- *Somatization disorder* is a condition of recurrent and multiple somatic complaints of several years' duration for which medical attention has been sought but no physical basis for the disorder has been found.
- *Conversion disorder* is a psychological disorder marked by symptoms affecting motor or sensory function mimicking a neurological or general medical disease.
- *Hypochondriasis* is a chronic, abnormal concern about one's health marked by the false belief of suffering from some disease, despite medical reassurance to the contrary.
- *Pain disorder* is a psychological disorder in which the patient unintentionally experiences pain in the absence of physiologic findings.

Sexual and Gender Identity Disorders

phil/o	attraction to, love

Sexual disorders are either sexual dysfunctions or paraphilia. **Sexual dysfunctions** (dĭs-fŭnk'shŭnz) are characterized by disturbances in both sexual desire and the psychophysiological changes that typify the sexual response cycle. As a result, the individual experiences marked distress and interpersonal difficulty.

Paraphilia (păr"ă-fĭl'ē-ă) are characterized by recurrent, intense sexual urges, fantasies, or behaviors. Consequently, clinically significant distress or impairment in social, occupational, or other important areas of functioning are experienced. Examples include exhibitionism, pedophilia, sexual sadism, and transvestic fetishism.

Gender identity disorders are characterized by persistent discomfort with one's sex. The individual has a strong and persistent cross-gender identification. The DSM-IV-TR cautions that

> notations of deviance, standards of sexual performance, and concepts of appropriate gender role can vary from culture to culture. (p. 493)

Sleep Disorders

Several different stages of sleep recur at fairly regular cycles throughout the sleep period: wakefulness, drowsiness, moderate sleep, deep sleep (whose cycle length decreases with age). **Sleep disorders** result in the disruption of one or more sleep stages. They include: insomnia, sleep apnea, narcolepsy, nightmares and night terrors, sleepwalking, and bruxism.

Eating Disorders

An **eating disorder** may be characterized by a compulsion to either eat or avoid eating. Three of the most common forms of eating disorders are anorexia nervosa, bulimia nervosa, and binge eating.

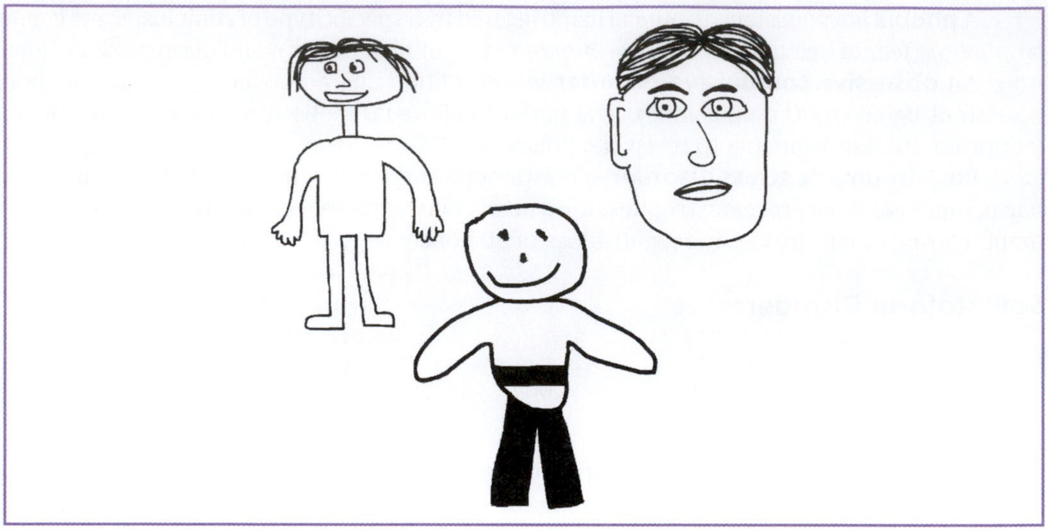

FIGURE 21-2
Samples of Persons Drawn by Different Individuals

In anorexia, the individuals chose to starve themselves. Figure 21-2 shows the consequences of such action. In bulimia, the individual eats a large quantity of food and then vomits before the food can be digested. The third type, binge eating disorder, exists when an individuals consumes huge amounts of food and is unable to stop or be in control of their eating. This results in morbid obesity, diabetes, hypertension, and cardiovascular disease. These three types of eating disorders affect every part of a person's life.

Impulse-Control Disorders

-mania	excessive preoccupation

The essential feature of **impulse-control disorders** is the failure to resist the temptation to perform an act harmful to the individual or to others. The individual experiences an increase in tension or arousal before committing the act and then feels relief as the act is committed. Following these acts, the individual may or may not feel regret. Examples of this disorder are: intermittent explosive disorder (impulsive destruction of property), kleptomania (stealing an object with no thought of gain), pyromania (setting of fires), and pathological gambling.

AXIS II: PERSONALITY DISORDERS AND MENTAL RETARDATION

Axis II is for reporting personality disorders and mental retardation. Using a separate axis for these disorders ensures that consideration will be given to issues that might otherwise be overlooked when attention is directed to Axis I disorders. A description of these disorders follows.

Personality Disorders

Personality disorders may interfere with an individual's behavior and interactions with other individuals. At the root is the inability to deal with the demands or the limitations of the world. Unfortunately, the individual may not recognize why these problems exist and probably considers them to be the fault of others. A brief description of some personality disorders follows.

Paranoid personality disorder exists when a patient considers himself or herself endowed with unique and superior abilities. In some cases, the paranoia is characterized by delusion of persecution.

Schizoid personality disorder is characterized by individuals who are usually loners and lack close friendships. They are indifferent to either praise or criticism and appear to have little need for any association with others.

Antisocial personality disorder (commonly called sociopathy) is characterized by repeated violation of the rights of others, unlawful behavior, and lack of remorse. This lack of concern for society's rules and expectations invariably results in law-breaking activities by the individual.

Borderline personality disorder is characterized by persons who have chronic problems such as moodiness, sadness, fearfulness, and interpersonal problems. They have difficulty maintaining a positive self-image and sometimes are impulsive to the point of engaging in damaging behavior.

Histrionic personality disorder is present when individuals with this disorder tend to be self-centered and constantly striving to gain attention. Emotions tend to be expressed in an exaggerated and highly intensive manner. Consequently the individual experiences unsatisfying and very volatile or unstable relationships.

Narcissistic personality disorder is present when a person seeks the admiration of others, but is indifferent to their needs. There is an exaggerated sense of importance and power leading the individual to assume a position of uniqueness. When the individual is rejected for such an attitude, excessive anger or shame may be displayed.

Dependent personality disorder is present when an individual cannot meet the ordinary demands of life. The individual perceives the self as helpless and allows others to assume responsibility for important decisions.

Obsessive-compulsive personality disorder is characterized by two key behaviors: inflexibility and a drive for perfection. An individual with this disorder tends to be overly concerned with details and rules and often loses sight of the overall purpose of an activity. Because work is considered more important than relationships, these individuals are perceived as being cold or indifferent.

Passive-aggressive personality disorder is demonstrated when an individual procrastinates about or ignores obligations to avoid fulfilling these responsibilities. The individual tends to work slowly or to deliberately perform poorly when the assigned task is not personally desirable. The blame for resulting problems is placed on others.

Mental Retardation

Mental retardation is a general term for a wide range of conditions—*not* diseases—that result in below-normal intellectual function. Causes for the disorder may derive from either internal or external factors. Retardation ranges from mild, requiring little adaptation, to profound, requiring special care and almost total supervision. There is no absolute measurement for retardation. When a child shows continued problems with language and motor skill development or social or emotional immaturity, an intelligence test may be administered on an individual basis.

AXES III, IV, V: THE REMAINING AXES

The remaining axes deal with current medical, psychosocial, and environmental problems. They attempt to provide the clinician's perception of the individual's overall status.

Axis III: General Medical Conditions

Axis III reports on general medical conditions that may have a bearing on the diagnosis or treatment of any mental disorder. The patient is encouraged to provide detailed responses and leave the determination of the relevancy of any condition to the health care provider.

Axis IV: Psychosocial and Environmental Problems

Axis IV reports psychosocial and environmental problems that may affect the diagnosis, treatment, and prognosis of a specific mental disorder. Psychosocial and environmental problems include a variety of factors such as social environment, education, occupation, housing, economic situation, and the legal system.

Axis V: Global Assessment of Functioning

Axis V reports the clinician's judgment of the patient's overall level of functioning and is useful in planning treatment, measuring its impact, and predicting its outcome.

THE TREATMENT PROCESS

A patient seeks help from or is referred for consultation with a psychiatrist or psychologist. Evaluating the problem begins with a diagnostic interview. From the information in the interview, the mental health professional determines whether clinical testing is necessary. Finally, an appropriate treatment is selected.

DIAGNOSTIC INTERVIEWS

Psychiatric/psychological evaluations, like medical evaluations, are critical to understanding the patient's problem because historical events provide the foundation for current behavior and attitudes. Both attempt to provide information that will aid in the diagnosis of a problem and suggest an appropriate treatment plan. The approach presented here is one that is commonly used.

1. **Identifying Characteristics**
   The patient's name, age, gender, marital status, occupation, and source of referral are determined.
2. **Presenting Problem**
   The problem is stated in the patient's own words.
3. **History of Present Illness**
   Symptoms and behavioral changes are chronologically recorded.
4. **Personal History**
   The patient is asked about the stages of life from infancy.
5. **Previous Medical History**
   Previous physical and psychiatric illnesses are noted.
6. **Personality Prior to Illness**
   Questions are asked about social relationships at home, work, and in the community; activities and interests; moods; religious and moral standards; ambitions; and drinking and smoking habits.
7. **Family History of Close Relatives**
   Information about family history of close relatives is essential since often there can be a predisposition to certain conditions.
8. **Mental Status**
   The interviewer makes an assessment of the patient's mental status, which is usually recorded under the following headings.
   - Appearance and behavior
   - Stream of talk—logical, relevant, realistic conversation
   - Thought content—any special preoccupations, misinterpretations, delusions
   - Perceptual abnormalities
   - Mood and affect
   - Concentration, insight, and motivation
   - Cognitive functions—level of consciousness, memory and orientation, general information, intelligence
   - Suicidal/homicidal ideation
   - Strengths and weaknesses

After the mental health professional reviews the data gathered, a decision is made as to whether additional psychological or clinical testing is necessary or what therapeutic intervention is most likely to be beneficial.

CLINICAL TESTS

Of the many clinical tests used by psychologists, the most frequently administered are personality, intelligence, neuropsychological, and projective tests. **Personality tests** quantify and/or describe personality structure and emotional functioning. This allows inferences and predictions to be made about an individual's adjustment to surrounding conditions. **Intelligence tests** quantify intellectual processes and the corresponding brain function. They provide an estimate of the person's intellectual capacity. **Neuropsychological** (nū"rō-sī"kō-lŏj'ĭ-kăl) **tests** allow more distinct deductions to be made about neurological impairment and about relationships between an impairment and intellectual, emotional, personality, and integrative functions. **Projective tests** use abstract patterns, cartoons, or unstructured stimuli to determine underlying personality traits, feelings, or attitudes. Examples of some commonly administered tests in each category are listed below.

Personality Tests

Personality, the relatively stable and predictable part of a person's thoughts and behavior, can be described as the way a person thinks, feels, and behaves. It includes conscious attitudes, values, and styles, as well as unconscious conflicts and defense mechanisms. Personality is evaluated with the following tests (among others).

Test	Description
Millon Clinical Multiaxial Inventory-III (MCMI-III)	self-report instrument for assessing DSM-IV-TR-related personality disorders and clinical syndromes
Millon Adolescent Clinic Inventory (MACI)	self-report instrument for assessing an adolescent's personality pattern along with self-reported concerns and clinical syndromes
Minnesota Multiphasic Personality Inventory-2 (MMPI-2)	most widely used test for adults that is designed to assess a number of the major patterns of personality and emotional disorders
Minnesota Multiphasic Personality Inventory-Adolescent (MMPI-A)	an empirically based measure of adolescent psychotherapy derived from the original MMPI test, which evaluates similar problems
Sixteen Personality Factors Questionnaire (16PF)	measures sixteen primary personality factors and five global factors that are more gender-, culture-, and race-neutral than previous versions

Intelligence Tests

Intelligence may be defined as the ability to comprehend something based on a combination of reasoning, memory, imagination, and judgment. The measurement of intelligence is called intelligence quotient (IQ). It is a numerical expression of the relationship of chronological age to mental age as ascertained by a specific test. Verbal aptitude, numerical skill, spatial relationships, perception, memory, and reasoning are capabilities most often examined. Other factors, such as determination, perseverance, artistic talent, creativity, and imagination, do not easily lend themselves to measurement and are generally not included in tests of intelligence.

Intelligence may be evaluated with these and other tests.

Test	Description
Wechsler Adult Intelligence Scale-III (WAIS-III)	evaluates adult intelligence
Wechsler Intelligence Scale for Children—Fourth Edition (WISC)	evaluates the intellectual ability of a child
Wechsler Preschool and Primary Scale of Intelligence—Revised (WPPSI-III)	assesses intelligence of children from approximately 3 to 7 years of age
Stanford-Binet (SB5)	assesses intelligence

Neuropsychological Tests

Neuropsychological tests are often referred to as "tests for brain damage." This field developed as a result of collaboration among neurologists, neurosurgeons, psychiatrists, and psychologists. Neuropsychological assessment has now grown to the extent that it is applied to areas that go well beyond clinical investigation of brain-damaged individuals.

Some neuropsychological tests are described in the following table.

Test	Description
Bender-Gestalt	graphomotor test of an individual's ability to copy figures; helps detect deficiencies in perception, movement, or coordination
Luria-Nebraska Neuropsychological Battery	comprehensive assessment of cortically-mediated functions, including sensory motor, language, calculation, memory, and concept formation skills
Wechsler Memory Scale—Revised	assesses memory for verbal and figure stimuli, meaningful and abstract material, and delayed as well as immediate recall

Projective Tests

Examples of tests using abstract stimuli to determine basic personality traits, feelings, or attitudes are listed below.

Test	Description
Children's Apperception Test (CAT)	assesses personality, level of maturity, and psychological health of children ages 3-10
Draw a Person Test	scoring system to meet the need for modernized, recently normed, and objective evaluation applied to human figure drawings produced by children and adolescents (see Figure 21-3)
Rorschach Technique	test in which a patient's description of a series of inkblots can be used to evaluate personality structure for clinical assessment and diagnosis
Thematic Apperception Test (TAT)	test that uses ambiguous pictures to stimulate stories, which enable a therapist to evaluate personality structure and reveals some of the dominant drives, emotions, sentiments, and conflicts of a personality

PSYCHOTHERAPEUTIC TECHNIQUES

Mental disorders require individually prescribed treatment. Therapeutic techniques for treating psychiatric illnesses are psychotherapy, psychotherapeutic medications, and electroconvulsive therapy.

Psychotherapy

The goal of **psychotherapy** (sī-kō-thĕr'ă-pē) is to treat mental illness using a variety of therapies which can take place in a variety of ways. For instance, psychodynamic therapy involves either one-on-one or group interactions and uses discussion, explanation, relaxation, exploration, and support techniques. Group therapy is conducted under the guidance of a therapist with six to ten patients. The group meets regularly to discuss their problems and is based on the belief that members with like problems can assist each other in confronting old habits and behaviors and developing new skills and behaviors. Group therapy may last for just a few sessions dealing with a specific problem, or it may be long term and open ended without specific problem focus.

Behavior therapies deal with techniques to change behavioral difficulties and are all based on learning theory. Focus is on the problem behavior rather than on an underlying specific psychological disorder. Symptoms are overcome through desensitization (repeated exposure) to situations about which the patient is concerned.

Other adjunctive therapies include techniques such as anxiety management training, social skills training, assertiveness training, biofeedback, and musical therapy.

Cognitive therapy is short-term psychotherapy to treat both depression and anxiety by acting on the belief that psychological disturbances result from faulty ways of thinking. The role of the therapist is to help restructure the patient's distorted perceptions through the use of verbal and behavioral modification techniques.

Brief therapy, or **solution-based therapy**, is a short-term therapy—usually limited to six to ten sessions—and is focused on a specific, observable problem. The goal is skill development. The assessment of the problem starts with what the patient believes should be changed. The therapist devises a solution based on what is working or not working for the patient. The current focus is on brief therapy rather than **psychoanalysis** (sī"kō-ă-năl'ĭ-sĭs), a lengthy and costly process which attempts to make the patient aware of unconscious conflicts and resolve them.

Regardless of the method selected for treatment, psychotherapy cannot change the patient's environment, but it can help the individual to cope more effectively with that environment, to evaluate personal priorities and stress responses, and to understand and accept oneself.

Psychotherapeutic Medications

There are three basic psychotherapeutic medications: antianxiety agents, antipsychotic agents, and antidepressants.

Antianxiety (ăn"tī-ang-zī'ĕ-tē) **agents** lessen anxiety in mild to moderate states of emotional upset. They also act as muscle relaxants. Examples of commonly used antianxiety agents are listed below.

Trade Name	Generic Name
Atarax, Vistaril	hydroxyzine
Ativan	lorazepam
BuSpar	buspirone
Klonopin	clonazepam
Librium	chlordiazepoxide
Tranxene	clorazepate dipotassium
Valium	diazepam
Xanax	alprazolam

Antipsychotic (ăn"tī-sī-kŏt'ĭk) **medications** reduce excitement and control hostile, aggressive behavior in schizophrenic patients. These medications provide a calming effect that makes the patient more responsive to therapy. Some examples are listed below.

Trade Name	Generic Name
Abilify	aripiprazole
Clozaril	clozapine

continues

Trade Name	Generic Name
Geodon	ziprasidone
Haldol	haloperidol
Invega	paliperidone
Loxitane	loxapine
Prolixin	fluphenazine
Risperdal	risperidone
Seroquel	quetiapine fumarate
Zyprexa	olanzapine

In the case of severe affective disorders such as bi-polar disorder, an illness is controlled with lithium medications (Eskalith, Lithane, Lithonate, Lithotabs). Those who cannot tolerate lithium may be helped by certain anticonvulsant drugs such as carbamazepine (Tegretol).

Antidepressants (ăn"tĭ-dē-prĕs'sănt) reverse depressive symptoms and produce feelings of well-being. Tricyclic antidepressants such as amitriptyline (Elavil), imigramine (Tofranil), and protriptyline (Vivactil) are all used in the treatment of severe depression; monoamine oxidase (MAO) inhibitors are ordered for patients who do not respond to tricyclic antidepressants. In addition to amphetamines, Central nervous system stimulants like selective serotonin reuptake inhibitors (SSRI) (Paxil, Prozac, Zoloft) and serotonin-norepinephrine reuptake inhibitors (SNRI) (Cymbalta, Effexor), which both work on serotonin and norepinephrine, are prescribed to produce mood elevation.

Names for some commonly used antidepressants are identified below.

Trade Name	Generic Name
Anafranil	clomipramine
Celexa	citalopram
Cymbalta	duloxetine
Depakote	divalproex sodium
Effexor	venlafaxine
Elavil	amitriptyline HCl
Lamictal	lamotrigine
Pamelor	nortriptyline
Paxil	paroxetine
Prozac	fluoxetine
Remeron	mirtazapine
Tofranil	imipramine HCl
Wellbutrin	bupropion
Zoloft	sertraline

Other medications that are used specifically for attention-deficit disorder are Cylert (pemoline), Ritalin (methylphenidate), and Adderall (amphetamine mixed salts).

Electroconvulsive Therapy

Electroconvulsive therapy is used for major depressive episodes that have been unresponsive to medications. The patient is given a barbiturate and muscle relaxant prior to application of a brief, low-grade electrical current that is passed through pads attached to the head. The treatment usually provides results very quickly, often within a few days. In most situations this therapy can be used with minimal side effects.

ABBREVIATIONS

These are some abbreviations commonly used by mental health professionals.

ADHD	attention-deficit hyperactivity disorder
CA	chronological age
DTs	delirium tremens
ECT	electroconvulsive therapy
GAD	generalized anxiety disorder
IQ	intelligence quotient
MA	mental age
MACI	Millon Adolescent Clinical Inventory
MCMI-III	Millon Clinical Multiaxial Inventory-III
MDD	major depressive disorder
MMPI-2	Minnesota Multiphasic Personality Inventory-2
MMPI-A	Minnesota Multiphasic Personality Inventory-Adolescent
OCD	obsessive-compulsive disorder
PTSD	post-traumatic stress disorder
SAD	seasonal affective disorder
SB5	Stanford-Binet, Fifth Edition
TAT	Thematic Apperception Test
WAIS-III	Wechsler Adult Intelligence Scale-III
WBST	Wonderlic Basic Skills Test
WISC-IV	Wechsler Intelligence Scale for Children, Fourth Edition
WPPSI-III	Wechsler Preschool and Primary Scale of Intelligence—Third Edition

INTERNET ASSIGNMENT

The National Institute of Mental Health (NIMH) at **www.nimh.nih.gov** is one of the National Institutes of Health organizations. The mission of the NIMH is to diminish the burden of mental illness through research. Their web site states that "this public health mandate demands that we harness powerful scientific tools to achieve better understanding, treatment, and eventually prevention of mental disorder." The site offers public information about the symptoms, diagnosis, and treatment of mental illness. Brochures and information sheets, reports, press releases, fact sheets, and other education materials are offered. Selecting Health and Outreach offers options to learn more about mental health topics and to identify available publications or clinical trials. Selecting MH Cornerstone from the list at the left of the homepage brings up mental health information related to the U.S. Department of Health and Human Services research, programs, policies, and media campaigns. A topic search list is included.

ACTIVITY

Access the National Institute of Mental Health at **www.nimh.nih.gov**. Select Health and Outreach. This section offers information from NIMH about the symptoms, diagnosis, and treatment of mental illnesses. Select one of the links and report your findings to your instructor.

Review *Mental Health*

- The field of mental health includes psychiatrists and psychologists who are concerned with the diagnosis, treatment, and prevention of mental illness.
- Five axes delineate mental disorders and the factors that impact their presence in a patient's life. They are: clinical disorders, personality disorders and mental retardation, general medical conditions, psychosocial and environmental problems, and global assessment of functioning.
- Psychological treatment can involve several techniques: psychotherapy, psychotherapeutic medication, and electroconvulsive therapy.
- Treatment is usually determined on the basis of an interview and various psychological tests (personality, intelligence, neuropsychological, and projective).

Key Terminology Review

Word	Definition
Advanced Practice Nurse (APN)	registered nurse with an advanced degree (MS or PhD) within a specific specialty; also called an Clinical Nurse Specialist (CNS) or Nurse Practitioner
alcoholism	chronic and often progressive disease resulting when alcohol is used regularly and excessively
antianxiety agent	medication that lessens anxiety in mild to moderate states of emotional upset
antidepressant	medication that reverses depressive symptoms and produces feelings of well-being
antipsychotic medication	medication that reduces excitement and controls hostile, aggressive behavior in schizophrenic patients
anxiety disorder	tension about an unidentified anger and fear relating to a specific cause
attention-deficit hyperactivity disorder (ADHD)	disorder characterized by a habitual inability to pay attention for more than a minute or two
bipolar disorder	manic-depressive illness; extreme and unpredictable mood swings from emotional highs (euphoria) to emotional lows (despair)

continues

Word	Definition
brief therapy (or solution-based therapy)	short-term therapy that focuses on a specific, observable problem with the goal of developing a skill to solve it
cognitive therapy	therapy that focuses on helping a patient reconstruct faulty thinking instead of emotions
communication disorder	disorder characterized by failure to use speech sounds correctly or slow speech development
delirium	condition characterized by a disturbance of consciousness and a change in cognition that develops over a short period of time
dementia	condition characterized by multiple cognitive deficits that include impairment in memory; leads to a progressive, generally irreversible decline in mental function
depressive disorder	mood disorder characterized by mild to severe symptoms affecting sleep, appetite, concentration, and interest in life; may be endogenous, situational, or seasonal
detoxification	medically supervised treatment program to counteract or destroy toxic properties in the body
disruptive behavior disorder	disorder characterized by behavior that violates the basic rights of others and includes negative, hostile, and age-inappropriate behaviors
eating disorder	a condition characterized by a compulsion to either eat or avoid eating
electroconvulsive therapy	therapeutic technique used for major depressive episodes that have been unresponsive to medications
gender identity disorder	disorder characterized by persistent discomfort with one's gender
impulse-control disorder	disorder characterized by the failure to resist an impulse, drive, or temptation to perform an act that is harmful to the individual or to others
intelligence test	test that quantifies intellectual processes and the corresponding brain function
learning disorder	disorder found in children with normal health and intelligence but who have problems with the ability to learn
mental disorder	clinically significant behavior associated with distress, disability, increased risk of suffering death, pain, disability, or important loss of freedom
mental health	a relative state of mind in which a healthy individual is able to cope with and adjust to the events of life in a way that maintains mental stability
mental retardation	condition resulting in below-normal intellectual functioning
mood disorder	disorder occurring when a prolonged emotion pervades an individual's entire mental life
motor skills disorder	disorder characterized by motor coordination that is substantially below that expected for a person of a given age and intellectual level
neuropsychological test	test that allows more distinct inferences to be made about neurological impairment and relationships between an impairment and intellectual, emotional, personality, and integrative functions

continues

Word	Definition
obsessive-compulsive	condition characterized by unrealistic thoughts (obsessions) and disorder behaviors (compulsions) in spite of the patient's awareness that they are inappropriate
panic attack	normal physical reaction to a life-threatening situation although no such situation is present
paraphilia disorder	characterized by recurrent, intense sexual urges, fantasies, or behaviors that include unusual objects, activities, or situations
personality disorder	disorder that may interfere with an individual's behavior and interactions with other individuals because of an inability to deal with the demands or the limitations of the world
personality test	test that quantifies and/or describes personality structure and emotional functioning
pervasive development disorder	syndrome that begins in infancy and applies to a child who is unresponsive to other people, including its parents
phobia	persistent, irrational fear triggered by a specific type of stimulus
post-traumatic stress disorder	anxiety disorder characterized by an acute emotional response to a traumatic event or situation involving severe emotional stress
projective test	test that uses abstract or unstructured stimuli to determine underlying personality traits
psychiatrist	medical doctor with several additional years of training in the methods of psychotherapy, neurology, and pharmacology
psychiatry	medical specialty that deals with the diagnosis, treatment, and prevention of mental disorders
psychoanalysis	therapy that attempts to make patients aware of unconscious conflicts that are at the root of their illness
psychologist	nonmedical person with a doctorate in psychology
psychotherapy	method used to treat mental illness using a variety of techniques
schizophrenia	disorder characterized by withdrawal from reality into a fantasy world
sexual dysfunction	disorder characterized by disturbance in sexual desire and in the psychophysiological changes that characterize the sexual response cycle resulting in marked distress and interpersonal difficulty
sleep disorder	irregularities in the sleep cycle
somatoform disorder	disorder that suggests a general medical condition, but when no general medical condition fully accounts for the physical symptoms
substance-related disorder	disorder that results in psychological and/or physical dependence on alcohol and drugs

Terminology Review Exercises

DEFINITIONS

Define the following terms.

1. psychiatry
____
2. learning disorder
____
3. impulse-control disorder
____
4. attention-deficit hyperactivity disorder
____
5. antidepressant medication
____
6. mental disorder
____
7. obsessive-compulsive personality disorder
____

COMPLETION

Complete the following statements.

1. The principal classification guide of mental disorders for mental health professionals is ____________________.
2. Application of the five axes to the planning and implementing of treatment for a patient is referred to as ____________________.
3. The DSM-IV-TR coordinates closely with ____________________.
4. Axis II mental disorders are ____________________ disorders, as well as mental retardation.
5. The relative state of mind in which individuals who are healthy are able to cope with all of the events of life, good or bad, in a way that allows their personalities to remain intact and even to grow emotionally is referred to as ____________________.
6. A disorder characterized by withdrawal from reality into a fantasy world is ____________________.
7. The four types of tests most commonly used by psychiatrists and psychologists to measure mental ability and status are: ____________________, ____________________, ____________________, and ____________________.
8. Treatment options for mental disorders include: ____________________, ____________________, and ____________________.
9. When an individual procrastinates about or ignores obligations to avoid fulfilling these responsibilities, the patient is said to have a ____________________.

MATCHING/DISORDERS

Match symptom or complaint with correct disorder.

1. _________ persistent discomfort with one's own sexuality
2. _________ below-normal intellectual functioning
3. _________ manic-depressive illness
4. _________ prolonged emotion pervading an individual's entire life
5. _________ persistent, irrational fear
6. _________ physical complaint with no apparent physical basis
7. _________ responding to a normal event as if it were an emergency
8. _________ helping patient to reconstruct faulty thinking
9. _________ child who is unresponsive to others, including family
10. _________ recurrent, intense sexual urges or fantasies

a. bipolar disorder
b. cognitive therapy
c. gender identity disorder
d. mental retardation
e. mood disorder
f. panic attack
g. paraphilia
h. pervasive development disorder
i. phobia
j. somatoform disorder

SHORT ANSWER

Provide an answer in your own words.

1. Explain the difference between dementia and delirium.

____

____

____

2. What is the major difference between a psychiatrist and a psychologist?

____

____

____

3. Explain the difference between psychoanalysis and brief therapy.

____

____

____

4. Explain the differences between antianxiety agents, antipsychotic agents, and antidepressants.

____

____

____

MATCHING/TESTS

Match the tests to their names.

1. _________ evaluates adult intelligence
2. _________ "inkblot" test
3. _________ graphomotor test that detects deficiencies
4. _________ most commonly used objective personality test
5. _________ intelligence test for very young children
6. _________ assesses DSM-IV-TR-related personality disorders and clinical syndromes
7. _________ comprehensive assessment of cortically-mediated functions
8. _________ uses human figure drawings of children to determine basic personality feelings
9. _________ uses ambiguous pictures to evaluate personality structure
10. _________ assesses memory for verbal and figure stimuli, delayed and immediate recall, and meaningful and abstract material
11. _________ evaluates intellectual ability of a child
12. _________ measure of adolescent psychotherapy derived from theoriginal MMPI test

a. Bender-Gesalt
b. Draw A Person
c. Luria-Nebraska Neuropsychological Battery
d. Millon Clinical Multiaxial Inventory-III
e. Minnesota Multiphasic Personality Inventory-2
f. MMPI-A
g. Rorschach Technique
h. Thematic Apperception Test
i. WAIS-III
j. Wechsler Intelligence Scale for Children—Fourth edition
k. Wechsler Memory Scale-Revised
l. WPPSI-III

ABBREVIATIONS

Identify each of the following abbreviations.

1. ADHD ______________________
2. CA ______________________
3. DTs ______________________
4. ECT ______________________
5. IQ ______________________
6. MA ______________________
7. OCD ______________________
8. SAD ______________________
9. TAT ______________________
10. WAIS-III ______________________

Word Element Review

Root	Meaning	Example	Definition
anxi/o	uneasy	**anxiolytic** (ăng"zī-ō-lĭt'ĭk)	mild sedative used for relief of anxiety
iatr/o	treatment, physician	**psychiatry** (sī-kī'ah-trē)	branch of medicine that deals with the causes, diagnosis, treatment, and prevention of mental illness
ment/o	mind	**dementia** (dĕ-mĕn'shē-ah)	mental deterioration due to organic brain disease
phil/o	attracted to, love	**philoneism** (fĭ-lō'nē-ĭsm)	excessive fondness for newness or change
phren/o	mind	**schizophrenic** (skĭz"ō-frĕn"ĭk)	mental disorder characterized by disturbances of thinking, mood, and behavior
psych/o	mind	**psyche** (sī"kē)	all that encompasses the mind and its processes
schiz/o	split	**schizoid** (skĭz'oyd)	traits of shyness, sensitivity, social withdrawal, and introversion
somat/o	body	**psychosomatic** (sī"kō-sō-măt'ĭk)	pertaining to the mind/body relationship

Suffix	Meaning	Example	Definition
-mania	excessive preoccupation	**kleptomania** (klĕp"tō-mā"nē-ah)	obsession to steal
-phobia	fear	**xenophobia** (zĕn"ō-fō'bē-ah) (*xeno* = "stranger")	abnormal fear of strangers
-phoria	feeling	**dysphoria** (dĭs-fō'rē-ah)	exaggerated feeling of depression and unrest without apparent cause
		euphoria (ū-fō'rē-ah)	exaggerated feeling of well-being

Word Element Practice Exercises

WORD ELEMENT AND DEFINITION

In each of the following terms, circle the word element that was presented in this chapter. Then define the term.

1. kleptomania (*klepto* = "steal")

   ____

2. xenophobia (*xeno* = "stranger")

   ____

3. dysphoria

   ____

4. anxiolytic

   ____

5. philoneism

   ____

6. psychosomatic

   ____

7. psychiatry

   ____

8. schizophrenic

   ____

9. psyche

   ____

SHORT ANSWERS

Supply a short answer to the following.

1. Name the three word elements that mean "mind."

   ____

2. Name a word element that refers to the body.

   ____

3. Name several word elements that refer to the quality of feeling.

   ____

4. Name the one word element that when joined with *psych* makes a word that identifies the branch of medicine dealing with mental illness.

   ____

5. Name the two word elements that can stand alone as words.

   ____

MATCHING

Match the word elements to their meanings.

1. _________ mind	a. anxi/o
2. _________ body	b. iatr/o
3. _________ uneasy	c. -mania
4. _________ feeling	d. ment/o, phren/o, psych/o
5. _________ excessive preoccupation	e. -phobia
6. _________ fear	f. -phoria
7. _________ treatment, physician	g. somat/o

WORD ELEMENTS

Provide the word element to complete the following words.

1. traits of shyness, sensitivity, social withdrawal, and introversion ______________________ oid
2. fear of strangers xeno ______________________
3. exaggerated feeling of depression and unrest without apparent cause dys ______________________
4. mental deterioration de ______________________ ia
5. exaggerated feeling of well-being eu ______________________

WORD ELEMENT MEANINGS

Give the meaning of each word element. Then use your dictionary to find a new word that contains each of the word elements. Specify whether the new word is a noun or an adjective by placing N or A in the last column.

Word Element	Meaning	Word	N or A
1. anxi/o	_________	_________	_________
2. iatr/o	_________	_________	_________
3. -mania	_________	_________	_________
4. ment/o	_________	_________	_________
5. phil/o	_________	_________	_________
6. -phobia	_________	_________	_________
7. -phoria	_________	_________	_________
8. phren/o	_________	_________	_________
9. psych/o	_________	_________	_________
10. schiz/o	_________	_________	_________
11. somat/o	_________	_________	_________

Dictionary Exercises

DICTIONARY EXERCISE 1

Use your dictionary to find the pronunciation and definition of the following words.

	Word	Pronunciation	Definition
1.	dissociation	____________	____________
2.	catatonia	____________	____________
3.	confabulation	____________	____________
4.	cyclothymia	____________	____________
5.	cyclothymic personality	____________	____________
6.	dysthymia	____________	____________
7.	hallucination	____________	____________
8.	hypnosis	____________	____________
9.	id	____________	____________
10.	mania	____________	____________
11.	enuresis	____________	____________
12.	ego	____________	____________
13.	encopresis	____________	____________
14.	narcolepsy	____________	____________

DICTIONARY EXERCISE 2

Rewrite the following sentences in your own words.

1. A strong feeling of *déjà vu* swept over her as she entered the conference room.

   ____

2. The idea was an *obsession*.

   ____

3. The doctor indicated that her father suffers from *anxiety*.

   ____

4. The psychiatrist knew that his patient's actions were the result of *narcissism*.

   ____

5. The patient's *superego* was not fully developed.

   ____

6. He was suffering from *post-traumatic stress syndrome*.

   ____

DICTIONARY EXERCISE 3

Match the terms to their meanings.

1. ________ affect
2. ________ illusion
3. ________ delirium
4. ________ psychomotor
5. ________ pyromania
6. ________ compulsion
7. ________ anorexia nervosa
8. ________ delusions
9. ________ senile
10. ________ hallucinogens
11. ________ bulimia nervosa
12. ________ dysphoria
13. ________ labile

a. misinterpreted sensory impression
b. abnormal drive to do something
c. psychosomatic eating disorder
d. false beliefs resulting from unconscious needs
e. emotional reactions associated with an experience
f. impulse-control disorder characterized by setting fires
g. relating to old age; exhibit symptoms of impaired memory or mental capability
h. acute, temporary disturbance of consciousness
i. drug that produces hallucinations
j. mental origin of muscular movements
k. recurrent episodes of binge eating
l. hopelessness
m. unstable

DICTIONARY EXERCISE 4

Pronunciation of the words below is provided. Using your dictionary, find the correct spelling and definition of each word.

	Word	Pronunciation	Definition
1.	________	ăm-nē'zē-ah	________
2.	________	aw'tĭzm	________
3.	________	ăp-nē'ă	________
4.	________	voy'ĕr-izm	________
5.	________	hī"pō-kŏn'drē-ah	________
6.	________	mū'tĭzm	________
7.	________	trănz	________
8.	________	brŭk'sĭzm	________
9.	________	bī"ō-fēd'băk	________
10.	________	sō"mah-tī-zā'shŭn	________
11.	________	ăp'ah-thē	________
12.	________	ăm-nēs'tĭk disorder	________
13.	________	ĭn-sŏm'nē-ah	________
14.	________	bē-rēv'mĕnt	________

*Study*WARE™ Connection

To take a practice quiz or play interactive games that reinforce the content in this chapter, go to your StudyWARE™ CD-ROM.

Listening Exercises

INSTRUCTIONS

1. Review the spelling, pronunciation, and meaning of the words provided in the preview.
2. Go to your StudyWARE™ CD-ROM and listen to **Listening Exercises 21-1 and 21-2**. Fill in the blank in the report as the word is dictated.
3. At the end of each activity, check your spelling against the preview words. They appear in the preview in the order in which they are encountered in each activity.
4. Review and practice the words you missed.
5. Look up words that are not familiar.

PREVIEW OF WORDS FOR LISTENING EXERCISES 21-1 AND 21-2

Word	Pronunciation	Meaning
Exercise 21-1: Progress Note		
phobic	fō'bĭk	irrational fear or aversion
relaxation responses		managing anxieties or phobias through the application of relaxation techniques to reduce tension
desensitization	dē-sĕn"sĭ-tĭ-zā'shŭn	treatment of phobias by intentionally exposing the patient to emotionally distressing stimuli
Exercise 21-2: Projective Test Analysis		
denial		defense mechanism where unpleasant realities are denied and unrecognized
repression		defense mechanism where a person avoids unpleasant situations by "forgetting" them
projection		unconscious defense mechanism where personal inadequacies are blamed on someone else

Listening Exercises 21-1 and 21-2

StudyWARE™ Connection

Listen to the following reports being read on your StudyWARE™ CD-ROM. Fill in each blank as the word is dictated.

Progress Notes

In today's session, the focus was on reduction of ____________________ responses related to flying. Ms. Chang had begun to practice the ____________________ we began to rehearse last session. Using the audio tape we made, she was able to gain some simple relaxation experiences. During the session today, we began developing a hierarchy of events leading up to actual flying itself to be utilized for the systematic ____________________. This list will need to be reviewed for the level of anxiety attached to each specific item.

Projective Test Analysis

The projective testing done on Mr. Ravioli suggests him to be a rather rigid, indecisive, cautious, and dependent person who defends against anxiety through the use of ____________________, ____________________, ____________________, and intellectualization. Generally, he views himself as living in an environment that is somewhat threatening, demanding, restraining, and unpredictable. Specifically, he appears to be apprehensive about close, interpersonal relationships, fear of loss of individuality, and fear of rejection. Because of this, he is restricted in his ability to express warm and tender emotions and instead copes by rigidly defining expectations and overcontrolling emotions and impulses. Under stressful situations, one would expect him to become preoccupied with rules and order and attempts to further impose these on others around him. In situations where he might assert himself, however, he is more apt to submit or passively accept things for fear of reprisal. Leadership abilities would therefore be limited.

CHAPTER 22

The Eye

"The keenest of all our senses is the sense of sight."

—Cicero

OBJECTIVES

When you have completed this chapter on the optic system, you should be able to

1. Spell and define major system components and explain how they operate.
2. Identify the meaning of related word elements.
3. Spell and define diagnostic procedures, diagnoses, treatment procedures, and abbreviations.
4. Spell the names of commonly used medications.
5. Use a dictionary as a tool in processing medical documents.
6. Hear how medical terminology is used in actual medical reports.

INTRODUCTION

The eye is the organ of sight. Combined with its accessory organs, this system is one of the most important sensory organs in the body. It warns of danger, gives a sense of direction, and aids in the performance of daily activities. Its care lies primarily in the hands of the ophthalmologist and the optometrist. An **ophthalmologist** (ŏf"thăl-mŏl'ō-jĭst) is a physician surgeon who specializes in the diagnosis and treatment of diseases of the eye. An **optometrist** (ŏp-tŏm'ĕ-trĭst) is a nonsurgeon specialist who tests the eye for visual acuity, prescribes corrective lenses, and recommends eye exercises. Recently, optometrists have been given privileges to prescribe medications and treat diseases of the eye.

LOCATION AND ACCESSORY STRUCTURES

blephar/o	eyelid	opt/o, optic/o	eye, vision
conjunctiv/o	conjunctiva	palpebr/o	eyelid
dacry/o	tear, tear duct	tars/o	eyelid
lacrim/o	tear	-tropia	to turn
-opia, -opsia	vision		

The eye is one of the few exposed organs of the body. However, it is well protected. The eyeball, located in the eye socket (or orbit), is embedded and cushioned in fat and connective tissue. Movement of the eyeball is controlled by six muscles. Figure 22-1 shows two of them: the **lateral** (1) and **medial** (7) **recti** muscles. The four other muscles are the **superior** and **inferior recti** and the **superior** and **inferior oblique**. The optic (ŏp'tĭk) nerve, ocular (ŏk'ū-lăr) muscles, and other nerves and vessels attach to the eyeball within the protection of the eye socket.

The front or anterior portion of the eyeball is covered by a very soft mucous membrane called the **conjunctiva** (kŏn"jŭnk-tī'vah) (14). The eyeballs and eye sockets are protected by the eyelids. These lids, and the eyelashes attached to them, protect the eyes from foreign materials. The shape of the eyelid is maintained by the **tarsal** (tahr'săl) **plate**.

Lacrimal and tarsal glands protect the eye. The **lacrimal** (lăk'rĭ-măl) **glands**, or tear glands, lie laterally and superiorly behind the shelter of the bones that form the eye orbit. Secretions (or tears) move by lacrimal ducts to the conjunctiva. Blinking spreads moisture over the eye to clean and lubricate it. These tears are drained into the nose by two small openings in the inner corners of the upper and lower eyelids called punctum. The nasolacrimal drainage system consists of the canaliculi, the lacrimal sac, and the nasolacrimal canal. That is why crying results in a runny nose.

Tarsal or **meibomian** (mī-bō'mē-ăn) **glands**, are located close to the inner surface of the eyelid and are embedded in the tarsal plates. The ducts of the meibomian glands lie in the eyelid margin and excrete oil that helps lubricate the eyelid and prevent the overflow of tears.

Above the eyes an additional row of hair forms the eyebrows (supercilia), which also aid in protection.

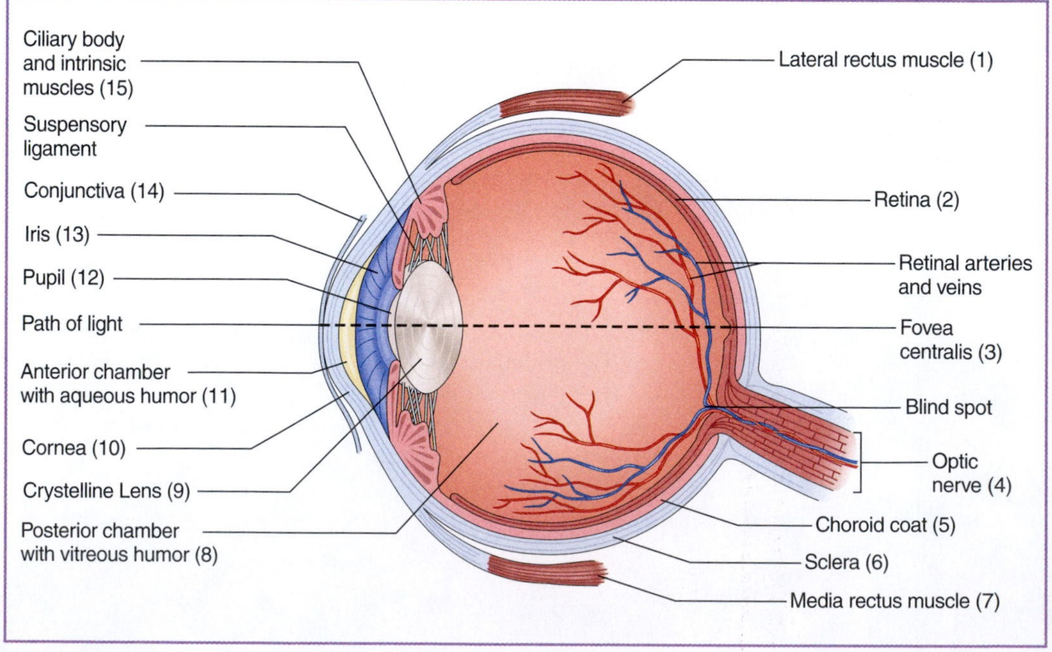

FIGURE 22-1
The Anatomy of the Eye, Transverse View

COMPOSITION OF THE EYE

aque/o	water	pupill/o	pupil
cor/o, core/o	pupil	retin/o	retina
corne/o	cornea	scler/o	sclera
ir/o, irid/o	iris	vitre/o	glassy
kerat/o	horny, cornea		

The eye is composed of three distinct layers known as **tunics**. Each of the tunics gives rise to various structures of the eye. The outermost tunic consists of the cornea (10) and the sclera (6). The **cornea** (kor'nē-ah) is the transparent anterior segment that allows light to pass directly through the eye. The **sclera** (sklē'rah) is the fibrous posterior segment that gives shape to the eyeball. It is also referred to as the white of the eye.

The middle tunic includes the choroid, the ciliary body, and the iris. The **choroid** (kō'roid) (5) is a thin, soft membrane that covers the posterior of the eyeball. It has a dark brown appearance caused by a black pigment that absorbs extra light. It also maintains the nutrition of the retina.

An extension of the choroid is the **ciliary** (sĭl'ē-ĕr"ē) **body** (15). This muscle connects to the iris, secretes aqueous humor, and flexes to bring the crystalline lens into focus on near or far objects—a process called **accommodation**.

The third structure of the middle tunic is the **iris** (13), the part that gives the eye its color. At its center is a round opening called the **pupil** (12) through which light enters the eye. The movement of the ring of muscle fibers that make up the iris determines the size of the pupil and therefore the amount of light admitted into the eye.

Just behind the iris is the capsular structure called the **crystalline** (krĭs'tah-līn) **lens** (9), which focuses light rays on the retina. The shape of the lens is altered by the action of the ciliary muscle. The crystalline lens also separates the anterior and posterior chambers of the eye. Circulating through both of these chambers is a clear, watery fluid called the **aqueous** (ā'kwē-ŭs) **humor** (11). In addition, the posterior chamber holds a transparent, semigelatinous substance called the **vitreous** (vĭt'rē-ŭs) **humor** (8).

The innermost tunic is the **retina** (rĕt'ĭ-nah) (2), which receives the images a person sees. Everything one sees comes to focus on the **fovea** (fō'vē-ah) (3). It is an area near the center of the retina that is smaller than a pinhead. The retina has specialized receptors, or nerve endings, known as **rods** and **cones**. The retina transmits visual impulses through the **optic nerve** (4) to the brain.

StudyWARE™ Connection

Play an interactive game labeling structures of the **Eye** on your StudyWARE™ CD-ROM.

HOW THE EYE WORKS

The image of an object reaches the eye in the form of light waves that are bent as they first pass through the cornea and then through the pupil, the opening in the iris. The ciliary muscle changes the shape of the crystalline lens to focus the image (now inverted) on the retina, as shown in Figure 22-2. Here light waves stimulate the rods and cones (the sensory receptors) where they are translated into nerve impulses. The nerve impulses are transmitted by the optic nerve to the occipital lobe at the back of the brain where we actually "see."

StudyWARE™ Connection

To watch an animation of how we see, go to your StudyWARE™ CD-ROM.

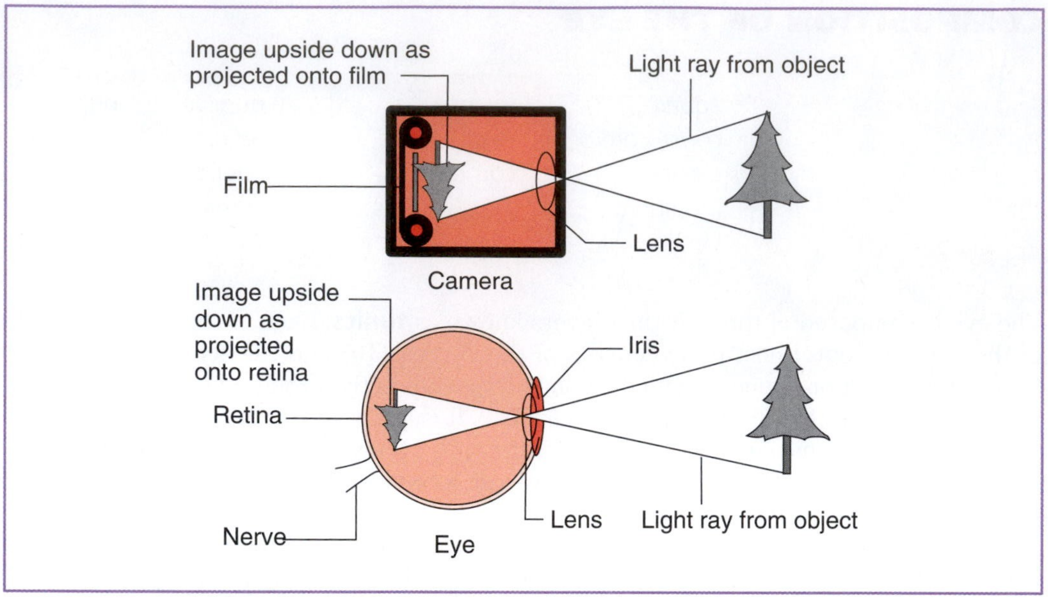

FIGURE 22-2
How the Eye Works

INTERNET ASSIGNMENT

NetWellness at **www.netwellness.org** is a web site whose purpose is to make consumer health information available to the public. It is sponsored by the University of Cincinnati, Case Western Reserve University, and The Ohio State University (OSU). NetWellness operates like a library in that it offers information, not medical advice. Links to other health related information that has been reviewed for quality, accuracy, and currency are provided and include:

- Adam Health Encyclopedia
- Clinical Trials.gov
- Drug information from MedMasters and USP DI Advice for the Patient
- MedlinePlus
- Merck Publications
- OSU patient education material
- PubMed
- Translations
- Your Child's Health

ACTIVITY

Access NetWellness at **www.netwellness.org**. Select Health topics from the list in the first box at the right side of the page. Scroll down Health Topics and select Eyes and Vision. Go to that screen and select Treatment from the horizontal bar. From the options provided in this section, select a link to your choice of topic. Review the type of information provided for your instructor.

Return to the home page and go to the Reference Library. From the references listed, select MedlinePlus. Select Drugs and Supplements from the list on the right side of the screen. Select one of the drugs presented in your text in Chapter 22 and click on the appropriate letter. Briefly review the content provided on this screen.

Now return to the home page and this time select OSU Patient Education. Select one of the topics from the list on the right side of the screen.

Finally, indicate which of the three sites would be most useful to you as a medical transcriptionist. Explain why briefly. Submit your findings to your instructor.

Review

The Eye

- The eye is protected by placement in a bony socket and a cushion of fat and connective tissue, covered by mucous membranes and eyelids, and assisted by lacrimal and tarsal glands that produce tears.
- The eye is composed of three tunics—the outermost tunic, consisting of the cornea and sclera; the middle tunic, consisting of the choroid, ciliary body, and iris; and the innermost layer, which is the retina.
- The eye receives an image and, through changes in the shape of the crystalline lens, focuses the image on the retina.
- Sensory receptors translated into nerve impulses are transmitted by the optic nerve to the brain—where we actually "see."

Key Terminology Review

Word	Definition
accommodation	process of bringing a lens into focus on near or far objects
aqueous humor	clear, watery fluid circulating in the anterior and posterior chambers of the eye
choroid	thin, soft membrane with a dark brown appearance that covers the posterior of the eyeball and maintains the nutrition of the retina
ciliary	body structure of the middle tunic that secretes aqueous humor and adjusts the lens in a process called accommodation
conjunctiva (*pl.* conjunctivae)	soft membrane that covers the front portion of the eyeball
cornea	anterior segment of the outermost tunic through which light enters the eye
crystalline lens	part of the eye that focuses light rays on the retina and is altered by the ciliary muscle
fovea	area near the center of the retina where everything seen comes to focus
iris	third structure of the middle tunic that gives the eye its color
lacrimal glands	tear glands

continues

Word	Definition
ophthalmologist	physician surgeon who specializes in the diagnosis and treatment of diseases of the eye
optic nerve	nerve that carries visual impulses to the brain
optometrist	nonsurgeon specialist who tests eyes for visual acuity, prescribes corrective lenses, and recommends eye exercises; recently given privileges to prescribe medications and treat diseases of the eye
pupil	rounded opening in the center of the iris
recti (superior, interior, lateral, and medial) and oblique (superior and inferior) muscles	six muscles that control the movement of the eyeball
retina	innermost tunic of the eye that receives visual images
rods and cones	specialized receptors, or nerve endings, within the retina
sclera	posterior segment of the outermost tunic known as the white of the eye
tarsal glands (meibomian glands)	glands located in the inner surface of the eyelid that lubricate the eyelid and prevent overflow of tears
tarsal plate	part of the eye that maintains the shape of the eyelid
tunics	layers of the eye that give rise to various structures of the eye
vitreous humor	transparent, semigelatinous substance in the posterior chamber of the eye

Key Terminology Practice Exercises

COMPLETION

Complete the following statements.

1. Structures of the outermost tunic of the eye are the ____________________ and ____________________.
2. The middle tunic of the eye has three structures; they are the ____________________, ____________________, and ____________________.
3. Focusing on near or far objects is referred to as ____________________.
4. The part of the eye that gives it color is the ____________________.
5. ____________________ change the shape of the crystalline lens by the process of accommodation.
6. The ____________________ is a transparent, semigelatinous substance in the posterior chamber of the eye.
7. We actually "see" in our ____________________.
8. The soft membrane covering of the eye is the ____________________.
9. There are muscles that hold the eye in place ____________________.
10. The innermost tunic of the eye is the ____________________.
11. Visual impulses are carried to the brain by the ____________________.
12. The rounded opening in the center of the iris is the ____________________.
13. The area near the center of the retina where everything we see comes to focus is the ____________________.

14. Clear, water fluid that circulates in both chambers of the eye is called ____________________.
15. The part of the eye that maintains the shape of the eyelid is the ____________________ plate.

SHORT ANSWER

Supply a short answer to the following.

1. Describe the protective devices of the eye.

____
____
____
____
____

2. Describe the difference between an ophthalmologist and an optometrist.

____
____
____
____
____

3. In your own words, summarize how the eye works.

____
____
____
____
____

MATCHING

Match the definitions of the components of the eye or accessory structures with the terms.

1. layers of the eye	a. accommodation
2. one of six muscles that control eyeball movement	b. aqueous humor
3. specialized receptors within the retina	c. choroid
4. focuses light rays on the retina	d. ciliary body
5. substance found in the posterior chamber	e. conjunctiva
6. maintains eyelid shape	f. cornea
7. process of bringing lens into focus on objects	g. crystalline lens
8. receives visual images	h. fovea
9. tear glands	i. iris
10. part of the eye that gives it color	j. lacrimal glands
11. light enters the eye through here	k. meibomian glands
12. opening in the center of the iris	l. optic nerve
13. part of the retina where what we see comes to focus	m. pupil
14. carry visual impulses to the brain	n. retina
15. white of the eye	o. rods and cones
16. soft membrane covering the front of the eyeball	p. sclera

17. clear fluid circulating in both chambers of the eye
18. maintains nutrition of the retina
19. adjusts lens by accommodation
20. another name for the tarsal glands

q. superior recti
r. tarsal plate
s. tunics
t. vitreous humor

Word Element Review

Root	Meaning	Example	Definition
aque/o	water	**aqueous humor** (ā'kwē-ŭs)	clear, watery fluid circulating through the anterior and posterior chambers of the eye
blephar/o	eyelid	**blepharectomy** (blĕf"ah-rĕk'tō-mē)	excision of an eyelid
conjunctiv/o	conjunctiva	**conjunctivitis** (kŏn-jŭnk"tĭ-vī'tĭs)	inflammation of the conjunctiva
cor/o, core/o	pupil	**corectasis** (kōr-ĕk'tah-sĭs)	dilation of the pupil
corne/o	cornea	**corneal** (kor'nē-ăl)	pertaining to the cornea
dacry/o	tear, tear duct	**dacryocystitis** (dăk"rē-ō-sĭs-tī'tĭs)	inflammation of the lacrimal sac
ir/o, irid/o	iris	**iridectomy** (ĭr"ĭ-dĕk'tō-mē)	surgical removal of the iris
kerat/o	horny, cornea	**keratoid** (kĕr'ah-toid)	resembling horny or corneal tissue
lacrim/o	tear	**lacrimotomy** (lăk"rĭ-mŏt'ō-mē)	incision of the lacrimal duct
ocul/o	eye	**ocular** (ŏk'ū-lăr)	pertaining to the eye
ophthalm/o	eye	**ophthalmalgia** (ŏf"thăl-măl'jē-ah)	pain in the eye
		ophthalmic (ŏf-thăl'mĭk)	pertaining to the eye
opt/o, optic/o	eye, vision	**optic** (ŏp'tĭk)	pertaining to the eye
palpebr/o	eyelid	**palpebrate** (păl'pĕ-brāt)	to wink
pupill/o	pupil	**pupillary** (pū-'pĭ-lĕr-ē)	pertaining to the pupil
retin/o	retina	**retinopathy** (rĕt"ĭ-nŏp'ah-thē)	any disease of the retina

continues

Word Element Review continued

Root	Meaning	Example	Definition
scler/o	sclera	**scleritis** (sklē-rī'tĭs)	inflammation of the sclera
tars/o	eyelid	**tarsus** (tahr'sŭs)	dense, white fibrous tissue forming the supporting structure of the eyelid
vitre/o	glassy	**vitreous humor** (vĭt'rē-ŭs)	transparent, semi-gelatinous substance in the posterior chamber of the eye
Suffix	**Meaning**	**Example**	**Definition**
-opia, -opsia	vision	**presbyopia** (prĕs-bē-ō'pē-ah)	impaired vision because of age
-tropia	to turn	**isometropia** (ī"sō-mĕ-trō'pē-ă)	equality of refraction in both eyes

Word Element Practice Exercises

CIRCLE AND DEFINE

Circle and define the word element in the following terms.

1. dacryocystitis ____________________
2. corectasis ____________________
3. ophthalmalgia ____________________
4. blepharectomy ____________________
5. presbyopia ____________________
6. palpebrate ____________________
7. tarsus ____________________
8. retinopathy ____________________
9. scleritis ____________________
10. iridectomy ____________________
11. keratoid ____________________
12. ophthalmic ____________________
13. isometropia ____________________
14. vitreous humor ____________________
15. aqueous humor ____________________
16. pupillary ____________________
17. optic ____________________
18. ocular ____________________
19. lacrimotomy ____________________
20. corneal ____________________

MATCHING

Match the word elements to their meanings.

1. ________ horny, cornea	a. conjunctiv/o
2. ________ retina	b. dacry/o, lacrim/o
3. ________ eyelid	c. scler/o
4. ________ cornea	d. cor/o, core/o, pupill/o
5. ________ eye, vision	e. vitre/o
6. ________ vision	f. aque/o
7. ________ pupil	g. corne/o
8. ________ eye	h. ir/o, irid/o
9. ________ sclera	i. kerat/o
10. ________ tear	j. retin/o
11. ________ glassy	k. opt/o, optic/o
12. ________ iris	l. -opia, -opsia
13. ________ conjunctiva	m. blephar/o, palpebr/o, tars/o
14. ________ water	n. ocul/o, ophthalm/o
15. ________ to turn	o. -tropia

SPELLING

Rewrite the misspelled words.

1. isometropea ____________________
2. blepherectomy ____________________
3. corectasis ____________________
4. palpebraite ____________________
5. ocular ____________________

WORD ELEMENT MEANINGS

Give the meaning of each word element. Then use your dictionary to find a new word that contains each of the word elements. Specify whether the new word is a noun or an adjective by placing N or A in the last column.

Word Element	Meaning	Word	N or A
1. aque/o	________	________	________
2. blephar/o	________	________	________
3. conjunctiv/o	________	________	________
4. cor/o	________	________	________
5. core/o	________	________	________
6. corne/o	________	________	________
7. dacry/o	________	________	________
8. ir/o	________	________	________
9. irid/o	________	________	________
10. kerat/o	________	________	________
11. lacrim/o	________	________	________
12. ocul/o	________	________	________

Word Element Practice Exercises continued

Word Element	Meaning	Word	N or A
13. ophthalm/o	________	________	________
14. -opia	________	________	________
15. -opsia	________	________	________
16. opt/o	________	________	________
17. optic/o	________	________	________
18. palpebr/o	________	________	________
19. pupill/o	________	________	________
20. retin/o	________	________	________
21. scler/o	________	________	________
22. tars/o	________	________	________
23. -tropia	________	________	________
24. vitre/o	________	________	________

Working Practice

DIAGNOSTIC PROCEDURES

Word	Pronunciation	Definition
General		
corneal topography	kŏr'nē-ăl tō-pŏg'ră-fē	computer-aided examination of the curvature of the cornea
electronystagmography	ē-lĕk"trō-nĭs"tăg-mŏg'ră-fē	method of recording the electrical activity of the extraocular muscles
electroretinogram (ERG)	ē-lĕk"trō-rĕt'ĭ-nō-grăm	recording of changes in electrical potential of retina after stimulation with light
fluorescein staining	floo"ō-rĕs'ē-ĭn	procedure using fluorescein-stained sterile filter paper strips to visualize a corneal abrasion
funduscopy	fŭn-dŏs'kō-pē	examination of fundus of eye with an ophthalmoscope (see Figure 22-3)

continues

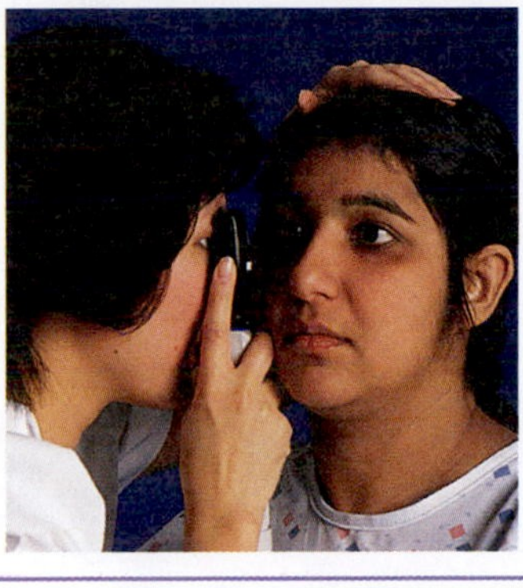

Source: Delmar/Cengage Learning

FIGURE 22-3
Funduscopy

DIAGNOSTIC PROCEDURES		
Word	**Pronunciation**	**Definition**
General (*continued*)		
gonioscopy	gō"nē-ŏs'kō-pē	examination of the angle of the anterior chamber with a gonioscope
ocular motility	ŏk'ū-lăr mō-tĭl'ĭ-tē	determination of the ability of the eye muscles to evaluation move in various gaze positions
ophthalmoscopy	ŏf-thăl-mŏs'kō-pē	visual examination of the interior eye
refraction/visual acuity	ah-kū-'ĭ-tē	determination of the amount of *nearsightedness (myopia), farsightedness (hyperopia)*, or *astigmatism* for the prescription of corrective lenses; uses Snellen's chart (see Figure 22-4)
slit lamp biomicroscopy	bī"ō-mī-krŏs'kō-pē	test that uses light emitted through a slit; used in combination with a biomicroscope to study the cornea, conjunctiva, iris, lens, and vitreous humor
tomography	tō-mŏg'ră-fē	method of measuring the optic nerve and retina using coherent light
tonometry	tō-nŏm'ĕ-trē	measurement of intraocular tension; increased tension may indicate the presence of glaucoma

continues

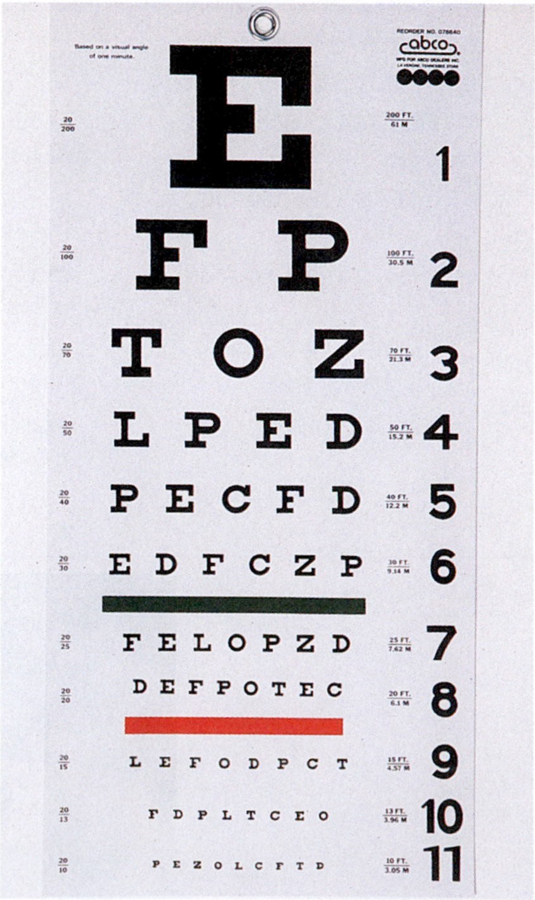

FIGURE 22-4
The Snellen Chart

Source: Delmar/Cengage Learning

DIAGNOSTIC PROCEDURES		
Word	**Pronunciation**	**Definition**
General (*continued*)		
visual field examination		measurement of the area within which objects may be seen when the eye is looking straight ahead; Goldmann perimeter visual field examination
Nuclear Medicine		
^{32}P scan		test using radioactive phosphorus to diagnose tumors
Radiology		
anteroposterior and lateral (AP & LAT)	ăn"tĕr-ō-pŏs-tēr'ē-or	x-ray procedure used to determine the presence of an intraocular foreign body
computer-assisted tomography (CAT)	tĕ-mŏg'rah-fē	procedure used to evaluate the optic nerve and orbital pathology
fluorescein angiography	floo"ō-rĕs'ē-ĭn ăn"jē-ŏg'răh-fē	test that uses retinal photography and an intravenous dye to reveal lesions of the retina and choroid
magnetic resonance imaging (MRI)		use of magnetism to create images on a computer screen to distinguish between normal and abnormal tissue changes
ultrasound		test used to locate tumors when there are vitreous, corneal, or lenticular opacities
Blood Tests		
erythrocyte sedimentation rate	ĕ-rĭth'rō-sīt sĕd"ĭ-mĕn-tā'shŭn	test used to determine the presence of temporal arteritis
white blood count and differential	dĭf"er-ĕn'shăl	test that counts the number of leukocytes and gives an estimation of the percentage of five types of white cells

DIAGNOSES		
Word	**Pronunciation**	**Definition**
Inflammation and Infection		
blepharitis	blĕf"ah-rī'tĭs	infection involving eyelashes and inflammation of both eyelid edges
chalazion	cah-lā'zē-ŏn	small, hard mass on the eyelid resulting from a plugged and infected meibomian gland
conjunctivitis	kŏn-jŭnk"tĭ-vī'tĭs	inflammation of the conjunctiva; pinkeye
corneal ulcer	kor'nē-ăl ŭl'sĕr	deep infection of the cornea

continues

DIAGNOSES		
Word	**Pronunciation**	**Definition**
Inflammation and Infection (*continued*)		
episcleritis	ĕp"ĭ-sklē-rī-tĭs	inflammation of the subconjunctival layers of the sclera
hordeolum (sty, stye)	hor-dē'ō-lŭm (stī)	localized inflammatory swelling of one of the sebaceous glands of the eyelid (see Figure 22-5)
iritis	ĭ-rē'ĭs	inflammation of the iris
keratitis	kĕr-ah-tī'tĭs	inflammation of the cornea
papilledema	păp"ĭl-ĕ-dē'mah	edema and inflammation of the optic nerve
scleritis	sklē-rī'tĭs	superficial or deep inflammation of the sclera
trachoma	trā-kō'mă	an infectious eye disease caused by *Chlamydia trachomatis*, a chronic condition that without treatment will lead to blindness
uveitis	ŭ-vē-ī'tĭs	inflammation of all or parts of the uvea
Conditions of the Eye		
age-related macular degeneration (ARMD)	măk'ū-lăr	impaired vision due to scar tissue produced by blood vessels in the macular region
amblyopia	ăm"blē-ō'pē-ah	lazy eye; vision in nondominant eye is poor
cataract	kăt'ah-răkt	clouding of the lens, which causes decreased vision (see Figure 22-6)
color blindness (monochromatism)		inherited disorder that affects the ability to distinguish between reds and greens
diabetic retinopathy	rĕt"ĭn-ŏp'ă-thē	disease of the retina caused by diabetes; may lead to blindness
diplopia	dĭp-lō'pē-ah	seeing two images of an object at the same time
ectropion	ĕk-trō'pē-ŏn	lower lid turns outward causing tears to run out instead of lubricating the eye

continues

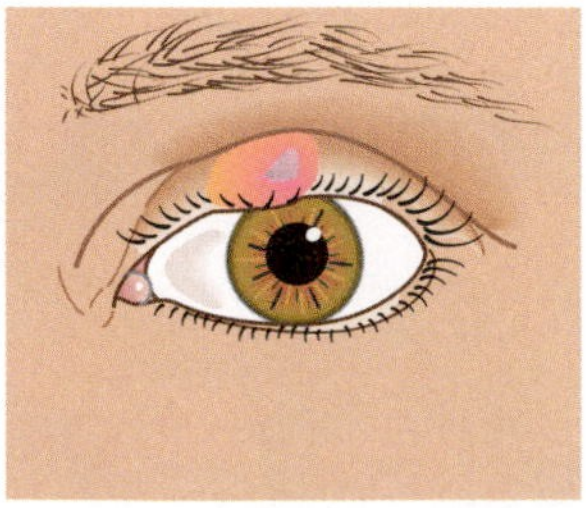

FIGURE 22-5 Hordeolum (stye)

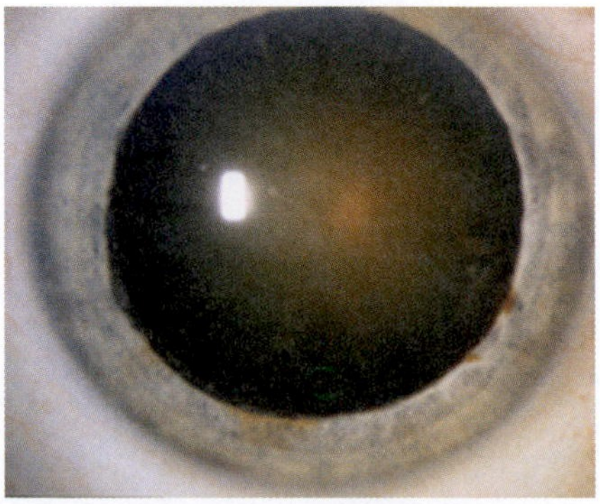

FIGURE 22-6 Cataract

DIAGNOSES		
Word	**Pronunciation**	**Definition**
Conditions of the Eye (*continued*)		
entropion	ĕn-trō'pē-ŏn	upper or lower lid turns inward and allows lashes to scratch the eyes
exophthalmia	ĕks"ŏf-thăl'mē-ă	abnormal protrusion of the eyeball
glaucoma	glaw-kō'mah	increased pressure in the eye; may be chronic or acute (see Figure 22-7)
hyphema	hī-fē'mă	bleeding into the anterior chamber of the eye as a result of an injury
keratoconus	kĕr-ă-tō-kō'nŭs	abnormal steepening of the cornea with blurring of vision, but no inflammation
nyctalopia	nĭk-tă-lō'pē-ă	night blindness
nystagmus	nĭs-tăg'mŭs	rapid, jerky eye movements
pterygium	tĕ-rĭj'ē-ŭm	triangular overgrowth of the cornea, usually the inner side, by thickened and degenerative conjunctiva
ptosis (blepharoptosis)	tō'sĭs (blĕf"ă-rō-tō'sĭs)	drooping of the upper eyelid (see Figure 22-8)

continues

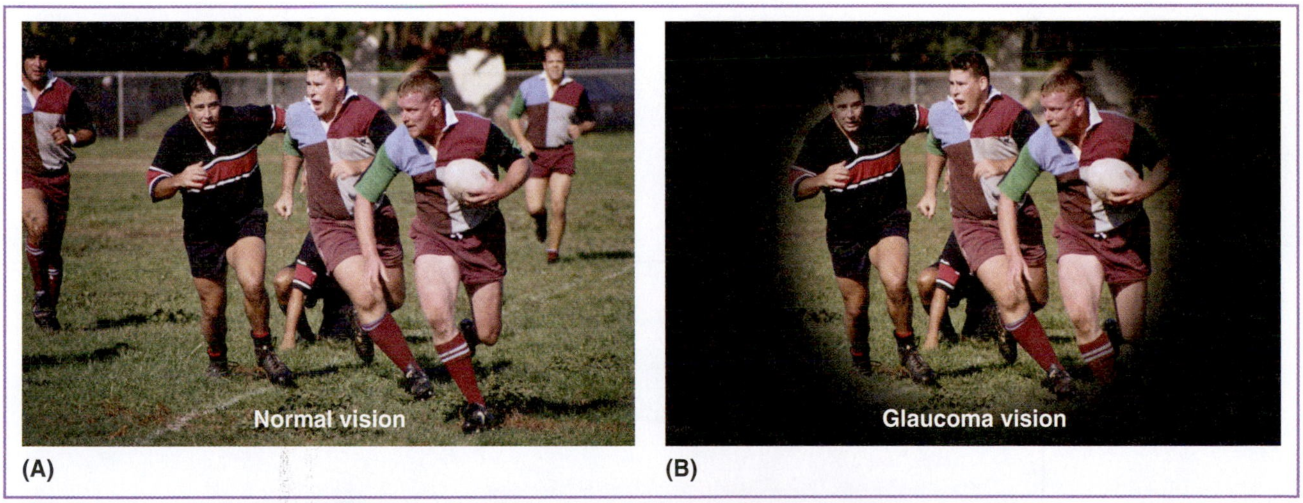

FIGURE 22-7 Decreased Vision with Glaucoma: (A) normal vision; (B) glaucoma vision.

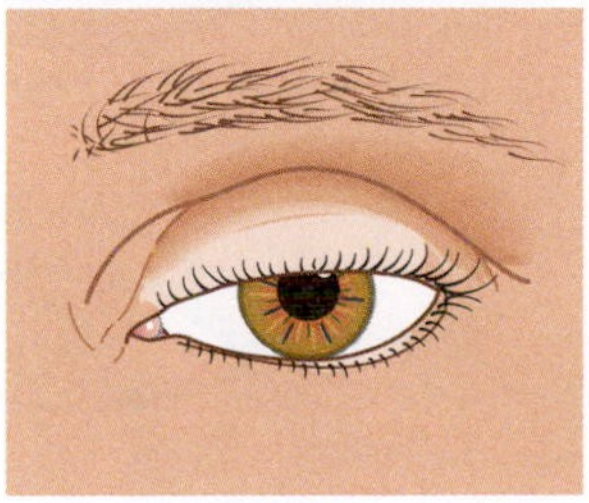

FIGURE 22-8
Ptosis

DIAGNOSES		
Word	Pronunciation	Definition
Conditions of the Eye (*continued*)		
retinoblastoma	ret"ĭ-nō-blăs-to'mah	malignant tumor of the eye
scotoma	skō-tō'mah	blind spot in the field of vision
strabismus	strah-bĭz'mŭs	abnormal eye alignments; esotropia, exotropia (see Figure 22-9)
Trauma		
blow out fracture		fracture of the floor of the orbit due to blunt trauma
commotion retina		confluent swelling of the retina due to trauma
corneal abrasion	kor'nē-ăl ă-brā'zhŭn	injury to cornea by foreign objects, poorly fitting contacts, extreme light, or physical injury
foreign body		foreign material in the eye
hyphema	hī-fē'mă	blood in the anterior chamber of the eye
retinal detachment	rĕt'ĭ-năl	separation of the inner layer of the retina from the choroid
retinal tear	rĕt'ĭ-năl tār	opening in the retina that allows leakage of vitreous humor
synechia	sĭn-ĕk'ē-ăh	an adhesion that develops after injury or surgery or secondary to cataracts, glaucoma, keratitis or uveitis

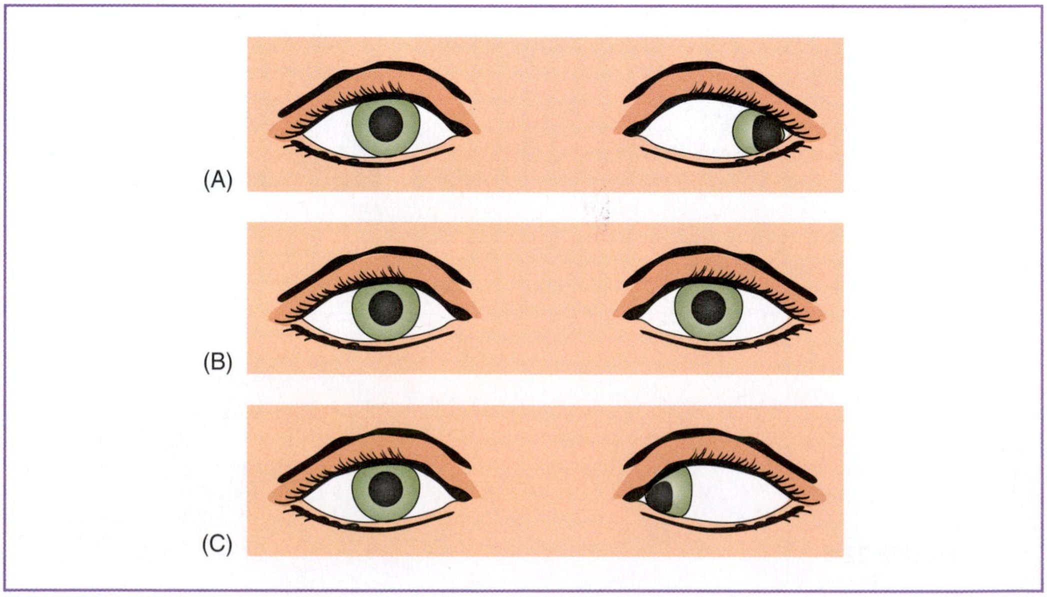

FIGURE 22-9 Strabismus: (A) exotropia (walleye); (B) normal pattern; (C) esotropia (cross-eye)

TREATMENT PROCEDURES		
Word	**Pronunciation**	**Definition**
blepharoplasty	blĕf'ah-rō-plăs"tē	surgical repair of the eyelids
corneal transplantation	kor'nē-ăl	replacement of the cornea from one person to another
cryopexy	krī'ō-pĕks-ē	use of intense cold to produce scar tissue that holds retina to underlying tissue
cryotherapy	krī-ō-thĕr'ah-pē	very cold probe is applied to scleral surface directly over the hole in the retina
cyclocryotherapy	sī"klō-krī"ō-thĕr'ah-pē	freezing of the ciliary body for treatment of glaucoma
dacryocystorhinostomy	dăk"rē-ō-sĭs"tō-rī-nŏs'tō-mē	surgical creation of an opening between the lacrimal sac and nasal cavity
ectropion correction	ĕk-trō'pē-ŏn	correction of an eversion, or outward turning, of the margin of the eyelid
entropion correction	ĕn-trō'pē-ŏn	correction of an inversion, or inward turning, of the margin of the eyelid
enucleation	ē-nū"klē-ā'shŭn	removal of the eye from its socket
evisceration	ē-vĭs"ĕr-ā'shŭn	removal of the contents of the eyeball (viscera), leaving the sclera
extracapsular cataract	ĕks"tră-căp'sū-lăr	removal of the anterior portion of the capsule and the extraction whole lens; an intraocular lens (IOL) is implanted (see Figure 22-10)
glaucoma operation	glaw-kō'mah	procedure that relieves increased intraocular pressure that has not been relieved by medications
intraocular lens implant	ĭn"tră-ŏk'ū-lĕr	surgical implantation of lens during cataract extraction
iridectomy	ĭr"ĭ-dĕk'tō-mē	excision of part of the iris; treats closed-angle glaucoma
keratoplasty	kĕr'ah-tō-plăs"tē	plastic surgery on the cornea; corneal grafting or transplant

continues

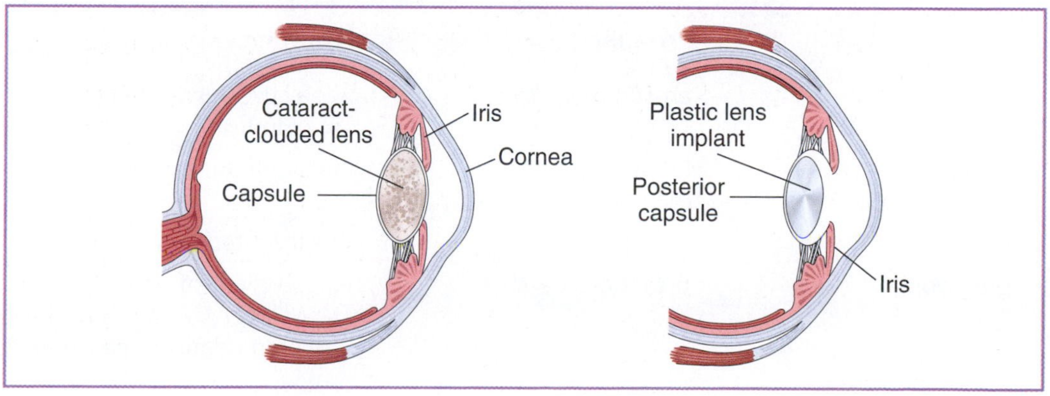

FIGURE 22-10
Cataract Extraction with Placement of Intraocular Lens

TREATMENT PROCEDURES		
Word	**Pronunciation**	**Definition**
laser-assisted in situ refractive keratomileusis (LASIK)	kĕr"ă-tō-mĭ-loo'sĭs	corrects near- and farsightedness and other errors by using a laser to sculpt corneal tissue after the creation of a corneal flap
laser iridotomy	ĭr"ĭ-dŏt'ō-mē	incision in the iris to relieve built-up pressure between the iris and lens
laser		use of a laser to treat a number of eye
photocoagulation	fō"tō-kō-ăg"ū-lā'shŭn	conditions such as diabetic retinopathy, acute and chronic simple glaucoma, retinal detachment, orbital and eyelid tumors, or secondary cataracts
limbal relaxing incision		surgical correction of astigmatism
nasolacrimal duct	nā"zō-lăk'rĭm-ăl	probing of the lacrimal drainage system probing
orbitotomy	or"bĭ-tŏt'ō-mē	orbital surgery
phacoemulsification	fak"ō-ē-mŭl'sĭ-fĭ-kā"shŭn	method to treat cataracts using ultrasound to destroy the cataract then aspirating the residue
photorefractive keratectomy (PRK)	fō"tō-rĭ-frăk'tĭv kĕr-ă-tĕk'tō-mē	procedure to shave off a few layers of corneal surface cells to flatten cornea and reduce nearsightedness (myopia) without a flap
retinal photocoagulation	rĕt'ĭ-năl fō-tō-kō-ăg-ū-lā'shŭn	a surgical procedure using a krypton, diode, or Yttrium-aluminum-garnet (YAG) laser to treat glaucoma, retinal detachment, diabetic retinopathy, or other conditions
scleral buckling	sklē'răl bŭk'lĭng	repair of retinal detachment
strabismus operation	strah-bĭz'mŭs	correction of squint or ocular misalignment; *resection* is strengthening of an ocular muscle; *recession* is weakening of an ocular muscle
trabeculectomy	tră-bĕk"ū-lĕk'tō-mē	surgical glaucoma diffusing procedure
trabeculoplasty	tră-bĕk"ū-lō-plăs"tē	laser glaucoma procedure
vitrectomy	vĭ-trĕk'tō-mē	removal of vitreous humor and its replacement with a clear solution

ERRORS OF REFRACTION		
Word	**Pronunciation**	**Definition**
astigmatism	ah-stĭg'mah-tĭzm	defective curvature of the cornea, resulting in blurry vision (see Figure 22-11B)
hyperopia (hypermetropia)	hī"per-ō'pē-ah (hī"per-mē-trŏ'pē-ah)	farsightedness (see Figure 22-12B)
myopia	mī-ō'pē-ah	nearsightedness (see Figure 22-12A)
presbyopia	prĕs"bē-ō'pē-ah	impairment of near vision in old age, resulting from loss of elasticity of the lens or accommodation (see Figure 22-11A)

FIGURE 22-11 Presbyopia and Astigmatism: (A) presbyopia (light rays focus behind the retina); (B) astigmatism (light rays focus on multiple areas of the retina)

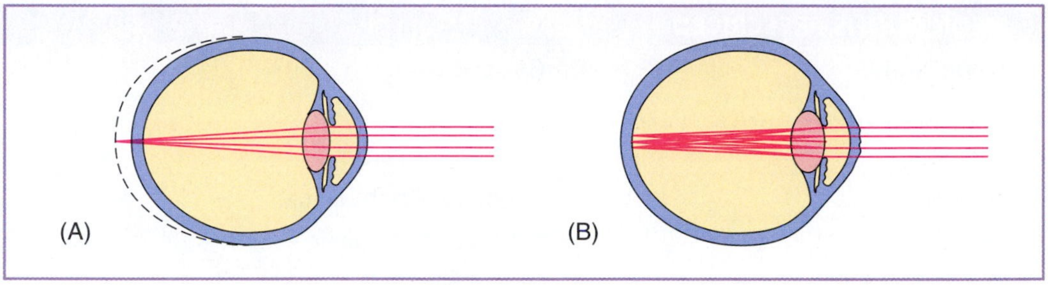

FIGURE 22-12 Myopia and Hyperopia: (A) myopia (nearsightedness), light rays focus in front of the retina; (B) hyperopia (farsightedness), light rays focus beyond the retina

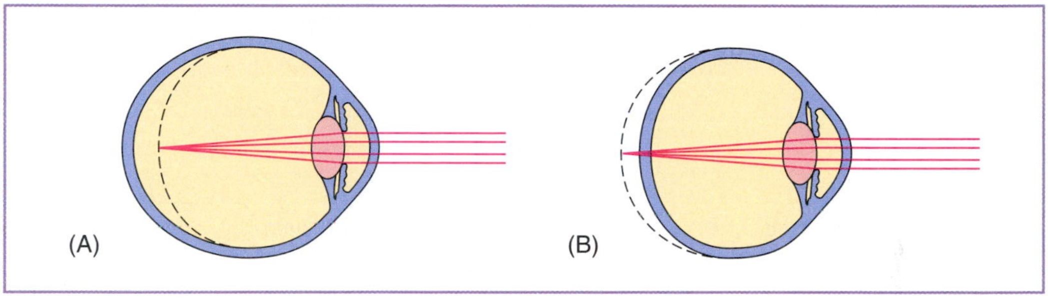

MEDICATIONS PRESCRIBED

Trade Name	Generic Name
Antibiotics/Antivirals	
AK-Tracin	bacitracin ophthalmic
Bleph-10	sulfacetamide ophthalmic
Ciloxan	ciprofloxacin ophthalmic
Genoptic, Garamycin, Gentak	gentamicin sulfate ophthalmic
Ilotycin, Roymicin	erythromycin ophthalmic
Neosporin, AK-Spore	gramicidin ophthalmic
Ocuflox	ofloxacin ophthalmic
Tobrex, Tobrasol, Tobralcon	tobramycin ophthalmic
Viroptic	trifluridine ophthalmic
Antibiotic/Steroid Combinations	
Blephamide, Cetapred, Vasocidin	sulfacetamide, prednisolone
Cortisporin Ophthalmic, Ocu-Cort, Neotricin HC	neomycin, polymyxin and hydrocortisone
Maxitrol, Neosporin Ophthalmic	neomycin, polymyxin, and dexamethasone ophthalmic
Mycitracin	neomycin, polymyxin, and bacitracin
Neodecadron	neomycin, dexamethasone
Tobradex	tobramycin, dexamethasone

continues

MEDICATIONS PRESCRIBED	
Trade Name	**Generic Name**
Glaucoma Treatment	
Alphagan	brimonidine tartrate
Betagan	levobunolol ophthalmic
Betoptic	betaxolol ophthalmic
Diamox	acetazolamide
Epifrin, Epinal, Glaucon	epinephrine bitrate
Isopto Carpine, Pilocar, Akarpine	pilocarpine ophthalmic
Miostat, Carboptic, Carbachol, Isopto, Carbachol	carbachol
Osmoglyn	glycerin
Propine, AK-Pro	dipivefrin ophthalmic
Timoptic Ocumeter, Betinol	timolol maleate ophthalmic
Trusopt	dorzolamide
Xalatan	latanoprost
Corticosteroids	
AD-DEX, Decadron Ocumeter, Dexasol, Maridex	dexamethasone ophthalmic
AK-Pred	prednisolone sodium phosphate ophthalmic
Econopred, Pred Mild	prednisolone acetate ophthalmic
FML, Eflone, Flarex, Fluor-Op	fluormetholone ophthalmic
HMS	medrysone ophthalmic
Vexol	rimexolone ophthalmic
Ophthalmic Agents	
AK-Con, Vasocon-A	naphazoline ophthalmic
Isopto Atropine, Atropine-1	atropine ophthalmic
Isopto Homatropine	homatropine ophthalmic
Anti-Inflammatory Drugs	
Acular	ketorolac ophthalmic
Ocufen	flurbiprofen
Voltaren	diclofenac sodium ophthalmic
Anti-Allergy Topicals	
Allerest	naphazoline ophthalmic
Patanol	olopatadine HCl
Zaditor	ketotifen fumarate

ABBREVIATIONS

accom	accommodation
AION	anterior ischemic optic neuropathy
ALT	argon laser trabeculoplasty
ARMD	age-related macular degeneration
BRAO	branch retinal artery occlusion
BRVO	branch retinal vein occlusion
CRAO	central retinal artery occlusion
CRVO	central retinal vein occlusion
EKC	epidemic keratoconjunctivitis; "pink eye"
Em	emmetropia (normal vision)
EOM	extraocular movement
ERG	electroretinogram
HRT	Heidelberg retinal tomography
HSV	herpes simplex virus
HZV	herpes zoster virus
IOL	intraocular lens
IOP	intraocular pressure
LASIK	laser-assisted in situ keratomileusis
LRI	limbal relaxing incision
OCT	optical coherence tomography
OD	*oculus dexter* (right eye)
ophth	ophthalmology
OS	*oculus sinister* (left eye)
OU	*oculi unitas* (both eyes)
PBK	pseudophakic bullous keratopathy
PERRLA	pupils equal, round, reactive to light and accommodation
PKP	penetrating keratoplasty (corneal transplant)
PRK	photorefractive keratectomy
REM	rapid eye movement
SLT	selective laser trabeculoplasty
VA	visual acuity
VF	visual field

IDENTIFICATION/DIAGNOSTIC PROCEDURES

Identify the following definitions.

1. visual examination of the interior eye ______________________
2. using radioactive phosphorus in the diagnosis of tumors of the eye ______________________
3. dye is used intravenously with photography to reveal lesions of the retina and choroid ______________________
4. examining the angle of the anterior chamber with a gonioscope ______________________
5. determines the ability of the eye muscles to move in various gaze positions ______________________
6. measurement of intraocular tension ______________________
7. determination of amount of myopia, hyperopia, or astigmatism ______________________
8. used to visualize a corneal abrasion ______________________
9. examines curvature of cornea ______________________
10. blood test to determine presence of temporal arteritis ______________________

DEFINITIONS

Define and provide the pronunciation for the following surgical procedures.

1. blepharoplasty ______________________
2. enucleation ______________________
3. keratoplasty ______________________
4. laser photocoagulation ______________________
5. strabismus operation ______________________
6. cryopexy ______________________
7. cyclocryotherapy ______________________
8. scleral buckling ______________________
9. laser-assisted in situ keratomileusis ______________________
10. ectropian correction ______________________

MATCHING

Match the following definitions with their meanings.

1. drooping of the upper eyelid	a. amblyopia
2. rapid, jerky, side-to-side eye movements	b. blepharitis
3. inflammation of the conjunctiva	c. cataract
4. clouding of the lens	d. chalazion
5. a blind spot	e. conjunctivitis
6. an enlarged meibomian gland on the eyelid	f. corneal abrasion
7. abnormal alignment of the eye	g. diabetic retinopathy
8. edema and inflammation of the optic nerve	h. diplopia
9. lazy eye	i. entropion
10. lid turns inward and allows lashes to scratch the eye	j. EOM
11. increased pressure in the eye	k. glaucoma
12. malignant tumor of the eye	l. keratitis
13. seeing two images at once	m. nystagmus
14. inflammation of the cornea	n. OD
15. inflammation of both eyelid edges	o. OS
16. localized swelling of a sebaceous gland in the eyelid	p. papilledema
17. triangular overgrowth of the cornea	q. PRK
18. injury to the cornea	r. pterygium
19. separation of the inner layer of the retina from the choroids	s. ptosis
20. disease of the retina that may lead to blindness	t. retinal detachment
21. abbreviation for right eye	u. retinoblastoma
22. abbreviation for visual acuity	v. scotoma
23. abbreviation for photorefractive keratectomy	w. strabismus
24. abbreviation for extraocular movement	x. sty, stye
25. abbreviation for left eye	y. VA

COMPLETION

Complete the following statements.

1. The surgical implantation of the lens during cataract extraction is a/n ______________________.
2. A method to treat cataracts using ultrasound is ______________________.
3. Surgical correction of astigmatism is ______________________.
4. A surgical procedure using a laser to treat glaucoma, retinal detachment, diabetic retinopathy, etc., is ______________________.
5. An abnormal steepening of the cornea is ______________________.
6. Night blindness is known as ______________________.
7. Bleeding into the anterior chamber of the eye is known as ______________________.
8. An abnormal protrusion of the eye is called ______________________.
9. An infectious eye disease caused by *Chlaymdia trachomatis* that without treatment can lead to blindness is ______________________.
10. A deep infection of the cornea is a/n ______________________.

11. A method of measuring the optic nerve and retina using coherent light is ____________________.
12. A method of recording the electrical activity of the extraocular muscles is ____________________.
13. The abbreviation for electroretinogram is ____________________.
14. The abbreviation for rapid eye movement is ____________________.
15. The abbreviation for limbal relaxing incision is ____________________.

Dictionary Exercises

DICTIONARY EXERCISE 1

Use your dictionary to find the pronunciation and definition of the following words.

	Word	Pronunciation	Definition
1.	canthus	____________	____________________
2.	cycloplegia	____________	____________________
3.	corneal dystrophy	____________	____________________
4.	floaters	____________	____________________
5.	orbital cellulitis	____________	____________________
6.	meibomian gland	____________	____________________
7.	melanoma of the eye	____________	____________________
8.	retrolental fibroplasia	____________	____________________
9.	vitreous hemorrhage	____________	____________________
10.	dacryorrhea	____________	____________________

DICTIONARY EXERCISE 2

Match the terms to their meanings.

1. __________ aphakia		a. inflammation of the optic nerve
2. __________ choroiditis		b. repair of the uvea
3. __________ coloboma		c. wasting away of the eye
4. __________ corneal ulcer		d. inflammation of the cornea
5. __________ exophthalmos		e. acute infection of the eye socket
6. __________ hemianopia		f. destructive lesion of the cornea
7. __________ keratitis		g. congenital defect in the development of the eye
8. __________ keratomycosis		h. abnormal protrusion of the eyeball
9. __________ mitosis		i. inflammation of the choroid
10. __________ mydriasis		j. pronounced dilation of the pupil
11. __________ optic atrophy		k. blindness in one-half of the visual field
12. __________ optic neuritis		l. a fungal growth on the cornea
13. __________ orbital cellulites		m. abnormal construction of pupil
14. __________ retrobulbar		n. behind the eyeball
15. __________ uveoplasty		o. absence of eye lens

DICTIONARY EXERCISE 3

Pronunciation of the words below is provided. Using your dictionary, find the correct spelling and definition of each word.

	Word	Pronunciation	Meaning
1.	________________	ā'kwē-ŭs	______________________________
2.	________________	dī-ŏp'tĕr	______________________________
3.	________________	dăk"rē-ăd-ĕn-ăl'jē-ah	______________________________
4.	________________	rĕt-ĭ-nī'tĭs pĭg-mĕn-tō'sah	______________________________
5.	________________	lĭm'bŭs	______________________________
6.	________________	rĕt"ĭ-nō'sĭs	______________________________
7.	________________	tahr'sŭs	______________________________
8.	________________	ū'vē-ah	______________________________
9.	________________	ăn-ī"sō-kō'rē-ă	______________________________
10.	________________	blĕf"ăr-ō-kăl'ă-sĭs	______________________________
11.	________________	mĭd-rē-ăt'ĭk	______________________________

DICTIONARY EXERCISE 4

Rewrite each sentence in your own words.

1. The cornea of the 72-year-old patient was marked by *arcus senilis*.

   ____

   ____

2. The doctor performed *cyclodiathermy*.

   ____

   ____

3. The problem was diagnosed as *ambiopia*.

   ____

   ____

4. Unfortunately, *iridodialysis* has occurred.

   ____

   ____

5. *Ophthalmoplegia* was the final diagnosis.

   ____

   ____

*Study*WARE™ Connection

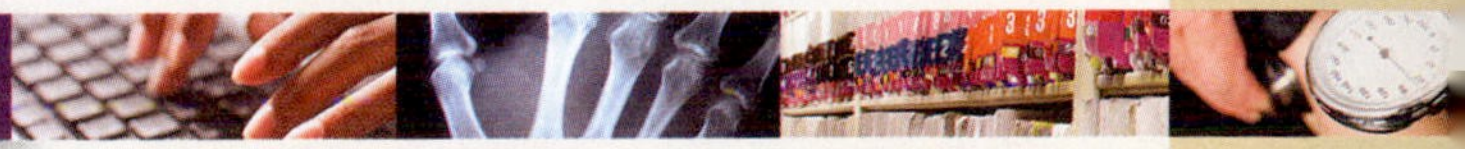

Take a practice quiz or play more interactive games that reinforce the content in this chapter, go to your StudyWARE™ CD-ROM.

Listening Exercise

INSTRUCTIONS

1. Review the spelling, pronunciation, and meaning of the words provided in the preview.
2. Go to your StudyWARE™ CD-ROM and listen to **Listening Exercise 22-1**. Fill in the blank in the report as the word is dictated.
3. At the end of the activity, check your spelling against the preview words. They appear in the preview in the order in which they are encountered in the activity.
4. Review and practice the words you missed.
5. Look up words that are not familiar.

PREVIEW OF WORDS FOR LISTENING EXERCISE 22-1

Word	Pronunciation	Meaning
phacoemulsification	fak"ō-ē-mŭl'sĭ-fĭ-kā"shŭn	a technique of cataract extraction that uses high-frequency ultrasound vibrations, irrigation, and suction
retrobulbar	rĕt"rō-bŭl'băr	behind the eyeball
scleral	sklĕ'răl	concerning the tough, white fibrous tissue covering the "white" of the eye
limbus	lĭm'bŭs	an edge; in this case, the edge of the cornea where it joins the sclera
capsulotomy	kăp"sū-lŏt'ō-mē	incision into a lens
lenticular	len-tĭk'ū-lăr	pertaining to the lens of the eye

Listening Exercise 22-1

*Study*WARE™ Connection

Listen to this report being read on your StudyWARE™ CD-ROM. Fill in each blank as the word is dictated.

Operative Report

PREOPERATIVE DIAGNOSIS: Senile nuclear sclerotic cataract, right eye.

POSTOPERATIVE DIAGNOSIS: Senile nuclear sclerotic cataract, right eye.

PROCEDURE: ____________________ with posterior chamber intraocular lens implantation, right eye.

INDICATIONS: Decreased vision due to cataract, right eye, affecting the patient's functional activities.

INFORMED CONSENT: The patient is alert, oriented, and understands the risks, benefits, and indications of the above procedure, and consents to the same.

PROCEDURE: After achievement of satisfactory ____________________ anesthesia, the patient was prepped and draped in the routine sterile manner. A wire lid speculum was placed in the right eye. A superior limbal peritomy was performed.

Cautery, as necessary, was achieved with bipolar cautery. A partial thickness ____________________ tunnel incision was advanced to the ____________________ through which the anterior chamber was entered with a 3.2-mm keratome. A separate stab incision was made at the six o'clock limbus. Under Amvisc Plus, an anterior ____________________ was performed with forceps. BSS was irrigated underneath the anterior capsule. Phacoemulsification was utilized to remove ____________________ nucleus. Remnant lenticular cortical material was removed with irrigation-aspiration device. The posterior capsule was polished with Graether collar button. A posterior chamber intraocular lens was implanted into the capsular bag. The intraocular lens used is the IOLAB model LI41U, power (-2) diopter. Remnant Amvisc Plus was removed with the irrigation-aspiration device.

The superior scleral wound was closed with a single interrupted 10-0 nylon suture. Cautery was utilized to reapproximate the conjunctiva. A subconjunctival injection with gentamicin was given in the inferior fornix. The eye was patched over Polysporin ointment and topical application of Iopidine.

The patient tolerated the procedure well. There were no operative complications. The patient left the operating suite in good condition.

______________________________ ____________________

Douglas R. Flannigan, MD Date

CHAPTER

23

The Ear, Nose, and Throat

"Nature has given man one tongue, but two ears, that we may hear twice as much as we speak."

—Epictetus

OBJECTIVES

When you have completed this chapter on the ear, nose, and throat systems, you should be able to

1. Spell and define major system components and explain how they operate.
2. Identify the meanings of related word elements.
3. Spell and define diagnostic procedures, diagnoses, treatment procedures, and abbreviations.
4. Spell the names of commonly used medications.
5. Use a dictionary as a tool in processing medical documents.
6. Hear how medical terminology is used in actual medical reports.

INTRODUCTION

The ear, nose, and throat contain receptor cells and structures that allow us to experience the senses of hearing, balance, smell, and taste. Physicians who specialize in the treatment of diseases and disorders of these organs and adjacent structures of the head and neck are called **otolaryngologists** (ō"tō-lăr"ĭn-gŏl'ō-jĭsts) (or otorhinolaryngologists). Head and neck surgery has recently been added to this specialty.

COMPONENTS OF THE EAR

acous/o	hearing	-cusis	hearing
audi/o, audit/o	hearing, sound	myring/o	eardrum
auri/o, auricul/o	ear	ot/o	ear
cochle/o	cochlea	tympan/o	eardrum

The ear is divided into three parts—the external ear, the middle ear, and the inner (internal) ear.

EXTERNAL EAR

As you will note in Figure 23-1, the external ear has two parts—the auricle and the **acoustic meatus** (mē-ā'tŭs), or opening that leads into the auditory canal. The **auricle** (aw'rĕ-kl), or **pinna** (pĭn'ah)(2) is the outermost portion of the ear. It is composed of an elastic cartilage that is covered with skin and a lobe (3) that extends from the lower portion of the auricle.

The external portion of the ear directs sound waves into the **external auditory canal** (4). This canal serves a double purpose. First, it guides sound waves to the **tympanic** (tĭm-păn'ĭk) **membrane** (eardrum) (1); second,

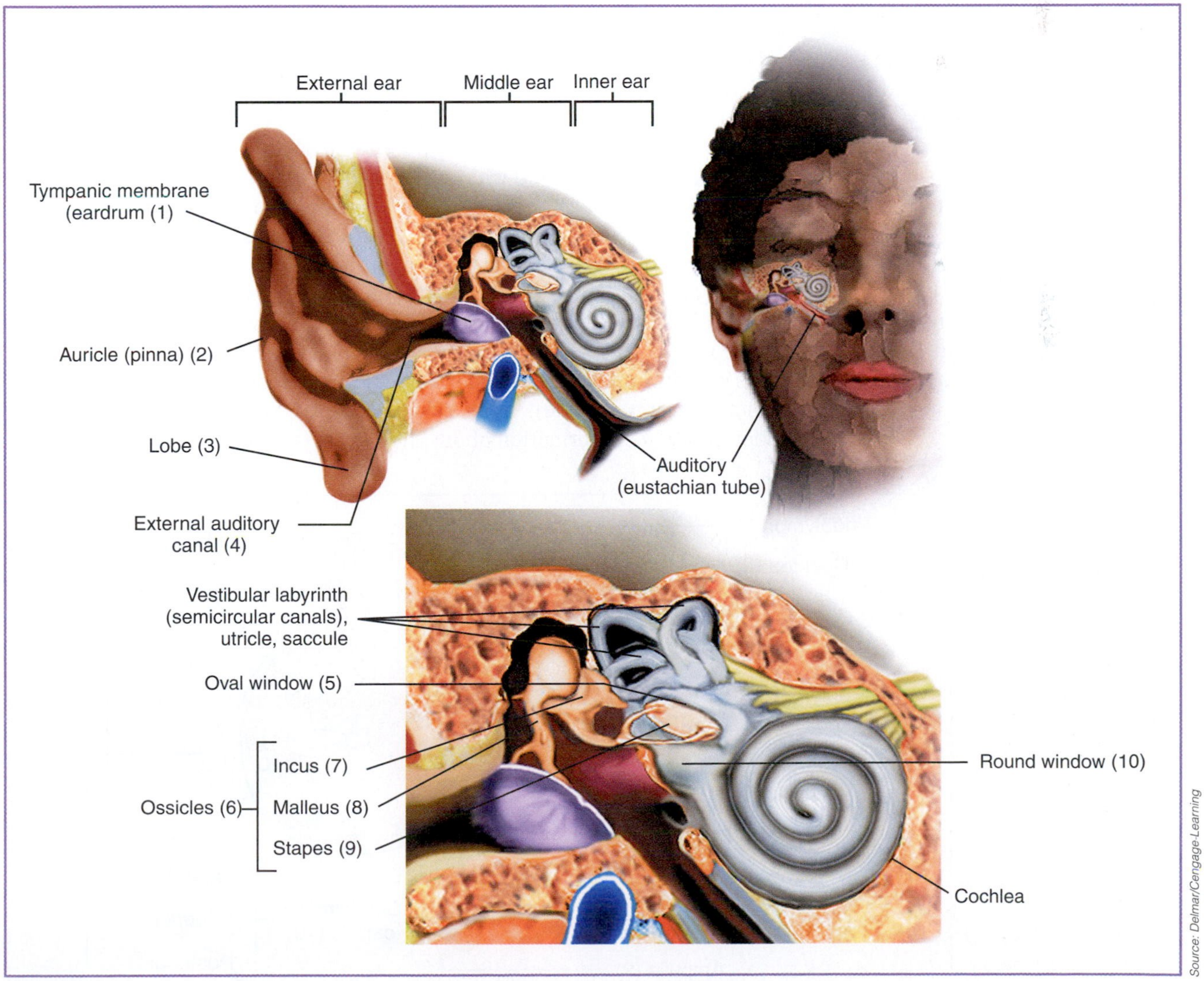

FIGURE 23-1 Structure of the Ear

it protects the internal structure of the ear. The fine hairs and cerumen in the canal assist in the protective function. **Cerumen** (sĕ-roo'mĕn) (referred to as earwax) is secreted by modified sebaceous glands. When sound waves reach the eardrum through the auditory canal, they are picked up by the tympanic membrane and the bones of the middle ear and transmitted to the inner ear.

MIDDLE EAR

The **middle ear** is an irregularly shaped, air-filled cavity within the temporal bone and is lined with mucous membranes. These mucous membranes are continuous with those that line the throat, which is why infections spread so readily to the middle ear. The air in the cavity comes from the nasal part of the pharynx through the auditory or **eustachian** (ū-stā'kē-ăn) **tube**. In this way, air pressure on both sides of the eardrum is equalized.

At one end of the cavity is the tympanic membrane (eardrum), and on the other end is a bone wall. This bone wall has two small membrane-covered openings called the **oval window** (5) and **round window** (10).

There are also three small bones or ossicles (6) in the middle ear. These are the **malleus** (măl'ē-ŭs) (hammer) (8), **incus** (ĭng'kŭs) (anvil) (7), and **stapes** (stā'pēz) (stirrup) (9). These three ossicles form a flexible bridge across the middle ear chamber and transmit sound waves to the internal ear in the following way. Since the malleus and the eardrum are in contact, a sound that sets the eardrum into motion is immediately transferred to the malleus. The motion of the malleus then moves the incus, which in turn moves the stapes. The vibrations of the footplate of the stapes are transmitted to the flexible membrane covering the oval window opening to the inner ear.

INNER EAR

The **inner ear**, shown in Figure 23-2, is the most complex structure of the ear. This structure, also called the **labyrinth** (lăb'ĭ-rĭnth), is divided into three fluid-filled areas—the **cochlea** (kŏk'lē-ah) (2), the **semicircular canals** (10), and the **vestibule** (vĕs'tĭ-bŭl) (6).

Delicate membranes lining the inner ear enable us to hear and maintain our balance. As was stated above, when the ear receives a sound, the stapes strikes against the oval window (8), which creates vibrations. The vibrations set off wavelike movements in the fluid of the inner ear. These fluid waves are cushioned and dampened by the round window (7). Waves in the inner ear travel through the cochlea (a snail-shaped structure), where the **organ of Corti** (kŏr'tē) is located. The organ of Corti contains the receptors for hearing—more than 20,000 sensory hair cells with additional supporting cells. As the waves travel through the cochlea, the hair cells vibrate. This stimulates the sensory fibers of the vestibulocochlear (vĕs-tĭb"ū-lō-kŏk'lē-ăr) nerve, which transmits the information to the brain.

The inner ear also controls the body's equilibrium. Near the cochlea are three semicircular canals, each containing a semicircular duct (11). Each duct contains an enlargement called an **ampulla** (ăm-pul'lah) (9), which in turn contains sensory cells that provide directional information about the body's position. For example, as the

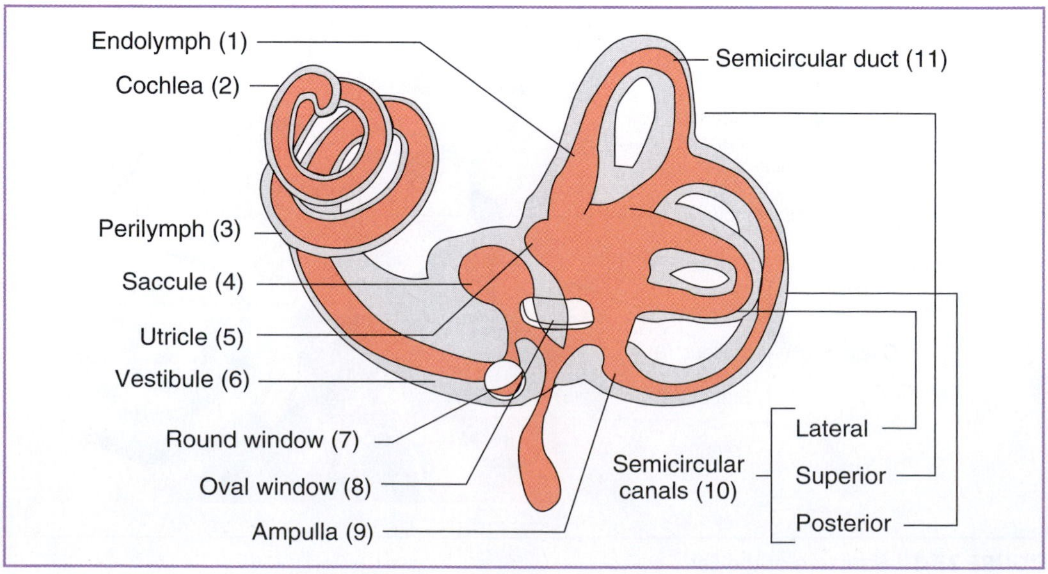

FIGURE 23-2
Inner Ear

Source: Delmar/Cengage Learning

head is turned, the fluid in the ducts flows to or from the ampulla, stimulating the sensory cells and telling the brain which way the head is moving.

The vestibule is a chamber between the cochlea and semicircular canals and separated from the middle ear by the oval window. This chamber is filled with a fluid called **perilymph** (pĕr'ĭ-lĭmf) (3) and separates the walls of the membranous labyrinth and the osseous labyrinth. The vestibule contains two membranous labyrinth enlargements called the **saccule** (săk'ūl) (4) and **utricle** (ū'trēk'l) (5). These, along with the semicircular canals, are structures of equilibrium. The membranous labyrinth is filled with a fluid called **endolymph** (ĕn'dō-lĭmf) (1). This entire complicated structure called the ear gives us the ability to hear sounds and to maintain our balance and equilibrium.

StudyWARE™ Connection

Play an interactive game labeling structures of the **Ear** on your StudyWARE™ CD-ROM.

Review *The Ear*

- The ear is a delicate instrument of hearing composed of the external, middle, and inner ears.
- The external ear conducts sound to the eardrum, which activates the three ossicles of the middle ear.
- Vibrations on the oval window leading to the inner ear stimulate the cochlea.
- The inner ear transmits sound wave information to the brain and senses movement and position to aid in the control of the body's equilibrium.

StudyWARE™ Connection

To watch an animation on how we hear, go to your StudyWARE™ CD-ROM.

COMPONENTS OF THE NOSE AND THROAT

gingiv/o	gum	or/o	mouth
gloss/o	tongue	-osmia	smell
lingu/o	tongue	phon/o	sound
mastoid/o	mastoid process	sial/o	salivary
odont/o	tooth		

The closely related senses of **olfaction** (ŏl-făk'shŭn) (smell) and **gustation** (gŭs-tā'shŭn) (taste) are located in the nasal and mouth area. The nose is composed of an external nose, a nasal cavity, and nasal sinuses.

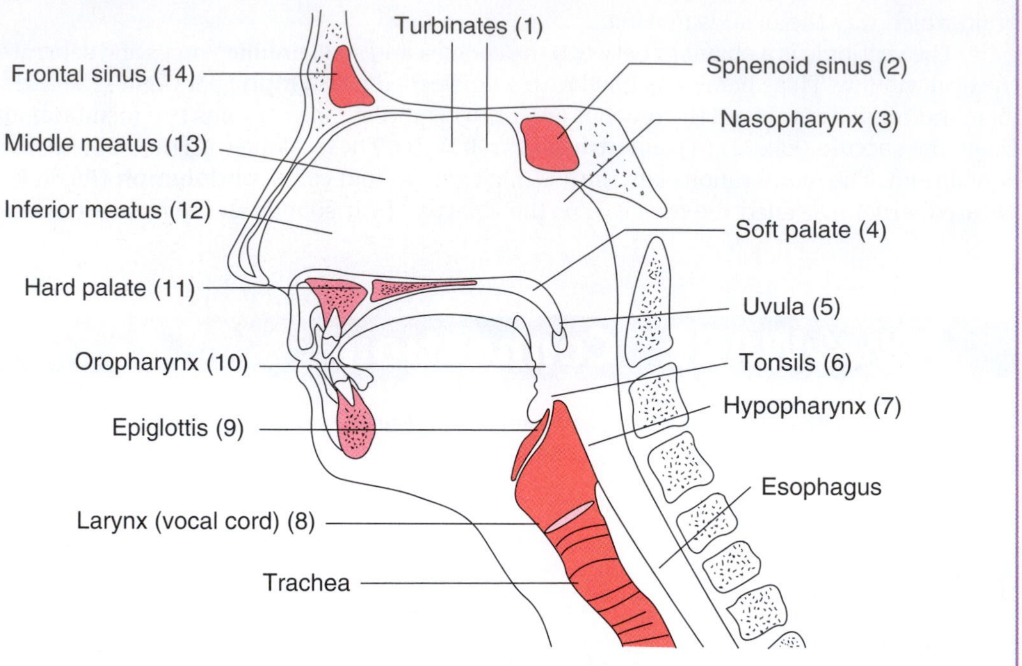

FIGURE 23-3 Structure of the Nose and Throat

EXTERNAL NOSE

The nose takes outside air as cold as –30°F and warms it to 98°F by the time it reaches the upper part of the throat. The bridge of the nose is formed of bone; the tip is built of cartilage and connective tissue. The **septum** (sĕp'tŭm) separates the nostrils into two cavities running from the floor of the skull to the base of the nasal cavity. The septum is made mostly of cartilage.

NASAL CAVITY

In Figure 23-3, note that the main cavity of the nose rests between the floor of the brain cavity and the roof of the mouth. The nasal **conchae** (kŏn'chē) are three scroll-shaped bones forming the nasal sidewall. The conchae are covered with moist membranes forming the turbinates. Essentially, these are the air conditioners of the nose because they provide moisture and warmth before the air reaches the lungs. Beneath the shelves formed by the **turbinates** (tŭr'bĭ-nāts) (1) are recesses called the superior (not shown), middle (13), and inferior (12) meatus.

The floor of the nasal cavity is formed by the bony **hard palate** (păl'ăt) (11) anteriorly and the muscular **soft palate** (4) posteriorly. Together the hard and soft palates separate the nasal cavity from the mouth.

The membranes in the nasal passage continuously secrete mucus and fluids. Coarse and fine hairs inside the nasal vestibule trap foreign particles, as does the sticky mucus of the internal nose.

NASAL SINUSES

Surrounding the nasal cavity within the skull is a series of air-filled spaces called **sinuses**. There are four major pairs of sinuses—frontal (14), sphenoid (2), maxillary (not shown), and ethmoidal (not shown). There is one of each pair on either side of the face. The sinuses serve as resonating chambers for the voice.

MOUTH

The tongue forms the floor of the mouth and is covered with numerous tiny projections called **papillae** (pah-pĭl'ē). These are often referred to as taste buds. Four tastes (sweet, salty, bitter, and sour) are identified in specific regions of the tongue, as shown in Figure 23-4. The receptor cells of the taste buds are in contact with the sensory nerve fibers, which run to the brain through the facial, glossopharyngeal, and vagus nerves.

Posterior and inferior to the mouth, the pharynx and larynx provide passages for food and air.

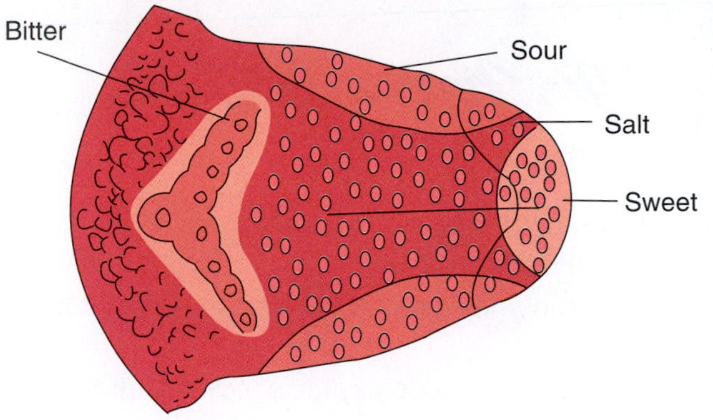

FIGURE 23-4 Taste Regions of the Tongue

PHARYNX

The hard palate, or roof of the mouth, merges with the soft palate and a small peninsula of tissue called the **uvula** (ū'vū-lah) (5), as shown in Figure 23-3. If the **tonsils** (6) are still intact, they can be seen as small rounded masses of lymphoid tissue on either side of the passageway into the throat. Saclike cavities called **crypts** (krĭpts) are present on the mucous membrane covering of the exposed surface of the tonsil.

Technically the **pharynx** extends from the base of the skull to the larynx (8). The pharynx is a common passageway for food from the mouth and for air from the nose. It consists of three sections—the nasopharynx, oropharynx, and hypopharynx (laryngopharynx). The **nasopharynx** (nā"zō-făr'ĭnks) (3) is the area that lies above the level of the soft palate and is covered by mucous membrane. It has five openings: two posterior nares or choanae (inner openings of the nostrils), two openings leading through the eustachian tubes to the middle ears (tori), and the downward opening to the oropharynx. On the posterior wall of the nasopharynx there is a localized accumulation of lymphoid tissue called the **adenoid** (ăd'ĕ-noyd).

The **oropharynx** (ō"rō-făr'ĭnks) (10) extends from the soft palate to the upper border of the epiglottis (9). The oropharynx has openings to the oral cavity, the nasopharynx, and the **hypopharynx** (hi"pō-făr'ĭnks) (7). The hypopharynx lies below the epiglottis and also has three openings—one from the oropharynx, one to the esophagus, and one to the larynx.

LARYNX

The **larynx** (lăr'ĭnks) (8) connects the laryngopharyngeal section with the trachea and is used for conduction of air to and from the lungs and speech and airway protection during swallowing. It is framed by nine cartilages—three paired and three unpaired. The cartilages are held together by ligaments and muscles. The most familiar one is the **epiglottis** (ĕp"ĭ-glŏt'ĭs) (9). It acts as a lid to prevent solids and fluids from entering the larynx, directing them instead to the esophagus. The opening through which air enters the larynx is the **glottis** (glŏt'ĭs), which consists of two mobile vocal cords. Air passing through the glottis causes the vocal cords to vibrate and produce sounds, which become the voice. If the mucous membrane of the glottis becomes irritated or inflamed, the ability of the vocal cords to vibrate is inhibited, and hoarseness may result.

INTERNET ASSIGNMENT

The National Institute on Deafness and Other Communication Disorders (NIDCD) is one of the National Institutes of Health. It is mandated to conduct and support research concerning normal and disordered processes of hearing, balance, smell, taste, voice, speech, and language. The Health Information section includes resources available as well.

ACTIVITY

Visit NIDCD at **www.nidcd.nih.gov.** Under Health Information, click on Hearing, Ear Infections, and Deafness. The next screen provides a list of Diseases and Conditions. Select any of the hyperlinks in the list. Provide a summary of the information included in bulleted form at your instructor's request.

Review

The Nose and Throat

- To reach the lungs, air first passes through a bone and cartilaginous structure composed of two nostrils and a nasal cavity lined with mucous membrane and protective hairs.
- Air continues on its journey through the pharynx, which consists of the nasopharynx, oropharynx, and hypopharynx.
- The larynx connects the laryngopharyngeal section with the trachea to conduct air to and from the lungs.

Key Terminology Review

Word	Definition
acoustic meatus	opening to the external or internal auditory canal
adenoid	localized accumulation of lymphoid tissue on the nasopharynx
ampulla	enlargement of the semicircular canal containing sensory cells that provide directional information about the body's position
auricle (pinna)	outermost portion of the external ear
cerumen	substance, also called earwax, that is secreted from the ear canal
cochlea	snail-shaped inner ear
crypts	saclike cavities contained in the mucous membrane covering of the exposed surface of the tonsil
endolymph	fluid that fills the membranous labyrinth
epiglottis	lid that prevents solids and fluids from entering the larynx, directing them to the esophagus instead
eustachian tube	auditory tube; ventilation pathway between the nasopharynx and The middle ear
external auditory canal	part of the ear that guides sound waves into the eardrum and protects the internal structure of the ear
glottis	opening through which air enters the larynx
gustation	sense of taste
hard palate	roof of the mouth, which separates the mouth from the nasal cavity
hypopharynx	portion of the pharynx that lies below the epiglottis and above the esophagus
incus	second of the three ossicles of the middle ear

continues

Word	Definition
inner ear (labyrinth)	complex structure of the ear that transmits sound waves to the brain as electrical impulses and controls equilibrium
larynx	structure that connects the laryngopharyngeal region with the trachea and is used to conduct air to and from the lungs and block food from entry into the trachea
malleus	first of the three ossicles of the middle ear
middle ear	irregularly shaped, air-filled cavity lined with mucous membranes; tympanic cavity
nasopharynx	space that lies above the level of the soft palate
nasal conchae	three scroll-shaped bones forming the lateral wall of the nasal cavity
olfaction	sense of smell
organ of Corti	organ that contains the receptors for hearing and is located within the cochlea
oropharynx	division of the pharynx that extends from the soft palate to the upper border of the epiglottis
otolaryngologist	physician who specializes in the treatment of diseases and disorders of the ear, nose, throat, and adjacent structures of the head and neck
oval window	small membrane-covered opening in the bone wall between the middle ear and inner ear through which sound is transmitted
papilla, *pl.* papillae	small projection on the tongue that is also known as a taste bud
perilymph	fluid in the vestibule that separates the membranous labyrinth and the osseous labyrinth
pharynx	passageway for food and air
round window	small, membrane-covered opening in the bone wall between the middle and inner ears
saccule	structure of equilibrium located in the vestibule
semicircular canals	structures of the inner ear that contain the fluid and sensory cells that provide information about equilibrium and movement
septum	bone and cartilage partition separating the nose into two nostrils
sinuses	series of air spaces surrounding the nasal cavity; major pairs are frontal, sphenoid, maxillary, and ethmoidal
soft palate	posterior portion of the floor of the nasal cavity that is involved in speech and swallowing functions
stapes	third of the three ossicles of the middle ear
tonsils	small, rounded masses of lymphoid tissue on either side of the passageway into the throat
turbinates	three scroll-shaped bones that form the sidewall of the nasal cavity; covered by mucous membrane
tympanic membrane	eardrum
utricle	structure of equilibrium located in the vestibule
uvula	small peninsula of tissue at the back of the mouth
vestibule	perilymph-filled chamber connected to the oval window that leads to the middle ear

Key Terminology Practice Exercises

COMPLETION

Complete the following statements.

1. The three parts of the ear are the ________________, ________________, and ________________.
2. The outermost portion of the ear is the ________________.
3. The canal leading to the eardrum is lined with ________________ and ________________ glands.
4. The bone wall in the middle ear has two windows; they are the ________________ and ________________.
5. The three ossicles in the middle ear are the ________________, ________________, and ________________.
6. The three areas of the labyrinth are the ________________, ________________, and ________________.
7. The part of the ear that controls equilibrium is the ________________.
8. The secretion of modified sebaceous glands is ________________.
9. The ________________ directs air so pressure is equalized on both sides of the eardrum.
10. The vestibule of the ear is filled with a fluid called ________________.
11. The three sections of the pharynx are the ________________.
12. The part of the ear that guides sound waves into the eardrum is the ________________.
13. The roof of the mouth is the ________________.
14. The structures of equilibrium located in the vestibule are the ________________.
15. The enlargement of the semicircular canal that contains sensory cells that provide directional information about body position is the ________________.
16. The physician who specializes in the disease and disorders of the ear, nose, and throat and adjacent structures of the head and neck is a/n ________________.
17. The bone and cartilage partition separating nose into two nostrils is the ________________.
18. The small, rounded lymphoid tissue masses on either side of the passageway into the throat are the ________________.
19. Cerumen secreted in the ear canal is more commonly known as ________________.

MATCHING

Match the terms to their meaning.

1. __________ eardrum
2. __________ inner ear
3. __________ organ that contains receptors for hearing in the inner ear
4. __________ sense of smell
5. __________ sense of taste
6. __________ small projections on the tongue
7. __________ lid on the larynx
8. __________ scroll-shaped bones forming the lateral wall of the nasal cavity
9. __________ separates the nasal cavity from the mouth
10. __________ series of air-filled spaces surrounding the nasal cavity
11. __________ localized accumulation of lymphoid tissue on the nasopharynx

a. acoustic meatus
b. adenoids
c. crypts
d. endolymph
e. epiglottis
f. glottis
g. gustation
h. labyrinth
i. larynx
j. nasal conchae
k. olfaction
l. organ of Corti

12. __________ opening through which air enters the larynx
13. __________ provides air conduction to and from the lungs, as well as speech and airway protection during swallowing
14. __________ fluid that fills the membranous labyrinth
15. __________ opening to the auditory canal
16. __________ small peninsula of tissue at the back of the mouth
17. __________ structure of equilibrium located in the vestibule
18. __________ passageway for food and air
19. __________ 3 scroll-shaped bones forming the sidewall of the nasal cavity
20. __________ saclike cavities in the mucous membrane covering of the tonsils

m. papillae
n. pharynx
o. sinuses
p. soft palate
q. turbinates
r. tympanic membrane
s. utricle
t. uvula

Word Element Review

Root	Meaning	Example	Definition
acous/o	hearing	**acousma** (ă-kooz'mah)	buzzing or ringing sound
audi/o, audit/o	hearing,	**audiogram** (aw'dē-ō-grăm")	graphic record of a test of hearing sound
		audiometer (aw"dē-ŏm'ĕ-ter)	apparatus for measuring hearing at different sound frequencies
auri/o, auricul/o	ear	**auricle** (aw'rĕ-kl)	projecting part of the ear outside the head
cochle/o	cochlea	**cochleitis** (kŏk-lē-īt'ĭs)	inflammation of the cochlea
gingiv/o	gum	**gingivitis** (jĭn"jĭ-vī'tĭs)	inflammation of the gums
		gingivosis (jĭn"jĭ-vō'sĭs)	condition or disease of the gums of the mouth
gloss/o	tongue	**glossal** (glŏs'ăl)	pertaining to the tongue
		hypoglossal (hī"pō-glŏs'ăl)	underneath the tongue
lingu/o	tongue	**lingual** (lĭng'gwăl)	pertaining to the tongue
		lingually (lĭng'gwăl-lē)	toward the tongue

continues

Root	Meaning	Example	Definition
mastoid/o	mastoid process	**mastoidectomy** (măs"toy-dĕk'tō-mē)	hollowing out of the mastoid process by various means to remove bony partitions forming mastoid cells
myring/o	eardrum	**myringoplasty** (mĭ-rĭn'gō-plăst"ē)	surgical repair of defects of the eardrum
odont/o	tooth	**odontogenic** (ō-dŏn"tō-jĕn'ĭk)	originating in the teeth
or/o	mouth	**circumoral** (sĕr"kŭm-ō'răl) **oral** (ō'răl)	around the mouth pertaining to the mouth
ot/o	ear	**otogenic** (ō"tō-jĕn'ĭk)	originating in the ear
phon/o	sound	**phonic** (fŏn'ĭk) **phonogram** (fō'nō-grăm)	pertaining to the sound of the voice record of any sound
sial/o	salivary	**sialolith** (sī-ăl'ō-lĭth)	stone in the salivary duct
tympan/o	eardrum	**tympanic membrane** (tĭm-păn'ĭk)	eardrum
Suffixes	**Meaning**	**Example**	**Definition**
-cusis	hearing	**presbycusis** (prĕs"bē-kū'sĭs)	sensory hearing loss due to aging
-osmia	smell	**anosmia** (ăn-ōz'mē-ah)	absence of the sense of smell

Word Element Practice Exercises

WORD ELEMENTS

Provide the correct word element to complete the following words.

1. pertaining to the tongue ____________________ al
2. pertaining to the mouth ____________________ al
3. record of a sound ____________________ gram
4. originating in the teeth ____________________ genic
5. surgical repair of defects of the eardrum ____________________ plasty
6. graphic record of a test of hearing ____________________ gram

7. pertaining to sound of voice ______________ ic
8. originating in the ear ______________ genic
9. condition or disease of the gums ______________ osis
10. inflammation of cochlea ______________ itis
11. buzzing or ringing sound ______________ ma
12. part of ear outside the head ______________ cle
13. removing bony portions forming mastoid cells ______________ ectomy
14. around the mouth ______________ oral
15. stone in the salivary duct ______________ olith
16. sensory hearing loss in the aging presby ______________
17. absence of sense of smell an ______________
18. eardrum ______________ ic membrane
19. record of any sound ______________ gram
20. toward the tongue ______________ ally

IDENTIFICATION

Identify the following definitions.

1. apparatus for measuring hearing at different sound frequencies ______________
2. eardrum ______________
3. stone in the salivary duct ______________
4. toward the tongue ______________
5. inflammation of the gums ______________
6. originating in the ear ______________
7. sensory hearing loss due to aging ______________
8. absence of sense of smell ______________
9. part of ear projecting outside head ______________
10. buzzing or ringing sound ______________
11. underneath the tongue ______________
12. around the mouth ______________
13. hollowing out mastoid process to remove bony partitions ______________
14. pertaining to the sound of the voice ______________
15. surgical repair of eardrum defects ______________
16. originating in the teeth ______________
17. pertaining to the tongue ______________
18. inflammation of the cochlea ______________
19. pertaining to the mouth ______________
20. inflammation of the gums ______________

SHORT ANSWER

Supply a brief answer to the following.

1. Name four word elements that mean hearing.

____

2. Name three elements that mean ear.

____

3. Name two elements that mean eardrum.

____

4. Name two elements that mean tongue.

____

5. Name three elements that mean sound.

____

WORD ELEMENT MEANINGS

Give the meaning of each word element. Then use your dictionary to find a new word that contains each of the word elements. Specify whether the new word is a noun or an adjective by placing N or A in the last column.

Word Element	Meaning	Word	N or A
1. acous/o			
2. audi/o			
3. audit/o			
4. auricul/o			
5. auri/o			
6. cochle/o			
7. -cusis			
8. gingiv/o			
9 gloss/o			
10. lingu/o			
11. mastoid/o			
12. myring/o			
13. odont/o			
14. or/o			
15. -osmia			
16. ot/o			
17. phon/o			
18. sial/o			
19. tympan/o			

DIAGNOSTIC PROCEDURES		
Word	**Pronunciation**	**Definition**
General		
audiometry	aw"dē-ŏm'ĕ-trē	use of an electronic device that delivers specific sound frequencies to determine a patient's hearing threshold
ear thermometry	thĕr-mŏm'ĕ-trē	measurement of the temperature of the tympanic membrane with a device that detects infrared radiation from the eardrum
impedance audiometry	ĭm-pēd'ăns ăw"dē-ŏm'ĕ-trē	evaluation of the middle ear function by measurement of the movement of the tympanic membrane and pressure in the middle ear
laryngoscopy	lăr"ĭng-gŏs'kō-pē	visual examination of the larynx with a laryngoscope or a mirror (see Figure 23-5)
myringotomy	mĭr"ĭn-gŏt'ō-mē	incision into the tympanic membrane for diagnostic evaluation (see Treatment Procedures)
otoscopy	ō-tŏs'kō-pē	visual examination of the ear with an otoscope
pneumatic	nū-măt'ĭk	air insufflation during an membrane movement; best way to diagnose middle ear effusion or infection
tuning fork test		test in which a tuning fork is placed near the ear to test for air conduction and in contact with the skull to test for bone conduction (Weber and Rinne tests) (see Figure 23-6)

continues

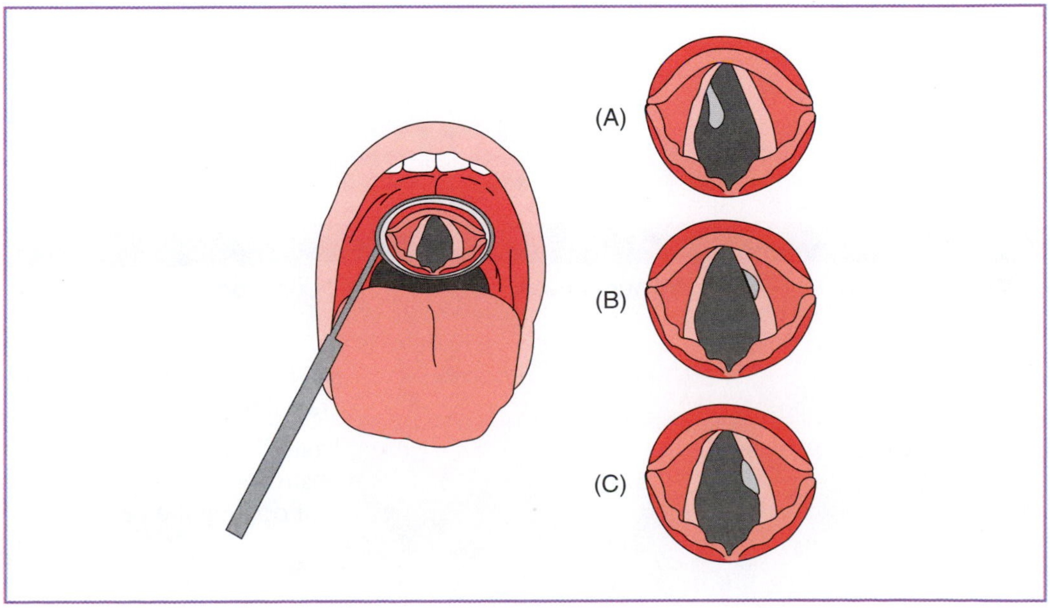

FIGURE 23-5 Laryngoscopy with Polyp: An indirect laryngoscopy is performed by using a small angled mirror, which provides a direct view of the vocal cords. (A) vocal cord polyp, (B) contact ulcer; (C) vocal cord cancer

Source: Delmar/Cengage Learning

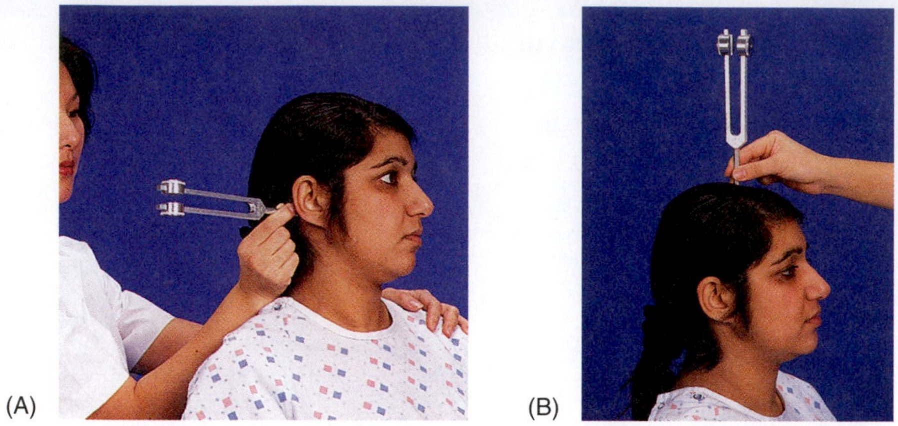

FIGURE 23-6 Tuning Fork Test: (A) Rinne test, (B) Weber test

Source: Delmar/Cengage Learning

DIAGNOSTIC PROCEDURES

Word	Pronunciation	Definition
Laboratory throat cultures (swabs or washings)		test in which secretions from inflamed areas are analyzed for presence of various pathogens by removing samples from these areas
nasal cultures (swab)		test in which secretions from the nares or meatus of the nose are checked for various pathogens
Radiology computer-assisted tomography (CAT)	tō-mŏg'-rah-fē	computer-reconstructed x-ray of a body section to look for abnormalities in the brain that may be causing of the skull visual, hearing, or other problems
magnetic resonant imagery (MRI)		use of radio waves and a strong magnetic field to make cross-sectional images of the body to reveal lesions and changes in organs and tissues
x-ray studies of the skull, mastoids, sinuses, and chest		standard views of the specific parts

DIAGNOSES

Word	Pronunciation	Definition
The Ear acoustic neuroma	ah-koos'tĭk nŭ-rō'mah	slow-growing benign tumor of the eighth cranial nerve
auditory canal obstruction		limited hearing because of cerumen obstruction, foreign bodies, or infections that occlude the ear canal

continues

DIAGNOSES		
Word	**Pronunciation**	**Definition**
The Ear (*continued*)		
benign paroxysmal positional vertigo (BPPV)	bē-nīn' păr"ŏk-sĭz'măl	recurrent episodes of brief vertigo occurring when the head is placed in certain positions and resolved when the head returns to normal position
cholesteatoma	kŏ"lĕ-stē"ah-tō'mah	destructive cyst of the middle ear and mastoid formed from chronic disease of the tympanic membrane
hearing loss		condition of reduced ability to perceive sound at its normal levels; non-age-related condition may be conductive, sensorineural, or mixed
• *conductive*		inability to conduct sound waves through the external ear canal to the tympanic membrane of the middle ear
• *presbycusis*	prĕz-bĭ-kū'sĭs	hearing loss caused by the normal aging process
• *sensorineural*	sĕn"sō-rē-nŭ'răl	hearing loss caused by nerve transmission failure within the inner ear, cochlea, or auditory nerve
impacted cerumen	ĭm-păk'tĕd sĕ-roo'mĕn	excessive accumulation of wax-like secretions from the glands of the external ear canal
labyrinthitis	lăb"ĭ-rĭn-thī'tĭs	inflammation of the inner ear causing hearing loss and vertigo (rare)
mastoiditis	măs"toyd-ī'tĭs	inflammation of the mastoid bone
Meniere's disease	mēn"ē-ārz'	episodic vertigo with hearing loss, ear fullness sensation, nausea, and tinnitus; may lead to progressive deafness
motion sickness		sensation of dysequilibrium that occurs when riding in autos, planes, boats, or amusement rides
otitis externa	ō-tī'tĭs ĕks-tĕr'nah	infection of the external ear canal; swimmer's ear
otitis media	ō'tī'tĭs mē'dē-ah	acute or chronic infection or inflammation of the middle ear occurring in the following two forms
• *serous otitis media*	sēr'ŭs	fluid in the middle ear following an infectious or inflammatory process (see Figure 23-7A)
• *suppurative otitis media*	sūp'ŭ-rā"tĭv	purulent fluid accumulation and infection build up in middle ear; may result in a ruptured eardrum (see Figure 23-7B)
otosclerosis	ō"tō-sklē-rō'sĭs	abnormal growth of bone at the stapes causing conductive hearing loss
ruptured eardrum		hole in the eardrum due to injury or infection

continues

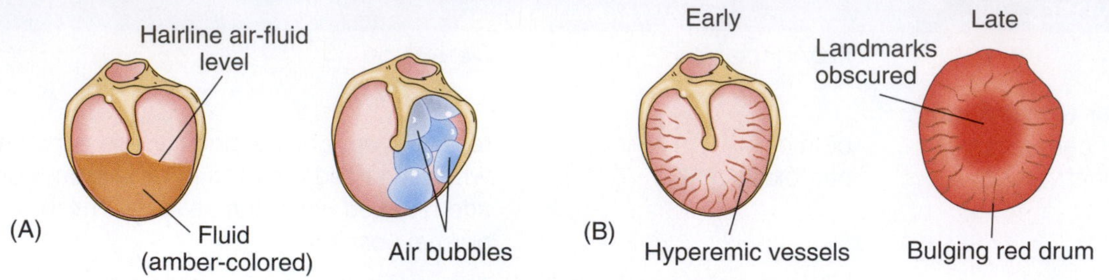

FIGURE 23-7 Otitis Media: (A) serous; (B) acute purulent (suppurative)

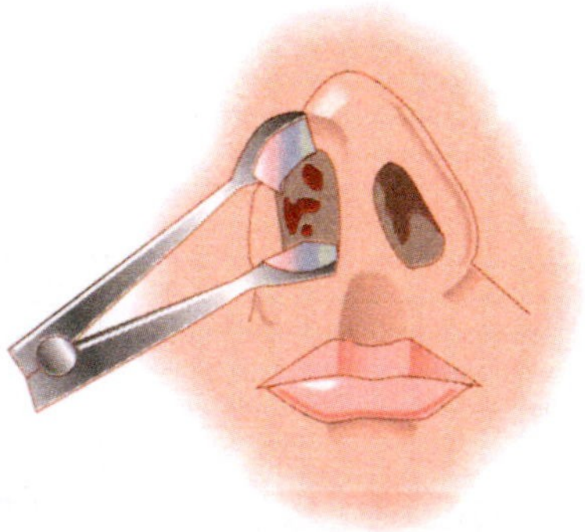

FIGURE 23-8 Rhinitis

DIAGNOSES

Word	Pronunciation	Definition
The Ear (*continued*)		
tinnitus	tĭn-ī'tŭs	perception of sound in the absence of stimuli
vertigo	vĕr'tĭ-gō	sensation of rotation or movement resulting from disease of the inner ear or disturbances of the vestibular centers or pathways in the central nervous system
vestibular neuritis	vĕs-tĭb'ū-lăr nū-rī'tĭs	inflammation of the vestibular nerve causing vertigo (common)
The Nose and Sense of Smell		
adenoid hyperplasia	ăd'ĕ-noyd hī"pĕr-plā'zē-ah	condition characterized by enlargement of the adenoidal structure due to lymphoid hyperplasia
epistaxis	ĕp"ĭ-stăk'sĭs	bleeding from the nose
nasal polyp	pŏl'ĭp	growth protruding from a mucous membrane in the nose
rhinitis: allergic, vasomotor, medicamentosus, viral	rī-nī'tĭs, văs-ō-mŏ'tor, mĕd"ĭ-kah-mĕn-tō'sŭs	inflammation and obstruction of the nose due to allergy, mucous gland imperfection, overuse of decongestant spray, or viral infection, respectively (see Figure 23-8)

continues

DIAGNOSES		
Word	**Pronunciation**	**Definition**
The Nose and Sense of Smell (*continued*)		
septal deviation	sĕp'tăl	condition when the partition between the two sides of the nose is out of alignment due to developmental abnormalities or trauma; may cause airway obstruction
sinusitis	sī-nŭs-ī'tĭs	inflammation of a sinus cavity; may be acute or chronic
The Tongue and Sense of Taste		
contact ulcers		traumatic ulcers that appear on vocal cords where larynx cartilages are in contact with each other on the endotracheal tube (see Figure 23-5B)
epiglottitis	ĕp"ĭ-glŏt-tī'tĭs	inflammation, most common in very young children, of lidlike cartilage covering the windpipe
laryngitis	lăr"ĭn-jī'tĭs	inflammation of the larynx
peritonsillar abscess	pĕr"ĭ-tŏn'sĭ-lăr	abscess formed between an infected tonsil and the surrounding soft tissue; known as quinsy
pharyngitis	făr"ĭn-jī'tĭs	inflammation of the pharynx
throat cancer		tumors on the vocal cords or in and around the larynx (see Figure 23-5C)
throat polyps	pŏl'ĭp	growth or mass protruding from a mucous membrane covering of the vocal cord (see Figure 23-5A)
tonsillitis	tŏn"sĭ-lī'tĭs	acute inflammation of the tonsils

TREATMENT PROCEDURES		
Word	**Pronunciation**	**Definition**
adenoidectomy	ăd"ĕ-noid-ĕk'tō-mē	surgical excision of the adenoids
antral window	ăn'trăl, ăn-trŏs'tō-mē	creation of an opening into the maxillary sinus or antrum (antrostomy)
cochlear implant	kŏk'lē-ăr	device implanted in the cochlea that improves hearing when a regular hearing aid is of no benefit
endoscopic sinus surgery	ĕn"dō-skŏp'ĭk	use of endoscope to perform surgery on a sinus cavity
laryngectomy	lăr"ĭn-jĕk'tō-mē	excision of the larynx (voice box), following which speech can be facilitated by using esophageal speech or an artificial voice aid—either neck type or an intra-oral device (see Figure 23-9)

continues

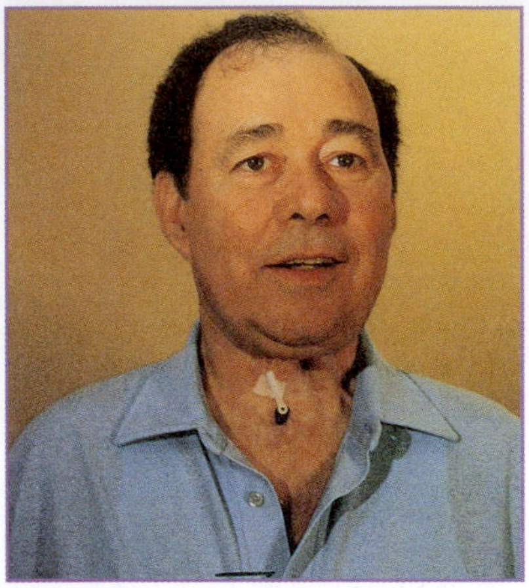

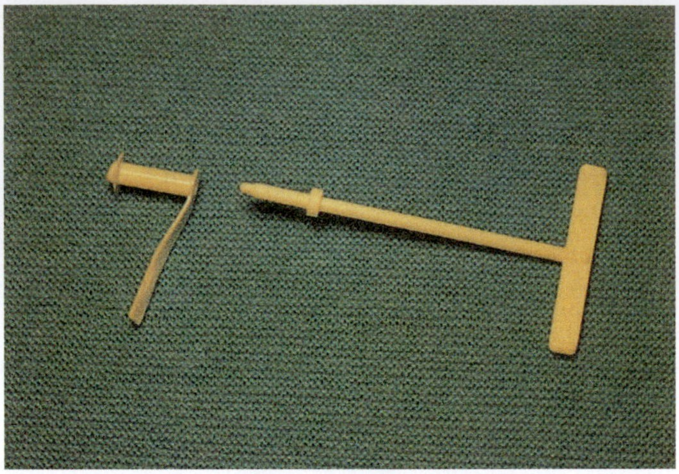

Source: Delmar/Cengage Learning

FIGURE 23-9 Voice Aids after Laryngectomy

TREATMENT PROCEDURES		
Word	**Pronunciation**	**Definition**
mastoidectomy	măs"toi-dĕk'tō-mē	surgical removal of mastoid cells
myringoplasty or tympanoplasty	mĭr-ĭn'gō-plăs"tē tĭm"păn-ō-plăs'tē	surgical repair of the tympanic membrane (eardrum) with a tissue graft
myringotomy (tympanostomy, tympanotomy)	mĭr"ĭn'gō"tō-mē (tĭm"păn-ŏs'tō-mē) (tĭm"păn-ŏt'ō-mē)	incision into the eardrum to relieve pressure or release fluid from the middle ear (see Diagnostic Procedures)
myringotomy with tubes		incision into the eardrum with the placing of a ventilation tube (see Figure 23-10)
otoplasty	ō'tō-plăs"tē	removal of a portion of the ear cartilage to bring the pinna or auricle nearer the head
polypectomy	pŏl"ĭ-pĕk'tō-mē	excision of polyps
rhinoplasty	rī'nō-plăs"tē	plastic surgery or reconstruction of the nose
septoplasty	sĕp"tō-plăs'tē	surgical procedure to realign the septum
stapedectomy	stā"pĕ-dĕk'tō-mē	surgical removal of the stapes and replacement with a prosthetic device (see Figure 23-11)
tonsillectomy	tŏn"sĭ-lĕk'tō-mē	surgical excision of the tonsils
tracheostomy	trā"kē-ŏs'tō-mē	creation of an opening into the trachea through the neck

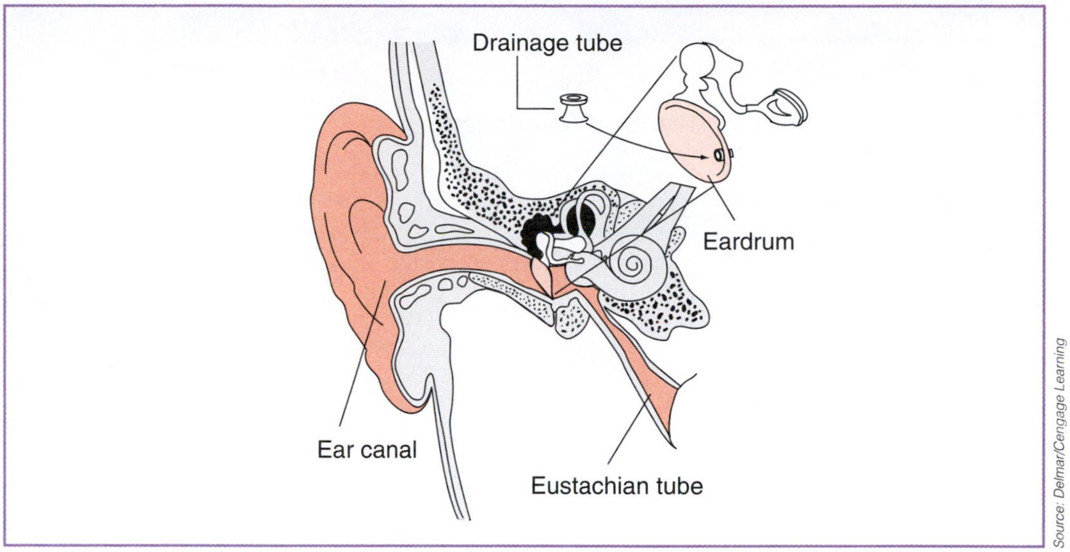

FIGURE 23-10 Myringotomy with Tubes

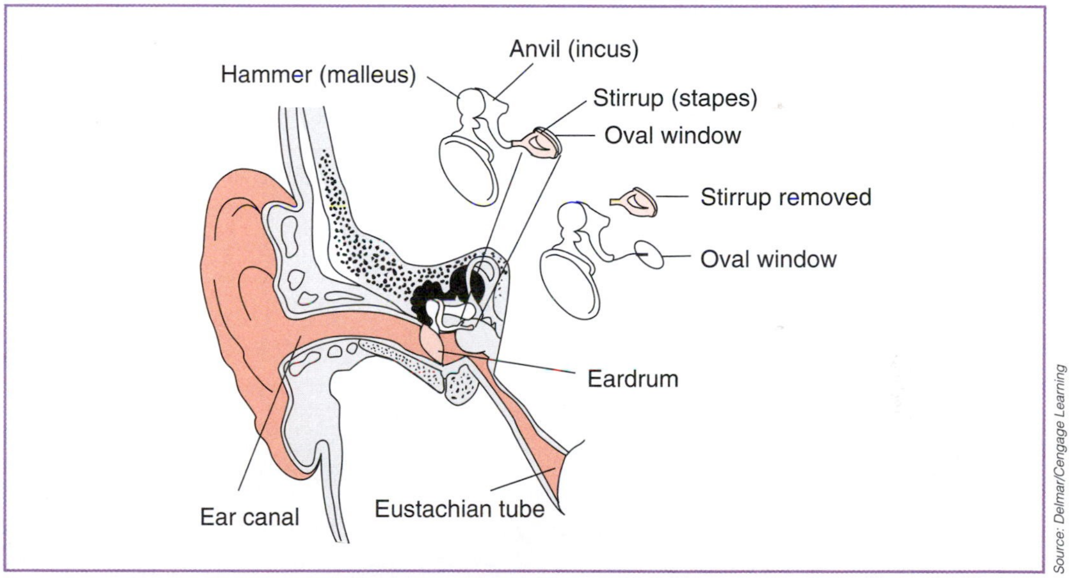

FIGURE 23-11 Stapedectomy

MEDICATIONS PRESCRIBED

Trade Name	Generic Name
Mouth and Throat	
Mycelex Troches	clotrimazole
Nilstat, Mycostatin, Bio-Statin	nystatin
Peridex, Periogard	chlorhexidine gluconate
Oral Antibiotics for ENT Disorders	
Amoxil, Biomox, Trimox	amoxicillin
Augmentin	amoxicillin and potassium clavulanate
Ceftin	cefuroxime axetil
E.E.S., Eryc, E-Mycin	erythromycin

continues

MEDICATIONS PRESCRIBED	
Trade Name	**Generic Name**
Oral Antibiotics for ENT Disorders (*continued*)	
Keflex	cephalexin
Omnipen, Principen, Totacillin	ampicillin
Suprax	cefixime
Otics	
Cerumenex	triethanolamine
Cortisporin Otic, Bacticort, Cortomycin	hydrocortisone, neomycin, polymyxin
Debrox	carbamide peroxide
Floxin Otic	ofloxacin
VoSol Otic	hydrocortisone, acetic acid
Antihistamines	
Allegra	fexofenadine HCl
Astelin	azelastine HCl
Atarax	hydroxyzine HCl
Claritin	loratadine
Deconamine SR	pseudoephedrine and chlorpheniramine
Optimine	azatadine maleate
Periactin	cyproheptadine HCl
Phenergan	promethazine HCl
Semprex-D	pseudoephedrine and acrivastine
Vistaril	hydroxyzine pamoate
Zyrtec	cetirizine HCl
Corticosteroids	
Beconase AQ, Vancenase	beclomethasone dipropionate
Flonase	fluticasone propionate
Nasacort	triamcinolone acetonide
Nasalide, Nasarel	flunisolide
Nasonex	mometasone furoate
Rhinocort	budesonide

ABBREVIATIONS	
AC	air conduction
AD	*auris dextra* (right ear)
AS	*auris sinistra* (left ear)
AU	*aures unitas* (both ears)
BC	bone conduction
BOM	bilateral otitis media
dB	decibel
ENT	ear, nose, and throat
ETD	eustachian tube dysfunction
Oto	otology
PE	tube pressure equalization tube
PTS	permanent threshold shift
T & A, T&A	tonsillectomy and adenoidectomy
TM	tympanic membrane
TTS	temporary threshold shift

Working Practice Review Exercises

MATCHING

Match the diagnoses to their meanings.

1. __________ episodic vertigo with hearing loss, nausea, and tinnitus; may lead to progressive deafness
2. __________ nosebleed
3. __________ growth protruding from a mucous membrane of the nose
4. __________ sensory hearing loss due to aging
5. __________ inflammation of air cells of the mastoid bone
6. __________ perception of sound in the absence of stimuli
7. __________ acute or chronic infection of the middle ear
8. __________ destructive cyst of middle ear and mastoid
9. __________ inflammation of inner ear causing hearing loss and vertigo (rare)
10. __________ fluid in the ear following an infectious or inflammatory process
11. __________ condition where the partition between the two sides of the nose is out of alignment

a. cholesteatoma
b. conductive hearing loss
c. epistaxis
d. labyrinthitis
e. mastoiditis
f. Meniere's disease
g. nasal polyps
h. otitis media
i. presbycusis
j. ruptured eardrum
k. septal deviation
l. serous otitis media
m. throat polyp
n. tinnitus
o. tonsillitis

12. __________ benign growth protruding from mucous membrane covering of the vocal cord
13. __________ acute inflammation of the tonsils
14. __________ inability to conduct sound waves through the external ear canal, tympanic membrane, or middle ear
15. __________ hole in the eardrum due to injury or infection

MEANING

Give the meaning of each of the italicized treatment procedures.

1. Ms. Macrino's hearing problem will be solved by a *stapedectomy*.
   ____
2. A *myringotomy* is commonly performed on little children.
   ____
3. Mr. Weber is scheduled for a *laryngectomy* tomorrow.
   ____
4. We do *antral windows* on Ms. Baxter tomorrow.
   ____
5. He debated whether he should have an *otoplasty*.
   ____
6. He has had a *polypectomy* three times.
   ____
7. The pediatrician finally suggested a *myringotomy with tubes*.
   ____
8. After the accident, she required *septoplasty*.
   ____
9. Her friend had an *endoscopic sinus surgery* that was quite successful.
   ____
10. Mrs. Obear was relieved when the otolaryngologist suggested a *tonsillectomy* for her son.
   ____

IDENTIFICATION

Identify the following definitions.

1. use of sounds to test a patient's hearing __________
2. detection of middle ear effusion or infection __________
3. visual examination of the ears __________
4. Rinne test or Weber test __________
5. detects tympanic membrane movement __________
6. visual examination of larynx __________
7. incision into tympanic membrane for diagnostic evaluation __________

8. test of secretions from nares for pathogens ______________________
9. standard views of specific parts ______________________
10. computer-reconstructed x-ray to look for abnormalities in the brain that may be causing problems ______________________

Dictionary Exercises

DICTIONARY EXERCISE 1

Use your dictionary to find the pronunciation and definition of each of the following words.

Word	Pronunciation	Definition
1. acoustic	______________	______________
2. anthelix	______________	______________
3. arytenoid	______________	______________
4. cleft palate	______________	______________
5. otomycosis	______________	______________
6. ossiculotomy	______________	______________
7. rhinophyma	______________	______________
8. torus palatinus	______________	______________
9. aural	______________	______________
10. purulent	______________	______________
11. auriculotemporal	______________	______________
12. barotitis media	______________	______________
13. deglutition	______________	______________

DICTIONARY EXERCISE 2

Match the terms to their meanings.

1. __________ located or performed behind the auricle of the ear
2. __________ benign tumor of the nose in puberty
3. __________ main division of the auditory nerve
4. __________ abnormal sound made by the larynx in spasm
5. __________ principal duct of the parotid gland
6. __________ bleeding from the ear
7. __________ differences in pressure on both sides of the eardrum
8. __________ dizziness due to disease of the ear
9. __________ relating to gum tissue

a. auditory vertigo
b. barotraumas
c. gingival
d. juvenile angiofibroma
e. laryngeal stridor
f. leukoplakia
g. NG
h. n.p.o.
i. otorrhagia

10. ________ one of the largest pairs of salivary glands		j. parotid gland
11. ________ precancerous lesion occurring anywhere in the mouth		k. periodontal disease
12. ________ inflammatory gum disorders		l. postauricular
13. ________ fungal infection in the mouth		m. Stensen's duct
14. ________ abbreviation for nothing by mouth		n. thrush
15. ________ abbreviation for nasogastric		o. vestibular nerve

DICTIONARY EXERCISE 3

Pronunciation of the words below is provided. Using your dictionary, find the correct spelling and definition of each word.

Word	Pronunciation	Definition
1. ________	fĕn"ĕ-strā'shŭn	________
2. ________	hī"pō-ă-kū'sĭs	________
3. ________	ō-tăl'jē-ah	________
4. ________	rī"nō-rē'ah	________
5. ________	nā"zō-mĕn'tăl	________
6. ________	kald'wĕl-lŭk' operation	________
7. ________	ō"tō-pī"ă-rē'ă	________
8. ________	săl-pĭng"gō-fă-rĭn'jē-ăl	________
9. ________	măk-rō'shē-ă	________
10. ________	mī-krō'shē-ă	________
11. ________	măs-tĭ-kā'shŭn	________
12. ________	ăf'thŭs stō-mă-tī'tĭs	________
13. ________	dĕn'tăl kār'ēz	________
14. ________	hĕr-pĕt'ĭk stō-mă-tī'tĭs	________
15. ________	bō'lŭs	________

*Study*WARE™ Connection

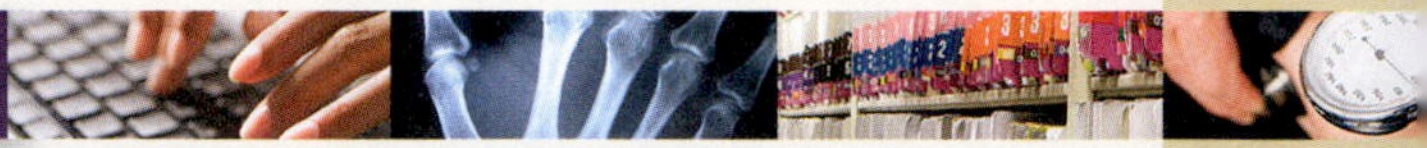

To take a practice quiz or play interactive games that reinforce the content in this chapter, go to your StudyWARE™ CD-ROM.

Listening Exercise

INSTRUCTIONS

1. Review the spelling, pronunciation, and meaning of the words provided in the preview.
2. Go to your StudyWARE™ CD-ROM and listen to **Listening Exercise 23-1.** Fill in the blank in the report as the word is dictated.
3. At the end of the activity, check your spelling against the preview words. They appear in the preview in the order in which they are encountered in the activity.
4. Review and practice the words you missed.
5. Look up words that are not familiar.

PREVIEW OF WORDS FOR LISTENING ACTIVITY 23-1

Word	Pronunciation	Meaning
sinusitis	sī-nŭs-ī'tŭs	inflammation of a sinus cavity
mucosal	mū-kō'săl	pertaining to mucous membrane
opacified	ō-păs'ĭ-fīd	made opaque—not penetrable by radiant energy
artifact	ăr'tĭ-făkt	a product produced by an external agent or action
nasopharynx	nā"zō-făr'ĭnks	the part of the pharynx above the soft palate
coronal	kō-rō'năl	pertaining to a crownlike structure

Listening Exercise 23-1

*Study*WARE™ Connection

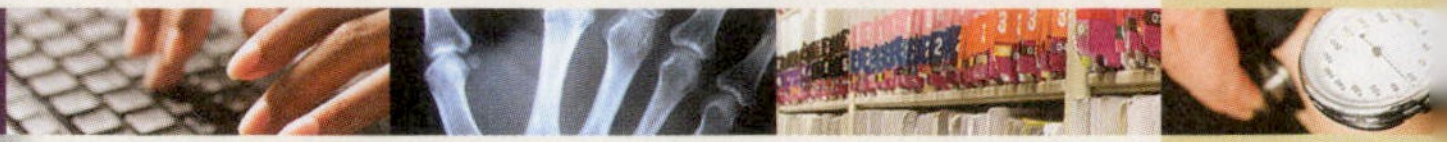

Listen to this report being read on your StudyWARE™ CD-ROM. Fill in each blank as the word is dictated.

Computed Tomograph of the Sinuses

History is that of a chronic _________________ with previous surgical intervention. A neo-synephrine study was performed.

FINDINGS:

Maxillary sinuses have some _________________ thickening and air-fluid levels. Front sinuses, ethmoid sinuses, right sphenoid sinuses, and portions of the left sphenoid sinus are nearly completely _________________ by soft tissue without definite evidence for expansion or erosion. A small fluid level is seen within the sphenoid sinuses. Dental amalgam creates what I believe to be significant _________________ along the posterior lateral walls of the maxillary sinuses, but certainly a subtle erosion there cannot be excluded as a result of that. Axial sections may be necessary if that is important to delineate clinically. I believe previous surgery involving the medial walls of both maxillary sinuses into the _________________ accounts for the lack of bony confines there. The osteomeatal complex certainly is compromised.

Rather prominent frontal sinuses are seen with respect to the capacity but they are completely occupied by soft tissue. The integrity of the posterior wall of the front sinuses is not able to be evaluated in the _________________ projection.

APPENDIX A Word Elements to Meanings

Word Element	Meaning
a-	no, not, without
ab-	away from, not
-ac	pertaining to
acous/o	hearing
acr/o	extremity
aden/o	gland
adip/o	fat
adnex/o	tie, connection
adren/o	adrenal gland
adrenal/o	adrenal gland
aer/o	air
agglutin/o	clumping, sticking
-al	pertaining to
albin/o	white
albumin/o	albumin
alg/o	pain; cold
alges/o	sensitivity to pain
-algia	pain
alveol/o	alveolus, air sac
ambly/o	dim, dull
ameb-	change
ameb/o	change
amni/o	amnion
amyl/o	starch
an/o	anal
an-	away from; no, not, without
ana-	against; back; backward; up
andr/o	male; man
angi/o	blood vessel
ankyl/o	crooked, bent
ant-	against
ante-	before; forward
anthrac/o	black
anti-	against
antr/o	chamber, cavity
anxi/o	anxious, uneasy
aort/o	aorta
append/o	appendix
appendic/o	appendix
aque/o	water
-ar	relating to; of; resembling
-arche	beginning; first
arter/o	artery
arteri/o	artery
arthr/o	joint
articul/o	joint
-ary	pertaining to
-asthenia	lack of strength, weakness

Word Element	Meaning
astr/o	star-shaped
astr-	star
ather/o	yellowish plaque; fatty substance
atri/o	atrium
audi/o	hearing; sound
audit/o	hearing; sound
auri/o	ear
auricul/o	ear
auto-	self
azot/o	nitrogen
bacteri/o	bacteria
balan/o	glans penis
bas/o	base; pertaining to a base
bi-	two
bil/i	bile
bilirubin/o	bilirubin
blast/o	embryonic; immature
-blast	immature
blast-	immature
blephar/o	eyelid
blephar-	eyelid
brachy-	short distance
brady-	slow
bronch/o	bronchus
bronchi/o	bronchus
bronchiol/o	bronchiole
bucc/o	cheek
burs/o	sac
calc/o	calcium
calci/o	calcium
cali/o	calyx
calic/o	calyx
capn/o	carbon dioxide
carcin/o	cancerous
carcin-	cancerous
cardi/o	heart
cardi-	heart
carp/o	wrist
cata-	down
caud/o	tail
cec/o	cecum
cel/o	abdomen
-cele	hernia
celi/o	abdomen
-centesis	puncture
cephal/o	head
cerebell/o	cerebellum

Word Element	Meaning
cerebr/o	brain
cervic/o	neck; cervix
cheil/o	lip
cheir/o	hand
chem/o	chemical, drug
chil/o	lip
chir/o	hand
chlor/o	green
chol/e	bile
chol/o	bile
cholangi/o	bile or hepatic duct
cholecyst/o	gallbladder
choledoch/o	bile duct
chondr/o	cartilage
cili/o	eyelid
cili-	eyelid
cirrh/o	tawny yellow
cleid/o	clavicle
coagul/o	clotting
-coccus	berry-shaped
cochle/o	cochlea
col/o	colon
coll/o	glue-like
colon/o	colon
colp/o	vagina
comat/o	deep sleep
conjunctiv/o	conjunctiva
contra-	against, opposite
corne/o	cornea; horny
coron/o	heart
cost/o	rib
crani/o	head, skull
crin/o	secrete
crin-	secrete
-crine	secrete
-crit	separate
cry-	cold
cry/o	cold
crypt/o	hidden
-cusis	hearing
cusis-	hearing
cut/o	skin
cutane/o	skin
cyan/o	blue
cyan-	blue
-cyesis	pregnancy
cyst/o	bladder, sac
cyt-	cell
-cyte	cell
cyt/o	cell
-cytosis	abnormal condition of cells
dacry/o	tear; tear duct
dactyl/o	finger; toe
dendr/o	branching
dendr-	branching
derm/o	skin
dermat/o	skin
-desis	binding; fixation
diaphor/o	profuse sweating

Word Element	Meaning
digit/o	finger; toe
dipl/o	double
dors/o	back
duct/o	carry
duoden/o	duodenum
dur/o	dura mater
dura-	hard
dynam/o	power
-dynia	pain
dys-	bad; labored
-eal	pertaining to
echo-	repeated sound
ect/o	outside
ect-	out; outside
-ectasia	dilation, expansion, stretching
-ectasis	dilation, expansion, stretching
-ectomy	excision, surgical removal
-ema	condition
-emesis	vomiting
-emia	blood condition
en-	in; within
encephal/o	brain
end/o	inside
endo-	within
enter/o	intestine
eosin/o	red
ependym/o	wrapping
epi-	above; upon
epididym/o	epididymis
epiglott/o	epiglottis
episi/o	vulva
eryth/o	red
erythr/o	red
esophag/o	esophagus
esthes/o	feeling; sensation
esthesi/o	feeling; sensation
eu-	good; normal
ex-	out; away from
fasci/o	sheet; band
fibr/o	fiber
fistul-	narrow opening
fluor/o	luminous
furc/o	division
-fusion	pour
gangli/o	swelling
gastr/o	stomach
gastr-	stomach
gemin-	two; twin
-gen	originate; produce
-genesis	formation
-genic	produced by
gingiv/o	gum
glauc/o	gray
gli/o	glue
-globin	protein
-globulin	protein
glomerul/o	ball, cluster
gloss/o	tongue
glott/o	glottis

Word Element	Meaning
gluc/o	sugar
glyc/o	sugar
gon/o	seed
-gram	record; picture; tracing
gran-	grain
granul/o	granule
-graph	instrument for recording
-graphy	processing of recording
gravid/o	pregnancy
-gravida	pregnant female
gynec/o	female
hallucin/o	hallucination
hem/o	blood
hemat/o	blood
hemi-	half
hemoglobin/o	hemoglobin
hepat/o	liver
hepatic/o	liver
hidr/o	sweat
hist/o	tissue
hydr/o	water; fluid
hydro-	water
hyper-	above; excessive; more than
hypn/o	sleep
hypo-	below; beneath; deficient; less than; under
hyster/o	uterus
-ia	condition, formation
-iac	pertaining to; relating to; of
-iasis	condition, formation
iatr/o	physician; treatment
-ic	pertaining to; relating to
-ical	pertaining to
ichthy/o	dry, scaly
-ile	pertaining to; capable
ile/o	ileum
ili/o	ilium
immun/o	immune, immunity; protection
in-	into; inward; not
infra-	beneath
inter-	between
intra-	within
irid/o	iris
is/o	equal, same
iso-	equal
ischi/o	hip
iso-	equal, same
-itis	inflammation
jaund/o	yellow
jejun/o	jejunum
kary/o	nucleus
kerat/o	cornea; horny
ket/o	ketone bodies
keton/o	ketone bodies
kines/o	movement
-kinesia	movement
-kinetic	movement
kyph/o	humpback
lacrim/o	tear

Word Element	Meaning
lact/o	milk
lamin/o	lamina
lapar/o	abdomen
laryng/o	larynx
later/o	side
lei/o	smooth
leiomy/o	smooth or nonstriated muscle
lept/o	slender, thin
leuk/o	white
leuk-	white
ligament/o	ligament
lingu/o	tongue
lip/o	fat
lith/o	stone
lob/o	lobe; section
-logist	specialist in the study of
-logy	study of
lord/o	swayback
-lucent	shine
lumb/o	loin; lower back
lute/o	yellow
lymph/o	lymph
lymphaden/o	lymph nodes
lymphangi/o	lymph vessel
-lysis	breakdown; destruction; loosening; setting free
-lytic	pertaining to destruction or loosening of
macro-	large
macul/o	spot
mal-	bad
-malacia	softening
malign-	bad
mamm/o	breast
-mania	excessive preoccupation
mast/o	breast
mastoid/o	mastoid process
maxill/o	upper jaw bone
meat/o	meatus
medull/o	soft inner part; medulla
mega-	large
-megaly	enlargement
melan/o	black
men/o	menses
mening/o	meninges; membranes around the central nervous system
ment/o	mind
meso-	middle
meta-	beyond; change
metr/o	uterus
micr/o	small size; microscopic
micro-	small
mon/o	single
morph/o	form; shape
multi-	many
muscul/o	muscle
mut/a	genetic change
mutagen/o	causing genetic change
my/o	muscle

Word Element	Meaning
myc/o	fungus
mydr/o	widen; enlarge
myel/o	bone marrow; spinal cord
myring/o	eardrum
narc/o	stupor
nas/o	nose
necr/o	death
neo-	new, recent
ne/o	new
nephr/o	kidney
neur/o	nerve; nervous system
neutr/o	neutral
noct/i	night
nulli-	no, none, not
nyct/o	night
ocul/o	eye
odont/o	tooth
-oid	like; resembling
-ologist	specialist in the study of
-ology	study of
-oma	tumor
oment/o	covering
onc/o	tumor
onych/o	nail
oophor/o	ovary
-opaque	obscure
ophthalm/o	eye
-opia	vision
-opsia	vision
opt/o	eye; vision
optic/o	eye; vision
or/o	mouth
orch/o	testis
orchi/o	testis
orchid/o	testis
-ory	pertaining to, relating to
-ose	pertaining to; glucose
-osis	condition
-osmia	smell
ossicul/o	ossicle
oste/o	bone
-ostomy	creation of a new opening
ot/o	ear
-otomy	incision into
-ous	pertaining to; possessing; full of
ov/i	egg
ov/o	egg
ovari/o	ovary
ovul/o	egg
oxy-	rapid; sharp; acid
palpebr/o	eyelid
pan-	all
pancreat/o	pancreas
papill/o	papillary, nipple-like; optic disk
-par	bear; birth; labor
par-	bear; other than
para-	abnormal; beside
-para	to bear; birth; labor
parathyroid/o	parathyroid glands
-paresis	partial paralysis; slight paralysis
pariet/o	wall of an organ; cavity
-parous	to bring forth; bear
-part	birth; labor
part-	bear
-partum	birth; labor
path/o	disease
-pathy	disease
pect/o	breast; chest
pector/o	breast; chest
ped/o	foot
-penia	decrease; deficiency
-pepsia	digestion
peri-	about; around; surrounding
pericardi/o	pericardium
peritone/o	peritoneum
-pexy	surgical fixation
phac/o, phak/o	lens of the eye
phag/o	eat; swallow
-phagia	eating; swallowing
pharmac/o	drug, medicine
pharyng/o	pharynx; throat
-phasia	speech
phil/o	attracted to; love
-philia	attraction for
phleb/o	vein
-phobia	fear
phon/o	sound
-phonia	voice; sound
-phoresis	carrying; transmission
-phoria	feeling
phot/o	light
phren/o	diaphragm; mind
physi/o	nature
pil/o	hair
plas/o	formation
-plasia	development; growth; formation
-plasm	growth; formation
-plasty	surgical correction
-plegia	paralysis
pleur/o	pleura; rib; side
-pnea	to breathe
pneum/o	lung; air
pneumon/o	lung; air
pod/o	foot
-poiesis	formation
-poietin	substance that forms pus
poli/o	gray
poly-	many
polyp/o	polyp
pont/o	pons
post-	after; behind
-praxia	action
pre-	before; in front of
presby/o	old age
primi-	first
pro-	before; favoring; in front of
proct/o	anus and rectum
prol-	offspring

Word Element	Meaning
prostat/o	prostate gland
psych/o	mind
-ptosis	prolapse; downward
-ptysis	spitting up
pulmon/o	lung
pupill/o	pupil
py/o	pus
pyel/o	trough; basin; pelvis
pyl/o	pylorus
pylor/o	pylorus
radi/o	ray; x-ray
radic/o	root
radicul/o	nerve root
rect/o	rectum
ren/o	kidney
retin/o	retina
retro-	backward, behind
rhabdomy/o	skeletal or striated muscle
rhin/o	nose
-(r)rhage	bursting forth; excessive flow
-(r)rhagia	bursting forth; excessive flow
-(r)rhaphy	suture of
-(r)rhea	flow, discharge
-(r)rhexis	break, burst, rupture
sacr/o	sacrum
salping/o	tube
-salpinx	uterine tube
sangui/o	blood
sarc/o	flesh
schiz/o	split
scintill/o	spark
scirr/o	hard
scirr-	hard
scirrh/o	hard
scler/o	sclera
-sclerosis	hardening
scoli/o	crooked, bent
-scop	look
-scope	instrument for visual examination
-scopy	visual examination
scot/o	darkness
scrot/o	bag, pouch
seb/o	fatty substance
sem-	half
semen	seed
semi-	half
semin/o	seed
sial/o	salivary
sigmoid/o	sigmoid colon
somat/o	body
-somnia	sleep
spas/o	draw; pull
spas-	to draw or pull tight
-spasm	sudden, involuntary muscular contraction
sperm/o	spermatozoa
spermat/o	spermatozoa
sphen/o	wedge

Word Element	Meaning
sphygm/o	pulse
spir/o	to breathe; breathing; coil
splen/o	spleen
splen-	spleen
spondyl/o	vertebra
squam/o	scale
staped/o	stapes; stirrup
-stasis	stop; control
steat/o	fat, lipid
-stenosis	tightening; structure
steth/o	chest
-sthenia	strength
stom/o	mouth
stomat/o	mouth
-stomy	creation of a new opening
strept/o	twisted
strict/o	drawing tight; narrowing
sub-	under; below
sud/o	sweat
sudor/o	sweat
super-	above; in the upper part of
supra-	above; over
-supression	to stop
sym-	together; with
syn-	together; with
syncop/o	to cut off; cut short
synov/o	synovial membrane
syring/o	tube
tachy-	fast; rapid
tars/o	of or pertaining to the foot; eyelid
tele/o	distant
tele-	distant
ten/o	tendon
tend/o	tendon
tendin/o	tendon
tens/o	stretch
test/o	testes; testicles
thalam/o	thalamus
thec/o	sheath
thel/o	nipple
therap/o	treatment, therapy
-therapy	treatment
therm/o	heat
thorac/o	chest
-thorax	chest
thromb/o	clot; lump
thym/o	thymus
-thymia	mind
thyr/o	thyroid gland
thyroid/o	thyroid gland
-tic	pertaining to
-tocia	labor; birth
tom/o	cut
-tome	instrument to cut
top/o	place
tox/o	poison
toxic/o	poison
trache/o	windpipe

Word Element	Meaning
trans-	through; across
traumat/o	wound; injury
-tresia	opening
tri-	three
trich/o	hair
-tripsy	crushing; friction
-trophy	development; growth
trophy-	development; nourishment
-tropia	turn
-tropin	growth; development; nourish; stimulate
turbin/o	shaped like a top
tympan/o	eardrum
ultra-	beyond
umbilic/o	navel
ungul/o	nail
uni-	one
ur/o	urinary tract; urine
-uresis	urination
uret/o	urinary tract; urine
ureter/o	ureter
urethr/o	urethra
-uria	condition of the urine; urination

Word Element	Meaning
urin/o	urinary tract; urine
uter/o	uterus
uve/o	uvea; vascular layer of the eye
vag/o	vagus nerve
vagin/o	vagina
valv/o	valve
valvul/o	valve
vas/o	vessel; duct
vascul/o	vessel
ven/o	vein
ventricul/o	ventricle
-version	act of turning
vertebr/o	vertebra
vesic/o	bladder
vesicul/o	seminal vesicles
vestibul/o	entrance
viscer/o	internal organ
vitr/o	glass
vitre/o	glassy
viv/o	life
vulv/o	vulva
xanth/o	yellow
xer/o	dry

APPENDIX B Meanings to Word Elements

Meaning	Word Element
abdomen	cel/o, celi/o, lapar/o
abnormal	para-
abnormal condition of cells	-cytosis
about	peri-
above	epi-, hyper-, super-, supra-
acid	oxy-
across	trans-
act of turning	-version
action	-praxia
adrenal gland	adren/o, adrenal/o
after	post-
against	ana-, ant-, anti-, contra-
air	aer/o, pneum/o, pneumon/o
air sac	alveol/o
albumin	albumin/o
all	pan-
alveolus	alveol/o
amnion	amni/o
anal	an/o
anus and rectum	proct/o
anxious	anxi/o
aorta	aort/o
appendix	append/o, appendic/o
around	peri-
artery	arter/o, arteri/o
atrium	atri/o
attraction for	-philia
attraction to	phil/o
away from	ab-, ex-
back	ana-
backward	ana-, retro-
bacteria	bacteri/o
bad	dys-, mal-, malign-
bag	scrot/o
ball	glomerul/o
band	fasci/o
base	bas/o
basin	pyel/o
(to) bear	-par, -para
before	ante-, pre-, pro-
beginning	-arche
behind	post-
below	sub-, hypo-
beneath	hypo-, infra-
bent	ankyl/o, scoli/o
berry-shaped	-coccus
beside	para-

Meaning	Word Element
between	inter-
beyond	meta-, ultra-
bile	bili/o, chol/e, chol/o
bile duct	cholangi/o, choledoch/o
bilirubin	bilirubin/o
binding	-desis
birth	-par, -para, -tocia
black	anthrac/o, melan/o
bladder	cyst/o, vesic/o
blood	hem/o, hemat/o, sangui/o
blood condition	-emia
blood vessel	angi/o
blue	cyan/o, cyan-
body	somat/o
bone marrow	myel/o
bone	oste/o
brain	cerebr/o, encephal/o
branching	dendr/o, dendr-
break	-rrhexis
breakdown	-lysis
breast	mamm/o, mast/o
breast (chest)	pect/o, pector/o
(to) breathe	-pnea, spir/o
breathing	spir/o
bring forth	-parous
bronchiole	bronchiol/o
bronchus	bronch/o, bronchi/o
burst	-rrhexis
bursting forth	-(r)rhage, -(r)rhagia
calcium	calc/o, calci/o
calyx	cali/o, calic/o
cancerous	carcin/o, carcin-
carbon dioxide	capn/o
carry	duct/o
carrying	-phoresis
cartilage	chondr/o
causing genetic change	mutagen/o
cavity	antr/o, pariet/o
cecum	cec/o
cell	cyt/o, -cyte
cerebellum	cerebell/o
cervix	cervic/o
chamber	antr/o
change	ameb/o, ameb-, meta-
cheek	bucc/o
chest (breast)	pect/o, pector/o, steth/o, thorac/o, -thorax

Meaning	Word Element
clavicle	cleid/o
clot	thromb/o
clotting	coagul/o
clumping	agglutin/o
cluster	glomerul/o
cochlea	cochle/o
coil	spir/o
cold	cry/o
colon	col/o, colon/o
condition	-ema, -iasis, -osis
condition of the urine	-uria
conjunctiva	conjunctiv/o
connection	adnex/o
control	-stasis
cornea	corne/o, kerat/o
covering	oment/o
creation of a new opening	-ostomy, -stomy
crooked	ankyl/o, scoli/o
(to) crush	-tripsy
crushing	-tripsy
(to) cut	tom/o
(to) cut off	syncop/o
cut short	syncop/o
darkness	scot/o
death	necr/o
decrease	-penia
deep sleep	comat/o
deficiency	-penia
deficient	hypo-
destruction	-lysis
development	-plasia, -trophy, -tropin
diaphragm	phren/o
digestion	-pepsia
dilation	-ectasia, -ectasis
dim	ambly/o
discharge	-rrhea
disease	path/o, -pathy
distant	tele/o, tele-
division	furc/o
double	dipl/o
down	cata-
downward	-ptosis
draw	pas/o
drawing tight	spas-, strict/o
drug	pharmac/o
dry	ichthy/o, xer/o
duct	vas/o
dull	ambly/o
duodenum	duoden/o
dura mater	dur/o
ear	auri/o, auricul/o, ot/o
eardrum	myring/o, tympan/o
eat	phag/o
eating	-phagia
egg	ov/i, ov/o, ovul/o
embryonic	blast/o
enlarge	mydr/o

Meaning	Word Element
enlargement	-megaly
entrance	vestibul/o
epididymis	epididym/o
epiglottis	epiglott/o
equal	is/o, iso-
esophagus	esophag/o
excessive	hyper-
excessive flow	-rrhage, -rrhagia
excessive preoccupation	-mania
excision	-ectomy
expansion	-ectasia, -ectasis
extremities	acr/o
eye	ocul/o, ophthalm/o, opt/o, optic/o
eyelid	blephar/o, blephar-, cili/o, cili-, palpebr/o, tars/o
fallopian tube	salping/o
fast	tachy-
fat	adip/o, lip/o, steat/o
fatty substance	ather/o, seb/o
favoring	pro-
fear	-phobia
feeling	esthes/o, esthesi/o, -phoria
female	gynec/o
fiber	fibr/o
finger	dactyl/o, digit/o
first	primi-
fixation	-desis
flesh	sarc/o
flow	-rrhea
fluid	hydr/o
foot	ped/o, pod/o
foot, of or pertaining to	tars/o
form	morph/o
formation	-ia, -iasis, -genesis, plas/o, -plasia, -plasm-, -poiesis
forward	ante-
friction	-tripsy
fungus	myc/o
gallbladder	cholecyst/o
genetic change	mut/a
gland	aden/o
glans penis	balan/o
glass	vitr/o
glassy	vitre/o
glottis	glott/o
glue	gli/o
glue-like	coll/o
good	eu-
grain	gran-
granule	granul/o
gray	glauc/o, poli/o
green	chlor/o
growth	-plasia, -plasm, -trophy, -tropin
gum	gingiv/o
hair	pil/o, trich/o
half	hemi-, sem-, semi-

Meaning	Word Element
hallucination	hallucin/o
hand	cheir/o
hard	dura-, scirr/o, scirrh/o, scirr-
hardening	-sclerosis
head	cephal/o, crani/o
hearing	acous/o, audi/o, audit/o, -cusis
heart	cardi/o, cardi-, coron/o
heat	therm/o
hemoglobin	hemoglobin/o
hepatic duct	cholangi/o
hernia	-cele
hip	ischi/o
horny	corne/o, kerat/o
humpback	kyph/o
ileum	ile/o
ilium	ili/o
immature	blast/o, -blast, blast-
immune	immun/o
immunity	immun/o
in	en-
in front of	pre-, pro-
in the upper part of	super-
incision into	-otomy
inflammation	-itis
injury	traumat/o
inside	end/o
instrument for recording	-graph
instrument for visual exam	-scope
instrument to cut	-tome
intestine	enter/o
into	in-
iris	ir/o, irid/o
jejunum	jejun/o
joint	articul/o, arthr/o
ketone bodies	ket/o, keton/o
kidney	nephr/o, ren/o
labor	-par, -part, -partum, -tocia
labored	dys-
lack of strength	-asthenia
lamina	lamin/o
large	macro-, mega-
larynx	laryng/o
lens of the eye	phac/o, phak/o
less	mi/o
less than	hypo-
life	viv/o
ligament	ligament/o
light	phot/o
like	-oid
lip	cheil/o
lipid	steat/o
liver	hepat/o, hepatic/o
lobe	lob/o
loin	lumb/o
look	-scop
loosening	-lysis
love	phil/o
lower back	lumb/o
luminous	fluor/o
lump	thromb/o
lung	pneum/o, pneumon/o, pulmon/o
lymph	lymph/o
lymph nodes	lymphaden/o
lymph vessel	lymphangi/o
male	andr/o
many	multi-, poly-
mastoid process	mastoid/o
meatus	meat/o
medulla	medull/o
membranes around the central nervous system	mening/o
meninges	mening/o
menses	men/o
microscopic	micr/o
middle	meso-
milk	lact/o
mind	ment/o, phren/o, psych/o, -thymia
more than	hyper-
mouth	or/o, stom/o, stomat/o
movement	cine/o, kines/o, -kinesia, -kinetic
muscle	muscul/o, my/o
muscle, nonstriated or smooth	leiomy/o
muscle, striated or skeletal	rhabdomy/o
nail	onych/o, ungul/o
narrow opening	fistul-
narrowing	strict/o
nature	physi/o
navel	umbilic/o
neck	cervic/o
nerve	neur/o
nerve root	radicul/o
nervous system	neur/o
neutral	neutr/o
new	neo-
night	noct/i, nyct/o
nipple	thel/o
nipple-like	papill/o
nitrogen	azot/o
no	a-, an-, nulli-
none	nulli-
nonstriated muscle	leiomy/o
normal	eu-
nose	nas/o, rhin/o
not	a-, ab-, an-, in-, nulli-
nourish	-tropin
nucleus	kary/o
obscure	-opaque
of or pertaining to the foot	tars/o
offspring	prol-
old age	presby/o
one	uni-
opening	-tresia

Meaning	Word Element
opposite	contra-
originate	-gen
ossicle	ossicul/o
other than	par-
out	ect-, ex-
outside	ect/o, ect-
ovary	oophor/o, ovari/o
over	supra-
pain	-algia, -dynia
pancreas	pancreat/o
papillary	papill/o
paralysis	-plegia
paralysis, slight	-paresis
parathyroid glands	parathyroid/o
pelvis	pyel/o
pericardium	pericardi/o
peritoneum	peritone/o
pertaining to	-ac, -al, -ar, -ary, -eal, -iac, -ic, -ical, ose, -ous, -tic
pertaining to a base	bas/o
pertaining to destruction or loosening of	-lytic
pharynx	pharyng/o
physician	iatr/o
picture	-gram
place	top/o
pleura	pleur/o
poison	tox/o, toxic/o
polyp	polyp/o
pons	pont/o
pouch	scrot/o
pour	-fusion
power	dynam/o
pregnancy	gravid/o, -cyesis
pregnant female	-gravida
primitive cell	blast/o
process of recording	-graphy
produce	-gen
produced by	-genic
profuse sweating	diaphor/o
prolapse	-ptosis
prostate gland	prostat/o
protection	immun/o
protein	-globin, -globulin
pull	spas/o, spas-
pulse	sphygm/o
puncture	-centesis
pupil	pupill/o
pus	py/o
pylorus	pyl/o, pylor/o
rapid	oxy-, tachy-
ray	radi/o
recent	neo-
(a) record	-gram
rectum	rect/o
red	eryth/o, erythr/o
repeated sound	echo
resembling	-oid

Meaning	Word Element
retina	retin/o
rib	cost/o, pleur/o
root	radic/o
rosy	eosin/o
rupture	-(r)rhexis
sac	burs/o, cyst/o
sacrum	sacr/o
salivary	sial/o
same	is/o, iso-
scale	squam/o
scaly	ichthy/o
sclera	scler/o
secrete	-crine
section	lob/o
seed	gon/o, semen, semin/o
self	auto-
seminal vesicles	vesicul/o
sensation	esthes/o, esthesi/o
sensitivity to pain	algesi/o
separate	-crit
setting free	-lysis
shape	morph/o
shaped like a top	turbin/o
sharp	oxy-
sheath	thec/o
sheet	fasci/o
(to) shine	-lucent
short distance	brachy-
side	later/o, pleur/o
sigmoid colon	sigmoid/o
single	mon/o
skeletal muscle	rhabdomy/o
skin	cut/o, cutane/o, derm/o, dermat/o
skull	crani/o
sleep	hypn/o, -somnia
slender	lept/o
slight paralysis	-paresis
slow	brady-
small	micro-
small size	micr/o
smaller	mi/o
smell	-osmia
smooth	lei/o
smooth muscle	leiomy/o
soft inner part	medull/o
softening	-malacia
sound	audi/o, audit/o, phon/o, -phonia
spark	scintill/o
specialist in the study of	-logist, -ologist
speech	-phasia
spermatozoa	sperm/o, spermat/o
spinal cord	myel/o
spleen	spleen/o, splen-
split	schiz/o
splitting	-ptysis
spot	macul/o
stapes	staped/o

Meaning	Word Element
star	astr-
star-shaped	astr/o
starch	amyl/o
sticking	agglutin/o
stimulate	-tropin
stomach	gastr/o, gastr-
stone	lith/o
stop	-stasis, -suppression
strength	-sthenia
stretch	tens/o
stretching	-ectasia, -ectasis
striated muscle	rhabdomy/o
structure	-stenosis
study of	-logy, -ology
stupor	narc/o
substance	-in, -ine
substance that forms pus	-poietin
sudden involuntary muscle contraction	-spasm
sugar	gluc/o, glyc/o, -ose
surgical correction	-plasty
surgical fixation	-pexy
surgical removal	-ectomy
surrounding	peri-
suture of	-rrhaphy
swallow	phag/o
swallowing	-phagia
swayback	lord/o
sweat	hidr/o, sud/o, sudor/o
swelling	gangli/o
synovial membrane	synov/o
tail	caud/o
tawny yellow	cirrh/o
tear	dacry/o, lacrim/o
tear (to rip)	-spadia
tear duct	dacry/o
tendon	ten/o, tend/o, tendin/o
testes	test/o
testicles	test/o
testis	orch/o, orchi/o, orchid/o
thalamus	thalam/o
therapy	therap/o
thin	lept/o
three	tri-
throat	pharyng/o
through	trans-
thymus	thym/o
thyroid gland	thyr/o, thyroid/o
tie	adnex/o
tightening	-stenosis
tissue	hist/o
toe	dactyl/o, digit/o
together	sym-, syn-

Meaning	Word Element
tongue	gloss/o, lingu/o
tooth	odont/o
tracing	-gram
treatment	iatr/o, therap/o, -therapy
trough	pyel/o
tube	salping/o, syring/o
tumor	-oma, onc/o
(to) turn	-tropia
(act of) turning	-version
twin	gemin-
twisted	strept/o
two	bi-, gemin-
under	hypo-, sub-
uneasy	anxi/o
up	ana-
upon	epi-
upper jaw bone	maxill/o
ureter	ureter/o
urethra	urethr/o
urinary tract	ur/o, uret/o, urin/o
urination	-uresis, -uria
urine	ur/o, uret/o, urin/o
uterine tube	-salpinx
uterus	hyster/o, metr/o, uter/o
uvea	uve/o
vagina	colp/o, vagin/o
vagus nerve	vag/o
valve	valv/o, valvul/o
vascular layer of the eye	uve/o
vein	ven/o, phleb/o
ventricle	ventricul/o
vertebra	spondyl/o
vessel	vas/o, vascul/o, vertebr/o
vision	-opia, -opsia, opt/o, optic/o
visual examination	-scopy
voice	-phonia
vomiting	-emesis
vulva	episi/o, vulv/o
wall of an organ	pariet/o
water	aque/o, hydr/o, hydro-
weakness	-asthenia
wedge	sphen/o
white	albin/o, leuk/o
widen	mydr/o
windpipe	trache/o
with	syn-
within	en-, intra-
without	a-, an-
wound	traumat/o
wrapping	ependym/o
wrist	carp/o
x-ray	radi/o, roentgen/o
yellow	jaund/o, lute/o, xanth/o
yellowish plaque	ather/o

APPENDIX C Abbreviations

Note: Italicized words and phrases are Latin.

17-KS 17-ketosteroids
17-OHCS 17-hydroxycorticosteroids
2hPPG . . . . . 2-hour postprandial glucose
^{67}Ga . . . . . radioactive isotope of gallium
^{99m}Tc . . . . . radioactive isotope of technetium
^{99m}Th . . . . . radioactive isotope of thallium
^{131}I . . . . . radioactive isotope of iodine
^{201}Th . . . . . radioactive isotope of thallium
μm^3 . . . . . cubic micrometers

A_{1C}, Hb A_{1C} . . . . . glycosylated hemoglobulin
A&P, P&A . . . . . auscultation and percussion
AB . . . . . abortion
Abdo, ABDO, abd . . . . . abdomen; abdominal
ABG, AGBs . . . . . arterial blood gas(es)
a.c., A.C. . . . . . *ante cibum* (before meals)
AC . . . . . air conduction
ACAT . . . . . automated computerized axial tomography
ACE inhibitors, ACEI . . . . . angiotensin-converting enzyme inhibitors
accom . . . . . accommodation
ACJT . . . . . acromioclavicular joint
ACL . . . . . anterior cruciate ligament
ACTH . . . . . adrenocorticotropic hormone
AD . . . . . *auris dextra* (right ear)
ad lib. . . . . . *ad libitum* (at pleasure)
ADH . . . . . antidiuretic hormone
ADHD . . . . . attention-deficit hyperactivity disorder
A/G . . . . . albumin globulin ratio
AI . . . . . aortic insufficiency
AIDS . . . . . acquired immune deficiency; acquired immunodeficiency syndrome
AION . . . . . anterior ischemic optic neuropathy
AKI . . . . . acute kidney injury
alb . . . . . serum albumin
alk phos . . . . . alkaline phosphatase
ALL . . . . . acute lymphocytic leukemia
ALT . . . . . alanine aminotransferase; argon laser trabeculoplasty
AMA . . . . . American Medical Association
AMI . . . . . acute myocardial infarction
AML . . . . . acute myelogenous leukemia
ANA . . . . . antinuclear antibody
ANCA . . . . . antineutrophil cytoplasmic antibody
anti-TPO . . . . . thyroid peroxide antibodies
AP . . . . . anteroposterior; from front to back
APAP . . . . . acetaminophen
ARB . . . . . angiotensin receptor blocker(s)
ARC . . . . . AIDS-related complex
ARD . . . . . acute respiratory disease
ARDS . . . . . acute respiratory distress syndrome
ARF . . . . . acute renal failure; acute respiratory failure
ARMD . . . . . age-related macular degeneration
ART . . . . . assisted reproductive technology
AS . . . . . *auris sinistra* (left ear); aortic stenosis
ASA . . . . . acetylsalicylic acid (aspirin)
ASCP . . . . . American Society of Clinical Pathologists
ASD . . . . . atrial septal defect
ASHD . . . . . arteriosclerotic heart disease
AST . . . . . aspartate aminotransferase
AU . . . . . *aures unitas* (both ears)
AV, A-V . . . . . atrioventricular (node); arteriovenous

Ba . . . . . barium
baso . . . . . basophil(s)
beta-HCG . . . . . beta human chronic gonadotropin
BBB . . . . . blood-brain barrier; bundle branch block
BC . . . . . bone conduction
BE . . . . . barium enema
b.i.d. . . . . . *bis in die* (twice a day)
BMT . . . . . bone marrow transplantation
BOM . . . . . bilateral otitis media
BP . . . . . blood pressure
BPH . . . . . benign prostatic hypertrophy
BRAO . . . . . branch retinal artery occlusion
Bronch . . . . . bronchoscopy
BRVO . . . . . branch retinal vein occlusion

BSS . . . . balanced salt solution
BUN . . . . blood urea nitrogen
BV . . . . bacterial vaginosis
BW . . . . body weight
bx, BX . . . . biopsy

c . . . . with
C . . . . Celsius
C-section, CS . . . . cesarean section
C&S . . . . culture and sensitivity
C1, C2, etc. . . . . cervical vertebrae
Ca . . . . calcium
CA . . . . chronological age
CABG . . . . coronary artery bypass graft
CAD . . . . coronary artery disease
CAPD . . . . continuous ambulatory peritoneal dialysis
cap, caps . . . . capsule(s)
CAT . . . . computerized axial tomography; computerized-assisted tomography
cath . . . . catheter; catheterization
CAVH . . . . continuous arteriovenous hemofiltration
CBC . . . . complete blood count
cc (cm^3) . . . . cubic centimeter
CC . . . . chief complaint
CCPD . . . . continuous cycling peritoneal dialysis
CCU . . . . coronary care unit
CDC . . . . Centers for Disease Control (and Prevention)
CEA . . . . carcinoembryonic antigen
CGL . . . . chronic granulocytic leukemia
cGy . . . . centigray
CHD . . . . coronary heart disease
CHF . . . . congestive heart failure
Chol . . . . cholesterol
CID . . . . cytomegalic inclusion disease
CIN . . . . cervical intra-epithelial neoplasia (cervical dysplasia)
CIS . . . . carcinoma in situ
CK . . . . creatine kinase
CKD . . . . chronic kidney disease
CLL . . . . chronic lymphocytic leukemia
CML . . . . chronic myelogenous leukemia
CMV . . . . cytomegalovirus
cm . . . . centimeter
cm^3 . . . . cubic centimeter
CNS . . . . central nervous system
CO_2 . . . . carbon dioxide
CoA . . . . coarctation of the aorta
COLD . . . . chronic obstructive lung disease
COPD . . . . chronic obstructive pulmonary disease
CP . . . . cerebral palsy
CPAP . . . . continuous positive airway pressure
CPK . . . . creatine phosphokinase
CPR . . . . cardiopulmonary resuscitation
CRAO . . . . central retinal artery occlusion
creat . . . . creatinine
CRF . . . . chronic renal failure
CRH . . . . corticotropin-releasing hormone
CRRT . . . . continuous renal replacement therapy
CRVO . . . . central retinal vein occlusion
C-spine . . . . cervical spine film
CS, C-section . . . . cesarean section
CSF . . . . cerebrospinal fluid
CT . . . . computed tomography
CTA . . . . clear to auscultation
CST . . . . contraction stress test
CTS . . . . carpal tunnel syndrome
CTT . . . . computerized transaxial tomography
CVA . . . . cerebrovascular accident; costovertebral angle
CVD . . . . cardiovascular disease
CVS . . . . chorionic villus sampling
CVVH . . . . continuous venovenous hemofiltration
Cx . . . . cervix
cysto . . . . cystoscopy

D&C . . . . dilatation (dilation) and curettage
DAT . . . . diet as tolerated
dB . . . . decibel
DEA . . . . Drug Enforcement Administration
decub . . . . decubitus ulcer (bed sore)
DERM, derm . . . . dermatology; dermatologist
DES . . . . diethylstilbestrol
DEXA . . . . dual-energy x-ray absorptiometry
DHEA . . . . dehydroepiandrosterone
DI . . . . diabetes insipidus
DIC . . . . disseminated intravascular coagulation
diff . . . . differential blood count
dipj . . . . distal interphalangeal joint
disp . . . . dispense
DLE . . . . discoid lupus erythematosus
DM . . . . diabetes mellitus
DMARD . . . . disease-modifying antirheumatic drug
DNA . . . . deoxyribonucleic acid
D.O., DO . . . . Doctor of Osteopathy; Doctor of Ophthalmology
DOE . . . . dyspnea on exertion
dr . . . . dram
DRE . . . . digital rectal examination
DSA . . . . digital subtraction angiography
DSM-IV-TR . . . . *Diagnostic and Statistical Manual of Mental Disorders*
DST . . . . dexamethasone suppression test
DT, DT = s, DTs . . . . delirium tremens
DTR . . . . deep tendon reflex

DUB . . . . dysfunctional uterine bleeding
DVI . . . . digital vascular imaging
DVT . . . . deep vein thrombosis
DX, Dx . . . . diagnosis

ECC . . . . extracorporeal circulation; endocervical curettage
ECG . . . . electrocardiogram
ECHO . . . . echocardiography
ECT . . . . electroconvulsive therapy
EDB . . . . expected date of birth
EEG . . . . electroencephalogram
EFM . . . . electronic fetal monitoring
EGD . . . . esophagogastroduodenoscopy
EIA . . . . enzyme immunoassay
EKC . . . . epidemic keratoconjunctivitis; "pink eye"
EKG . . . . electrocardiogram
Em . . . . emmetropia (normal vision)
EMG . . . . electromyography; electromyogram
ENT . . . . ear, nose, and throat
EOM . . . . extraocular movement
eos, eosins . . . . eosinophil(s)
ERCP . . . . endoscopic retrograde cholangiopancreatography
ERG . . . . electroretinogram
ESRD . . . . end stage renal disease
ERT . . . . estrogen replacement therapy
ESR . . . . erythrocyte sedimentation rate (Sed rate)
ESWL . . . . extracorporeal shock wave lithotripsy
ETD . . . . eustachian tube dysfunction
ETT . . . . exercise tolerance test

F . . . . Farenheit
FANA . . . . fluorescent antinuclear antibody
FBS . . . . fasting blood sugar
FDA . . . . Food and Drug Administration
Fe . . . . iron
FH . . . . family history
FHR . . . . fetal heart rate
FHT . . . . fetal heart tones
fl. dr. . . . . fluid dram
fl. oz. . . . . fluid ounce
FSH . . . . follicle-stimulating hormone
FT_3, Free T_3 . . . . free triiodothyronine serum
FT_4, Free T_4 . . . . free thyroxine serum
FTI, FT_4 Index . . . . free thyroxine index
Fx . . . . fracture

g . . . . gram
G . . . . gravida (pregnant)
g/dl . . . . grams per deci-liter
Ga . . . . gallium
GAD . . . . generalized anxiety disorder
GBM . . . . glomerular basement membrane
GERD . . . . gastroesophageal reflux disease
GFR . . . . glomerular filtration rate
GGT . . . . gamma-glutamyl transpeptidase
GH . . . . growth hormone
GI . . . . gastrointestinal
GIFT . . . . gamete intrafallopian transfer
GIT . . . . gastrointestinal tract
glu. . . . . glucose
gm. . . . . gram
gm% . . . . grams percent
GnRH . . . . gonadotropin-releasing hormone
GPA . . . . gravida, para, abortion
gr. . . . . grain
gtt. . . . . *guttae* (drops)
GTT . . . . glucose tolerance test
GU . . . . genitourinary
GVHD . . . . graft-versus-host disease
gyn . . . . gynecology

H&P . . . . history and physical
Hb . . . . hemoglobin
Hb A_{1C}, A_{1C} . . . . glycosylated hemoglobulin
hCG, HCG . . . . human chorionic gonadotropin
HCl . . . . hydrochloride; hydrochloric acid
Hct . . . . hematocrit
HCTZ . . . . hydrochlorothiazide
HD . . . . hemodialysis
HDL . . . . high-density lipoprotein
HEENT . . . . head, eyes, ears, nose, throat
Hgb . . . . hemoglobin
HGH . . . . human growth hormone
HIV . . . . human immunodeficiency virus
HJR . . . . hepatojugular reflux
HMO . . . . health maintenance organization
HNP . . . . herniated nucleus pulposus
HPF . . . . high-power field
HPI . . . . History of Present Illness
HPV . . . . human papillomavirus
HRT . . . . hormone replacement therapy; Heidelberg retinal tomography
h.s. . . . . *hor somni* (at bedtime)
HSV . . . . herpes simplex virus
Hx, hx . . . . history
HZV . . . . herpes zoster virus

I . . . . iodine
I&D . . . . incision and drainage
I/A . . . . irrigation/aspiration
IABP . . . . intra-aortic balloon pump
IBC . . . . iron-binding capacity
IBD . . . . inflammatory bowel disease
IBS . . . . irritable bowel syndrome
ICD . . . . internal cardioverter-defibrillator
ICD-9 . . . . *International Statistical Classification of Diseases and Related Health Problems*
ICSI . . . . intracytoplasmic sperm injection
ID . . . . intradermal

IDDM . . . . insulin-dependent diabetes mellitus, Type IDM
IgA, IgD, IgE, IgG, IgM . . . . immunoglobulins
IGF-I. . . . . insulin-like growth factor I
IL-2. . . . . interleukin-2
IM . . . . intramuscular(ly)
inj . . . . injection
IOL . . . . intraocular lens
IOP . . . . intraocular pressure
IPD . . . . intermittent peritoneal dialysis
IPPB. . . . . intermittent positive pressure breathing
IQ . . . . intelligence quotient
ITP . . . . idiopathic thrombocytopenia
ITT . . . . insulin tolerance test
IU/L . . . . international units per liter
IUD. . . . . intrauterine device
IV . . . . intravenously
IVC . . . . inferior vena cavae; intravenous cholangiogram
IVF . . . . *in vitro* fertilization
IVP . . . . intravenous pyelogram

JVD. . . . . jugular venous distention

K. potassium
K^+ . . . . potassium ion (potassium electrolyte)
KOH . . . . potassium hydroxide
Kt/V . . . . way of measuring dialysis adequacy or clearance
KUB . . . . kidney, ureter, and bladder

L. liter
L1, L2, etc.. . . . . lumbar vertebrae
L&D . . . . labor and delivery
LASIK. . . . . laser assisted in situ keratomileusis
LD. . . . . labor and delivery
LDH . . . . lactic dehydrogenase
LDL . . . . low-density lipoprotein
LE. . . . . lower extremity
LE cell . . . . lupus erythematosus cell
LH. . . . . luteinizing hormone
LHRH. . . . . luteinizing hormone-releasing hormone
LMP . . . . last menstrual period
LP. . . . . lumbar puncture
LPF. . . . . low-power field
LRI . . . . limbal relaxing incision
LSD . . . . lysergic acid diethylamide
LTH . . . . lactogenic hormone (prolactin)
LVAD . . . . left ventricular assist device
lymph. . . . . lymphocyte

MA . . . . mental age
MACI . . . . Millon Adolescent Clinical Disorder
MAOI . . . . monoamine oxidase inhibitor
MCH. . . . . mean corpuscular hemoglobin
MCHC. . . . . mean corpuscular hemoglobin concentration
MCMI-III. . . . . Millon Clinical Mutiaxial Inventory-III
MCV . . . . mean corpuscular volume
MDD. . . . . major depressive disorder
MEA . . . . multiple endocrine adenomatosis
MEN. . . . . multiple endocrine neoplasia
mEq . . . . milliequivalent
mEq/L . . . . milliequivalent per liter
mg. . . . . milligram
mg% . . . . milligrams percent
MI . . . . mitral insufficiency; myocardial infarction
ml, mL . . . . milliliter
mm . . . . millmeter
mm/Hg . . . . millimeters of mercury
mm^3 . . . . cubic millimeters
mMol, mMole, mM . . . . millimole
MMPI-2 . . . . Minnesota Multiphasic Personality Inventory-2
MMPI-A . . . . Minnesota Multiphasic Personality Inventory-Adolescent
MMSE . . . . Mini-Mental Status Examination
mono . . . . monocyte
MPGN. . . . . membranoproliferative glomerulonephritis
MR . . . . mitral regurgitation
MRI. . . . . magnetic resonance imagery; magnetic resonance imaging
MS . . . . multiple sclerosis; mitral stenosis
MSH . . . . melanocyte-stimulating hormone
MT . . . . medical technologist
MT (ASCP) . . . . Registered Medical Technologist
MUGA . . . . multiple-gated acquisition scan
MVP . . . . mitral valve prolapse

Na. . . . . sodium
Na^+ . . . . sodium ion (sodium electrolyte)
NB . . . . newborn
NF. . . . . *National Formulary*
NG . . . . nasogastric
NG tube . . . . nasogastric tube
NGU . . . . nongonococcal urethritis
NHL . . . . non-Hodgkin's lymphoma
NIDDM. . . . . noninsulin-dependent diabetes mellitus, Type II DM
NIMH . . . . National Institute of Mental Health
NKHHC . . . . nonketotic hyperglycemia-hyperosmolar coma (syndrome)
NMR. . . . . nuclear magnetic resonance
NPO . . . . nothing by mouth

NSAID . . . nonsteroidal anti-inflammatory drug
NT . . . nastotracheal intubation

O_2 . . . oxygen
O&P . . . ova and parasite (test)
OB . . . obstetrics
OCD . . . obsessive-compulsive disorder
OCT . . . optical coherence tomography; oxytocin challenge test
OD . . . *oculus dexter* (right eye)
ophth . . . ophthalmology
ortho . . . orthopedics
OS . . . *oculus sinister* (left eye)
OT . . . oxytocin
OTC . . . over the counter
Oto . . . otology
OU . . . *oculi unitas* (both eyes)
oz . . . ounce

P . . . para (number of births); phosphorus
P&A, A&P . . . auscultation and percussion
PA . . . posteroanterior; from back to front
PAC . . . premature atrial contraction
Pap test . . . Papanicolaou test
PAP . . . prostatic acid phosphatase
Para 2-0-1-2 . . . 2 full-term infants, 0 premature, 1 abortion, 2 live births
PAT . . . paroxysmal atrial tachycardia
Path . . . pathology
PBK . . . pseudophakic bullous keratopathy
PBSC . . . peripheral blood stem cell(s)
PBSCT . . . peripheral blood stem cell transplantation
p.c., P.C. . . . *post cibum* (after meals)
PCD . . . pacemaker cardiac defibrillator
PCI . . . percutaneous coronary intervention
PCP . . . phencyclidine
PD . . . peritoneal dialysis
PDA . . . patent ductus arteriosus
PDR . . . *Physicians= Desk Reference*
PE . . . pulmonary embolism
PE, PX . . . physical examination
PE tube . . . pressure equalization tube
PERRLA . . . pupils equal, round, react to light and accommodation
PET . . . positron emission tomography
PFT . . . pulmonary function test
PH . . . past history
Pharm.D. . . . Doctor of Pharmacy
phos . . . phosphorus
PI . . . present illness
PICC . . . peripherally inserted central venous catheter
PID . . . pelvic inflammatory disease
PKD . . . polycystic kidney disease
PKP . . . penetrating keratoplasty (corneal transplant)
PMH . . . past medical history
PMN . . . polymorphonuclear neutrophil
PMNL . . . polymorphonuclear neutrophil leukocyte
PMS . . . premenstrual syndrome
PND . . . paroxysmal nocturnal dyspnea
p.o., PO . . . orally
Poly . . . polymorphonuclear
polys . . . polymorphonuclear leukocytes
POR (POMR) . . . problem oriented (medical) record
PPD . . . purified protein derivative
PPM . . . permanent pacemaker
PR . . . rectally
PRA . . . plasma renin activity
PRK . . . photorefractive keratectomy
PRL . . . prolactin level
p.r.n., PRN . . . *pro re nata* (as required)
ProTime . . . prothrombin time
PSA . . . prostate specific antigen
Pt, pt . . . patient
PT . . . prothrombin time; protime
PTA . . . percutaneous transluminal angioplasty
PTC . . . percutaneous transhepatic cholangiography
PTCA . . . percutaneous transluminal coronary angioplasty
PTH . . . parathyroid hormone; parathormone
PTHC . . . percutaneous transhepatic cholangiography
PTS . . . permanent threshold shift
PTSD . . . post-traumatic stress disorder
PTT . . . partial thromboplastin time
PUVA . . . psoralen ultraviolet A range
PVC . . . premature ventricular contraction
PVD . . . peripheral vascular disease
PX, PE . . . physical examination

q.4h . . . *quaque quarta hora; quaque 4 hora* (every 4 hours)
q.d. . . . *quaque die* (everyday)
q.h. . . . *quaque hora* (every hour)
q.i.d. . . . *quater in die* (4 times/day)
q.o.d. . . . every other day

RA . . . rheumatoid arthritis
rad . . . radiation absorbed dose
RAI . . . radioimmunoassay
RAIU . . . radioactive iodine uptake
RBC . . . red blood cell; red blood cell count
RDA . . . recommended daily allowance
RDS . . . respiratory distress syndrome

REM ....rapid eye movement
RF......................rheumatoid factor
RFA ....radiofrequency ablation
Rh......................Rhesus factor
RIA.....................radioimmunoassay
RLE ....right lower extremity
RNA ....ribonucleic acid
ROM.....................range of motion
ROS ....review of systems
R.Ph....................registered pharmacist
RPGN....................rapidly progressive glomerulonephritis
RPR ....rapid plasma reagin
RTA ....renal tubular acidosis
RTOG....................radiation therapy oncology group
RUE ....right upper extremity
RX, Rx ....treatment; prescription

S̄.......................without
SA, S-A.................sinoatrial (node)
SAD ....seasonal affective disorder
SB5.....................Stanford-Binet fifth series
SBFT ....small bowel follow-through
SBS.....................small bowel series
SC......................subcutaneous
Sed rate ....sedimentation rate
SH......................social history
SIADH ....syndrome of inappropriate antidiuretic hormone
sig., Sig. ....let it be labeled
SIL ....squamous intra-epithelial lesion (cervical dysplasia)
SL......................sublingual(ly)
SLE.....................systemic lupus erythematosus
SLEDD...................sustained low-efficiency daily dialysis
SLT.....................selective laser trabeculoplasty
SOAP ....subjective; objective; assessment; plan
SOB ....shortness of breath
sol, soln ....solution
SOR ....source oriented record
spec ....specimen
SPECT...................single-photon emission computed tomography
SPEP ....serum protein electrophoresis
SPF.....................sun protection factor
SQ......................subcutaneous(ly)
SRS.....................stereotactic radiosurgery
SSRI ....Selective Serotonin Reuptake inhibitor
stat., STAT.............*statim* (immediately)
STD ....sexually transmitted disease
STI ....sexually transmitted infection
subcu, subcut, subq, SC, SQ ....subcutaneous
supp ....suppository
susp ....suspension
syr.....................syrup

T&A ....tonsillectomy and adenoidectomy
T1, T2, etc. ....thoracic vertebrae
T_3, T3 ....triiodothyronine
T_4, T4 ....thyroxine
tab, tabs ....tablet(s)
TAT.....................Thematic Apperception Test
TB......................tuberculosis
TBG ....thyroid binding globulin
T bili ....total bilirubin
Tc ....technetium
TENS ....transcutaneous electrical nerve stimulation
TFT ....thyroid function test
Th......................thallium
THR ....total hip replacement
TIA.....................transient ischemic attack
t.i.d. ....*ter in die* (3 times/day)
tinc....................tincture
TIPS....................transjugular intrahepatic portosystemic shunt
TKR ....total knee replacement
TM ....tympanic membrane
TMJ ....temporomandibular joint
top ....topically
TP......................serum total proteins
TPN ....total parenteral nutrition
TPR ....temperature, pulse, and respirations
tr......................tincture
TRF ....thyrotropic-releasing factor
TRH ....thyrotropin-releasing hormone
TRUS ....transrectal ultrasound
TSH ....thyroid-stimulating hormone
TSS.....................toxic shock syndrome
TTS.....................temporary threshold shift
TUIP....................transurethral incision of the prostate
TUMT....................transurethral microwave thermotherapy
TUNA....................transurethral needle ablation
TURP....................transurethral resection of the prostate

UA ....urinalysis
UC ....urine culture
UE ....upper extremity
UGI.....................upper gastrointestinal (series)
ung ....ointment, unguent
URI.....................upper respiratory infection
URR ....urea reduction ratio
US, U/S.................ultrasound
USP ....*United States Pharmacopeia*
UTI.....................urinary tract infection
UV......................ultraviolet

V/Q scan................ventilation-perfusion scan
VA......................visual acuity
vag.....................vaginally

VCE . . . . videocapsule endoscopy
VCUG . . . . voiding cystourethrogram
VD . . . . venereal disease(s)
VDRL . . . . Venereal Disease Research Laboratories
VF . . . . visual field
VMA . . . . vanillylmandelic acid
VSD . . . . ventricular septal defect
VT . . . . ventricular tachycardia

W/D . . . . well developed
W/N . . . . well nourished
WAIS-III . . . . Wechsler Adult Intelligence Scale-III
WBC . . . . white blood cell; white blood cell count
WBST . . . . Wonderlic Basic Skills Test
WISC-IV . . . . Wechsler Intelligence Scale for Children-Fourth Edition
WPPSI-III . . . . Wechsler Preschool and Primary Scale of Intelligence-Third Edition

x . . . . times, multiplied by

ZIFT . . . . zygote intrafallopian transfer

APPENDIX D Medications

Trade Name	Generic
C	morphine
C	nitrous oxide (N_2O)
5-FU	fluorouracil
A/T/S	topical erythromycin
A-Hydrocort	hydrocortisone topical
Abilify	aripiprazole
Abbokinase	urokinase
Abraxane	paclitaxel
Accupril	quinapril
Accutane	isotretinoin
Achromycin V	tetracycline
Aciphex	rabeprazole sodium
ACTH	adrenocorticotropic steroid
Acthar	corticotropin
Acticin	permethrin
Actigall	ursodeoxycholic acid
Activase	alteplase
Actonel	risedronate sodium
Actos	pioglitazone
Acular	ketorolac ophthalmic
AD-DEX	dexamethasone ophthalmic
Adrenalin	epinephrine
Adriamycin	doxorubicin hydrochloride
Advair	fluticasone propionate and salmeterol
Advil	ibuprofen
Afrin	pseudoephedrine
AK-Con	naphazoline ophthalmic
AK-Pred	prednisolone sodium phosphate ophthalmic
AK-Pro	dipivefrin opthalmic
AK-Spore	gramicidin ophthalmic
AK-Tracin	bacitracin ophthalmic
Akarpine	pilocarpine ophthalmic
Albuterol	albuterol
Aldactazide	spironolactone and HCTZ
Aldactone	spironolactone
Aldomet	methyldopa
Alesse	levonorgestrel
Aleve	naproxen
Allegra	fexofenadine hydrochloride
Allerest	naphazoline ophthalmic
Aloxi	palonosetron
Alpha	Keri
Alphagan	brimonidine tartrate
Alternagel	
Alupent	metaproterenol sulfate
Amaryl	glimepiride

Trade Name	Generic
Ambien	zolpidem tartrate
Amcil	ampicillin
Amethopterin	methotrexate
Aminophylline	aminophylline
Amoxil	amoxicillin
Amphogel	
Ampicill	ampicillin
Ampicillin	ampicillin
Anacin	acetaminophen and APAP
Anafranil	clomipramine
Anaprox	naproxen sodium
Anaspaz	hyoscyamine sulfate
Anexsia	hydrocodone with acetaminophen
Ansaid	flurbiprofen
Antepar	piperazine citrate
Antiminth	pyrantel
Antivert	meclizine
Anturane	sulfinpyrazone
Anzemet	dolasetron
Apresoline	hydralazine hydrochloride
Aranesp	darbepoetin alfa
Arimidex	anastrozole
Aristocort	triamcinolone acetonide
Armour Thyroid	desiccated thyroid, thyroid extract
Artane	trihexyphenidyl
aspirin	acetylsalicylic acid and ASA
Astelin	azelastine hydrochloride
Atacand	candesartan cilexetil
Atarax	hydroxyzine hydrochloride
Ativan	lorazepam
Atromide-S	clofibrate
Atropine-1	atropine ophthalmic
Atrovent	ipratropium
Augmentin	amoxicillin and potassium clavulanate
Avandia	rosiglitazone
Avastin	bevacizumab
Aveeno	Bath
Avonex	interferon beta
Axid	nizatidine
Aygestin	norethindrone acetate
Azelex	azelek acid
Azmacort	triamcinolone
Azo Gantrisin	sulfisoxazole and phenazopyridine
Azulfidine	sulfasalazine

Trade Name	Generic
Bacid	lactobacillus
Baciguent	bacitracin
Bacticort	neomycin, polymyxin, hydrocortisone
Bactrim	trimethoprim and sulfamethoxazole
Bactroban	mupirocin topical
Balnetar oil	
Bancap-HC	hydrocodone with acetaminophen
Banophen	diphenhydramine
Baridium	phenazopyridine hydrochloride
BCNU	carmustine
Beclovent	beclomethasone
Beconase	beclomethasone dipropionate
Beconase AQ	beclomethasone dipropionate monohydrate
Beepen-VK	penicillin V and potassium
Benadryl	diphenhydramine
Benemid	probenecid
Bentyl	dicyclomine hydrochloride
Betaderm	betamethasone
Betadine	povidone iodine
Betagan	levobunolol opthalmic
Betapen-VK	penicillin V and potassium
Betaseron	interferon beta
Betinol	timolol maleate ophthalmic
Betoptic	betaxolol opthalmic
Biaxin	clarithromycin
Bicillin	penicillin G and benzathine
Bicitra	sodium citrate, citric acid
BiCNU	carmustine
Bio-Statin	nystatin
Biomox	amoxicillin
Blenoxane	bleomycin sulfate
Bleph-10	sulfacetamide
Blephamide	sulfacetamide, prednisolone
Blocadren	timolol
Bonine	meclizine
Boniva	ibandronate
Brethine	terbutaline
Bronkaid	epinephrine
Brycanyl	terbutaline
Bumex	bumetanide
BuSpar	buspirone
Butisol	butabarbital
Byetta	exenatide
Cafergot	ergotamine and caffeine
Calan	verapamil
Calciferol	vitamin D preparations
Calcimar	calcitonin
Calderol	calcifediol
Caltrate	oyster shell calcium
Camptosar	irinoteca
Copaxone	glatiramer acetate
Carafate	sucralfate
Carbachol	carbachol
Carbocaine	mepivacaine hydrochloride
Carboptic	carbachol
Cardene	nicardipine
Cardizem	diltiazem hydrochloride
Cardura	doxazosin mesylate
Cascara Sagrada	
Casodex	bicalutamide
Catapres	clonidine hydrochloride
Cathflo Activase	alteplase
CCNU	lomustine
Ceclor	cefaclor
CeeNu	lomustine
Ceftin	cefuroxime axetil
Cefzil	cefprozil monohydrate
Celebrex	celecoxib
Celestone	betamethasone
Celexa	citalopram
CellCept	mycophenolate mofetil
Cenestin	conjugated estrogens
Cerubidine	daunorubicin
Cerumenex	triethanolamine, chlorobutanol
Cetacaine	tetracaine
Cetapred	sulfacetamide, prednisolone
Chronulac	lactulose
Ciloxan	ciprofloxacin
Ciobrevate	clobetasol topical
Cipro	ciprofloxacin
Citracal	calcium citrate
Citrucel	
Claritin	loratadine
Claritin D	loratadine and pseudoephedrine sulfate
Cleocin	clindamycin
Climara	estradiol
Clindex	clidinium and chlordiazepoxide
Clinoril	sulindac
Clinoxide	clidinium and chlordiazepoxide
Clomid	clomiphene citrate
Clozaril	clozapine
Cogentin	benztropine
Colace	docusate sodium
Colestid	colestipol
Colchicine	colchicine
Colyte	
Compazine	prochlorperazine maleate
Cordarone	amiodarone hydrochloride
Cordran	flurandrenolide topical
Cordrol	prednisone
Cormax	clobetasol topical
Cort-Dome	hydrocortisone acetate
Cortaid	hydrocortisone topical
Cortef	hydrocortisone
Cortisporin	neomycin, polymyxin, hydrocortisone
Cortomycin	neomycin, polymyxin, hydrocortisone
Cortone	cortisone
Cortrosyn	cosyntropin (synthetic corticotropin)

Trade Name	Generic
Cotrim	trimethoprim and sulfamethoxazole
Coumadin	warfarin sodium
Cozaar	losartan
Creon	pancreatin
Crestor	rosuvastatin
Crixivan	indinavir sulfate
Cutivate	fluticasone propionate
Cycloflex	cyclobenzaprine hydrochloride
Cyklokapron	tranexamic acid
Cymbalta	duloxetine
Cystospas	hyoscyamine sulfate
Cytomel	liothyronine sodium
Cytotec	misoprostol
Cytoxan	cyclophosphamide
Dantrium	dantrolene sodium
Darvocet	propoxyphene napsylate
Darvon	propoxyphene
Daypro	oxaprozin
DDAVP	desmopressin acetate (vasopressin)
Debrox	carbamide peroxide
Decadron	dexamethasone
Decadron Ocumeter	dexamethasone ophthalmic
Deca-Duraboli	nandrolone
Deconamine SR	pseudoephedrine and chlorpheniramine
Delatestryl	testosterone enanthate
Deltasone	prednisone
Demulen	
Depakene	valproic acid
Depakote	divalproex sodium
Depo-Provera	medroxyprogesterone acetate
Dermacin	fluocinonide topical
Dermatop	prednicarbate topical
Desmopressin AC	desmopressin acetate
Desogen	
Detrol	tolterodine tarte
Dexasol	dexamethasone ophthalmic
Dexedrine	dextroamphetamine sulfate
DHT, Dht	dihydrotachysterol
DiaBeta	glyburide
Diabinese	chlorpropamide
Diamox	acetazolamide
Didronel	etidronate
Differin	adapalene
Diflucan	fluconazole
Dilantin	phenytoin
Diovan	valsartan
Diprivan	propofol
Diprolene	betamethasone dipropionate
Diprosone	betamethasone dipropionate
Ditropan	oxybutynin chloride
Diuril	chlorothiazide
Dolacet	hydrocodone and APAP
Donnatal	atropine, scopolamine, hyoscyamine, phenobarbital
Donnazyme	pancreatin
Dovonex	calcipotriene

Trade Name	Generic
Dramamine	dimenhydrinate
DTIC-Dome	dacarbazine
Dulcolax	bisacodyl
Duphalac	lactulose
Duricef	cefadroxil
Duvoid	bethanechol
Dyazide	triamterene and hydrochlorothiazide
E.E.S.	erythromycin
E-Mycin	erythromycin
Econopred	prednisolone acetate ophthalmic
Effexor	venlafaxine
Eflone	fluorometholone ophthalmic
Elamite	permethrin
Elavil	amitriptyline hydrochloride
Eldepryl	selegiline
Elimite	permethrin
Eloxatin	oxiliplatin
Elspar	asparaginase
Emcyt	estramustine
Emend	aprepitant
Emgel	topical erythromycin
Enbrel	etanercept
Enduron	methyclothiazide
Entex	guaifenesin and phenylephrine
Epifrin	epinephrine bitrate
Epinal	epinephrine bitrate
Epivir	lamivudine
Epogen	epoetin alfa (man-made)
Erbitux	cetuximab
Ergotrate	ergonovine
Ergostat	ergotamine tartrate
Eryc	erythromycin
Eryped	erythromycin ethylsuccinate
Esidrex	hydro-chloro-thiazide
Estrace	estradiol
Estraderm	estradiol
Ethrane	enflurane
Eulexin	flutamide
Eurax	crotamiton
Evista	raloxifene hydrochloride
Excedrin	acetaminophen, APAP and caffeine
Exelderm	sulconazole nitrate
Ex-Lax	
Exosurf	colfosceril palmitate
Famvir	famciclovir
Fareston	toremifene
Fastin	phentermine
Feen-a-mint	
Feldene	piroxicam
Femara	letrozole
Feosol	ferrous sulfate
Fergon	ferrous gluconate
Ferosul	ferrous sulfate
Ferralet	ferrous gluconate
Ferrlecit	ferric gluconate
Ferro-Sequels	
Fioricet	caffeine, butalbital and APAP

Trade Name	Generic
Fiorinal	caffeine, butalbital and ASA
Flagyl	metronidazole
Flarex	fluorometholone ophthalmic
Fleet Preparation	
Flexeril	cyclobenzaprine
Flonase	fluticasone propionate
Florinef	fludrocortisone
Flovent	fluticasone propionate
Floxin Otic	ofloxacin
Fludara	fludarabine
Fluex	fluocinonide topical
Fluonid	halothane
Flurosyn	fluocinolone acetonide
Fluor-Op	fluorometholone ophthalmic
Fluothane	fluocinonide topical
FML	fluorometholone ophthalmic
Folex	methotrexate
Forane	isoflurane
Fortaz	
Forteo	teriparatide ceftazidime
Fortovase	saquinavir mesylate
Fosomax	alendronate
Fosrenol	lanthanum carbonate
Fragmin	dalteparin
Fulvicin P/C	griseofulvin
Furadantin	nitrofurantoin
Gantrisin	sulfisoxazole
Garamycin	gentamicin sulfate
Gastrocrom	cromolyn sodium
Gaviscon	
Gemzar	gemcitabine
Genoptic	gentamicin sulfate
Genotropin	somatropin
Gentacidin	gentamicin sulfate
Gentak	gentamicin sulfate
Geodon	ziprasidone
Glatiramer acetate	copaxone
Glaucon	epinephrine bitrate
Gleevec	imatinib mesylate
GlucaGen	glucagon
Glucagon	glucagon
Glucophage	metformin
Glucotrol	glipizide
Glucovance	glyburide and metformin
Glynase	glyburide
Glyset	miglitol
Golytely	
Grisactin	griseofulvin
Grisfulvin V	griseofulvin
Gyne-Lotrimin	clotrimazole
Halcion	triazolam
Haldol	haloperidol
Halotestin	fluoxymesterone
Haltran	ibuprofen
Hectorol	doxercalciferol
Heparin	heparin
Herceptin	trastuzumab
Hexadrol	dexamethasone
Hivid	zalcitabine

Trade Name	Generic
HMS	medrysone ophthalmic
Humabid	guaifenesin
Humalog	insulin lispro
Humatrope	somatropin
Humulin (L, N, R, or U)	human insulin
Hycamtin	topotecan
Hydrea	hydroxyurea
Hydrocet	hydrocodone and APAP
Hydrocortone	hydrocortisone
HydroDIURIL	hydrochlorothiazide
Hygroton	chlorthalidone
Hyperstat	diazoxide
Hytone	hydrocortisone topical
Hytrin	terazosin hydrochloride
Iberet-Folic-500	
IFEX	ifosfamide
Ilotycin	erythromycin
Immunex	aminocaproic acid
Imodium	loperamide
Imuran	azathioprine
Inderal	propranolol
Indocin	indomethacin
Infed	iron dextran
Inocor	amrinone lactate
Intal	cromolyn Na
Intron A	interferon alfa
Intropin	dopamine
Invase	saquinavir mesylate
Invega	paliperidone
Isoptin	verapamil
Isopto Homatropine	homatropine opthalmic
Isopto Aropine	atropine opthalmic
Isopto Carbachol	carbachol
Isopto Carpine	pilocarpine ophthalmic
Isuprel	isoproterenol
IVIG	intravenous immune globulin
Januvia	sitagliptin
K-Lor	potassium chloride
K-Tab	potassium chloride
Kay Ciel	potassium chloride
Kayexalete	sodium polystyrene sulfonate
Keflex	cephalexin
Kefzol	cefazolin
Kenalog	triamcinolone acetonide
Ketalar	ketamine hydrochloride
Klonopin	clonazepam
Klor-Con	potassium chloride
Kwell	crotamiton
Kytril	granisetron
Lactinex	lactobacillus
Lamictal	lamotrigine
Lamisil	terbinafine
Lanoxin	digoxin
Lantus	insulin glaring
Lasix	furosemide
Lescol	fluvastatin
Leucovorin Calcium	folinic acid
Leukeran	chlorambucil
Leukine	sargramostim (GM-CSF)

Trade Name	Generic
Levaquin	levofloxacin
Levbid	hyoscyamine sulfate
Levophed	norepinephrine bitartrate
Levothroid	levothyroxine sodium
Levoxyl	levothyroxine sodium
Levsin	hyoscyamine sulfate
Levsinex	hyoscyamine sulfate
Lexapro	escitalopram oxalate
Librax	clidinium and chlordiazepoxide
Librium	chlordiazepoxide
Lidex	fluocinonide topical
Lignocaine	lidocaine
Lioresal	baclofen
Lipitor	atorvastatin calcium
Lo/Ovral	
Locoid	hydrocortisone topical
Lodine	etodolac
Loestrin	
Lomotil	diphenoxylate and atropine
Loniten	minoxidil
Lopressor	metoprolol
Loprox	ciclopirox topical
Lopurin	allopurinol
Lorcet	hydrocodone and acetaminophen
Lorelco	probucol
Lortab	hydrocodone and acetaminophen
Lotrimin	clotrimazole topical
Lotrisone	betamethasone and clotrimazole
Lovenox	enoxaparin
Levoxyl	levothyroxine sodium
Loxitane	loxapine
Lozol	indapamide
Lubath	
Lugol's Solution	iodine and potassium iodide
Lupron	leuprolide acetate
Lyrica	pregabalin
Lysodren	mitotane
Maalox	
Macrodantin	nitrofurantoin
Mandol	cefamandole
Mannitol	mannitol
Marcaine	bupivacaine hydrochloride
Maridex	dexamethasone ophthalmic
Materna 1-60	
Matulane	procarbazine
Maxitrol	neomycin, polymyxin, dexamethasone opthalmic
Maxivate	betamethasone dipropionate
Medrol	methylprednisolone
Megace	megestrol acetate
Menest	esterified estrogen
MESNEX	mesna
Mestinon	pyridostigmine bromide
Metamucil	psyllium preparations
Metaprel	metaproterenol
Methergine	methylergonovine maleate
Mevacor	lovastatin
Mexate	methotrexate
Mexiletine	mexiletine hydrochloride
Miacalcin	calcitonin salmon
Miacalcin nasal spray	calcitonin salmon
Micro-K	potassium chloride
Micronase	glyburide
Midamor	amiloride hydrochloride
Midol	ibuprofen
Milk of Magnesia (MOM)	
Minipress	prazosin hydrochloride
Minocin	minocycline
Miostat	carbachol
Mircette	
Mitrazol	miconazole
Monistat	miconazole
Monistat 7 Vaginal Cream	miconazole nitrate
Monistat-Derm	miconazole
Monocid	cefonicid
Motrin	ibuprofen
Mustargen	mechlorethamine
Mutamycin	mitomycin
Mycelex	clotrimazole topical
Mycelex Troches	clotrimazole
Myciguent	neomycin sulfate
Mycitracin	polymyxin B, neomycin, bacitracin
Mycolog-II	nystatin
Mycostatin	nystatin
Myfortic	mycophenolic acid
Mylanta	
Myleran	busulfan
Mysoline	primidone
Naftin	naftifine topical
Nalfon	fenoprofen calcium
Naprosyn	naproxen
Nasacort	triamcinolone acetonide
Nasalcrom	cromolyn sodium
Nasalide	flunisolide
Nasarel	flunisolide
Nasonex	mometasone furoate
Natabec Rx	
Natalins	
Navelbine	vinorelbine
Neodecadron	neomycin, dexamethasone
Neoral	cyclosporine
Neosar	cyclophosphamide
Neosporin opthalmic	neomycin, polymyxin B, bacitracin
Neosporin G.U. irritant	neomycin, polymyxin B
Neotricin HC	neomycin, polymyxin, hydrocortisone
Nesacaine	chloroprocaine hydrochloride
Neulasta	pegfilgrastim
Neupogen	filgastrim (G-CSF)
Neurontin	gabapentin
Nexavar	sorafenib
Nexium	esomeprazole magnesium

Trade Name	Generic
Niaspan	nicotinic acid
Nicobid	nicotinic acid
Nicolar	nicotinic acid
Niferex-PN Forte	
Nilstat	nystatin
Nipride	nitroprusside sodium
Nitrostat	nitroglycerine
Nizoral	ketoconazole
Nolvadex	tamoxifen
Nordette	
Norditropin	somatropin
Norinyl	
Norlestrin	
Noroxin	norfloxacin
Norpace	disopyramide phosphate
Norvasc	amlodipine
Norvir	ritonavir
Novantrone	mitoxantrone
Novocaine	procaine hydrochloride
Novolin (N, L, or R)	human insulin
Novolog	insulin aspart
Nutracort	hydrocortisone topical
Nutropin	somatropin
Ocu-Cort	neomycin, polymyxin, hydrocortisone
Ocufen	flurbiprofen
Ocuflox	ofloxacin opthalmic
Ogen	estropipate
Omnipen	ampicillin
Oncovin	vincristine
Optimine	azatadine maleate
Orapred	prednisolone
Orasone	prednisone
Organidin	iodinated glycerol
Orinase	tolbutamide
Ortho-Est	estropipate
Ortho-Cyclen	
Ortho-Novum	
Ortho Tri-Cyclen	norgestimate/ethinyl estradiol
Orudis	ketoprofen
Oruvail	ketoprofen
OSCal	oyster shell calcium
Osmoglyn	glycerin
Ovral Oxandrin	
Oxandrolone	
Oxistat	oxiconazole topical
Oxsoralen	methoxsalen
OxyContin	oxycodone
P.T.U.	propylthiouracil
Pacerone	amiodarone hydrochloride
Pagitane	cycrimine hydrochloride
Pamelor	nortriptyline
Panadol	acetaminophen and APAP
Pancrease	pancrelipase, pancreatic preparations
Paraplatin	carboplatin
Parisdol	ethopropazine hydrochloride
Parlodel	bromocriptine mesylate
Patanol	olopatadine hydrochloride
Paxil	paroxetine
Pediapred	prednisolone
Pediatric Gentamicin	gentamicin sulfate
Pen-Vee-K	penicillin V and potassium
Pentothal Sodium	thiopental sodium
Pepsid	famotidine
Pepto-Bismol	bismuth subsalicylate
Percocet	oxycodone and acetaminophen
Perdiem	
Pergonal	menotropins
Periactin	cyproheptadine hydrochloride
Peri-Colace	casanthranol and docusate sodium
Peridex	chlorhexidine gluconate
Periogard	chlorhexidine gluconate
Permax	pergolide mesylate
Persantine	dipyridamole
Phenergan	promethazine hydrochloride
Phenobarbital	phenobarbital
PhosLo	calcium acetate
Pilocar	pilocarpine ophthalmic
Pitocin	oxytocin
Pitressin	vasopressin
Platinol	cisplatin
Platinol-AQ	cisplatin
Plavix	clopidogrel bisulfate
Polocaine	mepivacaine hydrochloride
Polycillin	ampicillin
Pontocaine	tetracaine
Prandin	repaglinide
Pravachol	pravastatin sodium
Precose	acarbose
Pred Mild	prednisolone acetate ophthalmic
Prelone	prednisolone
Premarin	conjugated estrogens
Premphase	conjugated estrogens and medroxyprogesterone
Prempro	conjugated estrogen and medroxyprogesterone
Prevacid	lansoprazole
Prevalite	cholestyramine
Prilosec	omeprazole
Primatene	epinephrine
Principen	ampicillin
Prinivil	lisinopril
Pro-Banthine	propantheline bromide
Probalan	probenecid
Procardia	nifedipine
Procrit	epoetin alfa
Profasi HP	chronic gonadotropin
Prograf	tacrolimus
Prolixin	fluphenazine
Pronestyl	procainamide hydrochloride
Propine	dipivefrin ophthalmic
Prosed (various)	methenamine, phenyl salicylate, atropine, hyoscyamine, benzoic acid, and methylene blue
Prostigmin	neostigmine bromide
Protonix	pantoprazole

Trade Name	Generic
Proventil	albuterol
Provera	medroxyprogesterone acetate
Provil	ibuprofen
Prozac	fluoxetine
Purinol	allopurinol
Pyridiate	phenazopyridine hydrochloride
Pyridium	phenazopyridine hydrochloride
Questran	cholestyramine
Quinidex	quinidine
Rapamune	sirolimus
Reclast	zoledronic acid
Regitine	phentolamine mesylate
Reglan	metoclopramide
Relafen	nabumetone
Remeron	mirtazapine
Remicade	infliximab
Renacidin Irrigation	citric acid, magnesium carbonate, gluconodelta-lactone
Renagel	sevelamer
Renova	tretinoin
Rescriptor	delavirdine
Retavase	reteplase
Retin A	tretinoin
Retrovir	zidovudine
Revlimid	lenalidomide
Rezine	hydroxyzine
Rheumatrex	methotrexate
Rhinocort	budesonide
Riopan	
Risperdal	risperidone
Ritalin	methylphenidate
Rituxan	rituximab
Robaxin	methocarbamol
Robimycin	erythromycin
Robinul	glycopyrrolate
Rocaltrol	calcitriol
Rocephin	ceftriaxone
Roferon-A	interferon alfa
Rolaids	calcium carbonate and magnesia
Roxanol	morphine
Roymicin	erythromycin ophthalmic
Rufen	ibuprofen
Rythmol	propafenone hydrochloride
S.S.K.I.	potassium iodide saturated solution
Sandimmune	cyclosporine
Sandostatin	octreotide acetate
Sansert	methysergide maleate
Seasonale	
Semprex-D	pseudoephedrine and acrivastine
Senokot	
Sensorcaine	bupivacaine hydrochloride
Septra	trimethoprim and sulfamethoxazole
Serevant	salmeterol
Seroquel	quetiapine fumarate
Shohl's solution	sodium citrate, citric acid
Silvadene	silver sulfadiazine

Trade Name	Generic
Simron	ferrous gluconate
Sinemet	carbidopa, levodopa
Slo-bid	theophylline
Slo-Niacin	nicotinic acid
Slo-Phyllin	theophylline
Slow Fe	ferrous sulfate exsiccated
Slow-K	potassium chloride
Solu-Cortef	hydrocortisone
Solu-Medrol	methylprednisolone
Soma	carisoprodol
Somnothane	halothane
Spectazole	econazole topical
Spiriva	tiotropium
Sporanox	itraconazole
Sprycel	dasatinib
Starlix	nateglinide
Stimate	desmopressin acetate
Streptase	streptokinase
Sublimaze	fentanyl citrate
Sudafed	pseudoephedrine
Sulfamylon	mafenide acetate
Sumycin	tetracycline
Suprane	desflurane
Suprax	cefixime
Surfak	docusate calcium
Survanta	beractant
Sustiva	efavirenz
Sutent	sunitinib malate
Symmetrel	amantadine
Synalar	fluocinolone acetonide
Synarel	nafarelin acetate
Synthroid	levothyroxine sodium
T-Stat	topical erythromycin
Tagamet	cimetidine
Tambocor	flecainide acetate
Tapazole	methimazole
Tarceva	erlotinib
Taxol	paclitaxel
Taxotere	docetaxel
Tegison	etretinate
Tegretol	carbamazepine
Temodal	temozolomide
Temovate	clobetasol topical
Ten-K	potassium chloride
Tenormin	atenolol
Tequin	gatifloxacin
Terazol Vaginal Cream	terconazole
Testoderm	testosterone
Thalomid	thalidomide
Theo-clear	theophylline
Theo-Dur	theophylline
Thyrogen	thyrotropin alfa
Thyrolar	liotrix
Tigan	trimethobenzamide
Timoptic Ocumeter	timolol maleate ophthalmic
Tobradex	tobramycin, dexamethasone
Tobralcon	tobramycin opthalmic
Tobramycin	aminoglycosides
Tobrasol	tobramycin opthalmic

Trade Name	Generic
Tobrex	tobramycin opthalmic
Tofranil	imipramine hydrochloride
Tolectin	tolmetin sodium
Tolinase	tolazamide
Topicort	desoximetasone topical
Toprol XL	metoprolol succinate
Torecan	thiethylperazine
Torisel	temsirolimus
Totacillin	ampicillin
Tramadol	ramadol
Tranxene	clorazepate dipotassium
Trental	pentoxifylline
Trexall	methotrexate
Tri-Norinyl	
Tri-Phasil	
Tricor	fenofibrate
Trimox	amoxicillin
Trusopt	dorzolamide
Tykerb	lapatinib
Tylenol	acetaminophen and APAP
Tylenol with Codeine	acetaminophen with codeine
Ultane	sevoflurane
Ultram	tramadol
Ultrase	pancrelipase
Ultravate	halobetasol propionate
Urecholine	bethanechol
Urispas	flavoxate
V-Cillin K	penicillin V potassium
Vagifem tablets	estradiol
Valisone	betamethasone valerate
Valium	diazepam
Valtrex	valacyclovir
Vancenase	beclomethasone dipropionate
Vanceril	beclomethasone
Vancocin	vancomycin hydrochloride
Vancoled	vancomycin hydrochloride
Vaponephrine	epinephrine
Vasocidin	sulfacetamide, prednisolone
Vasocon-A	naphazoline ophthalmic
Vasotec	enalapril maleate
Vectibix	panitumumab
Velban	vinblastine sulfate
Velcade	bortezomib
Venofer	iron sucrose
Ventolin	albuterol
VePesid	etoposide
Vermox	mebendazole
Vexol	rimexolone ophthalmic
Viagra	sildenafil citrate

Trade Name	Generic
Vibramycin	doxycycline
Vicodin	hydrocodone and acetaminophen
Videx	didanosine
Vincasar	vincristine sulfate
Viracept	nelfinavir mesylate
Viramune	nevirapine
Virilon	methyltestosterone
Viroptic	trifluridine opthalmic
Vistaril	hydroxyzine pamoate
Vitamin B12	cyanocobalamin
Vivelle	estradiol
Vivelle-Dot	estradiol transdermal system
Voltaren	diclofenac sodium ophthalmic
VoSol otic	hydrocortisone, acetic acid
Vytorin	ezetimibe
Welchol	colesevelam
Wellbutrin	bupropion hydrochloride
Westcort	hydrocortisone valerate
Wycillin	penicillin G and procaine
X-prep	
Xalatan	latanoprost
Xanax	alprazolam
Xeloda	capecitabine
Xylocaine	lidocaine
Yaz	
Yocon	yohimbine
Yutopar	ritodrine
Zaditor	ketotifen fumarate
Zantac	ranitidine
Zarontin	ethosuximide
Zaroxolyn	metolazone
Zemplar	paracalcitol
Zenate	
Zerit	stavudine
Zestril	lisinopril
Zetar	
Zetia	ezetimibe
Ziagen	abacavir
Zithromax	azithromycin
Zocor	simvastatin
Zofran	ondansetron hydrochloride
Zoladex	goserelin
Zoloft	sertraline
Zovirax	acyclovir
Zyban	bupropion hydrochloride
Zyloprim	allopurinol
Zyprexa	olanzapine
Zyrtec	cetirizine

Index

Note: Page numbers referencing figures are bolded.

B

H

Q

R

T

U